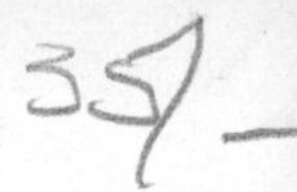

MODERN NURSING

THEORY AND PRACTICE

MODERN NURSING
THEORY AND PRACTICE

By

WINIFRED HECTOR, M.Phil.

Principal Tutor, St. Bartholomew's Hospital, London

FIFTH EDITION

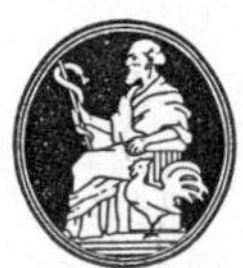

LONDON
WILLIAM HEINEMANN MEDICAL BOOKS LTD

First published 1960
Reprinted with revisions 1961
Second Edition 1962
Reprinted 1962
Reprinted 1963
Reprinted 1964
Reprinted 1965
Third Edition 1965
Reprinted 1966
Reprinted 1967
Fourth Edition 1968
Reprinted 1969
Fifth Edition 1970

SBN 433 14206 5

By the same author,
Textbook of Medicine for Nurses
Food for the Diabetic

By the same author, in association with
GORDON BOURNE, F.R.C.S. (ENG.), F.R.C.O.G.,
Modern Gynæcology with Obstetrics for Nurses
Fourth Revised Edition 1969

Printed in Great Britain
by The Whitefriars Press Ltd., London and Tonbridge

PREFACE TO FIFTH EDITION

Colleagues and students are thanked for suggestions and advice about this edition, which contains new material on central venous pressure, spina bifida, renal biopsy, the management of chronic renal failure, epilepsy, electroencephalography, pacemakers, and the preservation of health in old age. Rewriting has been required in many sections, and Mrs. Audrey Besterman is thanked for the new illustrations. I am grateful to Miss J. A. Clark, Miss Roche, and Mr. C. W. S. Manning, F.R.C.S., for help with the subjects on which they are experts.

September, 1970. W. E. Hector

PREFACE TO FIRST EDITION

During the last quarter of a century a profound change has taken place in the work of nurses. Some diseases that were once incurable have yielded to new medical and surgical advances ; some that used to run a prolonged course are speedily controlled ; others that necessitated hospital care can now be treated at home. Many nursing procedures have been superseded and are now mainly of historical interest, and in their place have arrived new techniques, new and powerful, but dangerous, drugs to administer, new operations with which to assist. Many patients to whom at one time we were only able to give comfort, we may expect to help to make well.

This has involved widening our horizons and looking outside the hospital to the community from which our patients come and trying to understand the personal and economic pressures that may have contributed to their illnesses, and whether we can help to prevent them falling ill again.

It is however in hospitals and among the sick that nurses in training gain the knowledge, skill and technical efficiency that enable them to undertake their preventive work. This book aims to describe the procedures which the nurse may have to undertake or prepare for, and how to perform them. Some of the problems and challenges to be found in different branches of nursing are suggested, and in addition it is hoped to show that the nurse in hospital may send her patient home better equipped to maintain himself in health.

I am indebted to a very large number of nurses, doctors, and other workers in the health field, who have given me during my years of nursing information, help, ideas and ideals. I would especially mention the sisters who have welcomed me into their wards and made all their experience available. A teacher must ensure that the methods she is advocating are not only sound in theory, but are the most effective and acceptable in practice, and I am grateful for the opportunities I am afforded of working with the sisters and their students in the wards. I must also remember the many hundreds of students I have taught, since it is by listening to them as well as talking to them that my ideas on their needs have been formulated for this book. While expressing my gratitude to those named below, there are many others I would have liked to mention had space allowed.

Miss Helen Dey, C.B.E., R.R.C., was my Matron when I started nursing and she encouraged me to begin teaching ; I owe her more than I can say.

The consultant staff of St. Bartholomew's Hospital have been the kindest and most helpful of colleagues, whom I thank most sincerely for all they have taught me.

The following have given me their advice and opinions on sections of the text : Miss L. Arrow, Divisional Nursing Officer, London County Council ; Miss K. D. Bartlett ; Miss J. A. Clark ; Mr. W. D. Coltart, M.B., B.S., F.R.C.S. ; Miss G. Elles ; the late Mr. J. R. Elliott, Ph.C., M.P.S. ; Miss A. E. Evrall ; Miss E. M. Hall ; Miss M. F. Haworth ; Miss E. Jones ; Miss K. Knapman ; Miss A. Morris, of St. Mark's Hospital ; Mr. J. E. A. O'Connell, M.S., F.R.C.S. ; and Miss T. Wareham, M.C.S.P.

In addition, I would especially like to acknowledge my debt to Mr. Norman K. Harrison, who photographed the nursing procedures with great patience as well as his usual skill ; to Mr. R. N. Lane, who took endless trouble over the line drawings ; and to Miss N. E. Hunton, who typed the manuscript.

Dr. Johnston Abraham and Mr. Owen R. Evans, of William Heinemann Medical Books Ltd., have encouraged me to write this book and have seen it smoothly through the press. I am indebted to them for much personal kindness.

W. E. H.

January, 1960.

CONTENTS

CHAPTER 1

PEOPLE AS PATIENTS AND NURSES

A VERY large number of young girls in this country and in others with a similar social and cultural structure think at some time that they would like to be nurses and, although for many this is a youthful phantasy that is eventually discarded, some keep this wish steadfastly, and in their later schooldays work to equip themselves with knowledge that will help them in their chosen career. All of them, when they think of nursing, picture themselves as tending the sick, usually in hospital, and though our concept of nursing is rapidly broadening to include the prevention of illness, it is in our hospitals that nurse-training is given, and by the bedside that professional skills and attitudes are learnt.

It has been thought necessary in the past to warn nurses that the inmates of a ward are not " cases "—peptic ulcers and acute abdomens —but patients. Such an idea would today seem outdated. The sick persons whom we tend are primarily people, who have a past which may have led up to their present illness, and a future which may be greatly influenced by it. The word " patient " is one that describes a transitory phase in a person's life, and most nurses will at some time in their lives be patients as well.

Consideration of the type of illness seen in hospitals will show that half of them are disorders of the mind or spirit, necessitating treatment in a mental hospital. Many more may show organic disease, which is believed to be the result of the personality pattern and the way in which it responds to strain ; peptic ulcer, toxic goitre and ulcerative colitis are examples of such body-mind or *psychosomatic* interaction. Some conditions appear purely organic and physical, but even these may, if inspected more closely, prove not entirely accidental. In the United States recently an equal number of patients with cardio-vascular conditions and of people with a fracture were asked if they had ever been involved in an accident. Less than 1% of the cardio-vascular group said yes, but 72% of those with fractures had had two or more. This group had evidently a preponderance of people whose temperament led them into physical hazards or occupations where there was a risk of injury.

All nurses, therefore, and many patients, reach hospital as the result of their nature and environment and, before considering their technical relations, some thought should be given to the influences that mould each one of us into the form we eventually show. It would be pretentious to term so slight a review " psychology ", but it is an indication of the factors that psychologists believe are important in mental and social development.

NORMAL DEVELOPMENT

The baby at birth is helpless, capable only of vague movements and of sucking, and it passes through a well-marked series of physical changes as it grows older. Everyone recognizes that there is a normal age at which it can lift its head, stand up, walk and talk. It is not so widely recognized that there are phases of behaviour and psychological and social development that are just as characteristic of different ages, and just as important to adult development as physical growth.

Every baby is born with a hereditary pattern. The colour of the eyes and hair, the general physical type, the possible attainments in height and intelligence are innate. In addition, it is born into an environment that will profoundly affect its development. The child may be an only one or one of a big group ; belong to a wealthy or under-privileged family ; lose one or both parents in infancy ; live on a farm or in a slum. No child has the same environment as any other ; even in a family the oldest and the youngest grow up in quite different circumstances.

At birth and in the succeeding months the baby's main source of activity and pleasure is its mouth and psychologists refer to this stage of development as the oral one. Sucking is the baby's great source of satisfaction, not only because it results in the disappearance of hunger, but because it is pleasant in itself. Many mothers look back with nostalgia during later phases of childhood to this time when the baby was dependent, helpless, looking to her for its entire satisfaction. As the months pass, the baby begins to distinguish her from himself and from other people, and his need for her becomes all-important. To be separated from her or from a satisfactory mother-figure is believed to be a potent cause of difficulty in establishing social relations later in life.

By about the second year this oral phase is passing ; the baby no longer examines articles with its mouth. He is actively running about, exploring his environment and his relations with his mother. He is now discovering that it pleases his mother if he is " clean," and that his excretions, for which he has no natural distaste until he is made to acquire one, can arouse disgust if deposited in what adults consider unsuitable places. He becomes irritable and aggressive, given to tantrums and gusts of anger, refusing to sleep at night, or to eat what his mother thinks is suitable food. His problems and his mother's are often increased by the arrival of a new baby, whom he sees as a rival for his mother's affection. The mother finds it hard to understand how the placid, happy baby has turned into a naughty, cross child who refuses to use his pot, and appears to reject her love as well as the food she offers him. This is the so-called anal phase of development, and it is a stage that is trying to all concerned. However, it must be lived through successfully if the child is to attain an independent adult attitude and leave behind the passive oral infantile phase.

By the age of three or four toilet training has been achieved, and the child enters on the " genital " phase of development, in which he begins to ask questions on sexual topics, and on the relations between his parents. Boys see in their father a rival for their mother's love, and this is the time when they get up in the night and want to be taken into mother's bed. Difficulties pass, however, as the boy tries to copy the father he perceives to have gained his mother's love. Children of both sexes copy the ideals of their parents and build them up into those concepts to which they refer moral issues, and which we think of as the conscience.

At five a child goes to school and begins to enlarge his social experience, and can now measure himself against children of his own age in physical and mental skills, and find his place, sometimes with difficulty. Children of slightly less than average intelligence may find themselves left behind in class work, and may try to compensate for their intellectual lack by bullying the little ones, and will need sympathetic handling.

Children now tend to separate into one-sex groups. Boys form gangs engaged in play as cowboys, Indians, or soldiers, and learn the principles of group loyalty, while girls form their own societies with secret discussions from which boys are excluded ; some girls will always be found who try to join the boys' groups, of which they are jealous, and who try to emulate the boys' physical prowess.

The teen-ages are difficult for many boys and girls. At the time of puberty they have entered the reproductive period of life, but social custom and ethical standards forbid the exercise of their powers until they are of an age to bear the responsibilities of them. They are alternately impatient and resentful of parental control, and anxious about the time ahead when they must leave school and decide how they are to earn their own living. Their experiments in clothes and friendships may cause their parents no little dismay, but tastes must be determined by trial and error, and if there is a secure and happy home from which these forays into new territory can be made no harm will result.

The choice of a career is often a difficult one ; social prestige is closely connected with it, and all need to feel that they are using all their abilities, but not trying to reach a position that they cannot hold without strain. Parents must be careful not to bring pressure on a child to follow a career that is of their own choosing rather than his. This particularly applies to medical families, in which the sons are often made to feel that if they do not become doctors they will disappoint their fathers. It should never be tacitly assumed that a son must succeed his father.

Adult life is occupied with the choice and marriage of a mate, rearing a family in whom the above-mentioned cycle of events is repeated, pursuing a career and in the development of a social conscience. The child's loyalties do not extend beyond his family, his gang and his school, but adult sympathies take in the social group, the country and even the whole of mankind. Those who have not married may find satisfaction in work that allows them to extend to the young, the sick or the under-privileged the love that they would have bestowed on a family. The psychologists, who tell us that the outlines of the character are complete by the age of seven, sometimes sound as if life were rather uneventful after that age, but it is of course in the adult period of life that the greatest satisfaction is to be attained when emotional life is at its fullest, pleasure in work at its greatest and the place in the community assured.

After the age of 50 a readjustment of values has to be made. Children will have left home, the end of the working life is approaching and people may feel that life is going to be more lonely and restricted in future. Retirement from business should be planned in advance and undertaken at the correct time, when the wage-earner feels glad to surrender full-time employment and able to accept a life of lessened activity as his physical and mental powers decrease.

REACTIONS TO ILLNESS

The main impressions that nurses retain of their patients is of the courage, dignity and good humour with which they meet hospital situations that involve pain, anxiety and physical indignity, but the reactions they display are very varied. Those of children and the aged are discussed in other chapters, and here we consider the adults.

We have suggested that illness can be produced by the personality and the stresses to which it is subject ; the reverse is also true—that illness can have a profound effect on the personality. It disrupts the normal life, upsets plans, may cause financial loss, and causes loss of self-esteem and self-confidence. If it entails admission to hospital it always produces fear, as we realize when we think of our own reactions to minor procedures. Fear in connection with serious operations is normal, but even small ones cause much vague anxiety about the anæsthetic and its consequences, and whether one will behave well. Fears about work are less pressing now than they used to be, but prolonged illness always leads to loss of money. Women with families think about their children, and their welfare while mother is away.

In addition to these, patients feel apprehension on less obvious but very real grounds—how they will react to the lack of privacy in a general ward, whether they will see or hear distressing things, whether they will have to use a bedpan, or be subjected to procedures that may be embarrassing, even if they are not painful. While most of the anxieties are relieved quickly by kindly and thoughtful attention by the nurses, there is no doubt that hospitalization is fear-provoking.

The pattern of ward life inevitably reminds a patient of his infancy, with the sister as a kind but powerful mother-figure. The grown man finds himself helpless in bed, bathed by a stranger for the first time since childhood and receiving enquiries about his bowel actions. Some relapse with ease into the dependant oral attitude of their earliest days, receiving attention passively and eating whatever is given them. Such an attitude may be very convenient for the nurses during an acute illness, but it may be difficult to wean the patient from it during convalescence. Old people especially may regress to a childish attitude, enjoying being petted and jealous of attention to others. Others bitterly resent their helplessness, and try to compensate for their physical weakness by aggressive complaints and fault finding.

Illnesses often have a characteristic emotional tone. Euphoria is a groundless sense of well-being sometimes seen in advanced tuberculosis, and in patients who are having morphine ; nurses should not be deceived into thinking that there is any real improvement in the condition. Hysterical illness is often accompanied by a bland indifference to the alarming, if functional, symptoms displayed. Apathy may be the mood of the patient who has received some great physical shock—the loss of a limb, or a sudden paralysis ; his apparent absence of feeling is because he cannot yet bring himself to contemplate the magnitude of his calamity.

But illness has also its compensations—flowers, gifts, letters, visits from friends, skilled care, and the sense of being the centre of interest. This is all too clearly seen in the delight people take in recounting tales of their operations. It is not surprising that some abandon their illness with some reluctance, and the convalescent who makes what the nurse considers unreasonable demands on her time is wistfully trying to hold on to the privileges that he no longer enjoys.

Many people need to be encouraged into convalescence, and time should be found to show pleasure at their progress, and to suggest how pleasant it will be to take up normal life again. The breezes of the outside world seem a very cold wind to someone who has spent a long time in the sheltered life of a hospital ward. In some cases, too, the patient's fears of the outside are only too justified. Such illness as tuberculosis or epilepsy shake the self-confidence and cause great mental insecurity, which is not always helped by the attitude of work-mates. The appearance is of great importance in enabling one to face life with equanimity, and a limp or a visible scar may be a handicap economically as well as emotionally. Women are often very unhappy about the appearance of a thyroidectomy scar just after operation, but can be truthfully assured that this will speedily settle into a line at the base of the neck only visible at close quarters.

The thoughtful nurse who notices these varying reactions to illness will realize that she herself will one day be ill and respond to it in one of the ways that she notices in her patients, and will hope to behave with the courage and humour and adult insight that so many are able to display.

NURSES

Those who are in a position to choose their work look for an occupation which will fulfil their emotional needs and allow them to exercise their intellectual and manual abilities. Nurses are no exception to this rule, and although people who have no inclination to the care of the sick may consider it exacting and hard, the nurse knows that there is no reason to admire her for doing it, because it gives her satisfaction.

The instinct that prompts young people to do nursing is the parental one—the instinct to care for the young which is extended in civilized communities to cover the helpless and the sick. Girls often make their choice for emotional reasons when quite young, but it is important that when they reach the age to begin it that the choice of their heart should be confirmed by the head, or disillusionment will follow. Nursing involves exacting personal service to people who are not always grateful or courteous, not only by day but at night and at weekends when her friends in other occupations are free for social pleasures. Nevertheless, it provides challenging and enthralling work to many girls, who mostly marry at the end of their training and extend to their own children the care they have learned for others, and often as well manage to spare time from their homes for some nursing. Those who do not marry have a profession which will occupy heart and mind and spirit most happily.

Men do not commonly think of nursing as a career at an early age; they arrive at it as a result of their experience of life, their contact with sickness, their realization of the needs of the community and their own possibilities. Parental instincts operate in men as powerfully as in women, and can be as happily employed in nursing.

The would-be candidate for nursing who reads some accounts of the qualities required for such work must feel daunted, in spite of the evidence of many quite ordinary people engaged on it with satisfaction to themselves and their patients. In fact, many very widely differing temperaments are seen among nurses, but there are some qualities that all must possess.

The first is a liking for people, so that service is offered, not with condescension, but with warmth and tolerance that makes social intercourse easy. One of the first things that a student learns in hospital is to extend this feeling impersonally and impartially to all without becoming so emotionally absorbed in her patients' troubles that she is less capable of caring for them effectively. Intuitive sympathy with her fellows will make her observant of their needs and ready to satisfy them.

The second is physical health, since nursing involves physical work which is often quite heavy, and working in conditions where infection is greater than in most environments. The health is in many ways a reflection of the mental outlook, and repeated minor illnesses are often an indication of unhappiness, so that ailments which would be disregarded by one who is at ease in her occupation become for the less well-adjusted an opportunity for retreat from reality. Student nurses' health is a matter of much concern to hospital authorities, who take the greatest care to prevent the major illnesses that attack the young, such as tuberculosis.

Manual dexterity is a *sine qua non* in a profession where people are lifted and handled, delicate instruments cleaned and adjusted, and hypodermic injections given. Given these three qualities, a girl may engage in bedside nursing in the simpler tasks with every confidence that she and her patients will be happy. If she desires, however, to possess a professional qualification and to perform the more complicated tasks implicit in modern nursing, she must have something else.

She must have good average intelligence and an adequate education that will enable her to cope without strain with complicated techniques, a bewildering variety of drugs, many of which are dangerous, and examinations in the scientific bases of her calling. If her endowment or schooling do not enable her to manage these adequately she may not only imperil lives, but will be anxious and insecure. Perhaps intelligence is the more important of the two, but a good education enriches the personality and the capacity for enjoyment off duty as well as on.

The crowning quality which the nurse must have and carefully maintain in all circumstances, is integrity. The traits previously described have been physical or mental, but in addition the nurse must have moral and spiritual wholeness. Her profession exposes to her the weaknesses, shames and humiliations of her patients; it lays a physical strain on the meticulous performance of routines; it makes her responsible for the safety and even the lives of others, and she must be capable of carrying this burden with faithful assurance. She must not be moved by hope of gain, the temptations of interesting gossip, from the loyal and meticulous performance of her duties.

ETHICS

Every nation has its standards of right behaviour to which all its good citizens adhere ; they are learned from the parents by precept and example and are maintained by social approval. Ethical standards are higher than legal ones. Assault or theft are illegal ; lying, adultery and discourtesy are not, but they are offences against ethical standards.

The professional man or woman aims to maintain the accepted standards of the community, but is, in addition, bound in honour to observe the special ethical rules that his or her professional body believes to be binding on all right-thinking members of that profession. The International Council of Nurses has promulgated a code of nursing ethics, to which countries all over the world subscribe. It should be a thrilling thought to the nurse that in countries old or new, socially advanced or desperately struggling upwards, white or coloured, Christian, Mohammedan and Buddhist, that in this welter of diverse cultures nurses can stand together and declare their belief in a common code of professional behaviour.

There are fourteen points in the Code, and they run as under :

1. *The fundamental responsibility of the nurse is threefold : to conserve life, to alleviate suffering and to promote health.* In the last war, terrifying and tragic wrongs were done to millions of innocent people, and even medical men were swept along by national neurosis to work in concentration camps. It may even be that times will come again when nurses will have to remind themselves of where their duty to humanity lies. Their mission to promote health as well as to nurse the sick stands at the head of their rules of conduct.

2 *The nurse must maintain at all times the highest standards of nursing care and of professional conduct.* All of us are capable of recognizing the best when we see it, and should steadfastly set ourselves to emulate it.

3. *The nurse must not only be well prepared to practise, but must maintain her knowledge and skill at a consistently high level.* Her duty to her profession is not ended when she has finished her training and taken her examinations ; she must add new knowledge to her store of understanding, read journals and books, incorporate modern techniques in her practice, and maintain her work at a high level.

4. *The religious beliefs of a patient must be respected.* The world is getting smaller and Christian, Jew and Mohammedan meet and mingle as patients and nurses and must in that relation recognize the sincerity and personal sanctity of each other's religious convictions.

5. *Nurses hold in confidence all personal information entrusted to them.* This means not only the facts that patients may divulge, but all details of medical histories and diagnoses that they learn in the course of their work.

6. *A nurse recognizes not only the responsibilities but the limitations of her or his professional functions; recommends or gives medical treat-*

ment without medical orders only in emergencies and reports such action to a physician at the earliest possible moment.

Nurses are constantly consulted by people about their ailments, minor and major, from the moment they begin training, and must be very wary of giving any advice, except that a doctor be consulted. Our training does not enable us to diagnose illness, but only to observe the symptoms that may indicate the need for medical advice. Rash suggestions or treatment can lead to loss of time in consulting a doctor.

7. *The nurse is under an obligation to carry out the physician's orders intelligently and loyally and to refuse to participate in unethical procedures.*

No nurse is an automaton in the performance of her duties ; she understands the physician's aims, reports fully to him, and expects his confidence in return. The second part of the sentence might refer to illegal abortion, sometimes carried out under a cover of respectability in nursing homes. Once a nurse feels that she is being asked to take part in such work, she cannot continue in it. The fact that one is working under a doctor's direction does not mean that the conscience is surrendered to his keeping.

8. *The nurse sustains confidence in the physician and other members of the health team; incompetence or unethical conduct of associates should be exposed but only to the proper authority.*

The first part of this is one that every nurse is happy to do. She not only actively supports and speaks well of the physician, but is careful not to imply that there are any other methods of treatment which she has seen used successfully. Even such negative statements may lead a patient to feel that better treatment is possible. Unethical conduct in an associate is fortunately an experience that few encounter, but a nurse who does so may wonder if in private practice, what is the proper authority. If she is wise enough to belong to her professional body, she will know where to turn for advice.

9. *A nurse is entitled to just remuneration and accepts only such compensation as the contract, actual or implied, provides.*

Gifts, in money or kind, should not enter into the nurse-patient relation. Patients in hospital who tender presents may do so in the hope of favours or better treatment. Were this true, it would be the saddest of all reflections on the nurse, and even if it is false, the patient and his fellows may believe it to be true which is almost as bad. Such presents are in the nature of tips, and though their giving is prompted by gratitude their acceptance is not consonant with the dignity of a professional nurse.

10. *Nurses do not permit their names to be used in connection with the advertisement of products, or with any other forms of self-advertisement.*

The temptation to do this may not appear very great in this country, but the names and pictures of many well-known people may be seen in magazines and on television recommending branded goods, and it is not difficult to see that matrons and others might be asked to lend their support to medical products, and neither is it difficult to see why this should be refused.

11. *The nurse co-operates with and maintains harmonious relation-*

ships with members of other professions and with her or his professional colleagues.

All of us need the support of the community in which we live, in the narrowest and the broadest sense, and confidently expect it in return for the help and kindly courtesy we extend to others.

12. *The nurse in private life adheres to standards of personal ethics which reflect credit upon the profession.*

The standards of nursing conduct to which we aspire are based on our personal beliefs and conduct. Our behaviour should be such that other nurses are proud to have us linked with them in the public view.

13. *In personal conduct nurses should not knowingly disregard the accepted patterns of behaviour of the community in which they live and work.*

After training the nurse may find her work takes her to other parts of the world, to live in cultures other than her own. She must not by behaviour which might seem normal in her own country give offence to others of different views.

14. *A nurse should participate and share responsibility with other citizens and other health professions in promoting efforts to meet the health needs of the public—local, state, national and international.*

We are members of a community greater than the one in which we live, and have colleagues who share our hopes and understand our difficulties working all over the world. It is the greatest comfort and support to belong to a profession whose standards we strive to maintain, and in which we can always find fellowship and understanding.

CHAPTER 2

SOME SOCIAL ASPECTS OF DISEASE

THE social structure of countries everywhere is constantly affected by change. Wars in small countries may involve large ones far away; recessions in trade and currency devaluations bring unemployment and falling living standards. Increasing industrial output or discovery of oil brings prosperity that may lead to inflation. Waves of migration and fluctuations in the birth rate may occur. The nurse who is a thoughtful citizen will see that apart from these there are two influences of importance to her changing the society in which she lives and works; one is medical and the other political.

Medical advances during this century have virtually abolished some infections (such as erysipelas and gas gangrene) and deficiency states (like scurvy and rickets). Efficient treatment has enormously reduced the mortality of tuberculosis, many specific fevers, and pneumonia. While efficient treatment for the venereal diseases now exists, all countries are anxious about the rising incidence which has resulted from changing sexual customs. Active immunization against measles is now widely used, and the severe complications like otitis media and broncho-pneumonia can be cured. Since many of the deaths from infection used to occur in children and young people, the expectation of life has considerably increased. This does not mean that more people are reaching an exceptional age, but that more survive to reach their seventies, so that the population contains more elderly people than formerly, a fact of great importance in fixing levels of Retirement Pensions and of contributions.

Such medical advances have meant that beds that were formerly used for people with tuberculosis or the specific fevers can now be used for other types of patient, including the increasing number of aged.

While curative medicine has made great advances, even greater possibilities exist in the field of prevention. Smallpox and diphtheria can be prevented by inoculation, and there is every hope that poliomyelitis has also been conquered. It may seem that it is mainly the infectious diseases that may be prevented, but this is not so. Cancer of the lung has been shown to be related statistically to heavy cigarette smoking, and a campaign among the young to reduce smoking may be a factor in reducing the incidence of this terrible condition. A heavy toll of life is taken annually in road accidents, and though a reduction in this figure might seem a civil problem, doctors are concerned in the relation of taking alcohol with car accidents, and the circumstances that make drivers accident-prone. Anxiety about pollution of water and soil by sewage, pesticides and industrial waste, and of the air by smoke and sulphur dioxide is world wide.

Accidents in the home to the very young and the aged produce an even higher mortality, and doctors and nurses who see so many young children with burns and scalds and old people with fractures know the circumstances in which these most often occur and the measures that can be taken to provide greater safety in the home, such as the use of fireguards and non-inflammable night attire, and the avoidance of loose rugs and stair-rods.

A policy of prevention is economically attractive in that fewer hospital beds would be needed, but above all it will help to lessen the amount of individual pain and suffering from preventable disease. Such a patient ill in hospital is not merely costing the nation money in treatment and in lost working-time, but is undergoing an experience traumatic not only to him but to the family of which he is a unit.

The political tendency of the last century, and especially of the last fifty years, has been to give security to the under-privileged section of the community. The lowest-paid workers have always been most vulnerable to misfortunes. They have no reserves on which to call when illness results in loss of earnings, or old age prevents them working, and by a series of measures to which all parties have contributed, there has arisen in Great Britain the concept of the Welfare State that would provide basic security in times of illness or unemployment or age, which culminated in the passing of the Health Act in 1947.

Some diseases have been associated with occupations and income levels, and although coronary thrombosis and duodenal ulcer are relatively common among the better off, it is the people in the lowest income-brackets who have had the worst health in the country. The diseases associated with poverty are the deficiency states like scurvy or rickets ; infections, especially tuberculosis ; rheumatic fever ; venereal disease ; and such conditions as a high neonatal death rate.

Associated with poverty are these factors which contribute to the illnesses from which the underprivileged suffer, and which make their difficulties cumulative.

1. Poor diet. If money is short, the diet tends to be high in carbohydrate and low in protein and vitamin-containing foods.

2. Bad housing. Rents are high for even the poorest accommodation, which may be damp, cold and in ill-repair. Sanitary facilities and water supplies may be inadequate and vermin present, while overcrowding results in lower standards of hygiene and susceptibility to droplet infection. Health visitors and district nurses are not surprised that some families sink into apathy and squalor under their housing conditions, but are heartened by the struggle that so many families make to retain some standards under severe handicaps.

3. Insecurity of employment. The lowest paid worker is the unskilled labourer and he is the first to be discharged when seasonal work ends, or the economic wind blows cold. He has no savings to carry him over these emergencies.

4. Crime. There is a temptation to raise the family income by petty and then more serious crime. In the long run this usually means the family is left unprovided while the breadwinner goes to prison. Mother has to go to work, and the children are left unsupervised, so that there is truancy among school children, leading to juvenile delinquency that may be the beginning of a long acquaintance with the police.

5. Large families. These are common among the poorest families, who are least able to provide for them materially. There is no reason why a large family, even if poor, should not be happy as long as the mother remains healthy and able to care for them, but repeated pregnancies often result in chronic ill-health, fatigue and anæmia, that render her incapable of fulfilling her role.

6. Low intelligence. From the poorest-paid families the brightest and most ambitious graduate into the class of skilled workmen or of black-coated workers. The present educational and social system makes such a rise possible, so that the middle and professional classes are constantly being recruited from the wage-earning sections. Those who remain at the unskilled level consist to a greater amount than in other classes of the unfortunate, the handicapped or those of the lower intelligence levels.

It will be seen that these conditions are self-perpetuating in that children raised in them have difficulty in not conforming to their background, and that efforts to raise the living standards of a family may pay handsome dividends in the future of the country. The measures that are taken in this country are typical of its administrative methods in that the government, local authorities and voluntary organizations all play a part.

Nurses are aware of the legislation that directly affects them in their professional work, such as the Dangerous Drugs Act, 1953, and the Nurses Act, 1949, that protects their title as nurses. As citizens they must also realize that a great body of social legislation has been created since the last war that affects everyone and has moulded society into its present pattern. The theory underlying it is that the State must sustain and support its members who by reason of illness (physical or mental), injury, poverty, or unemployment are handicapped, until they are again self-supporting.

Some of these acts that have helped to create the concept of the Welfare State are the (1) National Insurance Acts, 1946–53, which provided National Insurance schemes for sickness and maternity benefits; retirement, widowhood, unemployment, occupational disease and injury benefits. Modifications have been made from time to time and these have been consolidated in the National Insurance Act, 1965. (2) The Children's Act, 1948, legislated for the welfare of boys and girls who have lost their parents or whose parents are unfit to care for them, and it was extended in respect of child protection by the Children's Act 1958. Allied to these Acts is the Adoption Act, 1958, and the Children and Young Persons' Act, 1933 to 1969. (3) The National Assistance Act, 1948, repeated all the Poor Law Acts, and laid the foundation of the modern approach providing assistance to those in need. Residential accommodation for the aged is still provided under the National Assistance Act, as is also aid for the handicapped, but financial help for those in need is now provided under the Ministry of Social Security Act, 1966. (4) Disabled Persons Employment Act, 1944, whose purpose is to registor disabled people, provide facilities for their rehabilitation and find them employment.

The National Health Service Act, 1946, and its later extensions provide the medical content which is needed in all these Acts. The provision of state benefits on medical grounds means that treatment must aim at shortening illness and where possible to prevent it. It is an enabling act, providing medical, hospital, dental and pharmaceutical services on a national scale. Everyone is entitled to receive the first two free, and the others at such small costs as are fixed from time to time. Broadly there are three sections to the Act :

1. Hospital and specialist services are administered by Regional Hospital Boards responsible to the Minister of Health. The regions differ in size according to their population, and each contains at least one Teaching Hospital with its own Board of Governors.

2. General practitioner, dental, ophthalmic and pharmaceutical services are administered by Executive Councils. There is such a council in every County or County Borough, so that its area is the same as that of the Local Health Authority.

3. Local Health Authority Services are administered by County Councils and County Borough Councils. No nurse has been long in her training hospital before she becomes aware of these services, whose aim is to reduce the number of people needing hospital care, or to receive patients leaving hospital, and continue their care. Her education includes talks by people engaged in Local Authority work, and visits to their district, and no one can fail to have her concept of nursing broadened, so that she sees it as a part of a wide scheme for the promotion of health.

The functions of the Local Authority under the various sections of the Act include the following :

1. To provide Health Centres for medical, dental, Local Authority Services and health education. The final shape of such centres has yet to be determined. Welfare Centres for well babies, antenatal mothercraft classes and similar work takes place. Development of Health Centres has been slow, but in recent years the situation has improved, and local authorities are now encouraged by grants from the Exchequer to go ahead with their plans.

2. To care for expectant and nursing mothers, and children up to the age of five who are not yet attending school.

3. To supply midwives and maternity nurses for domiciliary work in adequate numbers.

4. To engage health visitors. These do no actual nursing, but teach health education, and see that the families under their care are aware of the facilities at their disposal. A health visitor can be a friend as well as an adviser to her families. Increasingly, health visitors and district nurses are being attached to doctors' practices, so that a medical and nursing team work together and in consultation.

Tuberculosis still presents a problem in many areas, in spite of its reduced mortality. It is much feared by the general public, and its diagnosis may be a shattering blow to the patient. The tuberculosis visitor will call to give practical advice on sleeping accommodation, what to do about children, and money problems. Contacts will be examined for possible infection, and everything done to minimize the emotional and financial impact of the disease on the family unit. If treatment is to be given at home, the district nurse may call to give treatment such as streptomycin injections.

5. To provide home nursing facilities. District nurses care for the infirm, and people not ill enough to need admission to hospital, and at the request of hospital welfare departments or general practitioners

will carry out treatments such as dressings, or injections of insulin for diabetics, or mersalyl for those with chronic heart failure. She sees many sad and lonely people, and has a social as well as a nurse's functions to fulfil, for to many of her patients her visit is the big event, perhaps almost the only event, of the day.

6. To provide vaccination facilities against diphtheria and smallpox, and such other diseases as may be designated. Poliomyelitis is an example.

7. To provide an ambulance service to take acute cases to hospital, or others for physiotherapy and similar treatment.

8. To provide home helps, who are domestic workers. They can come while a mother is in hospital to work in the house or do the shopping, or to help the aged. Their presence may make it possible for a man temporarily deprived of his wife to keep his family at home rather than committing the children to the care of the local authority.

9. To provide facilities for the provisions of the Mental Treatment and Mental Deficiency Acts.

Provision is made for the health of school children under the Education Act, 1944. All children are examined on beginning and ending their school life, and once in between. The parents are encouraged to be present, and minor abnormalities and defects are looked for and corrected. The school nurse is present at these examinations, and in addition cares for the minor ailments of the pupil and tries to ensure their general cleanliness.

Schools are provided for such handicapped children as the deaf, the partially sighted and the educationally subnormal.

Total health depends not only on physical and mental wellbeing, but on successful social adjustment within the community, and acceptance of one's obligations to it. Apart from the statutory bodies mentioned, there are many voluntary organizations doing valuable work in connection with them.

There are religious bodies working for the welfare of their own people, such as the Jewish Board of Guardians, the Catholic Social Welfare Committee, and the Church of England Moral Welfare Council. Some care for certain groups, such as the Soldiers', Sailors' and Airmen's Families Association. Many, of which the Save-the-Children Fund and the National Adoption Society are examples, work for deprived children.

Maintaining the family unit intact is of fundamental importance to children and the Marriage Guidance Councils and Family Welfare Association give advice to couples in difficulties and try to help them solve them.

More working time is lost from nervous and mental illness than from any other cause, and the loss of money and the anxiety created within families by it is very great. The National Association for Mental Health provides an Advisory Service on all aspects of this problem. The Mental After-Care Association helps in the re-establishment in normal life of those who have suffered from mental illnesses.

Parents of children with special handicaps may form groups for exchange of information, mutual support, and presentation of their point of view to the authorities. Spastics, the backward child and the deaf have their own societies.

The Police Courts deal with people whose way of life has brought them into conflict with society. To help a first offender to stop becoming a second offender is obviously better than concentrating only on punishing him. If he is in prison he has to be kept at public expense, and frequently his family become a charge to the State. The Probation Officers do excellent work in this respect, and the Police Court Missions provide practical assistance to the needy who come within their scope.

The National Society for the Prevention of Cruelty to Children is thought of by the public mainly in connection with its police court work, but in fact it does, as its name implies, much preventive work that happily never results in prosecution. The large number of cases of cruelty occurring annually in this country is very sad, but many are due to mental illness or backwardness, or exhaustion and despair in the mother. Case work by the Society's officers can help both these disturbed parents and their offspring.

General advice about State services and legal points can be obtained from the Citizen's Advice Bureaux, and the Women's Royal Voluntary Services (who did such excellent work in the war) will provide practical help in many ways for community welfare.

The statutory workers are well acquainted with the voluntary organizations who supplement their work in so many ways, and collaborate closely with them. Nurses who are married, or retired, and have some spare time should consider helping in this field. We should be people with a highly developed social conscience, and men and women of good will are always needed in community service.

CHAPTER 3

WARD EQUIPMENT

ALL hospital patients spend part of their time in bed, and many are totally confined to it, so that beds are obviously of great importance. A standard pattern is shown in the picture. It is made of tubular steel for durability and ease of cleaning. The length is $6\frac{1}{2}$ ft. (1·95 m.) and the height 2 ft. (60 cm.). There are wheels for free movement, but the end of the bed rests on rubber feet, the wheels only being lowered when the bed is to be moved. A metal grid can be slanted forward over the mattress to support pillows when the patient is sitting up.

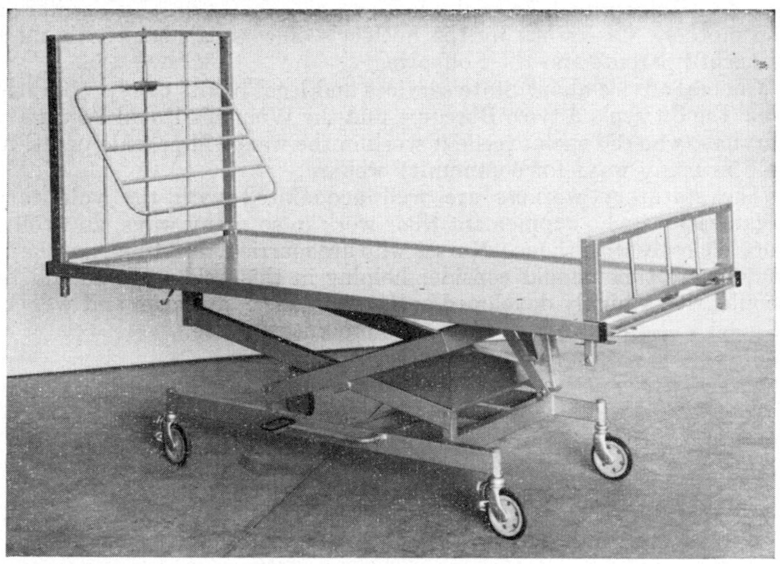

FIG. 1. The Nesbit-Evans King's Fund general purpose bed.

Modifications of this type exist for specialized use. The Nelson bed, for postural drainage of the chest, can be raised in the middle by turning a handle so that the patient's buttocks are higher than the head or feet, and fluid runs out of the bronchi by gravity. In cardiac beds, the end can be dropped so that the feet are dependent.

A working party established by the King's Fund to study the design of hospital bedsteads indicated that many improvements and much more sophisticated types of all-purpose beds were possible. Points that the working party made included the following:

1. Bedsteads should not accumulate an electrostatic charge, which may be painful for those who touch the bed, and offer explosion risks if anaesthetic gases are present.

2. The ideal bed is labour saving. One nurse should be able to operate any moving parts or accessories and methods of use of such parts should be obvious or easily learned.

3. The bed should move easily, but be capable of complete immobilization, so that patients should not be in danger if they lean against it.

4. The height should be variable, the high position being that at which nursing procedures can be comfortably performed, and the low

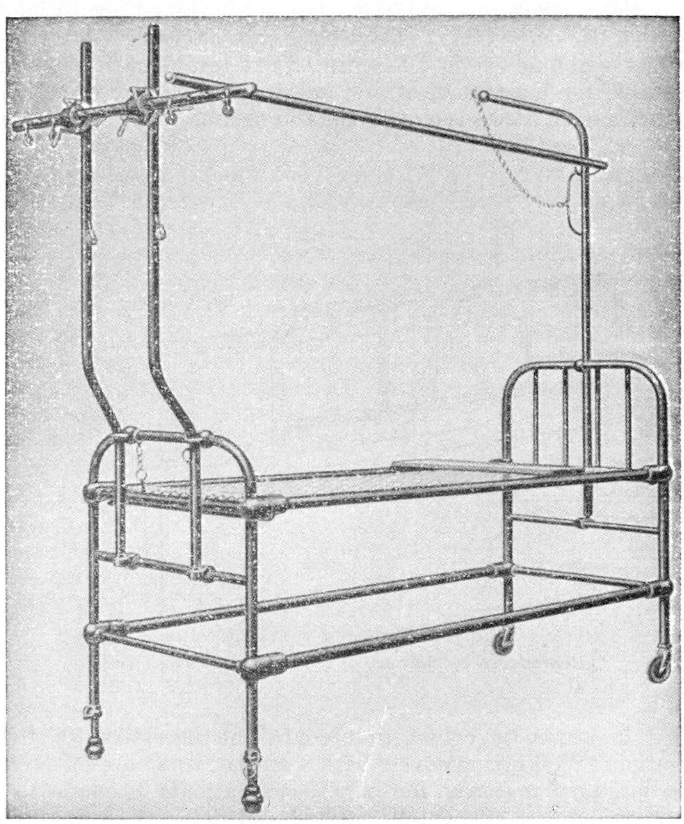

Fig. 2. A bedstead with overhead bars for the attachment of traction apparatus. The pulley attached to the lifting pole enables the patient to help in raising himself. (*Reproduced by courtesy of S. B. Whitfield (Sales) Ltd.*)

one that at which patients may safely get out of bed. Height adjustment should preferably be foot-operated.

5. The head of the bed should be detachable for ease in carrying out treatment.

6. The bed should be capable of tilting in either direction, and the method of operation should be labour-saving.

7. There should be a back support stable, and capable of being adjusted from either side of the bed. The method of operation should

not be strainful to the nurse. Most nurses would agree that most back rests are difficult to adjust, tend to slip, and can pinch the fingers.

8. A surface on which to strip the bedclothes is desirable.

9. Safety sides should be available, easily attached and removed.

(Design of Hospital Bedsteads. Published by King Edward's Hospital Fund for London, 1967. Price 15s.)

Mattresses can be made of hair, of latex or be interior-sprung. All should be used in a cover and protected from soiling, since they are not easy to clean efficiently and their life is shortened by disinfection. Latex foam is comfortable but apt to induce sweating which can be a serious cause of fluid loss in a dehydrated patient. Interior-sprung ones are suitable for most medical and surgical cases, but in orthopædic wards a firmer mattress is more generally useful. Mattresses should be enclosed in a plastic cover, to obviate the necessity for frequent disinfection. Well fitting covers with a zip fastening are effective.

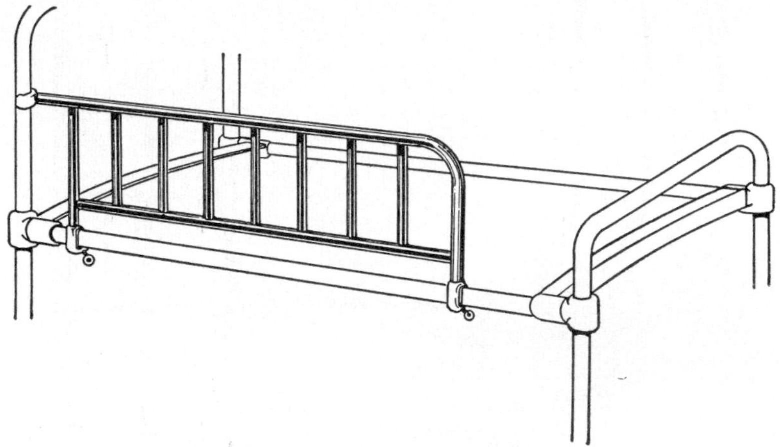

FIG. 3. Bedstead with side-rail.
(*Reproduced by courtesy of Hoskins and Sewell Ltd.*)

A proprietary mattress for paraplegic patients is made in small segments which are alternately inflated and deflated rhythmically by an electric motor, producing a "ripple" movement which prevents continuous pressure. The greatest care must be taken of these expensive mattresses in order to avoid punctures which will put them out of action.

Short plastic sheets covered with a draw sheet are used beneath the buttocks if the bottom sheet must be protected. The draw sheet can be pulled through at intervals to provide a fresh cool surface.

Pillows are filled with feathers or made of latex foam, and plastic covers are used beneath the outer one if there is any fear that they may be soiled by blood or discharge. Small pillows are useful for putting in the hollow of the back, or under the ankles to keep the heels from pressing on the bed.

It is often necessary to raise the foot and sometimes the head of the bed, and this is done with bed blocks of varying heights, or by steel frames with hooks on to which the bottom rung of the bed can be lifted. Sense should be used while lifting the bed on to the blocks, or the back may be strained. The nurses should stand with the weight evenly distributed between the feet and raise the bed by straightening the back and shoulders, not by flexing the elbows. Newer types of bed may be raised or lowered at one end by turning a handle, or moving a switch.

Latex foam cushions are used to protect from pressure the ischial tuberosities of people who are nursed sitting up. They must be protected against soiling, and the linen cover should be free from creases.

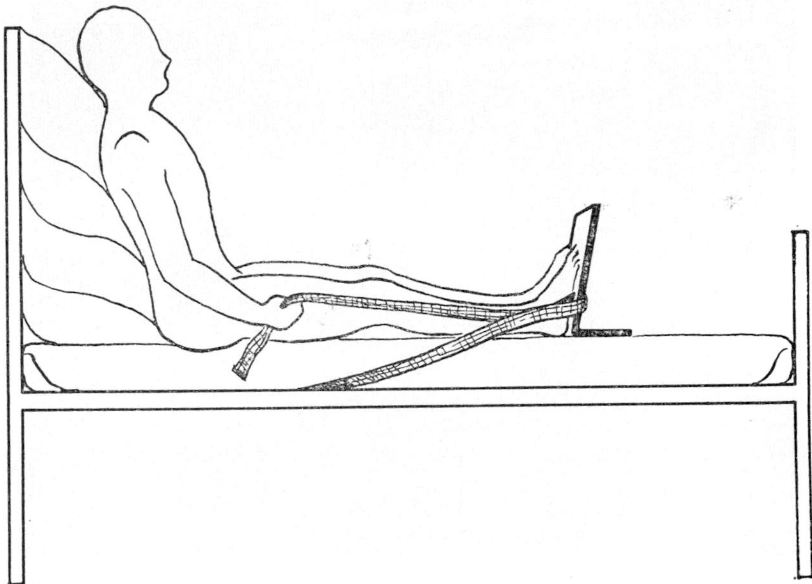

Fig. 4. A wooden foot-rest. The position is adjustable for a patient of any height, and it prevents the weight of the bedclothes from falling on the feet.

Those who are nursed in a sitting position can be supported with five or six pillows, or economy in pillows can be effected by using a back-rest. This may be a fitting on the bed or an adjustable wooden or metal frame with webbing stretched across it.

Cradles are devices for keeping the bedclothes from limbs that must be relieved of pressure—amputation stumps, legs with arterial disease, œdematous feet, or those liable to foot-drop—or from the trunk of those with fever. The traditional metal leg cradle could be improved in design, since minor injuries to limbs accidentally knocking against it can lead to serious results if the circulation is impaired ; its most useful position is with one side tucked under the end of the mattress. A variation of this pattern is illustrated, of which either the long or the short side of the cradle can be put under the end or side of the mattress. This kind can also be used instead of the body cradle, which is cumbersome and difficult to enclose in bedclothes of standard size.

Sandbags are used to immobilize limbs or support feet in a dorsi-flexed position, and it is best to keep them in jaconet covers, since if they are soiled the removal of their covers is a laborious business. A footboard is the most efficient device for foot support.

Blankets have received a good deal of attention from the pathologists, since they invariably become infected by any organisms that a patient may harbour and disseminate them into the air during bedmaking. Constant laundering of woollen blankets results in felting and shrinking,

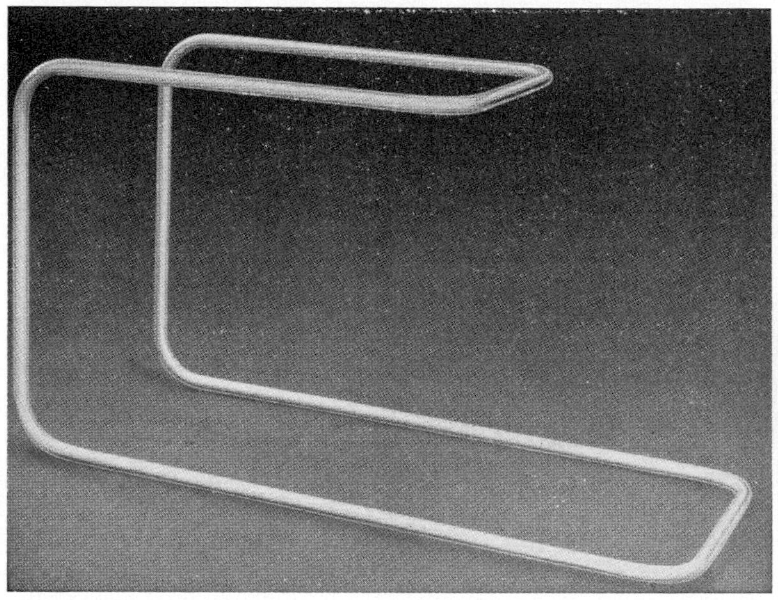

FIG. 5. A bed cradle, of which the long or short portion may be passed under the mattress, either at the foot or the side. (*Reproduced by courtesy of Hoskins & Sons Ltd.*)

however carefully it is done, and oiling techniques for minimizing the broadcasting of bacteria with the fluff are not satisfactory. Cotton cellular-weave blankets are warm though light, and can be regularly laundered. Blankets of man-made fibres can be washed without shrinking, and disposable blankets solve some problems.

Thin cotton or flannelette blankets are most useful in providing warmth without weight, and are much used next to people with bed cradles.

Sheets are of linen or cotton, but nylon and similar fabrics much used in the home are now appearing in hospital. Sheets should be of ample length, made of a fabric that is a poor heat conductor so that they do not feel chilly, and resistant to frequent laundering without shrinking. Draw-sheets are put transversely on the bed under the patient's buttocks and tucked in at each side. As their name implies, a portion can be drawn through from one side to another to provide a fresh part to sit on. While they must be long enough to perform this function, they should not be so long that the tuck-in is bulky enough to raise the edge of the mattress.

Electric blankets are used to warm beds, and there are few occasions on which it is necessary to use them except in an empty bed. Though so widely used in the home as well as in hospital, shocks or burns can occur with defective equipment, especially if it is allowed to become wet, and some hospitals like to have a signal on a bed that contains an electric blanket, to obviate the risk of a patient being laid on one. Before it is removed the switch should be turned off and the plug removed, and it must not be folded tightly in a way that might fracture the wiring. It should be inspected before being stored to see that the plug is uncracked, the points not loose and the flex unfrayed. Any that are not in perfect order should be sent to the electrician or the maker, and the removable cover should be frequently laundered.

Small electric pads are often given for pain in joints, but must not be supplied without instructions from the doctor, who should specify the degree of heat to be used and the length of time. They should have a jaconet cover under the removable one to prevent moistening by sweat.

Hot-water bottles have been to a great extent superseded by electric blankets as a means of heating beds, and a marked increase in the number of patients bringing legal actions against hospitals because of hot-water-bottle burns has caused reluctance to allow patients to have them at all, in spite of their universal use at home and the comfort they undoubtedly bring. Many normal people sustain burns at home through using uncovered bottles at too high a temperature and falling asleep in contact with them, and hospitals contain many people who are exceptionally vulnerable to such injury. It appears undesirable to give a hot-water bottle to anyone whose sensation is impaired (e.g. the paralysed or unconscious), whose circulation is defective (e.g. those with arterial disease), or who is in any way incapable of managing it effectively (e.g. infants, the aged, the confused or the heavily-sedated patient).

A large number of burns are due to overlooking a hot-water bottle that has been used to warm a bed and laying an unconscious patient on it after operation or on admission. This cause can be obviated by using distinctive coloured covers ; white flannel should never be used.

If a patient is to be given a hot-water bottle it must be a rubber one in good condition, two-thirds filled with water at about 70° C. (the temperature at which water is supplied from the tap in most hospitals) and totally enclosed in an efficient cover. Some use near-boiling water, but put it outside the blanket. Those who are not allowed a bottle can be offered socks or an extra blanket.

Metal and stone bottles are only used for warming empty beds. They should be completely filled with boiling water through a funnel, screwed up tightly, dried and tested for leakage before being put into a coloured cover and into the bed. The reason for not allowing patients to use them is that pressure from them on a limb may produce a lesion indistinguishable from a burn, even though their temperature is only moderate. Rubber bottles are treated similarly, but must not be completely filled, and it appears necessary to tell nurses that the air must be excluded, but not by pressing the bottle against the chest.

Bed tables are needed for those with congestive heart failure, who by fixing the shoulder girdle by resting the elbows on the table can assist their breathing. Others appreciate them for keeping books, flowers and handiwork on. They should not be left across the beds of restless patients who may kick them over. A plastic surface is labour saving, and some patterns have a rising centre section which supports a book at a convenient reading angle.

A locker stands by each bed, the interior holding the patient's personal belongings, and the top carrying drinks and other articles in constant use. Nurses would probably say that the ideal one has yet to be found, and that it must include some essential features. It must be capable of standing on either side of a bed and must have a section that can be drawn across the bed at mealtimes. Since most people in hospital get up, it must contain enough space for a dressing-gown, but the space must be sub-divided so that search for some articles does not involve turning over everything the patient possesses. The rail at the back must stand clear enough to enable a bath towel to be conveniently hung, and hooks for face flannels are desirable. Older ones had a portion that could be used for a temporary seat, and which was invaluable for placing a bed-pan while bedclothes were adjusted, but this useful feature seems to be disappearing.

MAKING BEDS

Skilful bedmaking contributes materially to the patient's comfort and, since the rounds of bedmaking twice a day take a fair amount of the nurse's time, an efficient and labour-saving technique is important. The traditional British method is described here, in which two nurses work together, while the climate and the temperature at which wards are kept mean that the top coverings are usually a sheet, two blankets and a counterpane. These are only local customs ; in America nurses make beds alone except for the seriously ill. In Scandinavia the top clothes consist of a feather quilt in a cotton cover, which considerably reduces the time spent on making beds, while in warm countries the use of blankets will be modified. Sheets with fitted corners are widely used in the home and, when these are marketed in a material suitable for hospital purposes, may prove valuable in promoting comfort and saving time.

The details of technique are worth while studying in order to find one that involves no unnecessary movement and strain, since even a few extra steps at each bed are wasteful of time and energy when twenty or thirty beds have to be made. Some important points are as follows :

1. A supply of sheets, pillowcases and ring covers should be available at hand so that each time it is found that some article needs changing another walk to the linen room is not involved.

2. Clothes should be stripped on to two chairs placed back to back, which will not topple under a weight of clothes and are of a height that does not involve stooping.

3. Clothes should be stripped in a style that involves no unnecessary movement either in removing or replacing them. Most people agree that folding into three is the most suitable, and there are two ways of doing this. Firstly, the bottom edge is folded inwards for one-third of the length of the sheet or blanket, then the top section is folded across it thus ⊃. This can be neatly and swiftly executed, but the bottom section is the middle one, and the sheet must be taken to the

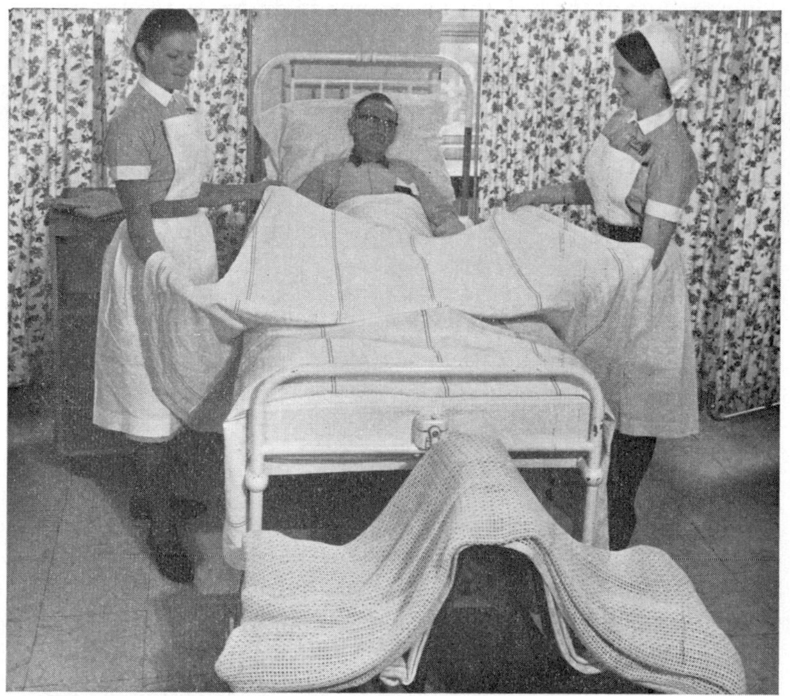

FIG. 6. Stripping a bed. The method shown is economical in movement.

middle of the bed, laid on it and unfolded, and then the nurse walks first to the foot, then to the head to tuck it in. Secondly, the sheet is folded thus ≶; now the bottom section is the lowest, and it can be laid on the foot of the bed and the end secured without walking more than a step.

4. If two nurses are working together, they should work directly opposite each other and in unison. Speed and neatness are not produced if one is tucking in the foot while the other is removing the pillows.

5. It is very easy to get absorbed in conversation with one's opposite number, but patients who are well enough greatly enjoy the opportunity

for talking to their nurses, and patients who are too ill to do so require the nurses' undivided attention.

Making an Empty Bed. The counterpane is folded and the top clothes loosened and stripped as described and laid over the chairs, the pillows being put on the seat of one of them. The drawsheet, plastic sheet, bottom sheet and long mackintosh follow in order, and the mattress is turned over and its cover straightened ; it must lie as close to the top rail as possible or the pillows will tend to slip down behind it.

The long mackintosh, if this is used, must completely cover the mattress, or it is ineffective. An under-blanket to cover this is not universally used but is very comfortable. The folded bottom sheet is laid on the foot of the bed, the upper margin drawn up the bed and the end of the sheet pulled taut beneath the mattress. The pictures illustrate the way in which the corner is mitred to secure a neat and firm end, and this corner is repeated at the top. One nurse picks up the plastic sheet and the other the drawsheet, which is tucked in with

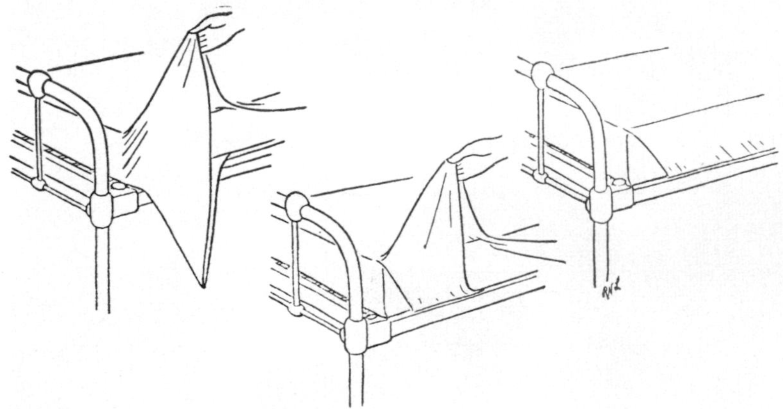

FIG. 7. Mitring the corner of a sheet. This method ensures that the bottom sheet remains taut.

the major part of the sheet on one side. The pillows are shaken up and put in position, and the ward will present a tidier appearance if all the closed ends of the pillows are placed facing down the room towards the door. Enough of the top sheet is folded in at the end to allow a turnover of about 18 in. (or the length of the forearm) at the top. The blankets are tucked in and mitred at the bottom, the upper corner of each is turned inwards and excess folded over so that a patient lying down has spare blanket to draw up over the shoulders. The counterpane usually has only a half-mitre fold at the bottom so that its edges are free ; excess at the top is turned under and secured and the sheet folded outside it. When finished it should be a neat rectangular shape with equal amounts of sheet and counterpane on each side. Many people would maintain today that making an empty bed is a task for domestic rather than nursing staff, and that the nurse's responsibility is merely to see that the bed is efficiently made.

Making an Occupied Bed. The counterpane and top blanket are removed, then the top sheet drawn out from beneath the second blanket so that for the rest of the procedure the patient is covered with a blanket, a necessary precaution against chilling in a "temperate" climate. The bottom clothes are tightened and the drawsheet pulled through. If the patient can roll, he is asked and helped to roll towards the nurse with the short end of drawsheet, while her colleague straightens the mackintosh, tucks in the end of the drawsheet and rolls the excess neatly into the centre of the bed against the buttocks of the patient, who is then rolled in the opposite direction. The first nurse draws through the sheet, stretching it as taut as possible and tucks it in. The patient is assisted to sit, and one nurse may have to support him while the other arranges the pillows. The top bedclothes are replaced without tension sufficient to restrict leg movement.

Admission or Duty Beds. A ward on duty for urgent or casualty admissions has one or two beds ready to receive such cases. Two old blankets or bath blankets are put into the bed so that patients in street clothes may be put to bed in them without soiling, and these blankets may be removed when the patient has been undressed and bathed. It is customary to warm these beds, and people who have made a journey by ambulance, often in fear or pain, appreciate a warm bed. If the ward is a surgical one where warmth is deprecated for shocked patients, the wishes of the surgeon are followed.

Positions in Bed

Beds are made for people, not for diseases ; we do not prepare a bed for congestive heart failure, but for a particular individual. The sections that follow are therefore only comments on the principles that underlie the positions in which people have to be nursed in bed. A good posture in bed is little different in its basic ideas from posture in ordinary life. One of the most important of this is that a good position of the spine, with the lumbar spine hollowed and the shoulders expanded will prevent fatigue and allow good respiratory movement which will in its turn improve the circulation.

Lying flat. Patients who are unconscious should be nursed in the horizontal position, lying on the side, so that neither the tongue nor secretions can obstruct the airway. It is therefore necessary to make provision against his rolling onto his back. The best way is to draw the lower arm behind the patient, and flex the upper leg a little more than the other. Putting a pillow behind the back is a less reliable means of maintaining this position.

People suffering from shock or the effects of hæmorrhage need to be in a position in which the brain can receive the best blood supply that the enfeebled circulation can provide. Not only is the patient laid flat, but the foot of the bed should be raised so that gravity can help the passage of the blood to the head.

Following some eye operations patients may have to lie flat, often for two or three weeks, and with the eyes covered. These must be made really comfortable if they are to rest, with a small pillow under the lumbar spine to support its hollow.

The heart may be affected by many disease processes such as diphtheria, acute nephritis, acute rheumatism or occlusion of a coronary artery. If acute heart failure is feared, the patient is nursed at rest, flat or semi-recumbent in order to minimize the work the heart has to do.

Sitting up. The same point about supporting the lumbar spine is to be observed in patients who must sit upright, and the pillows must be so arranged that the shoulders are expanded. People who have had abdominal operations are usually nursed sitting up so that good lung expansion is encouraged, while free movement of the diaphragm encourages return of blood to the heart from the abdomen and legs by drawing up the inferior vena cava.

People with congestive heart failure are usually so breathless that they must sit up. This is because the lungs are waterlogged, and when the patient sits up this fluid drains downward and makes breathing easier. The œdematous lungs are rather heavy and unelastic to expand, and often the patient is more comfortable if he can fix his shoulder girdle by resting his arms on a heart-table, and thus enable the accessory muscles of respiration, such as pectoralis major, to come into play. Someone leaning forward in this position will find his legs cramped, and uncomfortable, and it will be a relief if the end of the bed can be lowered a little so that the knees can be flexed.

Use of blankets. Sweating is a constant accompaniment of some diseases; acute rheumatoid arthritis and rheumatic fever are examples. Cotton nightclothes and sheets may feel chilly and uncomfortable if damp, and a light flannelette sheet or blanket next to the patient may be welcome. People who have a cradle in the bed to keep the weight of the bedclothes from their legs sometimes complain of lack of cosiness and a flannelette sheet is welcome. People with acute nephritis must be protected from skin-chill in order to avoid throwing additional strain on the kidneys. Some physicians like these patients to be nursed with a blanket next to them for this reason.

Fracture Beds. A broken leg, whether immobilized by a splint or in plaster, requires level support, and beneath a firm mattress are laid fracture boards to provide that support. If an above-knee plaster has been applied a pad or small sandbag should be provided to go under the knee and the ankle, a cradle keeps the bedclothes from pressing on the toes, and a blanket next to the patient ensures warmth. For the first twenty-four hours the end of the bed is kept open, so that the circulation of the toes can be checked. Details about the nursing of patients in plaster and in splints are given in Chapter 26.

If balanced traction is being used to treat a fractured femur on a Thomas's splint, the limb on its splint is supported clear of the bed, and the top clothes are divided into two halves, one of which covers the trunk and the other the uninjured leg. The bed itself is of the Pearson type, with an overhead beam from which the broken leg is suspended, while the foot of the bed is always raised. The bedclothes cannot of course be drawn up over the end of the bed ; one nurse lifts the sheet or blanket and passes it across the patient to her partner.

The upper clothes consist of a small blanket folded in two, and enclosed in a small sheet ; the lower may consist of another blanket (which is omitted in warm weather) and the counterpane.

The Prone Position. Patients may be nursed face downwards because of burns or injuries to the back, or for shorter periods to relieve pressure on the back, and careful arrangement of pillows is needed if the position is to be comfortable. A flock one is placed under the legs above the ankle so that the feet are dorsiflexed without pressure on the toes, and the knees can be slightly flexed. Another softer one is under the abdomen to prevent excessive and tiring hollowing of the lumbar spine. A third lies under the chest, and a fourth small one goes under the head, which is usually turned to one side or the other so that the cheek rests on the pillow. The arms are most comfortable lying on the bed with the forearms flexed and pronated, about the level of the head, but can be brought down to the sides for a change of position. There is little difficulty in nursing the young and supple prone, but older patients with more rigid spines can be most uncomfortable unless adjustments in the size and position of pillows are made intelligently.

Lifting and Turning Patients

During bedmaking, and often at intervals throughout the day, it is necessary to adjust the pillows and position of a patient who is being nursed in the sitting posture. The nurses face the top of the bed and each puts an arm under the patient's axilla while he puts a hand behind the shoulder of each nurse and is assisted to sit forward. It may be necessary for one to maintain him in that position, while the other adjusts the pillows. If it is desirable and possible for the patient to help himself, he is asked to put his hands on the bed slightly behind him, flex the knees and dig the heels into the bed, and lift himself while the nurses assist with an arm under the axilla. The exercise involved is valuable for some surgical patients, but they will need instruction into how to do it painlessly, with the head forward and the spine slightly flexed.

There are two ways of lifting the helpless patient, both needing some patience and understanding of body mechanics if nurse and patient are to find them easy and comfortable.

1. The nurses face up the bed and ask the patient to hook her upper arm over their shoulders, while they join hands beneath the thighs. The free hand is placed on the bed behind the patient or may grasp the bedhead. As before, the effort for the lift comes from the straightening of the thighs. This method (Australian) is mechanically more effective than the next, and does not involve such close proximity of the faces of nurse and patient.

2. The nurses stand facing each other with feet about 12 or 18 in. apart and slightly behind the patient, who is asked to fold her hands on her chest and to keep the head forward. The nurses join hands behind the patient at the level of the hip joint, and below the thighs rather nearer to the buttocks than the knees. The stronger or more experienced clasps the arm of her assistant just above the wrist on the outer side. The patient is asked to lean slightly back against the nurses'

hold and to keep the legs steady. The nurses stand with weight firmly distributed on both feet, and with hips and knees slightly flexed. The lift is accomplished by tightening the arms, and straightening the back and legs, and the patient is transferred to her new position. It must be noted that the motive power comes from the big muscles of the thighs ; if lifting of a heavy patient is attempted by using only the arms and shoulders efforts will be ineffectual and likely to strain the back.

Turning a helpless patient on to the side may be accomplished by

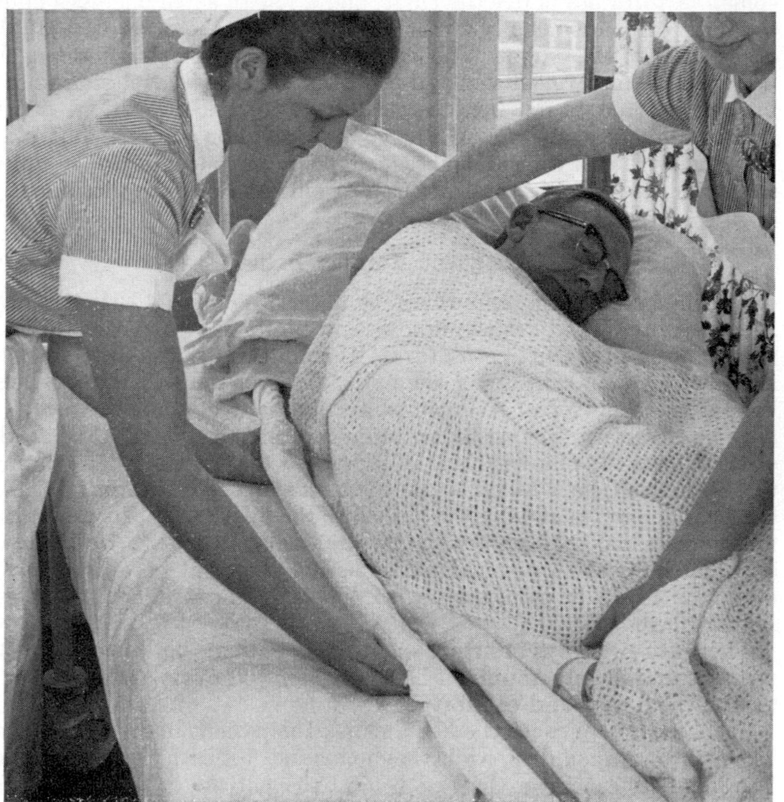

FIG. 8. Changing bottom sheet from side to side.

one nurse for someone light, but two are generally needed. The upper clothes are stripped or loosened so that the limbs can be easily controlled. An arm and a leg are drawn across to the side which the patient is to face ; one nurse draws over the shoulder, and the other rolls the pelvis. Both join arms below the hip joint and thigh, and lift the pelvis into the centre of the bed. The pillow is adjusted to its new position under the cheek, the arms are made comfortable and the upper leg slightly flexed.

Changing Bottom Sheets

The nurses bring to the bedside a clean bottom sheet and drawsheet, such other linen as may be required, and a linen bin. If the patient can be turned, the side to side method is the easier, but cardiac cases and those who cannot be rolled have their sheets changed from bottom to top. In either case the top clothes are stripped and the patient covered with a blanket. The bottom sheet and drawsheet are untucked.

Side to Side. All pillows but one or two are removed, and the nurse with the major portion of drawsheet assists the patient to roll towards her colleague. The drawsheet, plastic sheet and bottom sheet are

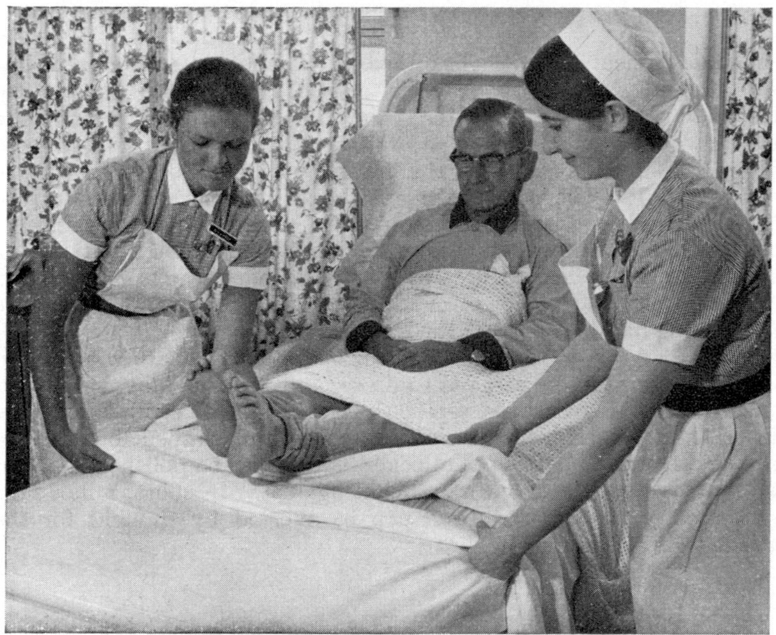

FIG. 9. Changing a sheet from bottom to top. This method is used for a patient who cannot be rolled from one side to another.

each rolled separately the length of the bed up to the patient's buttocks, the mattress cover and long mackintosh are straightened, and the clean bottom sheet tucked in at the side, bottom and top, then the free portion is rolled to lie alongside the used bottom sheet. The rolled part of the draw-mackintosh is unrolled again and the clean drawsheet tucked in at one side and the excess rolled up. The patient is turned on to the clean sheets, his pillow moved under his head, and the nurse who has made her half of the bed takes over the task of supporting the patient while her colleague removes the used draw-sheet, rolls up her half of the plastic sheet and takes out the used bottom sheet. The rolled clean clothes are then unfolded and the second half of the bed made.

Bottom to Top. It is easiestto lift the patient and take out the plastic sheet and sheet first. The bottom sheet is rolled up to the patient's buttocks, the clean one tucked in at the bottom, straightened beneath the legs and rolled up alongside the used one. The buttocks are lifted by clasping wrists beneath them, and with the free hand the nurses roll the dirty sheet and unroll the clean one, and lower the patient on to the clean one. One nurse now supports the patient in a sitting position while the other takes out the pillows and the used sheet, and unrolls and tucks in the top of the clean one. The pillows are re-adjusted, a clean plastic and draw sheet inserted, and everything drawn taut and tucked in.

Getting Up

When a patient is to get out of bed for the first time after an operation, the nurses must know if she is to stand or walk, or if she is to be lifted into a chair. If the latter is the case, a chair is brought to the bedside with an unfolded blanket over the seat and one of the patient's pillows. If it is a wheel chair the brake must be on, or another nurse must steady it. The patient is helped to swing her legs over the side of the bed, and her dressing gown and slippers (and socks if the temperature of the ward suggests it) are put on, and she is lifted into the chair in one of the ways described. The blanket is folded round her legs and a footstool may be provided. A watch must be kept to see that she is not reacting unfavourably to the new position.

Those who are getting up after an operation and are required to stand or walk must be assisted to do so, and for some days may need supervision and assistance especially if elderly. Hospital beds are higher than those at home, dressing gown and slippers have to be extracted from the bottom of a locker, floors may be polished, beds on castors may tend to move when leant against. In short, minor falls occur readily at this time, and can be averted by thought for the patient's difficulties.

CHAPTER 4

CLINICAL OBSERVATIONS

THE term " clinical observations " is apt to imply the noting of such facts as the temperature, pulse and respiration rate, but all nurses know that by the time they have made these observations they have also noticed a great many other things. If the patient is a new one, the nurse has noticed his attitude in bed, his colour, and his state of nutrition; whether he is aware of his surroundings, and if so whether he is reacting with fear, anxiety or indifference ; she has noticed the

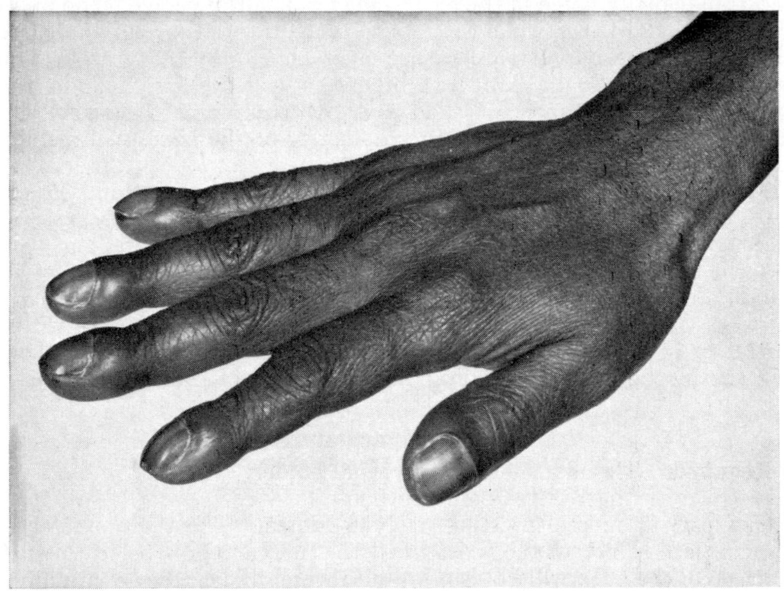

FIG. 10. Some clinical features that may be observed. Clubbing of the fingers in an Indian patient.

feel of his skin and his muscle tone, and perhaps has by his voice and conversation decided what part of the country he comes from, and formed an opinion on his educational status. She has not only to deal with a patient, but to form a relationship with a person, and she begins at once to estimate how best this can be done.

Colour. The skin may be *pale*, suggesting anæmia, shock or fear ; it may show *cyanosis* (blueness), indicating sub-oxygenation of the blood ; a *flush* may suggest that the temperature is high ; *jaundice* means yellowness, and is due to accumulation in the tissues of the pigments normally excreted in the bile. It ranges from a pale yellow only observable in the conjunctivæ, to a bronze-green staining of the whole skin.

Attitude. Patients with *colic*, whether of intestine, ureters or bile duct, tend to be restless with each attack of pain, groaning and sometimes vomiting.

Those with abdominal pain due to *peritonitis* tend to lie on the back with the hips flexed to slacken the tension of the abdominal muscles. Movement increases the pain, so they lie still, watching those around with alert anxiety. Patients with cerebral irritation often display dislike of light (*photophobia*). They lie on the side in an attitude of flexion, actively resenting any attempt to move or examine them.

TEMPERATURE

The normal body temperature is said to be 98·4° F. (36·9° C.), but the temperature varies in different parts of the body. The skin temperature (usually taken in the axilla) may in healthy people be no more than 97° F. (36·1° C.), while the mouth temperature is usually a degree higher, and the rectal temperature may be 99° F. (37·2° C.). The temperature is usually a degree higher in the evening than in the morning because of muscular and metabolic activity. The same site should always be used for the thermometer, or the chart will display unnatural variations.

The clinical thermometer is a mercury one, scaled from 95° to 110° F. or 35° to 43° C. A bulb at one end contains a reservoir of mercury, and above it is a kink to prevent the mercury falling back into the bulb once it has risen. Low-registering thermometers may also be obtained for use with patients whose temperature is artificially lowered. They are mercury thermometers, registering from 85° F. to 110° F. or 30 to 43° C. For such patients a rectal thermometer consisting of a thermocouple, self-recording, is more accurate and informative.

Axillary Temperatures

Required. Thermometer in individual holder.
Chart or temperature book.

The patient must be sitting or lying down. The thermometer is shaken with a flick of the wrist until the mercury falls below the 95° mark. On the back will be seen a figure which indicates the minimum time the thermometer takes to register, and this should be noted. The thermometer is inserted under the arm with the bulb in contact with the folds of the skin, care being taken that clothing does not intervene. The elbow is kept at the side and the forearm laid across the chest to retain the thermometer in position. It should be left there for half a minute longer than the minimum time marked on the thermometer; the interval is usually occupied in taking the pulse and respiration rate. The thermometer is removed and wiped, the level reached by the mercury is noted; then the thermometer is shaken and replaced in the carbolic. The temperature, pulse and respiration rate are recorded.

This method is not used if the patient is very thin, or if there is any local inflammation. Small children of one or two may resent having the arm held at the side, and the thermometer may then be placed in the groin, using the same technique as for the axillary method.

If the patient is unconscious or not well orientated, the thermometer must be held in position, a precaution taken whatever the site used.

Oral Temperatures

If ward temperatures are taken in the mouth, individual thermometers should be used; they may be stored dry or in glycothymoline, and sterilized in 70% alcohol on the patient's discharge. The bulb is placed under the tongue, and the patient asked to close the lips, but not the teeth. It is obviously not a method suited for any patient who cannot breathe through the nose, or anyone who is irresponsible because of his age or illness. Hot or cold drinks affect the mouth temperature, but the effect is short lived.

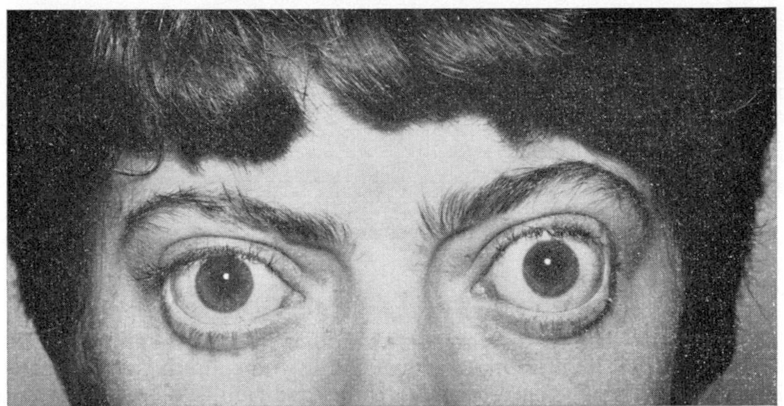

FIG. 11. Clinical sign Exophthalmos.

Rectal Temperatures

The rectal route is used for babies and for those subjected to low-temperature techniques. It is the most reliable site after head operations, and may be used if it is suspected that the patient is assisting the mercury to rise in some way. It is not uncommon for neurotic patients to feel that a rise of temperature would earn them the attention they feel they deserve, and a hot-water bottle, hot pipe or cup of tea may enable them apparently to obtain it. An unexpected rise unaccompanied by a proportionate elevation of the pulse should make the nurse take the temperature again, remaining with the patient. No comment should be made, but the doctor should be told.

Rectal thermometers should have round bulbs, to prevent their inadvertent use in other situations, and should be kept in individual jars of soft paraffin. When no longer needed they are washed with soap and water and steeped in 70% alcohol for half an hour.

When in use the bulb is inserted 1 in. into the anal canal and held there for the time indicated. A baby lies on the nurse's lap and she controls the feet with her left hand while holding the thermometer in the right.

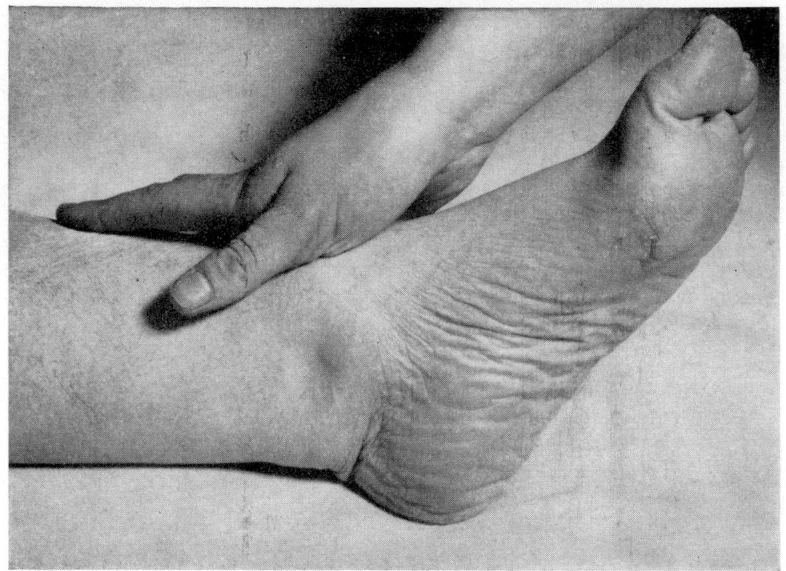

FIG. 12 Oedema of ankle.

Recording Temperatures

It is usual to record temperatures graphically on a chart by making a spot in ink at the appropriate level and in the column that indicates the time and date. Temperatures are by tradition taken morning and evening, and in hospital practice it is not usually possible to omit this even in convalescent patients without the risk of missing an indication of a complication sometimes. The temperature is taken four-hourly if it is abnormal, and is always recorded after operation and at such other times as the information proves useful. The dots on the chart are neatly joined by lines, and a tidy chart not only indicates the nurse's pride in her work, but is much easier for the doctor to read.

Terms have been applied in the past to different temperature ranges, but they are not generally useful, and it is much better to quote the actual temperature in a report. Pyrexia is a word used of any temperature rise ; hyperpyrexia means a high degree of fever, and is used of temperatures above 104° F. (40° C.).

An isolated temperature reading is of limited value ; a chart gives an informative picture, telling the degree of fever, if the tendency is increasing or decreasing, how big is the temperature range, and how fast it is rising or falling.

The quickest way in which a temperature can rise and fall is seen in the *rigor*. This incident is a sudden onset of fever in which the temperature may rise four or five degrees because of shivering, and fall again by reason of sweating. The whole episode may be over in half an hour. Rigors occur regularly in malaria ; at the onset of a few infections like *pyelitis* and *lobar pneumonia;* as a reaction to tbo

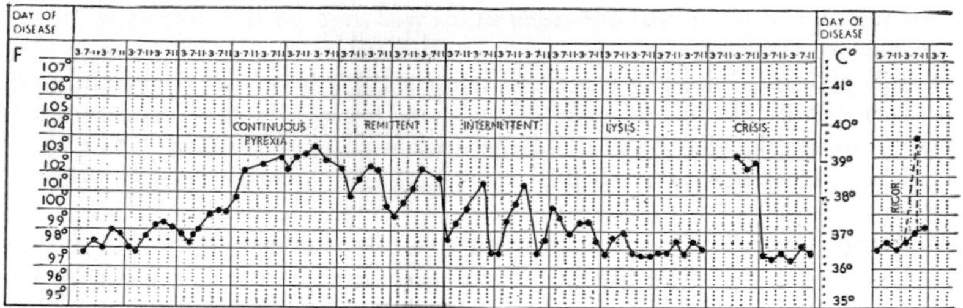

Fig. 13. Some temperature patterns.

injection of foreign protein, either intramuscularly or intravenously. Rigors are unusual in children, in whom fits occur instead.

The patient suddenly feels intensely cold, begins to shiver, and may vomit. His temperature is rising rapidly, and may reach 104° F. (40° C.) before the shivering ceases and he feels hot. Sweating begins at once and the fever subsides as quickly as it arose. During the " cold " or shivering stage (when the temperature is rising) the patient should be well covered and given warm drinks to help to get this distressing episode over quickly. Hot-water bottles are dangerous, since the patient cannot control his own actions, or appreciate temperature. As the shivering subsides blankets are gradually withdrawn, but bath towels and a dry blanket should be available. Not only will the pillow case be soaked, but the pillow too, and will need changing. The method of charting a rigor is shown in Fig. 13.

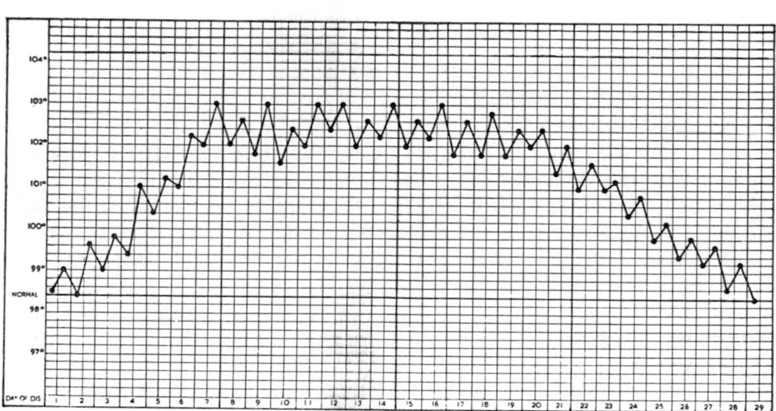

Fig. 14. Pel-Ebstein type of temperature.

The onset of a feverish episode is more commonly a gradual one, occupying several hours or even days. A high fever with not more than 2° F. variation in the day is termed *continuous pyrexia*. If there is a greater diurnal swing than this, but without a fall to normal, the term is *remittent pyrexia*. High fever with a descent to normal or below between the peaks of fever is very exhausting, involving alternate shivering as the temperature rises and sweating as it falls; *it is termed intermittent pyrexia.*

A fall of temperature to normal from a high level within an hour or two is a *crisis.* It is not now often seen, since effective treatment of lobar pneumonia altered the classic course of that disease. The more usual form of temperature fall is a gradual one, or lysis, taking a day or more.

A temperature pattern following a more prolonged course is the *Pel-Ebstein* curve. The temperature rises slowly over days, and takes a corresponding time to fall. It is sometimes seen in lymphadenoma, and the cause is unknown.

THE PULSE

The pulse is the wave of distension generated in an artery by the contraction of the heart, and it can be felt in any artery big enough, or near enough to the surface to be palpable. It is usually taken in the radial artery at the wrist, a place convenient both for patient and nurse. The anæsthetist often uses the temporal artery, just in front of the ear, or the facial artery where it crosses the mandible in front of the angle of the jaw. In states of shock or hæmorrhage when the radial pulse is imperceptible, the carotid pulse may be felt alongside the anterior border of the sternomastoid muscle.

All that is needed to take the pulse is a watch with a second hand big enough to be easily seen, the ability to observe accurately, and preferably the experience to interpret these observations and relate them to others that the nurse makes. An estimate of the pulse rate alone is of little value unless the other characters of the pulse are noticed.

The patient must be at rest, either sitting or lying down. It is convenient to have the forearm flexed across the chest, so that the respirations may be counted immediately after the pulse. The nurse uses the hand opposite to the one in which she is taking the pulse, so if she is using the patient's right wrist, she puts the tips of her left first three fingers along the line of the radial artery on the inner aspect of the wrist and her thumb behind it. She holds her watch in her free hand, and counts the rate for thirty seconds, doubling the answer to get the rate per minute. For as long as is necessary she considers the characters of the pulse described below. Having finished her observations she records the result.

The facts of anatomy and physiology that are especially relevant in considering the pulse are these :

1. Cardiac muscle fibres are united to each other so that the wave of contraction spreads rapidly over the heart.

2. Heart muscle has an inherent tendency to contract, and will do so in the absence of nerve stimuli. An isolated frog heart will contract rhythmically for some time if put into normal saline.

3. The heart is supplied with fibres from the vagus nerve that slow the rate, and by sympathetic fibres that quicken it.

4. Having contracted, heart muscles relax, and for a short time known as the *refractory period* will not contract again.

5. The contraction normally follows a regular path through the

heart. It is initiated in the sino-auricular node in the right auricle, passes over the auricles to the auroculo-ventricular node. From here the path by which the ventricles are stimulated to contract is the Bundle of His in the septum.

The points to be observed about the pulse are as follows :

1. **Rate.** The average adult rate is 72 beats per minute. In a baby it is 120 to 140, and at 12 years has fallen to 80.

2. **Rhythm.** This should be regular, the beats being evenly spaced.

3. **Volume.** This refers to the amount of blood distending the artery with each beat and only experience can tell the nurse if it is within normal limits.

4. **Tension.** This refers to the compressibility of the pulse, i.e. the ease or otherwise with which the flow can be interrupted by pressure. Unlike the other characters of the pulse, which are produced by the heart, tension is a property of the artery wall.

Changes in Rate

It is normal for the pulse rate to increase after exercise, during fever, and in emotional states like anger and fear. It is raised also in thyrotoxicosis, in shock and hæmorrhage ; in myocardial failure ; and by many drugs.

Tachycardia means a fast heart rate (above 120). Paroxysmal tachycardia is a condition in which there are attacks, of variable duration, in which the pulse rate is much increased.

Bradycardia means an abnormally slow heart rate. A slow pulse is seen in patients with raised intracranial pressure (concussion ; head tumour ; cerebrovascular accident) ; in heart block ; in those suffering from jaundice ; during the administration of some drugs, especially those of the morphine group, and digitalis.

Changes in Rhythm

Extra systoles are perhaps the commonest cause of upset of normal rhythm. An extra beat in interpolated, and is followed by a slight pause before normal rhythm is restored with a forcible beat. Extra systoles are serious if occurring very frequently, or in a heart known to be diseased.

Occasional extra systoles are not uncommon in convalescents, or in anyone after a heavy meal. Patients are often conscious of the heart-beat (palpitation) after an extra systole, and feel anxious about it.

In children the pulse may be noticed to decrease in rate and volume during inspiration, and to become quicker and fuller during expiration. This is *pulsus paradoxus*, and is not of pathological significance, but the changing rhythm makes it difficult to count, especially if the breathing is rapid.

A *dicrotic pulse* is one in which a normal character of the pulse is exaggerated. A pulse tracing shows a steep rise in pressure with each beat, and a more gradual falling away with a slight secondary rise (the dicrotic notch) due to the elastic recoil of the artery wall. Sometimes this dicrotic wave becomes palpable between the normal beats, though not so strong as they are.

Atrial fibrillation is a quite common and important cause of irregularity, often associated with organic heart disease like mitral stenosis, or as a sign of heart stress in thyrotoxicosis. The auricles cease their regular and co-ordinated contraction, and the muscle quivers as irregular and rapid waves flicker over it. Their function of filling the ventricles is inefficiently fulfilled, but more serious is the grossly irregular stimulation of the ventricles via the Bundle of His. This results in the heart becoming irregular both in its rhythm and in the force of its beats, some of which may be heard at the heart with a stethoscope, but are too weak to be felt at the wrist. This may be demonstrated by finding the apical and radial rates simultaneously. Two nurses are needed, of whom the senior listens to the apex beat with a stethoscope. She stands on the patient's right, while her assistant stands on the left to take the radial pulse, holding the watch in a position where both can see it.

The curtains are drawn if the patient is a woman, and the chest exposed. The earpieces of the stethoscope are adjusted in place; they should point forwards as the nurse puts it on. The apex beat normally lies about 3½ in. (9 cm.) from the midline just below the nipple level. If the heart is enlarged the beat may be heard much further to the left. The nurse satisfies herself that she is hearing it with maximum intensity, and then indicates to her assistant the time at which they will simultaneously begin to count. A half-minute is perhaps the best interval; counting the irregular and unpredictable pulse needs much concentration, and it is easy to lose one's place if a minute count is used. The apical figure is recorded above the radical one, e.g. $\frac{92}{78}$, and the difference between the two is the *pulse deficit*. When charting the pulse of such a patient, the apical rate should be marked in a different coloured ink above the pulse rate. As far as the physician is concerned, it is the rate and rhythm of the heart not of the pulse that determines treatment, and the doctor may request that the apex beat rather than the pulse that is recorded for his cardiac patients.

Coupling of the pulse means that the beats occur in pairs with a pause between. Since the usual cause is a relative overdose of digitalis, the rate is usually a slow one.

Heart block is a condition in which conduction down the Bundle of His is partially or completely interrupted. In partial heart block, every second, third or fourth stimulus may fail to pass from auricle to ventricle, so that ventricular contraction at these intervals is absent. This is an irregularity with a definite pattern.

Complete heart block results in the ventricles taking up their own slow rate independent of the auricles. The rhythm in such cases is regular, but bradycardia is marked.

Changes in Volume

The volume is less in shock, hæmorrhage, heart failure and in recovery states. It is increased by exercise, fever, and by raised intracranial pressure.

Changes in Tension

A child's pulse is soft and easily compressed, while that of an older person often becomes harder as the result of changes in the artery wall (arteriosclerosis).

Changes in any of these factors are not usually single. A *thready* pulse is one in which the rate is increased and the volume much reduced; it suggests the possibility of hæmorrhage. A *wiry* pulse is of high tension but low volume and is found in the arteriosclerotic. A patient with concussion often has a slow full pulse that is spoken of as *bounding*.

RESPIRATION

A newborn baby breathes from 32 to 50 times a minute, an adult 16 to 20. The pulse rate is usually about four times quicker than the respiration rate, and disturbance of this relation between them is characteristic of some diseases (e.g. lobar pneumonia). The muscles involved in inspiration are the intercostals (supplied by nerves from the thoracic part of the spinal cord) and the diaphragm (supplied by the phrenic nerves). This separate nerve supply means that in cases of injury or inflammation of the cord (as in fractures of the thoracic spine or poliomyelitis) it is possible for the intercostal muscles to be paralysed while the diaphragm is still working. Men breathe more with the diaphragm than women, who make relatively more use of the intercostals. Expiration is mainly due to the relaxation of these muscles decreasing the chest capacity and compressing the lungs. The respiratory centre is in the medulla and is stimulated by acid substances in the blood, carbon dioxide being the normal one. In times of stress, the accessory muscles of respiration like pectoralis major and sternomastoid come into play.

Normal respiration is regular in rhythm and almost noiseless and the chest movement, or excursion, falls within easily recognized limits. The rate and the excursion are both increased by exercise and by rise in the temperature, and by emotion.

Shallow breathing is noted in shock ; in pleurisy ; and in peritonitis. *Deep* breathing is characteristic of acidosis in uncontrolled diabetes. *Sighing* and *yawning* are signs of acute blood loss, and may be a valuable indication of internal hæmorrhage. *Stertorous* breathing is due to vibration of flaccid cheek and throat muscles, and is often noted in those unconscious after a stroke. *Wheezy* or *bubbly* breathing is due to secretions in the bronchi and is heard in bronchitis, pneumonia and bronchiectasis.

Changes in the rhythm are due to interference with the respiratory centre. *Grouped* respirations may be noticed in meningitis ; a few quick breaths are followed by a pause. *Cheyne-Stokes* breathing is a periodic type of breathing found in raised intracranial pressure of a serious degree ; in arteriosclerosis that impedes the blood supply to the medulla ; and in some terminal states. It is usually only noticed in sleep or unconsciousness. The breaths become gradually deeper and more rapid, then gradually decline in rate and amplitude, until breathing ceases for a few seconds. As carbon dioxide accumulates in the blood breathing recommences and the cycle is repeated. In post-craniotomy or concussion patients its onset is serious and must be reported at once, but patients with heart disease or chronic nephritis may exhibit this sign at night for quite long periods.

The following terms are often used in connection with respiration :

1. *Dyspnœa* is difficulty in breathing and occurs when air entry is obstructed or oxygenation of the blood impaired. Pneumonia, heart failure and carcinoma of bronchus or larynx are common causes. Where the airway is impeded, *stridor* or whistling noise is noticed. Dyspnœa is often accompanied by *cyanosis*, or blueness. This is first noticed in the lips, ears, fingers and toes. In children dyspnœa is accompanied by movements of the sides of the nose (alæ nasi).

2. *Orthopnœa* is inability to breathe except when sitting up, and is characteristic of congestive heart failure. Orthopnœic patients are often helped by resting the arms on a heart table. This fixes the shoulder girdle and enables the accessory muscles of respiration to come into play.

3. *Apnœa* is absence of breathing. The period during which in Cheyne-Stokes respiration there is no breathing is a period of apnœa.

4. *Hyperpnœa* is deep breathing, and has been referred to in connection with diabetic ketosis.

The patient with bronchial asthma has recurring bouts of respiratory difficulty due to spasm in the plain muscle of the bronchi. Typically it occurs at night. The patient wakes with a feeling of constriction and oppression in the chest, and sits up with his elbows an his knees, or sits across a chair with his arms on the back, so that he fixes his shoulder girdle and uses his accessory muscles. Inspiration is wheezy and difficult, but expiration is still more difficult and prolonged, the patient having to make a great effort to empty the chest through the constricted bronchi. Once the attack has been controlled, the patient usually sleeps till morning.

Acute dyspnœa, usually at night, is also seen in *cardiac asthma*, a condition having no connection with bronchial asthma except the unfortunate use of the same name. The patients suffering from it have left ventricular failure, and wake at night acutely dyspnœic, restless and often disorientated. Such attacks are a serious symptom of the heart disease that causes them.

Respiration is usually counted after the pulse while the nurse is holding the patient's wrist against his chest.

COUGH

A cough is a reflex act whose primary function is to protect the airway from the entry of foreign material. Its centre is in the medulla, and it is a primitive one which is one of the last to be extinguished as consciousness is lost. A cough begins with a deep inspiration ; the diaphragm is fixed, the glottis closed and a strong expiratory movement forces the cords apart and the breath is audibly expelled.

The causes of coughing are :

1. Irritation of the larynx by fluid or particles of food ; smoke, or fog ; chemical fumes like ammonia.

2. Inflammation of the larynx, trachea or bronchi (bronchitis, whooping-cough).

3. The presence of secretion in the airway (chronic bronchitis, bronchiectasis).

4. Irritation of the vagus nerve endings in the lung by pneumonia, tuberculosis, etc.

5. Pressure on the trachea or bronchi from without (e.g. by the enlarged thyroid, or mediastinal glands).

6. Nervous causes. Such a cough is common in anxious and inexperienced public speakers. Much coughing can be controlled, but all too rarely is, as can be observed in any concert hall.

Coughs may be classified as :

(*a*) *Dry*, if no sputum is produced. Such a cough serves no useful purpose in most cases, except as a symptom, and is usually controlled by means of a cough syrup or linctus.

(*b*) *Productive*, if sputum is expectorated. Where secretion is present in the respiratory tract it must not be allowed to accumulate, and treatment aims at encouraging easy expulsion of the sputum by expectorant mixtures, and sometimes by the help of the physiotherapist.

The points to be noted in connection with coughing are as follows :

1. The *time* at which it occurs, e.g. whether the patient is kept awake at night, or coughing is most frequent early in the morning after sleep, when sputum has tended to accumulate, or is only paroxysmal.

2. *Length of Attacks.* Some coughs, e.g. in tuberculosis, are persistent and exhausting, even if non-productive.

3. *Presence or Otherwise of Cyanosis.* Those with heart failure or pneumonia may become blue during coughing attacks.

4. *Presence or Absence of Pain.* Early acute laryngitis or tracheitis causes a dry cough obviously very painful to the sufferer. Acute pleurisy (as in lobar pneumonia, pulmonary infarct, tuberculous pleurisy) makes the patient endeavour to cut short the cough in order to avoid the painful pleural friction, and the suppressed cough is often followed by a groan

5. *The nature of the sputum*, if any. This is discussed in the next section.

6. *Any Special Characteristics.* The cough in acute laryngitis has a brassy, ringing note ; in a child it often heralds an attack of measles. In asthma it is tight and wheezy. Patients with *bronchiectasis* have spells of coughing with production of abundant sputum and cough-free intervals during which the sputum is accumulating again.

It must be remembered that coughing has a real therapeutic value in patients confined to bed, and is encouraged after operations (see p. 245) in order to expand the lungs, and improve the circulation.

Sputum

The material produced from the respiratory tract by coughing can be classified under these headings.

1. *Mucus.* This is the normal bronchial secretion, and is present

in excess in very early acute inflammation of the upper respiratory tract. Very soon it becomes cloudy as infection supervenes.

2. *Mucopus* occurs in the later stages of such infections, e.g. bronchitis.

3. *Pus.* In bronchiectasis or lung abscess pus may be coughed up.

4. *Blood.* Coughing up blood is called *hæmoptysis.* Small quantities of bright blood are sometimes produced in early pulmonary tuberculosis, a symptom alarming to the patient, but not a bad portent. Hæmoptysis of large amounts is also seen in the late stages of the disease, and in such cases is an unfavourable sign.

Morphine is commonly prescribed to check internal bleeding but is used with great caution for people with hæmoptysis, since it depresses the cough reflex by which the patient must get rid of the blood.

Cancer of the lung is often accompanied by hæmoptysis of variable amounts. In congestive heart failure and pulmonary infarct streaks of blood from the lungs are frequently seen in the sputum. The sputum in acute lobar pneumonia is a tenacious mucus coloured orange by red blood cells from the alveoli (" rusty " sputum).

Hæmoptysis is always frightening to the patient, who must be assured that the alarming significance attached to it by the lay public is not shared by doctors, and that it is a symptom that will disappear as treatment progresses.

5. *Watery sputum.* Acute œdema of the lungs may occur with left heart failure, and large quantities of fluid well up through the alveoli into the bronchi and are coughed up. Such attacks are more common at night, and can be dangerous unless the fluid can be expectorated.

6. *Saliva.* Those with an obstructive growth of the œsophagus are unable to swallow their saliva and must cough it up. This is very tiring, if the saliva is viscid, for a patient with a malignant disease. A good fluid intake, by whatever route is available, and plenty of mouth washes will help to keep the saliva fluid and therefore easier to expectorate.

Observations of the sputum include the *amount* ; the viscosity ; the *odour*, if any. Sputum from a lung abscess or in bronchiectasis may be very fœtid ; the presence of *blood.*

A suitable container for sputum must be provided and put within easy reach. China ones with a hole in the lid are unhygienic, noisy and not now frequently used. Small waxed cartons are light to handle and easy to dispose of by burning. Measurements of sputum are best done by weighing, but if cartons are used the amount in them can be seen by holding them to the light, and a graduated rod can be laid alongside to measure it. Transfer of sputum from its container to a measure involves atmospheric infection and should be avoided. In tuberculous wards a special routine for dealing with sputum is necessary and is discussed on p. 471.

THE URINE

Urine contains in solution all the by-products of body metabolism except carbon dioxide. In addition, substances not normally present, such as glucose, may appear in metabolic disorders, and such products of inflammation as pus and blood may also be found. Examination of the urine may yield information of the greatest value in diagnosis, and such examination should be made for all new patients on admission, and afterwards at such intervals as their condition suggests. It is especially important before an anæsthetic is given, since it is quite common to discover undiagnosed diabetes mellitus in people admitted with some other condition. While it is quite safe to operate on a diabetic with the proper precautions, it may be disastrous without them.

Amount. 1,500 ml. is the average amount secreted in twenty-four hours, but it varies greatly with the fluid intake and the external temperature. Increased output (*polyuria*) is noted in diabetes insipidus and uncontrolled diabetes mellitus. *Oliguria* or decreased urinary secretion is found in acute nephritis, congestive heart failure and dehydration. It is normal in the first twenty-four hours after operation, owing to increased output of anti-diuretic hormone from the pituitary due to the surgical stress.

Cessation of urinary secretion is *suppression*, or *anuria*. It may be caused by malignant pelvic growth involving both ureters, crushing injuries, acute nephritis, eclampsia, sulphonamide ureteric crystallization, and incompatible blood transfusion among others. Unless it can be corrected, anuria must prove fatal.

Retention of urine means that no urine is passed though it reaches the bladder. Acute retention arises suddenly and is intensely painful. Chronic retention is usually insidious in onset ; the patient fails to empty the bladder completely at micturition, and some remains (*residual urine*). This amount becomes gradually larger if the condition is undetected, until the bladder is grossly distended and atonic, and small amounts of urine are passed at frequent intervals—chronic retention with *overflow*. This is a dangerous condition leading to kidney failure unless treated early.

Reaction. Urine is normally acid to litmus (turns blue litmus paper red). It becomes alkaline on standing as the urea is decomposed by an organism in the air to form ammonia. This is the reason why specimens for examination should be fresh and kept covered. Urine may be alkaline if such substances as potassium citrate or sodium bicarbonate are being given, or in some urinary infections.

Specific Gravity. Urine is somewhat denser than water, 1·015 to 1·025 being the limits of the normal range. The early morning specimen is the most concentrated.

The specific gravity is increased when there is sugar in the urine (*glycosuria*), or when it is concentrated. It is decreased when it is dilute. The ability to vary the specific gravity of the urine by night and day, and in accordance with the temperature and the needs of the skin is a most important one, and is the basis of the water concentration and dilution test of kidney efficiency.

Colour. Urine is amber, darker when concentrated, paler when dilute. Blood colours it red if present in quantity, or gives it a smoky appearance if less is present. Bile pigments turn it a dark orange-brown. Methylene blue and indigo carmine are excreted in the urine and turn it greenish-blue.

The normal transparency of urine may be obscured by cloudiness which can be (*a*) organic (blood, pus, excess mucus) or (*b*) inorganic (phosphates usually). Phosphates tend to come out of solution when the urine is alkaline, and the addition of a few drops of acetic acid to a specimen will demonstrate the nature of this kind of cloudiness.

Infected urine is almost invariably hazy. If the infecting organism is *B. coli* the urine has a cloudy shimmer, and a fishy smell that is quite characteristic.

All substances that produce cloudiness in urine will form a deposit at the bottom of the specimen if left to stand.

Urine Testing

The tests given below should be done on a fresh specimen with clean equipment and careful attention to method and technique. Small faults in their execution may result in failure to demonstrate the presence of an important abnormality. These tests are meant to be performed on acid urine, and if it is not so a few drops of acetic acid should be added to make it so.

Reaction. One strip of red and one of blue litmus paper are dipped in the urine. Red litmus turns blue in alkaline solutions and blue litmus red in acid. If neither changes, the reaction is neutral.

Specific Gravity. This is measured with a urinometer, and the normal range is 1·015 to 1·025. The urinometer is floated in the specimen glass, and the figure level with the surface is read and recorded. If the amount of urine is small, it should be poured into the narrow glass vessel in which the urinometer is kept, and which allows the use of quite small volumes. A high specific gravity in an apparently dilute specimen suggests that sugar is present.

Reagent Strips

Urine testing has been simplified and speeded up by the introduction of chemical dip-and-read strips. These strips of paper have been impregnated with a substance which reacts with urinary constituents, and it is only necessary to dip them in urine, wait the prescribed time, and compare the colour produced with a chart.

Since the makers give instructions on each bottle as to how the tests are to be performed, these will not be repeated here. There are, however, some general rules about the use of such strips and tablets, which must be carefully followed to give a correct result. These tests give accurate answers only when used properly.

First, papers and tablets must be kept dry. Bottles must have the cap replaced as soon as a strip is extracted, must be screwed up tightly, and kept in a cool place. Secondly, the impregnated end must not be touched, or it may be contaminated and give a false positive. Thirdly, the instructions about the time that must elapse before reading the result must be allowed. This is especially important when more than one test is made on a single strip. A paper strip may test the pH of the urine, and for the presence of glucose, protein and blood. While the pH may be read at once, the result of the blood test is read at the end of a minute. The strips must not be left in the urine, or the reagents may dissolve away.

The ease with which these tests may be done means that they can be widely and freely used. A good example is "phenistix", a paper strip test for detecting phenylketonuria, due to an inborn error of protein metabolism. A child with this condition is usually mentally retarded unless fed with a phenylalanine-free diet. The condition is rare, but the result of an early diagnosis is so good that wide-spread testing is worth while. It can be done by pressing the test end of a strip against a wet napkin, and comparing any colour change with a chart.

In the next section, the chemical non-proprietary tests are retained for reference by nurses who need them.

Chemical Tests

Albumin. It is especially important that the urine is acid before the tests for albumin, and if the specimen is not clear some should be filtered.

(*a*) *Boiling Test.* A test tube is three-quarters filled, held by the lower end, and inclined over a small flame without shaking until the top inch boils. If the boiled portion is cloudy as compared with the lower, a drop of acetic acid is added. If the cloud disappears, it was of phosphates and is of no significance; if it remains it indicates the presence of albumin.

(*b*) *Salicyl-sulphonic Test.* Salicyl-sulphonic acid 25% is added drop by drop to about an inch of urine in a test tube, or 0·5 ml. of the reagent added to 5 ml. of urine. Cloudiness is a positive reaction.

(*c*) *Quantitative Test with Esbach's Solution.* A rough estimate of albuminuria may be formed by noting the density of the cloud formed in the above tests. In many conditions where protein is present in the urine it is, however, desirable to know exactly the amount present, and repeat this test regularly (perhaps daily) in order to assess progress. Patients with toxæmia of pregnancy and acute nephritis are instances.

Esbach's urinometer is a glass tube, graduated from 0 to 7, and marked with a "U" and an "R". The urine must be acid and is filtered if cloudy. Urine is poured into the tube up to the U, and Esbach's reagent added until the level reaches R. The rubber stopper is put in, the tube inverted a few times, and put into its wooden stand and left for twenty-four hours, without disturbance. The level of any white precipitate formed shows the amount of albumin in parts per 1,000. Dividing by 10 gives the percentage.

If the urine is very concentrated (i.e. if the amount of albumin is over 0·4%) the urine is diluted with equal parts of water, and the figure obtained multiplied by two to give the result. It may sometimes be necessary to use one part of urine to two of water and multiply the answer by three if very large amounts of albumin are present.

Sugar. (*a*) *Benedict's Solution.* To 5 ml. of Benedict's reagent in a test tube 8 drops of urine are added, and the mixture boiled for two minutes. If sugar is present, green, yellow or brick red colour change occurs, indicating increasing quantities of sugar. It is important to boil thoroughly and to record the colour that appears.

Salicylates and aspirin if taken in quantity may produce a false positive, which can be distinguished by the ferric chloride test described below.

(*b*) "*Clinitest.*" Five drops of urine and 10 drops of water are measured with a pipette into a test tube and a "clinitest" tablet added. Effervescence occurs and the tube must not be moved for fifteen seconds after it has ceased. The colour is then compared with a colour chart to read the result.

This method obviates boiling, and so is much the most convenient for diabetic patients who test their own urine.

Acetone and Diacetic Acid. These are products of faulty fat metabolism which are present in the blood, and excreted in the urine in cases of uncontrolled diabetes mellitus and acidosis. Some children who find difficulty in digesting fat readily display acetonuria.

(*a*) *Rothera's Test.* To about ½ in. of ammonium sulphate in a test tube is added about 5 ml. of urine and the two shaken up. Some crystals must remain undissolved at the bottom to show that the solution is saturated. A crystal or two of sodium nitro-prusside is added and well shaken. About 2 ml. of concentrated ammonia is run down the side of the tube to form a layer on the top of the urine, and if acetone is present a purple ring develops at the junction.

The depth of the colour and the speed with which it appears indicates the amount of acetone present. The test is a very sensitive one indeed, and a pink colour developing after a minute or two is of little significance.

(*b*) *Gerhardt's Test* for diacetic acid. To an inch of urine 10% ferric chloride is added drop by drop. The urine becomes cloudy as phosphates are precipitated, and then if diacetic acid is present a wine-red colour appears. This test is less sensitive than Rothera's and if positive indicates the presence of a fair amount of the acid.

The urine of a patient taking salicylic acid or aspirin gives a similar reaction, and if this is suspected the test should be performed on urine that has been boiled for five minutes. Diacetic acid is driven off by boiling, and if the test is positive after this the reaction is due to salicylates.

Blood. (*a*) *Guaiacum Test.* Two drops of tincture of guaiacum are added to an inch of urine and ozonic ether run down the side of the tube to form a layer on the top. A blue ring develops at the junction if there is blood present (hæmaturia). This is not a very sensitive test ; an examination of the centrifuged deposit with a microscope is required to detect small quantities of red blood cells.

Pus. Chemical tests are equally unreliable for pus in the urine (*pyuria*), and microscopic examination is necessary to detect small amounts. Equal quantities of urine (taken by pipette from the sediment at the bottom) and of liquor potassæ are well shaken together, and the mixture is poured from one tube to another, when it may be possible to detect that the mixture is "ropy" or gelatinous.

Bile Salts. Hay's Test. A pinch of powdered flowers of sulphur is dropped into the surface of the urine in a specimen glass. If bile salts are present the surface tension is reduced so that particles of sulphur fall through the urine and may be seen sinking to the bottom.

(*b*) *Iodine Test.* About 5 ml. of urine is poured into each of two test tubes, which are held side by side in one hand. Tincture of iodine is added drop by drop to one tube, shaking after each addition and comparing the result with the control. Development of a green colour is the positive reaction; 4 to 6 drops of iodine are usually enough to elicit this change if bile pigments are present.

Fouchet's Test. (c) Five ml. of 10% barium chloride are added to about 10 ml. of acid urine. It is shaken and filtered. The filter paper is unfolded and spread on a dry one and a drop of Fouchet's reagent allowed to fall on it. A green or blue colour shows the presence of bilirubin.

Chlorides. Chloride is always present in the urine, unless chloride deficiency in the tissues causes the kidney to stop excreting it. Intestinal obstruction, for instance, may cause a fall in the blood chloride through loss of it by vomiting or by gastric aspiration, and chloride may disappear from the urine. A quantitative test for chloride in the urine is therefore of assistance in diagnosing salt depletion. It is not of course as accurate as an estimation of the blood chloride, and may indeed be misleading if kidney function is not good, but it can be frequently and easily repeated by the nurse.

Equipment. Clean test tube.
Clean pipette with rubber bulb.
20% potassium chromate solution.
2·9% silver nitrate solution.
Distilled water for rinsing.

Method. Ten drops of urine are measured into the test tube. The pipette is thoroughly rinsed with distilled water and one drop of potassium chromate is added to the urine as an indicator. The liquid in the test tube is now a bright yellow. The pipette is thoroughly rinsed again and charged with silver nitrate. The same pipette is used in order to keep the drops constant in size. The silver nitrate is now added one drop at a time, shaking well after each drop and counting them. The end-point is a sudden and easily observed colour change to red. The number of drops taken to effect it is equivalent to the chloride present in grammes per litre. If the change occurs with the first drop, chloride is absent; 3–5 grammes per litre are usually the normal limits, but the doctor will want to know the amount of urine passed in twenty-four hours, and the specific gravity of the specimen in order to interpret the result.

FÆCES

The bowels are normally opened once or twice a day, and the material evacuated is the stool or fæces. The fæces of a baby are soft and yellow; in the adult they should be formed in consistency (neither hard nor fluid) and brown, because of the contained bile pigments. They are composed mainly of food residue, bacteria, salts and water. Food passes from the stomach to the ileo-colic sphincter in six to twelve hours and then moves slowly along the large intestine by mass peristalsis to the sigmoid colon, becoming more solid in transit as water is absorbed. The rectum is normally empty and fills once or twice a day, usually in response to the taking of food. This gastro-colic reflex is an important one in the establishment of rhythmic bowel habits and in the management of a colostomy. The sensation of fullness in the rectum should lead to its evacuation. Normal bowel action is promoted by a regular routine of evacuation, by a diet adequate in roughage and fluid to initiate peristalsis, and by good tone of the muscles of the abdomen and pelvic floor. Changes in bowel habit, especially in the elderly who have previously been regular, need investigation in order to exclude serious disease of the alimentary tract.

Constipation

Constipation means the passage of hard stools at longer intervals than usual. In the majority of cases the delay is in the rectum (*dyschezia*). Small hard masses of fæces are known as scybalæ and are often seen in a constipated stool. If dyschezia is allowed to go untreated, *impaction* of fæces may follow, when the patient's expulsive forces are no longer enough to evacuate the hard rectal contents. It is not infrequent in old people, and may occur in those with a fractured femur treated by a Thomas' splint or those in plaster hip spicas unless adequate attention is paid to the bowel habits.

Causes of Constipation. 1. *Intestinal Obstruction.* In acute obstruction there is absolute constipation once the bowel below the obstruction is empty. In chronic obstruction, as by carcinoma of rectum, there is increasing constipation of gradual onset, sometimes alternating with bouts of diarrhœa. These cases form a very small but important section of those complaining of constipation.

2. *Diet.* Lack of fluid and of roughage will cause constipation. Patients having a low-residue diet or having a restricted intake following operation are instances.

3. *Poor Muscle Tone.* Exercises may be beneficial.

4. *Neuromuscular Causes.* (*a*) *Dyschezia*, usually due to failure to respond to the normal stimulus to defæcation, so that the rectum becomes insensitive. Such patients need advice on diet, exercise and habits. An aperient is useful in the early stages of treatment but should not be taken over long periods in increasing doses. Liquid paraffin is especially dangerous in this respect ; the prolonged exposure of the rectal and anal mucosa to this lubricant is held by rectal surgeons to be responsible for many local ailments.

(*b*) *Spastic Constipation.* This is due to spasm of the colon, which can usually be felt through the abdominal wall and is associated with abdominal pain. Sufferers often believe, and so do their doctors, that they have appendicitis. A low residue diet, relaxation of nervous tension and explanation may improve the pain and constipation.

Diarrhœa

This is the frequent passage of fluid, bulky stools. The volume is increased because the water content is greater than usual. It is usually accompanied by waves of painful peristalsis, called *colic*, and can rapidly cause dehydration and if chronic may produce chemical imbalance through loss of salts, especially sodium.

Causes. 1. Dietetic indiscretion, especially in the soft-fruit season ; allergy to foodstuffs.

2. Infections as in dysentery or typhoid.

3. Ulcerative colitis. No infecting organism has yet been incriminated.

4. Nervous causes. It is quite a common manifestation of fear or anxiety.

A sudden attack of diarrhœa should be treated by rest in bed and warmth. Food should be withheld, but water may be given if there is no vomiting. If the diarrhœa persists or the temperature rises, a doctor should be called. If food poisoning is suspected, any food remnants should not be discarded in case a bacteriological examination is needed.

Abnormalities of Stools

The stools may be *black* if iron medicine is being taken ; *pale* or clay-coloured in obstructive jaundice ; *grey*, bulky and offensive in cœliac disease ; *green* in babies with intestinal upsets. *Melœna* is a term applied to the presence of altered blood in the stools. The stool is black, tarry and sticky, with the characteristic smell of blood. It is caused by bleeding from the upper intestinal tract and the blood is digested during its onward passage. If *bright* blood is mixed with the fæces, it has come from a lesion low down in the alimentary canal, probably from piles, or possibly a carcinoma of rectum. *Mucus* is not normally observable in the stools but may be obvious in pelvic abscess, fæcal impaction or ulcerative colitis. *Pus* is present in ulcerative colitis or if an abscess ruptures into the rectum. *Undigested food* indicates small intestinal hurry. *Sloughs* may be seen in the later stages of typhoid fever when they are separating from the typhoid ulcers. " Rice water " stools is a term used of the abundant pale watery stools of cholera. *Foreign bodies* that have been swallowed may be passed, safety pins being one of the commoner sort. All stools of a patient with a history of swallowing a foreign body must be inspected.

WORMS

1. *Thread-worm* (*Enterobius vermicularis*). This is the commonest intestinal worm in this country and not infrequently infects children. The male worm is inconspicuous, $\frac{1}{8}$ in. long, while the female is $\frac{1}{3}$–$\frac{1}{2}$ in. and looks like a short piece of white cotton. The eggs are laid on the perianal skin and are conveyed by the nails or fingers to the mouth and swallowed. None of the worms breed in the intestine, and as the life of the thread-worm is not more than six weeks all parasites in the intestine will die if auto-infection can be prevented for that period. Hygienic measures can by themselves produce a cure. Children may wear one-piece pyjamas and cotton gloves at night, or the hands restrained to prevent scratching. The nails must be kept short and clean and the hands washed after using the toilet and before taking meals. As other members of the family are likely to be infected, they should be given the same advice.

Drugs of the piperazine group are given by mouth to kill the adult worms. Anthelminthic enemata have been used but are not now ordered.

2. *Round-worms* (*Ascaris lumbricoides*). The eggs are swallowed in infected water or food, hatch in the small intestine and pass to the liver and thence to the lungs in the blood stream. The larvæ enter the trachea, and thence the œsophagus, and return to the small intestine to become adults. Auto-infection does not occur, and once the worms are expelled there should be no further trouble. Santonin, 60–200 mg. nightly, is given for three nights following a brisk purge. Tetrachlorethylene, 4–6 ml. for an adult, can be given once or twice with an interval of three days. It is better prescribed as a draught rather than in capsules for all intestinal parasites, since capsules may fail to dissolve in the duodenum where they are required. Hexylresorcinol in cachets can be given to adults, but not to children too young to swallow them whole.

3. *Tapeworms* (*Cestodes*). The cestodes have a complicated and precarious life, since two hosts are needed to bring them to maturity. The egg develops into a larva in an intermediate host and must then enter the tissues of its second host to reach maturity. Man is the host to the adult form of the beef tapeworm (5–6·5 m. long) and the fish tapeworm (up to 6 m. long), and the intermediate host to the dog tapeworm, while he may harbour both larval and adult worms of the pig tapeworm.

If an adult worm is present in the intestine, square segments full of mature ova are passed in the fæces as the segments ripen. Within the intestine will be a chain of ever-smaller segments arising from the head embedded in the duodenal mucosa, and until this head is detached there can be no cure for the unwilling host.

The patient must have a preliminary starvation period of forty-eight to seventy-two hours in which only bland fluids are given, so that the drug can come into contact with the parasite. Extract of male fern, 6–9 ml., is given early in the morning on an empty stomach and is followed by magnesium sulphate two hours afterwards. The stools are then strained through a black hair sieve in the hope of finding the head. If it does not appear, tetrachlorethylene can be tried as described for round-worms.

VOMIT

Vomiting is a reflex act, of which the centre lies in the medulla, and involves emptying the stomach and sometimes the upper part of the small intestine by reversed peristalsis. In its primitive form its purpose is to rid the stomach by the shortest route of harmful material. It is initiated by irritation of the stomach, chemical or bacterial ; by stimulation of the vomiting centre (e.g. by raised intracranial pressure, as in cerebral growths or injuries) ; by intestinal obstruction, in which it is a leading sign ; by nervous stimuli, such as severe pain, or even the sight or thought of something the patient finds revolting.

Vomiting is disagreeable even for a fit person, but an ill one may find it exhausting. If a patient feels sick the nurse should bring a bowl and, if there is time, paper handkerchiefs. The bed is screened, and the patient is helped into a comfortable position. Holding her forehead will make vomiting less of a strain. When it is over, the face is dried and the bowl removed. The amount is measured, and the nurse returns with a mouthwash and a clean vomit bowl if she deems it necessary. She allows the patient to rinse her mouth and settles her comfortably before withdrawing the curtains.

The points to be noted are :

1. The amount.

2. The presence or absence of nausea. Vomiting occurs with little or no nausea when a brain tumour is present.

3. The force with which the material is vomited. In congenital hypertrophic pylonic stenosis of infants this is sufficient to give it the name of *projectile vomiting*.

4. The material vomited :

(*a*) Stomach contents. Food is vomited if it has been taken recently, or mucus if the stomach is empty, as in sea-sickness.

(*b*) Bile. Clear greenish fluid from the duodenum is characteristic of post-operative vomiting.

(*c*) Intestinal contents. In intestinal obstruction fluid from the small intestine wells back into the stomach and brown opaque fluid with an intestinal smell (" fæculent vomiting ") is ejected.

(*d*) Blood. Vomiting of blood is *hæmatemesis*. It may come from a stomach lesion, such as a peptic ulcer, or from the œsophagus, as in œsophageal varices, or from blood swallowed, e.g. after tonsillectomy. If the bleeding is acute, the blood is vomited unchanged. If it is accumulating slowly, it is digested by the gastric juice to a dark brown sediment, known as coffee-ground vomit.

If a patient is admitted with suspected poisoning, a specimen of vomit must be saved in case it is needed to identify the poison.

ESTIMATION OF THE BLOOD PRESSURE

The blood pressure is the pressure within the arteries, measured in millimetres of mercury. It is at its highest (systolic) when ventricular contraction sends more blood into the arteries, and at its lowest (diastolic) when that force is spent. The normal range of systolic pressure is 110–130 mm. Hg, and the diastolic 70–90. The levels are influenced by emotion, by posture and by age, as well as by pathological processes, and a blood pressure that would be high for a child may be normal for a man of 50. The difference between the diastolic and systolic readings is the pulse pressure.

A fall in blood pressure is characteristic of shock, hæmorrhage, fainting and Addison's disease. A rise is seen in essential hypertension ; kidney disease, such as acute or chronic nephritis ; raised intracranial pressure, and toxæmia of pregnancy.

The apparatus used is a *sphygmomanometer*. This consists of a mercury manometer graduated in millimetres, an inflatable armband for compressing the brachial artery, and a rubber bulb with a release valve for blowing it up and letting it down. The armband is of non-stretch material containing a rubber bag from which lead two tubes, one going to the manometer and the other to the inflating bulb. The whole is contained in a long box which when opened has the mercury manometer in the lid. Other types of sphygmomanometer are in use, especially the aneroid type with a dial instead of a column of mercury.

These are portable but liable to error unless regularly checked.

The patient must be quietly at rest, sitting or lying down, and any apprehensions he may have should be dispelled or an unduly high reading will be obtained. The upper arm is exposed by removing the coat and rolling up the sleeve. The armband is placed around it with the bag over the internal aspect where the brachial artery lies, and the tubes to the front. The band is wrapped smoothly round and the end tucked in ; uneven pressure may be a source of error. The manometer is connected to it and should stand where the readings are visible to the operator but not to the patient, at about the level of the heart.

Palpatory Method. The radial pulse is palpated with the left hand, while with the right the bag is inflated. When the pulse has disappeared, the valve is slowly opened and the fall of the mercury level watched until the pulse is again felt at the wrist. This is the systolic pressure.

Auditory Method. A stethoscope is used for this method. With the left hand the chest-piece of the stethoscope is applied to the arm immediately below the armlet and the brachial artery is auscultated ; a rather muffled pulsation will be heard. The cuff is inflated well above normal levels (to about 200 mm.) or until no sounds are heard. The valve is opened and the mercury allowed to fall slowly. A faint tapping sound will begin and the mercury level is at once noted, as this is the systolic pressure. The mercury is allowed to continue its fall, and the sounds heard will change usually from a tapping to a loud knocking note. These changes can be disregarded ; the odd sound is because blood is pulsing into the artery at systole only, since the pressure of the cuff is still too high to allow continuous flow. The air is still allowed to escape, and soon the sounds change suddenly into the muffled murmur that was heard at first. This point marks the diastolic pressure. The pressure may be once more raised and the levels checked, but it causes discomfort and must not be unnecessarily repeated.

The pressure is recorded, the armlet removed and folded into the box. Patients should not be told their blood pressure unless the doctor wishes it. The nurse should thank her patient and add a reassuring word if it seems indicated.

If a series of blood-pressure readings are to be taken—e.g. after operation—the cuff should be left in position with the pressure at zero. This will lessen the disturbance involved to the patient.

CENTRAL VENOUS PRESSURE

In the large majority of patients, it is only necessary to take the arterial blood pressure, but in some (such as those who have undergone heart operations, or sustained severe injuries), it is necessary to know the venous pressure as well if the fluid balance is to be accurately adjusted. Only 15% of the blood volume is in the arteries, the rest is in the capillaries and veins.

Low arterial pressure may be due to a fall in the blood volume (as in hæmorrhage), or to poor heart action, or to a combination of both. If the low blood pressure is due to insufficient circulating fluid, giving intravenous fluid will improve his condition, but if it is due to a failing heart, giving fluid will embarrass the heart still further and make him worse. In patients like those mentioned above it is therefore highly desirable to know the venous pressure in order to decide on treatment.

Venous pressure must be estimated in a large vein in direct communication with the right atrium, and there must be no valve between the point of measurement and the heart. The external jugular vein can be used in an unconscious patient, but the internal jugular is more generally used. The head is lowered in order to congest the veins, and the jugular is pierced with a large intracath to which is attached an intravenous apparatus and manometer as shown in fig. 15. When the

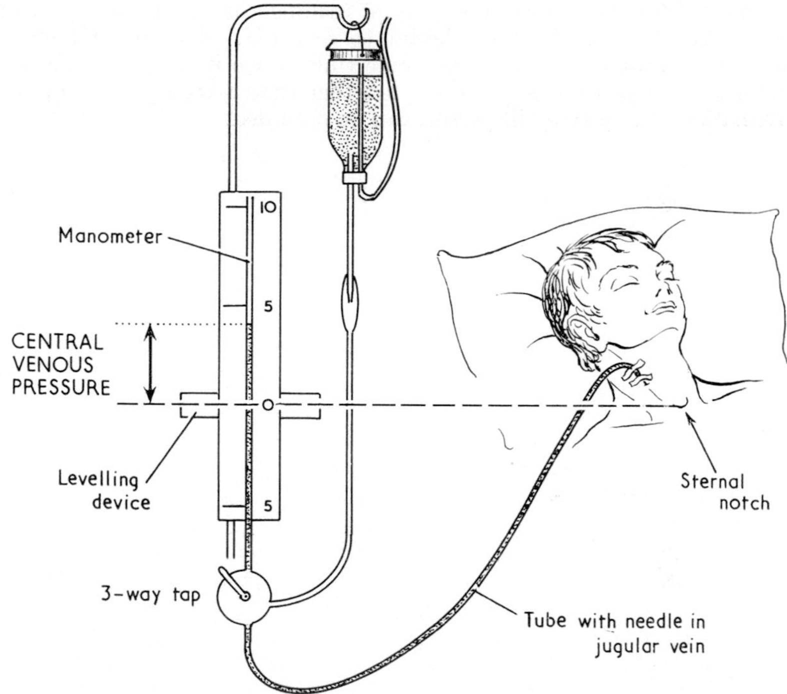

Fig. 15. Apparatus for estimating the central venous pressure.

pressure is not being read, fluid drips into the vein at a slow rate, and 1,000 units of heparin in each bottle will prevent clotting in the catheter.

If the reading is to be meaningful, the zero on the manometer scale must be at a constant point, and the sternal notch is a convenient one. Before taking the pressure, the zero is set by looking through the gun-sight, or whatever device is used for setting the scale. At the sternal notch the normal range of pressure is —1 to +10 cm. of water, about 0·5 cm. lower than the atrial pressure.

When the pressure is to be read, the procedure is as follows:—

1. The zero level is set.

2. The free-running of the infusion is checked.

3. The stop-cock is turned to direct fluid up the manometer to a height of at least 30 cm.

4. The stop-cock is turned so that the flow from the bottle is cut off, and fluid runs from the manometer into the vein. The level in the manometer will swing with the patient's breathing.

5. When the level is steady, the figure is read and recorded.

6. The stop-cock is turned to allow the fluid from the bottle once again to run slowly into the vein.

7. If there has been a change, the physician should be informed. He may have specified the levels at which he should be notified. In the absence of special instructions, c.v.p. readings of less than 1 cm. or more than 10 cm. of water should be reported. The arterial blood pressure is always taken at the same time, since it is by considering the arterial and venous pressures together that a true picture of the circulation of a gravely ill person can be obtained.

CHAPTER 5

THE PATIENT'S TOILET

SCRUPULOUS attention to the cleanliness of the skin is much appreciated by patients with a high standard of personal care, and is a useful way of teaching those without one. It raises the morale, is a good index to the efficiency of the nursing staff, and may help to prevent wound infection in surgical wards.

A daily bath for all patients is the ideal at which to aim, and if it can be taken in the bathroom so much the better. The nurse sees that the bath is clean and rinses it with a mop soaked in detergent, and then with hot water. She closes the window, runs the water and tests the temperature, which should be 40° C., and puts a stool beside the bath. Communal bath mats are best avoided, but if used should be clean daily. The patient and her toilet articles are taken to the bathroom and the towels hung on a warm rail. It may be necessary for the nurse to remain with and assist her patient, but in most cases she needs only to be within call. Bathroom doors should not be locked and hospitals should have an " Engaged " sign to hang on the handle. Should the patient feel faint in the bath, it is easier to lift her out if the bath is full of water.

BED BATH

A bath in bed may be the traditional " blanket bath," in which the patient lies between two blankets kept especially for the purpose, but this method presents difficulties in hospital. It is obviously desirable that each patient should have individual blankets, and few wards have facilities for storing these separately. If they are kept folded beneath the patient's mattress they do not add to comfort, and if damp are unhygienic. It is becoming common here as in other countries to use the patient's top blanket to keep her warm, and a bath towel to prevent the bedclothes getting wet.

Requirements. Bowl of hot water (105°–110° F.) (or 40°–44° C.). The quantity must be ample.
Soap.
Two flannels.
Nail brush.
Hand towel.
Bath towel.
Brush and comb.
Toothbrush and dentifrice or mouthwash and small bowl.
Nail scissors and receiver.
Spirit and powder.
Clean linen, if indicated, and linen bin.
Bucket and jug of hot water if running hot water is not available at hand.
Two bath blankets, if this method is used.

Method. The requirements are taken to the bedside and the curtains or screens are drawn. If the weather is not warm the windows are shut. The top clothes are stripped neatly on to a chair, leaving a blanket over the patient, and the nightdress removed. The bath towel is spread over the chest and the face washed with the flannel kept for the purpose and with soap. The flannel is kept well gathered in the hand, and pressure is firm but not heavy. The face is well rinsed and meticulously dried. Every young nurse suffers the humiliation of having the patient pick up the corner of the towel and do a little additional drying for herself, and resolves that it shall not happen again. The neck and ears are washed and dried.

The arms are washed one at a time, with especial care to the axillæ. If the nails need scrubbing this should be done before the whole arm is wetted. Nail trimming is best left until the end of the bath, when the night clothes have been put on. The chest and abdomen are washed next with the second flannel, and must be done speedily if chilling is to be avoided. The water should be changed at this point or the later stages of the bath will be uncomfortable. The umbilicus and the area beneath the breasts need special care, and talcum powder is useful if the breasts are heavy. The legs are exposed singly, the bath towel put beneath, and each well washed.

The patient is now turned on to her side away from the nurse, and the back from neck to buttocks well washed. The sacrum is the part of the body most likely to feel the effects of pressure from lying in bed, and application of spirit and powder after drying is common. The treatment of pressure areas is considered in detail on p. 57. With the patient still on her side and the upper thigh well flexed, the vulva, groins and cleft of the buttocks are washed and the groins powdered. If the patient is well enough to do this for herself, she may prefer to.

If the bottom sheet and drawsheet are to be changed it is done now ; if not, the drawsheet is pulled through. The patient's nightdress is put on, and a bedjacket is usually indicated. Finger and toe nails are trimmed and the teeth are cleaned, or the mouth attended to in the way described on p. 60. The hair is brushed and combed and the bed made up at once. If the patient does not feel warm and happy, the nurse's technique is at fault ; perhaps she was too slow or exposed her patient unduly, or used the water too cool, or failed to dry her thoroughly.

A man is bathed in the same way, but if he is unable to attend to the toilet of his genital area this should be performed for him.

BEDSORES

A bedsore is a loss of skin occurring in a patient confined to bed, and this term covers a wide variety of lesions with many different causes and methods of prevention and treatment. It is traditionally held to be a disgrace to the nurse in charge and, though in some cases it may be exceedingly difficult to prevent, a bedsore must at least be classed as a failure of nursing technique. These are the places where bedsores may occur :

1. *Pressure Sites.* These are the places where weight is borne heavily and the tissues are compressed between the bed and the underlying bone. The blood supply is interfered with and the skin gives way.

The most important of these areas is the skin overlying the ***sacrum***, the ***great trochanters*** and the ***heels***. In addition the point of the shoulder, the scapulæ, the elbows and the knees may be affected.

2. Where folds of skin are in *contact*, e.g. in the fold of the buttocks, and under pendulous breasts.

Certain kinds of patients are especially liable to bedsores :

(*a*) The *paralysed*. The skin deprived of its nerve supply is especially vulnerable and the patient can neither move to avoid pressure nor feel its effects. Sores in paralysed parts are called *trophic ulcers*. They arise with great speed, extend alarmingly and are difficult to prevent, but the work of units specializing in the care of those with spinal cord injuries has shown that they can be prevented or cured.

(*b*) The *heavy*, who carry much weight on their pressure areas. The œdematous are especially unfortunate in this respect.

(*c*) The *emaciated*, whose bones are near the surface.

(*d*) The *incontinent*, whose skin is excoriated by frequent soaking in urine or fæces.

(*e*) Sufferers from such diseases as *diabetes* or *cancer*, in whom the tissues are devitalized.

(*f*) Those in heavy *plasters*.

If a helpless person who has been lying on one side is turned to the other, a red area, perhaps with skin creases, is seen lying over the great trochanter. If it is gently and thoroughly massaged, the flush and the creases disappear. If a bedsore is threatening the flush is a cherry-red and does not disappear, and if preventive treatment is not effectively undertaken the skin breaks down and a raw area appears. It may remain superficial, or in a neglected or susceptible patient may enlarge and deepen, even to the extent of exposing the underlying bone.

Sometimes the skin becomes tender and fine peeling occurs which becomes worse over the pressure area until the skin is lost from it. In the fold of the buttocks linear cracks are seen.

Prevention of Bedsores. Many aspects of medical and nursing care are concerned in this. Measures by the doctor to relieve œdema, to raise a low hæmoglobin level or lower a high blood sugar are of the greatest help. A tradition of absence of bedsores in a ward or service (for instance, the District Nurses) is also a great incentive to vigorous efforts. The most important measures are:

(*a*) *Relief of pressure* by taking weight off the affected part, by regular turning; by the use of sorbo rings and ripple mattresses; by small pillows beneath the ankles to keep the heels off the bed; by well-made beds with taut drawsheets, free from crumbs; uncreased mackintoshes.

(*b*) *Cleanliness*. Sweat, urine, fæces must not be allowed to remain in contact with the skin.

(*c*) *Routine attention* to the pressure areas. The nurse takes to the bedside a washing bowl of warm water, surgical spirit and a container of starch powder. From the patient's locker she takes soap, the back flannel and towel. Screens are drawn and the patient turned, with assistance if necessary, to expose the buttocks. The state of the skin is carefully assessed, and if it is good the skin is well washed with soap and water and the flannel, paying special attention to the cleanliness of the folds between the buttocks and to its dryness afterwards. The hands are soaped and careful thorough massage given to the tissues over the sacrum and ischial tuberosities. The aim is not to give superficial friction but to stimulate the circulation by moving the skin on the subcutaneous tissues. The soap is washed off—it is a mistake to rub it into the skin and not rinse it off—and the skin patted quite dry, without harsh rubbing. A little spirit is poured into the palm and rubbed on to the skin till it dries, to harden it. A light dusting of powder should leave the skin clean, dry and refreshed. The drawsheet is pulled and the air ring turned over, or the cover smoothed. Other areas may need similar treatment.

This traditional form of treatment is very refreshing to those who are weary of lying in bed, but undoubtedly the most important part of it is the turning from one side to the other that accompanies it, and the smoothing of the undersheet. It also ensures that the pressure areas are regularly inspected, and signs of devitalization detected early. But if the skin is clean, it is doubtful if soap is needed more than once a day, and those with dry skins do not need spirit.

The skin of those who are incontinent should be protected from maceration by applying a barrier cream, and every effort should be made to keep the patient and his bedclothes clean and dry. Where possible, a more rational solution to the problem is to seek for and treat the cause of the incontinence. In old people, for instance, it may be due to apathy and lack of inducement to remain dry, and provision of more stimulation and regular offering of toilet facilities may raise the patient's morale.

The use of sheepskins beneath the buttocks to prevent pressure sores originated, not unnaturally, in Australia. Wool contains lanoline which lubricates the skin, and traps air which improves skin health. Wool does not wrinkle and good results have been reported from its use. Problems of washing and disinfection are avoided if small portions are used, and discarded when no longer needed. " Fleeces " of man-made fibres like acrilan have been marketed. These are washable, but lack the natural oils of wool.

Treatment of Pressure Sores

Once the skin is broken every effort must be made to heal it before the lesion gets bigger or infected. The most important point is that healing will never take place unless pressure on the part and friction can be avoided. As to the local applications needed, the large number used shows that there is no sovereign remedy. The type of sore, the patient and the cause of the skin loss must all be considered. A selection of popular remedies is given here.

Small cracks may be painted with a drying agent like Friar's Balsam, Whitehead's varnish, or Nobecutane. Elastoplast may be laid, without stretching, over small superficial areas of skin loss and left until it peels off. The surrounding skin must be healthy if this method is to be a safe one. If the pressure sore is in a place where it can be exposed to the air without a dressing, it may dry up quickly.

If the sore involves more than the superficial layers of the skin, it must be dressed with the usual non-touch technique and sterile lotions. Eusol is a popular one, or red lotion may be used on a deep sore to encourage granulation tissue formation.

Whatever treatment is used, all the usual measures to keep the skin intact elsewhere must be energetically undertaken, for if the skin is broken over one pressure point the patient will have to spend more time in positions which will expose other equally vulnerable areas to pressure.

CARE OF THE HAIR

The hair should be brushed and combed morning and evening. Men patients present no difficulty, but women need a style that they feel is attractive and at the same time is comfortable and practical for lying in bed.

A shampoo is not only a hygienic necessity for all but short-term patients, but provides a great lift to the morale. Many hospitals and nursing homes provide the service of a professional hairdresser, but if this is not available the nurse can wash her patient's hair effectively, even if her ability to set waves is not of professional standards.

If the patient can sit up in bed and lean over a bowl on a locker or heart table, the nurse can wash the hair in exactly the same way as she washes her own. If the patient is unable to do so, the nurse proceeds as follows :

Requisites. Bowl of water at 105° F. or 40° C.
Six-pint jug of water at same temperature.
Waterproof cape.
Two bath towels.
Hand towel.
Brush and comb.
Shampoo or soap solution.
Mackintosh.
Jaconet pillow-case.
Floor rug.

The trolley is taken to the right side of the screened bed and the mattress is drawn 2 ft. over the end of the bed, leaving the wires exposed at the top. In this space the bowl of hot water is placed on the mackintosh, with a floor rug on the floor beneath. The patient lies with a jaconet-covered pillow under her neck and her hair over the bowl. She has a cape across her chest, and if the bed head is removable it is a convenience in working. Her hair is wetted, thoroughly rubbed with a shampoo and rinsed with plenty of warm water, the bowl being emptied as necessary into the pail. When the hair is quite free of soap, it is wrapped in a bath towel and the bowl and mackintosh removed. The mattress is restored to position, and when the hair has been half-dried the clean towel is substituted, the hair set and dried with a hand drier. When the bed has been remade, the patient's brush and comb should be washed.

Pediculosis

Pediculus humanus is the human louse, which is one of the commoner parasites. When residing on the head it is often called *P. capitis.* The head-louse lays eggs (" nits ") which are attached to the hair close to the head, and from which the lice hatch in two to five days. The extent of the infection can be judged from the length of hair with nits attached and the area infected. In mild cases they may only be found behind the ears and in the occipital area, while in a severe case the hair may be grey with nits and teeming with lice. Scratching the head causes abrasions, which become infected, and enlargement of the lymph glands behind the ears and in the neck. Impetigo of the scalp in children is diagnostic of hair infestation. Inspection may be sufficient in some cases, but often it is necessary to use a fine comb.

Requisites Fine comb in small bowl of water.
Bowl of white wool swabs, 4 in. square.
Paper bag.
Patient's brush and comb.
Plastic or jaconet cape.
Cover.

The bed is screened and the cape adjusted around the shoulders. The hair must be combed quite free of tangles, or the process of fine combing will be painful. A parting is made just above one ear and the fine comb, moistened, is drawn through the hair from the roots to the tips, working from the front hair margin to the back. At intervals the comb is thoroughly wiped with a wool swab, which is inspected for lice before being discarded. The whole head is combed, making fresh partings at regular intervals. Children are especially liable to pediculosis, which can spread rapidly in a ward unless the source is detected on admission.

Treatment.

1. Lorexane No. 3 cream shampoo

Wet the hair with warm water. Massage 2 inches of shampoo into the scalp. Rinse and make a second application working up a good lather. Rinse thoroughly. Fine comb the hair while still wet. Dry the hair.

2. D.D.T. emulsion (Dicophane)

Disposable tray and gallipot, disposable 5 ml. teaspoon, pipette, comb. Protective for the shoulders. D.D.T. emulsion.

Comb the hair. Measure 3×5 ml. tsp. of emulsion into the gallipot. Make many partings in the hair, applying a few drops of the emulsion with the pipette and rub it into the scalp with the finger tips. Tidy the hair and leave for not less than 24 hours before washing the hair. Wash the non disposable equipment and patient's brush and comb in warm water containing detergent solution. The hair should be fine combed daily for a week. The nit cases will gradually be discarded. When a child is verminous it is usual for the Medical Social Worker to inform the Health Visitor in the home area who will advise on the treatment of the rest of the family.

Pediculus humanus vestimenti is the body louse. It lives on the body hair or in the clothing, around the seams of which the eggs are deposited. The female lays about 250 eggs which hatch in a week or a little more, and lice can live for a week without feeding. DDT powder is effective. The clothes must be disinfected by heat (54° C. is rapidly insecticidal). Ironing with a hot iron is also effective, but is a method only likely to be useful outside hospital.

Phthirius pubis is the crab louse, most often found in the pubis and perianal regions. DDT powder is used, and treatment may be more effective if the area is shaved.

Care of the Feet

The feet need special care because of these considerations :

(*a*) *Cleanliness.* They should be washed and dried thoroughly, especially between the toes. Cracking or peeling between the toes is a symptom of *athlete's foot* (tinea pedis), which should be treated, usually with an ointment such as Whitfield's or one containing undecylenic acid. If they are very dirty a soft nail brush and plenty of soap is usually effective.

(*b*) *Nails.* The nails should be trimmed regularly and cut straight across. Cutting out the corners of the nail will lead to ingrowing toe-nail.

(*c*) *Callouses.* A person with calloused feet who spends some time in bed finds that the hypertrophied skin becomes dry and cracked and tends to peel off. Such areas should be pared and may then have a little olive oil or castor oil rubbed in to soften them.

(*d*) *Pressure.* The heels of anyone lying helplessly in bed tend to become sore unless treated, but those of patients with arterial disease of the legs are especially vulnerable, and no pressure should be allowed on the heels of such patients. A small pillow or sorbo pad under the ankle should keep the heel off the bed. Heel rings, which are rolls of brown wool made into rings of an American doughnut shape and covered with open-wove bandage, are not advised. They are difficult to keep in place, and by pressing on the skin around the point of the heel they may diminish its circulation and hasten the skin loss they are designed to prevent.

(*e*) *Footdrop.* Every muscle has an antagonist which performs a contrary action. These muscle pairs are rarely of equal strength, since one usually has gravity to help it. The calf muscles, which plantarflex the foot, are much more powerful than those of the front of the leg, which dorsiflex it. If a patient lies helpless in bed for some time, the powerful gastrocnemius muscle may pull the anterior tibial muscle and its allies until they stretch, and the foot drops into a plantarflexed position, which will make subsequent walking difficult.

Footdrop must be prevented by supporting the feet of the helpless in a dorsiflexed position. A sandbag or a padded board can be used; pillows are rarely an effective support. If the patient can co-operate by active movements of the feet under the guidance of the physiotherapist it is of the greatest help. Bedclothes must not be allowed to rest on the feet to increase the plantarflexion, but must be supported on a cradle.

If footdrop occurs, physiotherapy should be given to restore the weak muscle. When walking recommences the foot must be supported by some device like a toe-raising spring. This is not very noticeable under trousers, but footdrop is one of the conditions which should be prevented rather than treated.

Care of the Mouth

The mouth is ordinarily kept fresh by morning and evening attention and the mastication of food. Eating solid food is important in this respect, and those who are unable to eat will need regular and careful treatment to keep the tongue clean.

The results of neglect of oral hygiene are offensive to the patient and his attendants. Lack of appetite (*anorexia*) always follows, and dental decay (*caries*) is hastened. Infections such as *thrush* (a fungus infection by *Oidium albicans*) or *Vincent's angina* (a bacterial oral infection) may occur, and one of the worst consequences is *parotitis*, or inflammation of the parotid gland. If saliva is not freely secreted, infection may ascend Stenson's duct, and an intensely painful swelling of the gland results. This often requires surgical incision to relieve the tension, which may otherwise damage the facial nerve, which divides within the gland. The incision follows the line of the jaw.

If a patient is unable to undertake the toilet of his own mouth, a treatment tray should be kept by his bed and the lips, tongue and teeth treated often enough to maintain a good standard of hygiene.

Equipment. Covered tray with gallipots of :

1. Sodium bicarbonate, 1 tsp. to 500 ml.
2. Compound glycerine of thymol.

A lubricant.
Swabs 1 in. square.
Receiver for used swabs.
Mouth-sticks.
Spencer Wells forceps.
Wooden spatula.

If dentures are worn, a mug of mouthwash and brush are needed. The dentures should be regularly cleaned and the patient encouraged to wear them when his condition warrants it.

Method. A swab (not too thick) is wound round the slightly open blades of the Spencer Wells forceps and the free end put between the blades and clipped into position. The blades are now covered, and the swab cannot escape. It is dipped in sodium bicarbonate solution and the tongue, gums and cheeks are thoroughly cleaned with a series of swabs. Swabs are dropped into the receiver as used with the help of the spatula. Mouth-sticks can be used for the teeth. Sodium bicarbonate is used for its mucus-dissolving powers and is followed by glycerine of thymol for its refreshing taste. Some lubricant will be needed to keep the lips moist, and the choice depends on the state of the mouth. Glycerine and borax is an old favourite, but borax is poisonous and plain glycerine may be preferred. Since it is hygroscopic, it keeps the lips moist for long periods, but if there are cracks it is painful, and liquid paraffin may be preferred. Yellow paraffin emulsion (" vaseline ") is stiffer and should be used if sordes (epithelial crusts) are present.

Many other measures can be used to suit the variety of circumstances. Chewing-gum is useful in certain cases to maintain a flow of saliva. Diluted unsweetened lemon juice or pineapple juice serves the same purpose. A dental spray or a Dakin's squirt is especially good if the mouth cannot be fully opened.

While treating the mouth, observation should be made, especially of the tongue and gums. Characteristic appearances of the tongue seen in some conditions are as follows :

1. Dry ; *dehydration.*
2. Dry and brown with a urinary smell ; *uræmia.*
3. Coated and offensive ; *acute abdominal conditions.*
4. Red and lacking in papillæ ; *pernicious anæmia.*

The gums may be the site of *gingivitis* (inflammation), *pyorrhœa* (suppurative inflammation) or *bleeding* (scurvy and the hæmorrhagic conditions). Bleeding gums cause great difficulty in treating the mouth, which is constantly offensive. Gentle and frequently repeated irrigation may be helpful. *Koplik's spots* are small red spots with a white head seen on the inner surface of the cheeks opposite the molar teeth before the eruption of the rash in *measles.* Inflamed tonsils may be noticed, or the sweet, fruity smell of the breath be noted when *acetone* is present (e.g. in *diabetic coma*).

CARE OF THE UNCONSCIOUS PATIENT

" Unconsciousness " is a term used with a variety of meanings. It may cover states ranging from *stupor*, in which a response can be elicited by some strong stimulus, to *coma*, in which no such response can be obtained. All details of toilet must be faithfully carried out, and may be summarized under these headings :

1. **Position.** It is easiest to prevent pressure sores if the patient can be nursed semi-recumbent and turned frequently from one side to the other. If it is necessary to keep the head and shoulders elevated (e.g. in raised intracranial pressure), the top of the bed may be raised on blocks. The patient should lie in a relaxed position, in which he could be comfortable if conscious, with the pillow adjusted under the cheek. Relatives are made happier in their anxious time if the patient appears comfortable.

Frequent turning will also help to prevent hypostatic pneumonia (p. 212).

2. **Toilet.** Regular blanket baths, treatment of pressure points, care of the mouth, feet and hair are obviously important. If incontinence is present, the sacral areas are best treated with zinc cream or a barrier cream which will help to waterproof the skin.

A drop of paroleine should be put daily into the eyes if they are not completely closed.

3. **Excretion.** Incontinence or retention of urine may occur, and the latter must not go unobserved. A distended bladder causes abdominal swelling, dull to percussion, and is often accompanied by much restlessness if the patient is not deeply unconscious. The frequent passage of small quantities of urine may show that retention with overflow has developed.

Fæcal incontinence is probably best managed by regular enemata or suppositories, which will partly prevent incontinence and also guard against unsuspected constipation. Bedlinen should be promptly changed when soiled.

4. **Nutrition.** If unconsciousness lasts more than a day or so, artificial feeding is needed, and nasal feeds (p. 179) are the most convenient. The dietitian should advise on a fluid diet adequate in calories, and vitamins should not be forgotten.

SANITARY ROUTINE

The prospect of using a bedpan is daunting to most people entering hospital, and the indication for its use has greatly declined. Many patients formerly confined totally to bed are now kept mobile and may use the lavatory. Others may be put on to a chair which can be pushed into the lavatory over the pan. Even quite ill people may use a commode beside the bed and find it less strain than a bedpan.

Portable commodes must have the brake firmly applied before the patient is installed, and should be turned to face the bed. The patient must be well supervised; it is not uncommon for patients to fall when attempting to rise or reach articles unaided, and precautions must be taken to avoid such accidents.

While sanitary rounds are in progress a screen is drawn across the ward door, and privacy is afforded individual patients by screens or curtains.

Bedpans are usually of metal, which is unbreakable, light and easily cleaned. A fitting metal lid or a disposable cover is provided.

A woman should be provided with a warm, dry bedpan, with toilet paper or brown wool. She is comfortably settled and, if fit, left alone. If not able to perform her local toilet, the nurse should bring brown wool and do it for her. The bedpan is taken to the sluice-room and wool removed into a bin with lavatory forceps before putting the bedpan into the flusher. This should be the enclosed cabinet type, with a steam jet as well as a flush of water. The makers of this type do not guarantee sterilization, but in fact bacteriological tests suggest that a high degree of safety is obtained.

A man who wishes to empty his bladder is given a urinal with a disposal cover, and screens are not necessary. If he wishes to open his bowels he is given a bedpan and urinal, and the bed is screened.

All patients should be given an opportunity to wash their hands after the use of the bedpan, and the ward should be well ventilated after the sanitary round.

Disposable bedpans and urinals require special apparatus for dealing with them and their contents. They are satisfactory in use and the chief problem in connection with them is finding adequate space to store the necessary stock.

CHAPTER 6

THE PATIENT'S FOOD

THE body is built from the food that it receives and, although our potentialities as to height and physique are inherited, the diet decides whether we will fulfil those potentialities. The food of a nation is decided partly by its climate (the Eskimo takes a diet higher in fat than could be tolerated in a warmer climate), partly by the economic level of the country and its resources. There are large areas of the world in which the diet of most of the population is deficient both in quality and quantity, and diseases due to these deficiencies are rife. In this country such diseases are rare today, but up to the First World War those caused by vitamin lack were common, and rickets had the distinction of being known as the English disease, and up to the Second World War the lowest-paid section of the community could not afford a good diet.

A growing child, an agricultural labourer and a City typist have obviously widely differing dietetic requirements, but all need in common the elements from which those diets are constructed, which are as follows :

1. **Proteins.** These are the nitrogen-containing foods which are necessary for all cell structure. The most valuable ones are animal products—lean meat, fish, cheese and eggs—and vegetable sources are peas, beans and nuts. Protein foods are the most expensive ones, and where money is short protein is also likely to be short in the diet.

2. **Fats.** Butter, milk, cheese and meat fat, margarine, olive and nut oils are sources of fat. Fat is a fuel food which when oxidized produces heat and energy and can be stored in a compact form for later use. For complete oxidation, foods from the next class must be taken with fat.

3. **Carbohydrates.** These are also fuel foods, and they fall into two important classes : (*a*) the *starches*, which are the bulky carbohydrates found in vegetables and cereals. Starches are the cheapest foods and form a high proportion of the diet when cost is important. (*b*) *Sugars*, including the disaccharides like cane sugar, and the simple monosaccharides, such as glucose and fruit sugar. They are compact and soluble sources of energy, very useful for enhancing the diet of those with no appetite for bulky foods.

4. **Salts.** *Iron* is needed for making red blood cells. Red meat is the best source, and green vegetables also provide some, while foods like dried fruit and sardines rather unexpectedly contain some because of their contact with the metal during processing. Iron is a mineral which is sometimes in short supply, especially for women, who have to make good the regular monthly loss of iron in menstruation. *Calcium* and *phosphorus* are required for making bones and so are needed in large amounts by children. Milk and cheese are the best sources. *Iodine* is found in sea fish and iodized table salts, and is required by the thyroid gland for making its hormone. *Sodium chloride* is the most abundant

salt in the body, but is so freely available that in temperate climates there is never any shortage, though in hot countries far from the sea it may be a valuable commodity. Other minerals are needed in small amounts which are easily supplied by a mixed diet.

5. **Roughage.** The indigestible cellulose found in vegetables provides the bulk to the diet which, although of no fuel value, helps to allay hunger and to stimulate peristalsis in the colon.

6. **Water.** 70% of the body weight is made up of water, and since water is being constantly lost from the skin and the kidneys it must be taken in amounts adequate to maintain the fluid content of the tissues.

7. **Vitamins.** Although the amounts needed of these accessory food factors are small, their presence is vital, as their name suggests, for health and growth. The letters by which they are usually known and a brief allusion to their sources and function is given below :

Vitamin A. *Sources.* Milk, butter, egg yolk, cheese, liver, vitaminized margarine. Its precursor, *carotene*, is the yellow pigment present in carrots, tomatoes, apricots and other yellow and red fruits.

Actions. Vitamin A forms part of the visual purple in the retina and is so necessary for sight in dim light. It is needed for healthy epithelium.

Vitamin B Complex. This group, at first thought to be a single vitamin, is now known to consist of quite a number. Only the ones now thought to be of major importance are mentioned, though from time to time discoveries may occur, as when vitamin B_{12} was found to be the missing blood-forming factor in pernicious anæmia.

Sources. In general the B group is found in liver, wheat germ, yeast, brown bread and lean meat.

Actions. B_1 is needed for carbohydrate metabolism, and if long absent from the diet *beri-beri* (with neuritis, œdema and heart failure) ensues. Lack of *vitamin* B_2 causes cracks and dermatitis around the mouth and nose. *Nicotinic acid* prevents the onset of pellagra (briefly characterized by dermatitis, diarrhœa and dementia). Vitamin B_{12} is the anti-anæmic factor which must be present in the liver if blood-cell formation is to be normal.

Much work is being done with the B vitamins in many connections. For instance, the psychiatrists are interested in their role in brain-cell metabolism and the possibility of its connection with mental disease, and the administration of isoniazid in the treatment of tuberculosis appears to interfere with the use in the body of *para-amino benzoin acid*, another member of the B complex.

Vitamin C. *Sources.* Citrus fruits, black currants, rose hips, potatoes and green vegetables.

Actions. It is necessary for health of connective tissues, blood capillaries and teeth and for the formation of red blood cells. In its absence scurvy develops, with bleeding into joints and the skin and anæmia. It is much used (as ascorbic acid) to hasten wound healing in surgical patients.

Vitamin D. *Sources.* Fish oils, summer milk and butter. It can be formed from the ergosterol present in the skin by the action of ultraviolet light.

Actions. Vitamin D, calcium and phosphorus are required for bone formation. If deprived of it babies develop *rickets,* and adults *osteomalacia* and severe bone weakness.

Vitamin E. The importance of this vitamin in the human diet has not been established, and its name, the "anti-sterility vitamin," is based only on the need of rats for its presence in the food.

Vitamin K. *Sources.* Green vegetables. It is synthesized in the bowel by the intestinal bacteria and is of much medical importance because the use of antibiotics to sterilize the intestine may induce a shortage.

Actions. It is the precursor of prothrombin, and if this substance falls below its normal blood value delay in blood-clotting power can lead to hæmorrhage.

CALORIE VALUES

Since carbohydrate and fat are fuel foods and protein can also be used in this way, the value of the diet as fuel can be expressed in terms of the amount of heat it will produce when burnt. The unit used is the Calorie (with a big C), and a Calorie is the amount of heat needed to raise the temperature of 1 kg. of water through 1° C. A gramme of either protein or carbohydrate yields about 4 C., and a gramme of fat 9 C.

Fuel is needed for three purposes :

1. To keep up the body temperature, which in temperate climates is well above that of the environment.
2. To maintain the vital functions like breathing and circulation.

These two headings comprise *basal metabolism,* and the amount needed for this is about 1,500 C. for an adult.

3. To enable the muscles to work.

Variations in the amount of food needed will obviously depend mostly on No. 3, but people may also vary in their basal metabolic rates, and reasons for this are discussed on p. 114. If food is taken in excess of Calorie needs it will be laid down as fat under the skin and in the mesentery. If the diet is deficient in Calorie value, weight will be lost as stored fat is utilized, and if the shortage continues muscles will waste as their proteins are oxidized for fuel.

FOOD IN HOSPITAL

It might seem that patients in hospital would need less food than normal, since their muscular expenditure is not great, and though this is true of some it is not a general rule. Many are underweight when they come for treatment, and many more have operations ahead during the course of which they will lose several pounds. It is also true that some people must not be allowed to cumber themselves with excess weight—those with arthritis or heart disease, for example—and may be much fitter if allowed to lose weight.

In a hospital ward the sister will have some patients with good appetites taking normal meals, and for these she will order from the main kitchen a *full diet.* Some will not be fit enough for this and may be ordered a *light diet,* with minced meat, chicken or fish supplying the protein, and jellies or milk puddings instead of the more substantial sweets given to those having a full diet. For some the nature of their illness requires considerable modification of their food, and these will be served from the kitchen, and the main varieties of special diets are discussed later.

Hospital catering has today reached a high standard, and complaints about inadequate or dull food are unusual. All food, however, must be cooked some time in advance and sent to the wards, so that vigilance is needed if meals are not to be less attractive in appearance and cooler in temperature than those the patient has at home. If meals are sent up in containers they usually need reheating in the wards before serving, though if heated trolleys are sent up to the wards this should not be necessary. Plates should be well warmed.

Before mealtimes a round should be done to see that all patients are ready. If meals are served on lockers, cutlery, bread and a drink should be laid ; if on trays, these should be complete with condiments. Food should be neatly served in average helpings, and there should be enough for everyone who desires more to have it.

Little cooking is now done in ward kitchens, and there is a tendency for housekeeping staff to take on the service of meals to those taking a normal diet. The nurse may make a few light dishes for patients unable to take the ward meals, and the suggestions that follow only relate to cooking as done under those circumstances. Nurses who cook for their patients in private practice will need a more extensive repertoire and should consult an invalid cookery book.

Making Drinks

Fruit squashes are obtainable in great variety and are supplied from the stores instead of the lemons from which it was once customary to make fruit drinks for the ward. Oranges are sometimes given by friends in greater amount than patients can eat, and the juice may then be squeezed and strained and given with an ice cube and sugar to taste.

Lemonade. The yellow part of the rind is peeled thinly off and simmered for a few minutes in a pint of water. A tablespoon of sugar and the juice of the lemon are added and the lemonade cooled and put in the refrigerator before serving.

Tea. All patients are connoisseurs of a good cup of tea. The water should be used as soon as it boils and the pot well heated beforehand. Those who like it without milk also like it quite weak.

Coffee. A hot dry jug should be used and the coffee put in (about 3 heaped dessertspoons to a pint of water). As soon as it boils, 3 pints of water are poured on and allowed to infuse for 5 minutes till the grounds settle, when the coffee is strained off. The milk must not be overheated until fragments of coagulated albumin appear. These are intensely distasteful to nearly everyone, and can be removed by straining should they occur.

If a coffee-flavoured milk drink is required, a cupful of milk can be brought to the boil, a teaspoonful of a coffee powder stirred in.

Cocoa. The required amount of powder is mixed to a paste with cold water and stirred into the milk. Cocoa improves with a little cooking and so is best made in a double saucepan.

Egg Flip. This high-Calorie drink can be served hot or cold and flavoured to suit the patient. The yolk and white of an egg are separated and the white beaten to a stiff froth. The yolk is put in a glass and beaten with 2 teaspoonfuls (or more) of sugar. Three ounces of boiling milk (or cold if preferred) are stirred in, and then the white of egg. Brandy is probably the most popular flavour, and if it is allowed ½ fl. oz. may be added to the egg yolk. Lemon juice or black-currant purée can also be used. Not all people like a frothy drink, and for a plain one an egg should be beaten with sugar and strained into a glass and hot or cold milk stirred carefully in till the glass is full.

Bread and Milk. This is popular with many invalids, especially the elderly. A slice of bread is cut into ½-in. cubes and put into a saucepan with the milk, which is brought just to the boil. Sugar or salt are added to taste and, if liked, a nut of butter.

Light Extras

Boiled Eggs. The egg is put into boiling water and is boiled for three and a half or four minutes by the nurse's watch, according to whether a light or medium set is required. If eggs are boiled in quantity at tea or breakfast time a saucepan with a wire basket is essential. The water will take a little time to boil again when the eggs have been put in and should be left in for four and a half minutes.

Poached Eggs. A pan of water is brought to simmering point while a slice of toast is made and buttered. Adding a little vinegar or lemon juice to the water will produce a better-shaped egg. The egg is broken in a cup and slipped into the water, which must be deep enough to cover it. When set it is lifted out and well drained before serving it on the toast. Eggs that are not absolutely fresh do not make an attractive shape when poached, and are better scrambled.

Scrambled Eggs. One or two eggs are beaten with salt and pepper and a tablespoonful of milk added for each egg. An ounce of butter is melted in an aluminium saucepan, the eggs are added and stirred continually over a low flame until thick. Take the saucepan off the flame before cooking is quite complete, since the saucepan retains enough heat to complete the process. Scrambled eggs can be served on buttered toast or with bread and butter separately.

Toast. Dry toast should be brown and crisp, and the heat of the grill should be adjusted so that the cooking time achieves this. If the flame is too low the toast is hard ; if too high it is browned while still soft inside. It should be stood on edge to cool to avoid toughness.

SPECIAL DIETS

For medical reasons, modifications may be made in the normal diet affecting its Calorie value, or the amount of protein, fat, carbohydrates, salts or roughage that it contains. Some people require dietetic restrictions for a short time only, while others, like the diabetic, must adhere to a diet throughout life. The dietitian must ensure that the omission of any article from the food does not entail the absence of some other important factor. For instance, a low fat diet may be lacking in the fat-soluble vitamins A and D.

The patient must be made to see the importance of his diet and his interest and co-operation gained. The word "diet" has a gloomy connotation, with a suggestion of scarcity and sparseness, and patients are always told what foods they may use freely, as well as the ones they must avoid. If the patient is a man, the co-operation of his wife must be ensured, since it is she who does the buying and cooking and will in the long run decide what her husband eats.

The diet must, too, be one that is adapted to the patient's social habits and his working conditions. It is useless to suggest that a policeman on his beat should have a mid-morning milk drink ; while if the diabetic takes out sandwiches for lunch, he is not sent home with a diet that entails meat and two vegetables for his midday meal.

Nurses must understand the principles of main diets so that they may answer the questions that are always asked, or refer them to the dietitian. The diabetic wants to know if he can eat diabetic chocolate without restriction ; the patient having a reducing diet asks if she can have a glass of sherry before dinner when she goes home ; the man having a low salt diet says he is tired of his breakfast egg, and may he have a kipper like the others are enjoying ? The dietitian visits the ward daily, and will answer any questions and is glad to hear of patients' likes and dislikes before planning their meals.

Calorie Modifications

Reducing Diets. Patients who are overweight are eating too much for their needs, and there is no exception to this rule. A few have glandular deficiencies which make those needs lower than those of most people, so that an average amount of food will allow them to put on weight. Any obese person can, however, lose weight by constantly taking a low-Calorie diet. The difficulty is that to many people large meals have become a habit and they feel constantly hungry without them, and to some food is one of the main pleasures of life. Lonely middle-aged women often become overweight by solacing themselves with food, especially sweets.

These patients must be given some stimulus to weight-losing that will atone for the foregone pleasure of eating. An improved figure, the ability to wear smarter clothes, the approval of friends, increased mobility, decreased strain on arthritic joints or ailing heart are examples of the inducements that can be offered. Out-patients must be seen regularly, weighed, and praised and encouraged.

Diets of less than 1,000 C. are mainly used for those in bed, since the patient will feel exhausted and vaguely ill as the result of living on her own fat. The 1,000 C. diet given below, will usually be found satisfactory. It contains enough bulk to satisfy hunger, but if the patient complains of this the doctor may order dextroamphetamine (" dexedrine ") to reduce appetite. Thyroid extract is never ordered for reducing purposes except for those people with thyroid deficiency, i.e. myxœdema. It produces tachycardia and sometimes atrial fibrillation in those with normal thyroids.

Reducing Diet (1,000 C.)

Allowed daily . 10 oz. milk.
3 thin slices of bread (3 oz.) or 3 Ryvita, or 3 water biscuits.
½ oz. butter or margarine.

Allowed ad lib. . Raw fruit, or fruit stewed with saccharine (except bananas, grapes, prunes, figs).
Vegetables (except potatoes, peas, beans and beetroot).
Consommé, Marmite, Oxo, Bovril, tea, coffee, fresh fruit, unsweetened drinks.

Not allowed . Sugar, sweets, ice-cream, alcohol, thick sauces and soups, nuts, pastry, fried foods, cakes and jam.

Menu

Breakfast . . Tea or coffee.
1 egg, or 3 oz. kipper or haddock.
1 oz. bread.
Butter from ration.
Fruit if desired.

Mid-morning . Tea. Fruit if hungry.

Dinner . . 2 oz. lean beef or mutton or 4 oz. chicken or herring or tinned salmon, or 6 oz. rabbit, tripe or white fish.
Vegetables. Fruit.

Tea . . . Tea.
1 oz. bread.
Butter from ration.
Tomatoes or salad if desired.

Supper . . Meat or fish as at lunch, or 1½ oz. cheese or 2 eggs.
Vegetables. Fruit.

If any milk remains, it may be taken at bedtime.

High Calorie Diet

A diet of more than normal calorie value is given to patients with thyrotoxicosis, whose raised metabolic rate increases their calorie needs, and to those underweight from disease or poor diet. The aim must be to omit high residue foods of little food value in favour of the more concentrated ones, and to introduce extra feeds between the main meals.

Fat in very large amounts cannot be included in spite of its high value, because it is nauseating, but it may be added where possible, e.g. on mashed potatoes or vegetables, or in scrambled eggs. Cream can be given on puddings, or on ice-cream or in coffee. Fruit drinks may have additional sugar, and lactose is less sweet than cane sugar, but will cause diarrhœa if given in excess.

Mid-morning milk drinks can have ½ oz. milk powder or Horlick's or Ovaltine added, and a buttered rusk or biscuit is offered. Cheese as well as pudding is given at dinner and supper. At teatime buttered toast with honey or jam is offered. Chocolate is a useful and concentrated source of calories, if it is not eaten in quantities that destroy the appetite for the main meals. Thyrotoxic patients must not have an abnormal amount of protein since this has a specific dynamic action in stimulating metabolism.

Anorexia nervosa is a condition in which a high calorie diet is needed because of the extreme emaciation. The appetite is completely lacking at the beginning of treatment, and the calorie intake must be built up gradually. As few people as possible should be concerned in the feeding of the patient.

Fat Modification

High fat or ketogenic diets used at one time to be given in the treatment of pyelitis, but with better treatment of infections this diet has become of historical interest only. The fat content of the diet cannot be raised at the expense of carbohydrates without causing acidosis and "biliousness."

A low fat diet is chiefly used in liver disorders. Acute hepatitis is treated with a diet low in fat, high in carbohydrate, and moderate (about 50 G.) in protein. Vitamin B supplements are required. The appetite is often very poor for the first few days, and a good fluid intake is a very important consideration. In most cases it is not a long-lasting condition, and dietetic restrictions can soon be relaxed.

Chronic hepatitis, however, may last for years. Fat in the diet is restricted, but plenty of carbohydrate is given, and protein must be in adequate supply (80–100 G. daily) in order to provide the damaged liver with an adequate amount of amino acids. Attention should be paid to the calorie value, which is difficult to keep at normal levels if fat is omitted. Vitamin tablets should be given.

Patients with chronic gall-bladder disease (cholecystitis) are frequently overweight, and complain of flatulent dyspepsia. The diet should, therefore, omit bulky starch foods, and be of a calorie value decided by the patient's weight. Fat must be reduced, but enough should be given (40–50 G.) to produce a flow of bile.

Foods Permitted in a Low Fat Diet. Very lean meat ; fish, except herrings, kippers and salmon ; cereals ; fruit ; vegetables (boiled) ; preserves (except lemon curd). Milk should be skimmed.

Foods not Allowed. Fat fish, cheese, eggs, fat meat, chocolate, cocoa, toffee, fried foods, roast potatoes, nuts, pastries, rich biscuits. Butter, cooking fats and mayonnaise.

Modification of Salt Intake

The retention of sodium in the tissues leads to retention of water as well, which becomes manifest as œdema. Whatever its cause, œdema is made worse by sodium retention, so that conditions characterized by œdema (such as congestive heart failure, and acute or subacute nephritis) are often treated by a low sodium diet. Since the commonest form in which this is taken is sodium chloride, salt is the substance which is most important to exclude. Such a diet is not a very appetizing one and patients need encouragement to persevere with it when they leave hospital.

In order to be effective, the sodium chloride intake must not exceed

500 mg. a day, and to achieve this salt-free bread and butter must be used. "Edosol" is a low-sodium milk that is very useful. Since the sodium ion is the important one in maintaining œdema, it must be remembered that sodium as its carbonate or bicarbonate must be excluded from the diet, and that, therefore, chocolate, syrup and cakes made with baking powder cannot be taken.

Low salt diets are sometimes ordered when cortisone or prednisolone is being given, to avoid the œdema that sometimes complicates treatment.

The Karell diet has been often used for patients with congestive heart failure. It consists of 800 ml. of milk per twenty-four hours, divided into four feeds. It is low in calorie value (460 C.) as well as in minerals, and is not used for more than a few days because of this. Low salt diets are often used for hypertension, but in spite of their popularity there is no conclusive evidence that the restrictions imposed have any directly beneficial effect, except that the diet is unappetizing and can lead to a fall in the weight.

Patients who have diarrhœa lose sodium in the stools and should have this loss made good. Half a teaspoonful of salt can be added to a pint of lemonade without being perceptible.

Calcium salts should be present in liberal amounts in the diets of those laying down bone, such as children and pregnant women, and are also needed by those with parathyroid deficiency. Those with an iron-deficiency anæmia need plenty of the iron-containing foods mentioned earlier in this chapter.

Modification of Protein Intake

A good protein intake is needed by those doing heavy muscular work, by convalescents who have lost weight, and by those who have had operations involving periods of intravenous feeding and restricted oral intake. It has also been referred to as important in the diet in chronic liver disease.

Since the products of protein metabolism are excreted in the urine as urea and uric acid, it is in kidney disease that consideration of the protein in the food is of major importance. Acute nephritis is a condition which is not long-lasting, and is characterized by kidney inflammation which results in greatly diminished urinary output, leading to œdema and a rising blood urea. The diet should, therefore, be salt-free, restricted in fluid content, and low in protein. For the first day or two an acutely ill patient may receive 500–1,000 ml. of well-sweetened orange juice and water, but as soon as the urinary output begins to rise fruit purées, milk, puréed vegetables and salt-free butter can be given. Milk puddings and jellies can be introduced, and moderate amounts of proteins other than milk can be added as the acute inflammation subsides.

The leading clinical features of subacute nephritis is albuminuria, leading to massive œdema, which is due to a fall in the plasma proteins. The blood urea is normal. The aim is to raise the level of the plasma proteins and reduce the œdema. If a protein value of 200 G. is desired, casilan (25 G. of protein per oz.) will have to be used to supplement it.

Patients with chronic renal failure awaiting dialysis require severe restriction of their protein intake and control of the sodium- and potassium-containing foods. There follow specimen instructions for such a patient.

You **must** *have* $1\frac{1}{2}$ *eggs a day.* This may be boiled, soft or hard, poached, fried, scrambled, as an omelette or in cooking, or in baking.

Breakfast. Fried tomatoes, mushrooms or apple rings with fried bread or crisp bacon fat. Low Protein bread, toasted if liked, with butter and marmalade. Weak tea, with milk from allowance, sugar if liked.

Midmorning. Weak tea or weak ground coffee, black or with milk from allowance. Low Protein biscuit or sandwich using Low Protein bread with jam.

Midday or Evening. 1 egg fried, scrambled, poached, boiled or as an omelette. Green or root vegetables or salad with oil and vinegar dressing. 6 oz. boiled potatoes, mashed with vegetable margarine, roast, fried or chipped or 3 oz. (cooked weight) boiled rice. Fruit with sugar or glucose, or Low Protein dish—see list and recipes.

Tea. Weak tea with milk from allowance. Low Protein bread with butter or vegetable margarine. Jam or honey. Low Protein cake, biscuit, jam tart or shortbread.

Supper or Midday. Low Protein savoury dish with $\frac{1}{2}$ egg. Vegetables or salad with oil and vinegar dressing. Low Protein bread and butter or unsalted margarine. Fruit, fresh or stewed with sugar, or tinned, with double cream if liked, water ice or iced lollie—no ice cream (unless Low Protein).

Bedtime. Fruit squash or remainder of milk in weak tea. Low Protein biscuit or sandwich if liked.

Daily Allowance. 3 oz. milk. 6 oz. cooked potato or 3 oz. (cooked weight) rice or $1\frac{1}{4}$ oz. rice (dry weight). $1\frac{1}{2}$ oz. butter. $1\frac{1}{2}$ eggs. Twice a week 1 egg may be changed for 1 oz. meat, chicken, cheese or $1\frac{1}{2}$ oz. fish. No more than 2 oz. double cream.

Low Protein Dishes

Do not use ordinary flour—use Rite Diet flour or wheat starch and vegetable margarine.

Savoury. Salt, pepper, herbs and spices may be used. Vegetable pie. Braised vegetables. Cauliflower fritters. Use wheat starch, seasoning and water as batter (see recipe). Sage and Onion stuffing, use Rite Diet Low Protein bread only. Vegetable stuffed marrow, or onions, using Rite Diet Low Protein bread crumbs. See recipes for suggestions.

Sweets. Fruit pies and crumbles. Jam or fruit sponge (egg from day's allowance). Sago pudding (milk from allowance). Fruit blancmange (use cream and water instead of milk). Fruit conde using cream and water instead of milk to cook the rice. Fruit charlotte using Rite Diet Low Protein bread crumbs. Jam tarts. Shortbread.

Avoid Rhubarb, dried fruit, fruit juices, citrus fruit. Tomato and mushroom more than once daily. Extra milk, egg, meat, fish, cheese. Extra potatoes, rice or butter. Ordinary bread, biscuits, cakes, flour, semolina. Oats, breakfast cereals. Peas, beans, lentils, nuts. Jellies, fruit gums. Chocolate, ice cream, yoghourt. Tinned and packet soups, meat and fish pastes. Salad cream and mayonnaise (home made only if the egg is from allowance). Instant or bottled coffee, meat and vegetable extracts, salt substitute.

You Need Not Restrict Sugar, glucose, jam, honey, marmalade, boiled sweets, barley sugar. Chewing gum, glace mints, mint creams, Kendal Mint Cake. Wheat starch, sago, cornflour, arrowroot, tapioca. Dripping, lard, vegetable margarine. Lucozade, coca cola, pepsi cola, White's lemonade, Tizer.

The Following are Available on Prescription

Bread. Your own doctor will receive a letter from this hospital asking him to give you a prescription for Rite Diet Low Protein Bread and flour. A local chemist will obtain the amount you require from Welfare Foods (Stockport) Ltd., Higher Hillgate, Stockport, Cheshire. The chemist can also obtain wheat starch from Energen Ltd., Ashford, Kent. Methyl Cellulose grade 20 powder B.D.H. is obtainable from your own chemist if you wish to make your own bread—see recipe sheet.

Hycal. Your own doctor will give you a prescription for Hycal which is available in strawberry, raspberry, blackcurrant, lime, lemon, orange and pineapple flavours. A chemist can obtain it from Beechams (Brentford) Ltd.

Caloreen. Is also available on presciption and the chemist will obtain it from Scientific Supplies Ltd., Liverpool.

Aproten Pasta. Also available on prescription and the chemist will obtain it from Carlo Erba (UK) Ltd., 28/30, Great Peter Street, S.W.1.

Low Protein Biscuits. Also available on prescription and the chemist will obtain them from Carlosta Ltd., 33, Ermine Road, S.E.13, and Liga Food Co., 23, Saxby Street, Leicester.

High and Low Residue Diets

The amount of bulk in the diet should be increased for those suffering from atonic constipation by adding fruits, vegetables and high residue cereals like bran. Those taking a reducing diet are also allowed these foods in order to allay hunger.

Low residue diets are principally of value in those suffering from hæmorrhage from the stomach, or those awaiting intestinal operations. Coarse, bulky foods should also be omitted from high calorie diets in which they may blunt the appetite for more nutritious foods. Patients who are not allowed whole fruits may usually be given their juices, and so are not deprived of the vitamin C they contain.

Patients with ulcerative colitis need a bland diet of the type described for peptic ulcer, but with added protein to make up for the protein loss as pus and blood in the stools. Casilan is valuable for this purpose, as the appetite is usually poor, and in a severe case meat is not tolerated. A fluid diet, as described on p. 82, may have to make up for the sodium loss.

Peptic Ulceration

Peptic ulcers occur in those parts of the digestive tract exposed to the action of the acid gastric juice, usually on the lesser curvature of the stomach or the first part of the duodenum. The aim is to give food that will not irritate the ulcerated mucous membrane mechanically, or stimulate the secretion of hydrochloric acid, but the most important point is that food should be taken in moderate quantities at frequent intervals so that the stomach is not empty for long times during which the gastric juice can act unopposed. Protein is necessary in good quantity because it delays the passage of food from the stomach, and sugar is a valuable source of calories. Roughage must be omitted as far as possible, and since this includes whole fruits, vitamin C will be short unless orange juice or ascorbic acid tablets are given.

For severe acute ulcer pain a continuous transnasal feed of milk by the drip method (p. 184) is an excellent treatment. Gradually the intake can be increased until a diet on the lines described below.

Specimen Diet for an Ambulant Patient

Foods not Recommended in Acute Stage. Alcohol. Smoking on an empty stomach. Highly seasoned foods. High residue foods like fruit and vegetables, nuts, jam with pips, brown bread, digestive biscuits, Shredded Wheat and All-bran. Rich foods like bacon, pork, fried foods, suet puddings or pastry.

Foods Allowed. Milky drinks and milk puddings, junket, jelly, blancmange, sieved porridge, eggs, chicken, lamb or liver, cream cheese, grated cheese, thin ham or tongue. Sieved greens, mashed potatoes and root vegetables. Sieved fruit, soft fruit without skins or pips. Honey, syrup and jellies.

Time	*Type of Food*
On waking	If some time elapses before breakfast, milk and a biscuit should be taken in bed.
Breakfast	Weak, milky tea. Smooth cereal with milk, egg, bread and butter and jelly.
Mid-morning	Milk, which may be flavoured, and biscuit.
Midday	Meat (minced, if the teeth are not good). Mashed potatoes, purée of vegetables. Milk pudding or light sponge. Fruit without pith or skin.
Tea	Milky tea, bread and butter, Madeira or similar cake.
5 p.m.	Milk and/or biscuit.
Evening	Cheese, egg or fish dish. Bread and butter. Milk as a pudding or drink.
Night	Milk drink and biscuit. If the patient wakes at night, he should take a milk drink to bed.

Vitamin C tablets or orange juice should be taken regularly.

Diet After Hæmatemesis

The improved mortality rates for those who have vomited blood are due to earlier replacement of lost fluid and minerals. Rest is needed for the stomach, but gastric contractions are less when the stomach contains bland food than when it is empty. While some physicians give a more generous diet than others, most allow the patient to drink N/5 saline freely, and take milky drinks, and some allow fo ds of purée consistency as soon as the patient feels able to take them, though those who are nauseated should not be pressed to eat.

Modification of Carbohydrate Intake: Diabetic Diets

The patient with diabetes mellitus has insufficient insulin secretion for his needs in metabolizing carbohydrate. As a result he suffers from a high blood sugar, glycosuria, thirst, loss of weight, and ketosis due to the production of keto-acids from improper fat metabolism. If untreated, a severe case will prove fatal from acidosis as ketones accumulate in the blood. Not all cases, however, are severe. In some, the insulin supply is adequate if the diet is moderate in calories and in carbohydrate. In others, the patient must be given insulin in quantities sufficient to deal with the carbohydrate in his diet. The management of these cases requires skill from the physician and dietitian, and insight from the nurse who is looking after the patient during the time when his insulin and dietetic requirements are being balanced.

Mild or Moderate Cases. Diabetes occurs in a mild form in middle-aged patients, and is often only discovered in the course of investigation of some other condition. Such people are usually overweight and frequently women. Insulin is often not needed provided the weight can be reduced, and a low carbohydrate diet adhered to. All sugar must be omitted and starch reduced as in all obesity diets. As the weight falls the sugar in the urine decreases and may eventually disappear.

Moderate or Severe Cases. These people, who are usually children and young adults, have insufficient insulin for their metabolic needs, and it must be given to them by injection. The management of the diabetic in hospital and his education for a normal life outside it, are described in Chapter 16. All that is given here are some of the principles used in constructing diabetic diets for a patient needing insulin. If he is receiving insulin he must have a diet matched to it; if he is given insufficient insulin, ketones will appear in the blood stream and diabetic coma will ensue, while if his insulin is excessive in relation to his carbohydrate intake, it will lower his blood sugar until hypoglycæmia (p. 203) and its attendant symptoms occur.

Some physicians advocate the free-diet treatment, in which the patient eats what he likes, and his insulin dosage is stabilized according to the severity of his disease. This relies on the fact that most people's calorie consumption is fairly constant. It is attractive to patients because they are not troubled with dietetic calculations, but in practice control of the blood sugar is not very good, and some of the long-term complications of diabetes, such as nephritis, seem to occur more commonly in people treated in this way.

The patient's carbohydrate needs are estimated, according to his age, weight and type of work, and as a rule only the carbohydrate need be weighed. A new diabetic is best stabilized in hospital, and usually begins with a diet with a carbohydrate intake of 150 G. and a calorie value of 1,500. His insulin is then adjusted until the urine is sugar free, and then the diet and the insulin are raised together until the diet is sufficient for the patient's needs in the outside world. The specimen diet given below is for 150 G. carbohydrate diet.

	Oz.		Carbohydrate	Total CHs in grammes
Breakfast : 4 portions	3½ 1	Milk in tea . . . . Bread . . . . Egg	5 15	20
Mid-morning: 2 portions	3½ ¼	Milk in coffee . . . Biscuit	5 5	10
Lunch : 9 portions	 3 7 ½	Meat Vegetables from "free" list Potatoes . . . . Fruit } . . . . Milk } pudding . . Cereal }	 15 10 10 10	45
Tea : 6 portions	3½ 1 ½	Milk in tea . . . Bread . . . . Egg and salad if desired Biscuits	5 15 10	30
Supper : 7 portions	3½ 1	Milk in tea or coffee. . Bread . . . . Fish . . . . . Vegetables from "free" list . . . . Fruit	5 15 15	35
Bedtime 2 portions	3½ ¼	Milk . . . . . Biscuit	5 5	10

EXCHANGE LIST FOR DIABETICS

Each of the following contains about 10 grams Carbohydrate

Bread

Brown or White	plain or toasted	½ slice of thick cut sliced large loaf	⅔ oz.
		⅔ slice of a thin cut sliced large loaf	⅔ oz.
		1 slice of a small sliced loaf	⅔ oz.

Cereal Foods

Allbran		3 level tablespoons	⅔ oz.
Biscuits	plain, semi-sweet, or small tea Matzos	2 biscuits	½ oz.
Custard Powder, Cornflower, Rice, Sago, Semolina, Tapioca	before cooking	2 heaped teaspoons	½ oz.
Chappatis		made from ½ oz. wheat flour	
Cornflakes, or other unsweetened breakfast cereal		3 heaped tablespoons	½ oz.
Cornmeal, Flour		1 level tablespoon	½ oz.
Macaroni, Spaghetti, Noodles	before cooking	1 heaped tablespoon	½ oz.
Porridge	cooked, made with water	4 level tablespoons	4 oz.
Rice	boiled	1 heaped tablespoon	1 oz.
Ryvita		1½ biscuits	½ oz.
Vitawheat		2 biscuits	½ oz.

Milk

Milk	fresh or sterilized	14 tablespoons (⅓ pint)	7 oz.
,,	condensed, sweetened	1½ tablespoons	⅔ oz.
,,	evaporated, unsweetened	6 tablespoons	3 oz.

Fruit

Stewed fruits should be cooked without sugar

Apples	raw with skin and core	1 medium	4 oz.
,,	baked with skin	1 medium	4 oz.
,,	stewed	6 tablespoons	5 oz.

Apricots	fresh with stones, stewed	3 large	6 oz.
,,	fresh with stones, raw	3 large	6 oz.
,,	dried, raw	6 halves	1 oz.
,,	dried stewed	6 halves	$2\frac{1}{2}$ oz.
Bananas	ripe without skin	1 small	2 oz.
,,	green	1 large	4 oz.
Cherries	raw with stones	20	4 oz.
,,	stewed with stones	3 tablespoons	4 oz.
Currants	dried	1 level tablespoon	$\frac{1}{2}$ oz.
Damsons	stewed with stones	10	5 oz.
Dates	with stones	4	$\frac{2}{3}$ oz.
,,	without stones	4	$\frac{1}{2}$ oz.
Figs	green, raw	1 large	4 oz.
,,	dried, raw	1	$\frac{2}{3}$ oz.
,,	dried, stewed	1	$1\frac{1}{2}$ oz.
Gooseberries	dessert, raw	12	4 oz.
Grapes	whole	10	2 oz.
Greengages	raw with stones	4	3 oz.
,,	stewed with stones	4	4 oz.
Melon	without skin	1 large slice	7 oz.
Nectarines	with stones	2	3 oz.
Oranges	without peel	1 large	4 oz.
Orange Juice	fresh or tinned, unsweetened	8 tablespoons	4 oz.
Peaches	fresh with stones	1 medium	4 oz.
,,	dried, raw	2 halves	$\frac{2}{3}$ oz.
,,	dried, stewed	2 halves	2 oz.
Pears	raw with skin and core	1 medium	4 oz.
,,	stewed	$2\frac{1}{2}$ halves	5 oz.
Pineapple	fresh, edible part	2 heaped tablespoons diced	3 oz.
Pineapple Juice	tinned, unsweetened	6 tablespoons	3 oz.
Plums	any dessert variety raw, with stones	3 large	4 oz.
,,	stewed with stones	5 medium	8 oz.
Prunes	dry, raw with stones	4 medium	1 oz.
,,	stewed with stones	4 medium	2 oz.
Raisins	dried	1 level teaspoon	$\frac{1}{2}$ oz.
Raspberries	raw	6 heaped tablespoons	6 oz.
,,	stewed	6 heaped tablespoons	6 oz.
Strawberries	fresh, ripe	15 large	6 oz.
Sultanas	dried	1 level tablespoon	$\frac{1}{2}$ oz.
Tangerines	without peel	2	4 oz.

The following fruits contain a small quantity of Carbohydrate, and may be eaten in moderate quantity without being counted in the diet: *Avocado rar, Blackberries, Blackcurrants, Grapefruit, Stewed Gooseberries, Loganberries, Redcurrants, Rhubarb, Whitecurrants.*

Nuts (Shelled)

Almonds			8 oz.
Barcelona Nuts			7 oz.
Brazil Nuts			8 oz.
Chestnuts			1 oz.
Hazel Nuts			5 oz.
Peanuts			4 oz.
Walnuts			7 oz.

Vegetables

Beans	baked, tinned	2 level tablespoons	2 oz.
,,	broad, boiled	2 level tablespoons	5 oz.
,,	butter, boiled	2 level tablespoons	2 oz.
,,	haricot, boiled	2 level tablespoons	2 oz.
Beetroot	boiled	3 heaped tablespoons	4 oz.
Carrots	boiled	4 heaped tablespoons	8 oz.
Corn	on the cob	½ large cob	3 oz.
Lentils	boiled	2 level tablespoons	2 oz.
Onions	fried	2½ heaped tablespoons	4 oz.
Parsnips	boiled	2 heaped tablespoons	3 oz.
Peas	fresh or frozen, boiled	4 heaped tablespoons	4 oz.
,,	tinned	2 heaped tablespoons	2 oz.
Plantains	boiled, steamed	the size of an egg	1¼ oz.
Potatoes	boiled	1 the size of an egg	2 oz.
,,	chips	4 large chips	1 oz.
,,	crisps	¾ of a 5d. packet	¾ oz.
,,	mashed	1 heaped tablespoon	2 oz.
,,	roast	1 small	1½ oz.
Sweet Corn	tinned	2 level tablespoons	1½ oz.
Sweet Potato	boiled	2 level tablespoons	1¼ oz.
Yam	boiled	2 level tablespoons	1½ oz.

Other vegetables and salads not on this list may be eaten without restriction.

Beverages

Bengers Food, Bournvita, Ovaltine, Horlicks	2 heaped teaspoons	½ oz.
Cocoa Powder	5 heaped teaspoons	1 oz.
Coca-Cola or Pepsi-Cola		3 oz.
Ale, strong		⅓ pt.
Beer, Draught Bitter		¾ pt.
Beer, bottled		1 pt.
Cider, bottled, dry		¾ pt.
,, bottled, sweet		½ pt.
Stout, bottled		½ pt.

Miscellaneous Foods

Lemon Curd		3 level teaspoons	¾ oz.
Jam, Honey, Marmalade, Syrup, Treacle		2 level teaspoons	½ oz.
Jelly	in packet, as purchased	1 small square (as in packet)	½ oz.
Ice Cream	plain	1 small cornet or 1 small brickette	2 oz.
Yoghourt	plain	1 carton	7 oz.
Sausages	cooked	2 sausages	3 oz.
Chipolatas	cooked	4 chipolatas	3 oz.

In an Emergency

Sugar or Glucose	2 heaped teaspoons or 3 small lumps	⅓ oz.

These figures are extracted from a leaflet published by the British Dietetic Association, and the British Diabetic Association, 3/6, Alfred Place, London, W.C.1, who publish this and other useful leaflets.

Fluid Diets

Many people at the onset of an acute illness, such as influenza, lose their appetite for solid food and take only fluids. This stage normally only lasts a day or two, and though fortified milk drinks should be encouraged, no alarm need be felt if the patient prefers fruit juices. Calorie value is **not** important as long as a good fluid intake is maintained. Some, however, are dependent on fluids for periods of weeks or months, and for these the considerations are quite different. The calorie value must be one that will enable the patient to maintain or increase his weight, and the vitamin intake must be adequate for its needs. Such a patient is the one with a gastrostomy, either temporarily following surgery of the œsophagus, or permanently for carcinoma of the œsophagus. A recipe like this one may be used:

Gastrostomy Feed

1 pint milk
2 oz. full-cream milk powder
2 oz. sugar
1 egg
¼ teaspoonful Marmite

The milk powder is stirred into the warm milk, the sugar and Marmite dissolved in it, and then the whole poured on to the beaten egg. This mixture contains 1,100 C., and enough is made up for daily needs and refrigerated. Few can tolerate more than 16 oz. at a time, and in case of cancer patients it is frequently much less. The fluid is stirred before measuring out the feed, which must be strained and warmed. Twice daily the feed should be followed by a fluid vitamin extract, e.g. Abidec.

A similar mixture may be used as a jejunostomy feed, but fat is not well tolerated, and the milk powder used should be skim. A teaspoonful or two of cornflour may be cooked with the milk to prevent regurgitation.

Nasal feeds need to be somewhat thinner, since they have to pass through a much finer tube. Complan, a proprietary feed that contains 2,000 C. per pound, is a very useful substance. Four ounces can be added to a pint of milk with which it combines well. If thin feeds cause diarrhœa, this method can be tried. 100 grams of Complan and the same of glucose are mixed with half a litre of cold water. 3 grams of methyl cellulose (celevac) are dispersed in boiling water and added to the Complan. The mixture is made up to one litre.

CHAPTER 7

ADMINISTRATION OF DRUGS

Drugs may be absorbed into the body by many routes, and the one chosen by the doctor in writing his prescription depends on convenience of administration, the speed of action desired, the nature of the drug, and the age and physical disabilities of his patient. There are some, too, like the insoluble sulphonamides and magnesium sulphate that are not absorbed into the tissues, but still exert a therapeutic effect. These are the routes by which drugs are given :

1. *By mouth.* This is the commonest and most convenient method. Some drugs, however, are destroyed in the stomach and can never be given by mouth. The sublingual method is to place a tablet under the tongue and allow it to dissolve.
2. *By injection.* Hypodermic, intramuscular and intravenous. The details of injection-giving are described in Chapter 8. It is efficient and quick in its effects.
3. *Per rectum.* If drugs cannot be given by mouth they may be absorbed from the rectum ; paraldehyde is often given thus. The dose usually needs to be double the amount effective by mouth.
4. *By inhalation*, e.g. anæsthetic gases ; amyl nitrite.
5. *By inunction*, or rubbing into the skin. The composition of the base will affect penetration. Mercury ointment was once used for syphilis, and testosterone may be given by inunction in ointment form.
6. *By intrathecal injection* when it is desired to bring the drug into direct contact with the meninges or the spinal nerves, e.g. streptomycin for tuberculous meningitis ; spinal anæsthetics.
7. *By ionization.* The drugs are introduced in ion form by an electric current, e.g. histamine.

DANGEROUS DRUGS ACT AND POISONS ACT

The storage and prescription of certain drugs is regulated by statute, and the nurse has legal obligations concerning them. In addition, every hospital has its own regulations concerning the administration of medicines controlled under these Acts, and these should be meticulously observed. A routine continually and faithfully followed in detail is a complete safeguard against an accident that might be tragic for patient and nurse.

The Dangerous Drugs Act regulates the use of certain powerful drugs of addiction, e.g.

Opium and its derivatives.
Morphine.
Cocaine.
Heroin (diamorphine).
Pethidine.
Methadone (" Physeptone ").
Cannabis indica.
Levorphanol (" Dromoran ").

Drugs controlled by this Act are labelled D.D.A. and must be kept in hospital in a locked cupboard not used for any other drugs, and the key must be kept on the person of the sister or nurse in charge. Dangerous drugs are ordered in a separate book, and a receipt for them is signed when they are delivered from the Dispensary. Prescriptions must be signed by the doctor's full name, and a record kept of their administration.

In private practice, the doctor's prescription must bear the name and address of the patient, and the prescription cannot be repeated without a new order. Doctors must keep a register of all the supplies of dangerous drugs he purchases.

The Poisons Act regulates in a similar way a large number of drugs divided into different schedules, of which Schedules I and IV are those that concern the nurse. Poisons must also be kept locked up, but in a separate cupboard from the dangerous drugs. Drugs controlled under it include :

The sulphonamides.
The barbiturates.
Digitalis preparations.
Atropine.
Codeine.
Ergot alkaloids.
Hyoscine.
Strychnine.

Drugs for external use as lotions or liniments should be in ribbed or fluted bottles, and appropriately labelled.

Penicillin and the other antibiotics are controlled by the Therapeutic Substances Act, 1956, since their indiscriminate sale to the public is obviously undesirable. As new drugs and antibiotics come into use they can be added to the appropriate section of these Acts if it seems desirable.

In addition to these legal obligations, each hospital has its regulations concerning the administration of dangerous drugs and poisons. They will include some or all of the following :

1. Two nurses should join in all steps described, and one should be a State Registered Nurse.
2. The written prescription is read, and all parts of it must be clearly understood.
3. The phial or bottle is taken from the locked cupboard and its label checked with the prescription.
4. The correct amount is measured out into the syringe or glass container.
5. The contents are rechecked with the prescription and the drug.
6. The cupboard is relocked.
7. Both nurses go to the patient and ensure that he is the one for whom the drug is intended. This is especially important on busy operating days, in casualty wards, and at night.
8. The nurse checking the procedure watches the administration.
9. Both sign the Drug Book before doing anything else.

Unfortunately, readers of the daily press must be aware that breakdowns in this routine occur with occasionally fatal results. Almost invariably these are due to failure to follow the rules, and it must again be stressed that the best protection for nurse and patient is a routine so consistently and conscientiously followed that it becomes a firmly established habit. Examination of the causes of mishaps shows that mistakes are most commonly made in these circumstances:

(*a*) Two or more injections are to be given, and two bottles are taken out of the cupboard at once. This is dangerous, as the wrong one may be used.

(*b*) A nurse is thinking about a patient who is gravely ill, and gives him an injection intended for someone else. The nurse checking the procedure must watch that the drug is delivered to the right person.

(*c*) Prescriptions are misread, and ounces may be given instead of drachms, or a pure drug given instead of a dilute mixture. Care and knowledge should prevent this, and prescribers should not use the pharmaceutical symbols for drachm (ʒ) or fluid ounce (℥) as these are easily confused. If in any doubt the nurse should ask the doctor or pharmacist for advice.

PREPARATIONS OF DRUGS

The following are common preparations :

Mixtures (draughts). Solutions or suspensions of drugs in water, often with a flavouring added. Suspensions must be well shaken, and taken as soon as they are poured out.

Tinctures. Solutions of drugs in spirit.

Linctuses. Syrupy preparations used for checking a cough. They must be given undiluted for best effect.

Pills. Solid preparations, sometimes sugar-coated, handed in a spoon and swallowed with a drink.

Tablets. Compressed drugs, given like pills. Tablets for sublingual use should be held under the tongue until dissolved, and not swallowed.

Capsules. Powdered drugs in thin gelatine cases. Unpleasant substances are often dispensed like this and the capsule must be swallowed whole and not chewed.

Cachets. Solid substances, often nauseous or insoluble, in a rice paper container. They should be slightly moistened immediately before swallowing. Children find difficulty with them, and they are not suitable for very young patients.

Powders. These may be stirred into water, or put on the tongue and swallowed with a drink.

Lozenges. Compressed drugs to be sucked for their local effect. A flavouring agent is usual.

Pastilles. Drugs for sucking in a flavoured gelatine base.

Mucilages. Their tacky consistency keeps these longer in contact with the mouth and throat, so they are used mainly for their local action.

Liniments. Drugs in oil or spirit for external use.

Lotions. Solutions or suspensions for external use. Other preparations used in skin diseases are described in Chapter 17.

Pessaries. Drugs in a gelatine or fatty base used in the vagina (see p. 291).

Suppositories. Similar preparations for rectal use.

PRESCRIPTIONS

It is a convenience to the prescriber and the dispenser to use one of the " official " preparations. The British Pharmacopeia (B.P.) includes a list compiled by the General Medical Council, with standard doses. The British Pharmaceutical Codex (B.P.C.) is a supplementary list compiled by the Pharmaceutical Society. The British National Formulary (N.F.) is a more recent introduction with the National Health Service, and new editions appear at fairly regular intervals. It is very widely used, and a copy should be in every ward. It contains chapters on drug actions of much interest to nurses, and a very useful list of alternative names of similar preparations, e.g. the different names under which identical drugs are manufactured.

Proprietary preparations are made by many firms under their own trade names, and many new and valuable drugs are introduced by the great drug houses who spend much money on research in connection with them. Eventually some of these become " official " remedies, and are then marketed under a new name and at a lowered price. It is naturally in the interests of economy in the Health Service to prescribe an " official " drug, but it is a great trial to doctors and nurses that having become familiar with a drug under one name they must subsequently learn to use another.

Latin Phrases and Abbreviations

Latin abbreviations are not recommended for use in prescriptions, but while their use is decreasing, they still occur frequently enough to make retention of the following section necessary for the present.

Abbreviation	*Latin*	*English*
aa	ab ana	of each
ac.	ante cibos	before meals
ad. lib.	ad libitum	to the desired amount
alt. die.	alternis diebus	on alternate days
aq. dest.	aqua destillata	distilled water
b.d. b.i.d.	bis die bis in die	twice a day
c.m.	cras mane	tomorrow morning
c.n.	cras nocte	tomorrow night
c	cum	with
co.	compositus	compound
ex. aq.	ex aqua	in water
ex. lact.	ex lacte	in milk
h.n.	hac nocte	tonight
h.s.	hora somni	at bedtime
m.	mane	in the morning
n.	nocte	at night
p.c.	post cibos	after meals
p.r.	per rectum	by rectum

Abbreviation	*Latin*	*English*
*p.r.n.	pro re nata	as required ; may be repeated at the customary intervals
q.h.	quartis horis	four hourly
q.i.d.	quater in die	four times a day
rep.	repetatur	let it be repeated
ss	semis	half
*s.o.s.	si opus sit	if required ; only one dose may be given
stat.	statim	immediately
t.d.s.	terdie sumendum	three times a day
t.i.d.	ter in die	three times a day

* In the minds of many doctors, no distinction is made between these two, and since they may be ambiguous the nurse must be sure that she understands the intention of the prescriber. Doctors are advised to avoid these terms.

MEASURING DRUGS

In Britain all drugs must now be dispensed according to the metric system.

Metric Weight

1,000 micrograms = 1 milligram.
1,000 milligrams = 1 gramme (G.).
1,000 grams = 1 kilogram.

Milligrams and grams are the weights used in dispensing. Parts are expressed in decimals, according to the metric usage, e.g. a milligram is 0·001 G. Great care must be taken not to confuse the grain (gr.) and gram (G.) abbreviations.

Metric Volume

1,000 millilitres (ml.) or 1,000 cubic centimetres (c.c.) = 1 litre

" Millilitres " are replacing " cubic centimetres " in medical use, as being a more rational measurement of volume.

Although the dispenser must use the metric system, it is still not illegal for the prescriber to use the apothecaries' measures, and in case the nurse encounters these, they are given below.

Apothecaries' Weights

20 grains (gr.) = 1 scruple.
3 scruples = 1 drachm (ʒ)
8 drachms = 1 ounce (℥).

Scruples are now not used at all, but grains and fractions of grains may still be met.

Imperial and Apothecaries' Fluid Measure

60 minims (♏) = 1 fluid drachm (ʒ).
8 fluid drachms = 1 fluid ounce (℥).
20 fluid ounces = 1 pint.
2 pints = 1 quart.
4 quarts = 1 gallon.

Equivalents

The equivalents given below are only approximate, but enable comparisons to be made.

English to Metric

Weight	1 grain	=	60 milligrams.
	$\frac{1}{4}$ gr.	=	15 mg.
	$\frac{1}{6}$ gr.	=	10 mg.
	1 ounce	=	30 grams.
Volume	15 minims	=	1 millilitre.
	1 fluid ounce	=	30 millilitres.
	1 pint	=	570 millilitres.

GIVING MEDICINES

Ward medicine rounds will be made after breakfast, lunch and supper for those drugs ordered three times a day after meals. Those given twice a day may be given on the first and last of these rounds, while four-hourly and before-meals medicine will be given at intermediate times. The nurse in charge will collect her medicine board, which is the list of ward prescriptions, kept carefully up to date. This ward list serves only to remind her of which medicines are due, and does not relieve her of the obligation of checking the medicines she gives with the patient's own prescription. She will need glasses, millilitre measures, china measures for oil, a jug of water, a bowl for washing glasses and a medicine cloth, spoons or watchglasses for offering pills, and any special requirements, e.g. in a children's ward, spoons for cod liver oil and malt and a separate container of water in which to put them after use. Even sweets are not unknown. Stock bottles of items such as vitamin tablets are added.

If the medicine to be given is a mixture, the nurse selects her bottle and a glass, and checks the patient's prescription. She shakes the bottle if it is a suspension, and inverts it to make sure that it is well mixed. She holds it with the label uppermost to prevent soiling it with drips, and removes the cap with the ulnar border of the left hand, holding it there while she raises the glass to eye level and pours out the dose. Fluids form a slightly curved surface in a small glass, and the lower level of this meniscus should be opposite the line marking the dose. Replacing the cap with the left hand, she gives her patient the glass, and sees that a sip of water is available. It is imperative that she watches it taken on the spot, for even adult patients will sometimes avoid taking drugs unless supervised. Pills, tablets and cachets are not touched with the fingers, but shaken out into a spoon or watch-glass. Liquid paraffin is given in a china measure.

Iron medicines stain the teeth and may be given through a straw, or a mouthwash and tooth brush supplied afterwards. Castor oil is not now often given, but should if prescribed be poured into an oil measure heated with boiling water to make the oil run more easily. Fruit juice or best of all (if it is allowed) a little brandy, can be added to disguise the taste. A biscuit eaten afterwards is a good method of getting the oily taste out of the mouth.

A

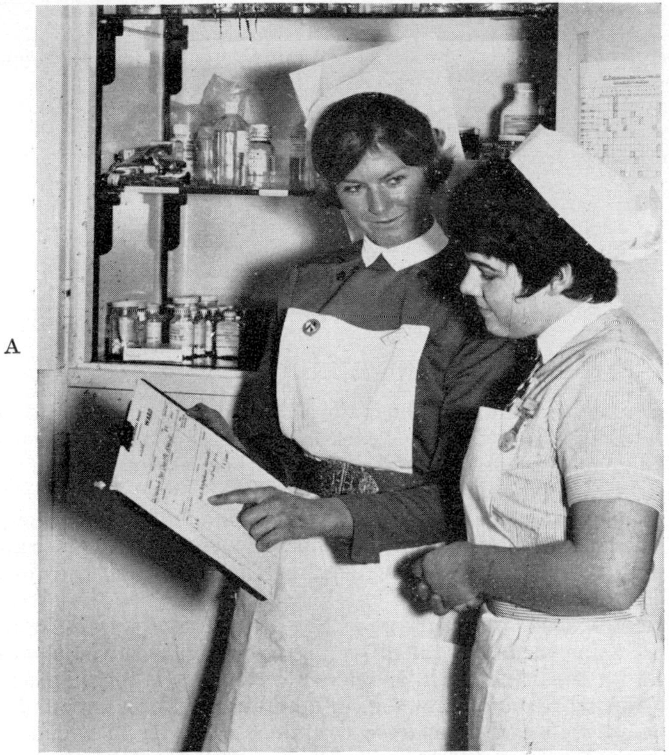

B

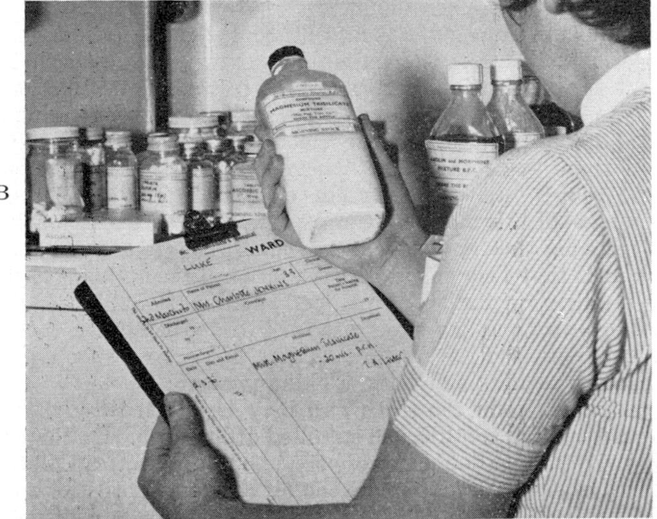

Fig. 16. Teaching a safe routine for administering drugs.
A. Read the prescription.
B. Read the label.

C

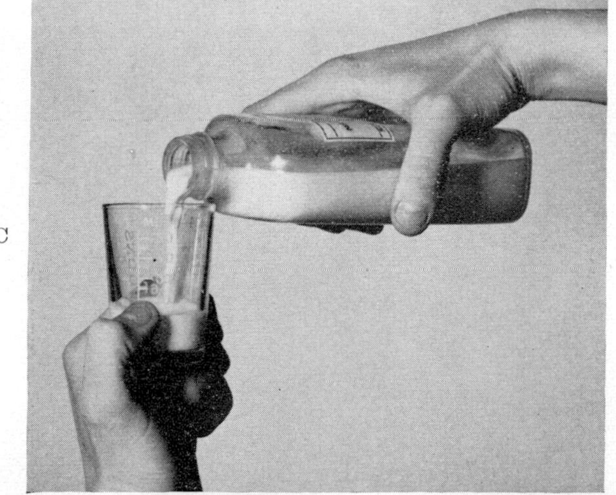

D

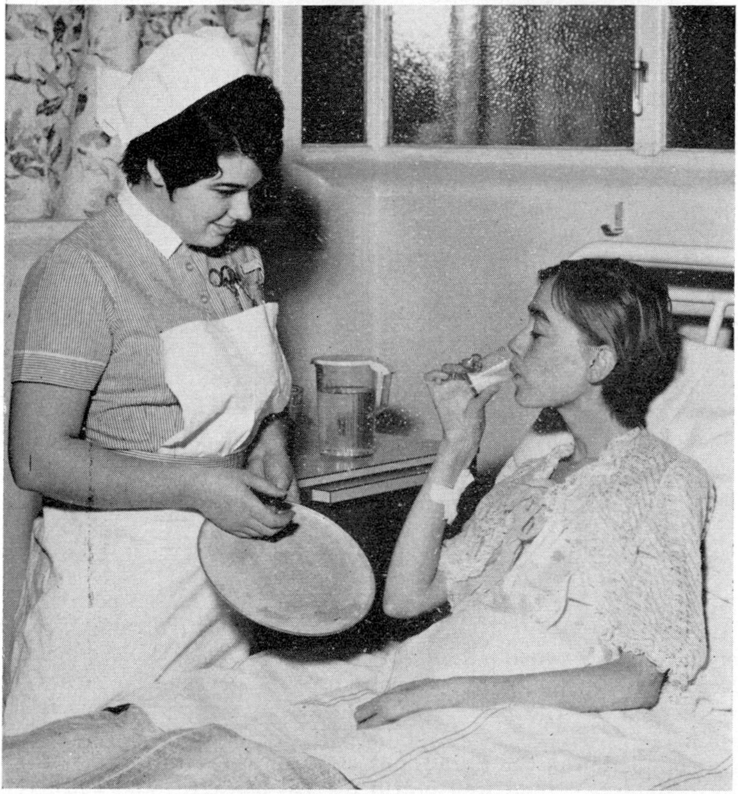

Fig. 16 (*cont*). Teaching a safe routine for administering drugs

C. **Measure out the correct amount.**
D. **Give it to the right patient.**

E

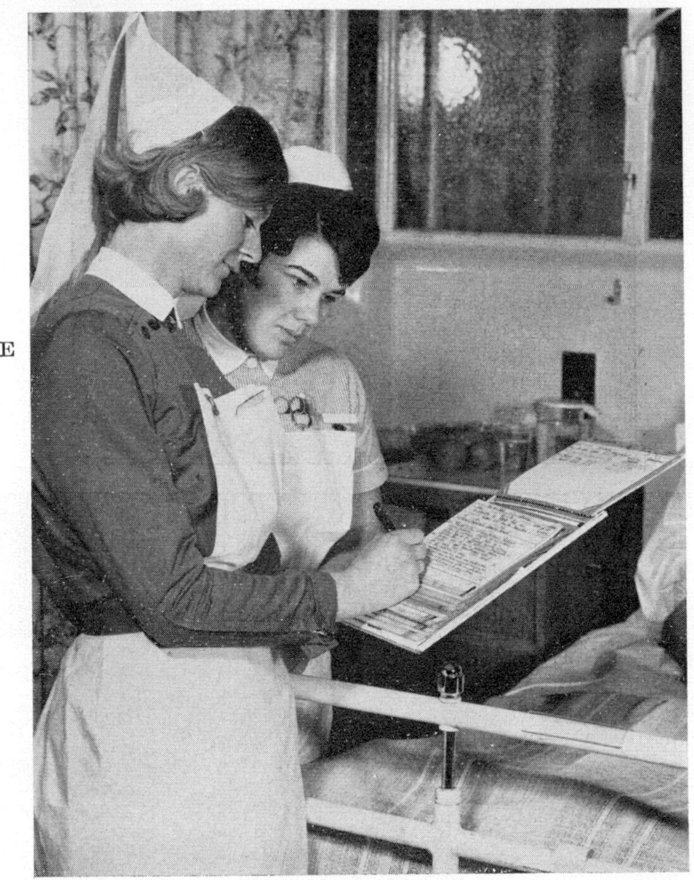

Fig. 16 (*cont.*). Teaching a safe routine for administering drugs.

E. Record its administration.

Medicines ordered before meals must be given at the correct times as these are most effective when the stomach is empty. Hypnotics should be given when all disturbing treatment is finished and the patient is ready for sleep. Special precautions may be needed with some drugs, e.g. the pulse should be taken before digitalis is given (p. 96).

On completion of the round, glasses are washed with hot water and soap or detergent, and well polished. Oil measures and cod-liver oil spoons are washed last. Empty boxes and bottles are put aside for replenishing.

MANAGEMENT OF THE MEDICINE CUPBOARD

Dangerous drugs and poisons are kept in their separate cupboards, and the amounts checked regularly to ensure that they agree with the stock supplied and the quantities used. Any discrepancies should be reported at once, and the security precautions reviewed. It should be an absolute rule that no nurse takes any medicine at all, however innocuous its nature, for her own use, and it would be wise if doctors did the same. Medical and auxiliary personnel who may be working under strain may find the temptation to take drugs increasingly difficult to resist. Addicts may also try to get possession of drugs if security is not good.

Drugs that have been ordered for a patient and discontinued should be returned to the dispensary, and not retained in the belief that they may be useful. If labels are detached or stained, the bottle should be sent to the pharmacist for relabelling. The outside of all bottles must be kept clean, and the shelves regularly washed. Drugs which need storing in a refrigerator should be kept there. As far as possible, medicines may be grouped according to their uses, e.g. aperients can be kept together. Those for external use are in distinctive bottles and must be kept apart. Some, like hydrogen peroxide, deteriorate in light and must be kept in brown bottles.

Some mixtures deteriorate quickly with time; penicillin is a common example, and if crystals appear in it, the mixture has become irritating and must not be used. Tablets may lose their potency or harden so that they do not dissolve in the alimentary tract. Insulin and adrenalin do not keep for long periods ; adrenalin is especially vulnerable when the bottle is half empty and air is present in quantity. If there is an expiry date on the bottle, it must be returned to the dispensary when the date is reached.

SOME GROUPS OF DRUGS

Alkaloids are potent nitrogenous substances of vegetable origin Their names typically end in -ine, and *morphine, atropine, strychnine* and *caffeine* are instances. Their dose is small because of their power.

Analgesics are pain relievers. They fall mainly into three groups : (*a*) morphine and other opium alkaloids ; (*b*) the antipyretics, represented by aspirin and sodium salicylate ; (*c*) other synthetic drugs like pethidine.

Morphine is exceedingly effective, but may have undesirable side effects, like depression of the respiratory centre, and vomiting. It must not be used if there is a risk of addiction developing.

Aspirin is safe and widely used, but it is irritating to the stomach and may cause severe reactions in asthmatics. Its soluble forms are more pleasant to take. *Sodium salicylate* is especially used in rheumatic fever, and is also a stomach irritant. Sodium bicarbonate is sometimes prescribed with it to lessen this effect and it should be given after meals, and the fluid intake kept high. Toxic signs like nausea, vomiting, tinnitus (ringing in the ears) and deafness may necessitate changing to calcium aspirin.

Codeine is a weak alkaloid of opium, with no tendency to cause addiction or depress respiration. The related *dihydro-codeine* is well absorbed by mouth, and is a useful analgesic for ambulant patients with mild pain, as is *paracetamol*.

Pethidine is widely used as a pre- and post-operative drug and as an analgesic, in doses of 50 or 100 mg. It is most effective as an intramuscular injection. Intolerance is unusual, but giddiness and tachycardia are sometimes met. Early hopes that it would be a less powerful drug of addiction than morphine have not been fulfilled. *Methadone* is another synthetic pain-reliever.

Antacids are substances that neutralize gastric acid. Weak alkalis like sodium bicarbonate can be used, but have the disadvantage of provoking further secretion of hydrochloric acid. Neutral substances like *magnesium trisilicate*, *aluminium hydroxide* do not have this side-effect.

Antibiotics are substances produced by micro-organisms, mainly moulds, which are active against other micro-organisms. The ones of interest in medicine are those effective against the bacteria that attack man.

The organisms especially sensitive to the original forms of penicillin were streptococci, gonococci, meningococci and pneumococci. The spirochæte that causes syphilis is sensitive, and it is in the treatment of venereal disease that penicillin has had one of its most spectacular successes. Staphylococci have proved increasingly capable of resisting it. The newer forms of penicillin mark an advance in one of three ways.

(*a*) They are not destroyed by gastric acid, and so can be taken by mouth, (e.g. Phenethicillin, Propicillin, Phenbenicillin).

(*b*) Some are active against intestinal organisms (e.g. Ampicillin).

(*c*) Some are able to destroy staphylococci (e.g. Cloxacillin, Methicillin).

Cephaloridine appears to be similar in its activity to this third group of penicillins and to be free of harmful side-effects.

Streptomycin is effective against many bacteria, including the colon organisms, which are resistant to most penicillins. Its most important use is in tuberculosis, and it is not as widely used as it might be in other infections because of its toxic effects, especially deafness and giddiness. Tubercle bacilli fairly rapidly become resistant to streptomycin, but this effect is delayed if isoniazid (I.N.A.H.) and/or para-amino salicylic acid are given with it.

Both penicillin and streptomycin are very prone to cause dermatitis in nurses and doctors who do not use the precautions in giving them described on p. 108. These reactions occur most often in those who have been long exposed to them, so that trained nurses are often affected. Students should always adopt the precautions indicated.

Viomycin is also effective against the tubercle bacillus, but is more toxic still, and is only prescribed for cases resistant to streptomycin.

Chlortetracycline (aureomycin), *oxytetracycline* (terramycin) and *tetracycline* are all chemically related, active against a wide range of organisms, including some viruses, and given by mouth. Nausea, diarrhœa and vomiting may occur, and if administration is continued, shortage of vitamins B and K may occur. Thrush of the mouth, rectal and vaginal mucous membranes may follow.

Chloramphenicol is also given by mouth and its most valuable action is against the typhoid bacillus and salmonella infections, and in certain forms of meningitis, since it penetrates the cerebro-spinal fluid better than most antibiotics. Nausea, vomiting and thrush infections of the mouth and anus may complicate its administration, but its most serious side-effect is aplastic anæmia, which though uncommon is usually fatal. Chloramphenicol is for this reason not used for trivial infections.

Erythromycin and *novobiocin* are similar in their action to penicillin, but organisms acquire resistance to them readily, and they are not used except in those cases in which penicillin is ineffective. Neomycin is often given by the mouth to suppress the bowel flora before operations on the colon; little is then absorbed.

Nystatin is used in the treatment of fungal infections (like thrush) of the mouth, anus or vagina. It is useful in preventing the overgrowth of such organisms which may be a problem during treatment with some of the other antibiotics. *Griseofulvin* is given by mouth to treat fungus infections of the skin.

Anti-coagulants decrease the clotting power of the blood. They are used frequently for people with deep venous thrombosis, to prevent pulmonary embolism, and are given for life to patients with artificial heart valves. Such patients must have the clotting power of the blood regularly examined, and should be asked to watch for and report bruising, nosebleeds or hæmaturia. Aspirin should not be given to those having anticoagulants, as it may cause gastric bleeding. Barbiturates reduce the power of anticoagulants.

Heparin is prepared from liver, and is given by intravenous or intramuscular injection. Its effects are soon felt, and its antidote is protamine sulphate. *Arven* is another intravenous anticoagulant.

Warfarin is given by mouth, and as it has a cumulative action, its dose must be carefully regulated. The antidote is vitamin K by intravenous injection.

Anti-histamine drugs are used in allergic conditions in which production of histamine in the tissues occurs. "*Benadryl*" was the earliest, and many proprietary drugs like "antistin" and "anthisan" are used. They are most effective in relieving hay fever and sensitivity rashes, and are of little use in asthma. They are extensively used in hospital to prevent reactions to transfusions. Drying of the mouth and sleepiness follow their use, and outpatients should be warned of this, especially if they are motorists.

Aperients or **laxatives** are opening medicines; *purgatives* have a stronger action, but any aperient in large enough dose will act as a purgative. A very large number exist, with a variety of actions, and care should be taken to select one suited for the purpose.

Some, of which *agar* is the type, add *bulk* to the stools, and are most useful for those with an inactive colon or a low residue diet. The most commonly used *lubricant* is liquid paraffin, which should be given in divided doses, or it may run through the colon and leak through the anal sphincter. If used habitually it is said to interfere with vitamin absorption.

The sulphates of magnesium and sodium are *saline* aperients. They attract water into the colon, and so produce a fluid stool, the magnesium sulphate being the stronger of the two. Salts should be given well diluted in hot water before breakfast.

The *vegetable* laxatives include rhubarb, senna, figs, cascara and aloes, and all are comparatively mild in ordinary dosage. Castor oil, once so widely prescribed, is not now often given except occasionally for cases of food poisoning. Bisacodyl (Dulcolax) can be given by mouth, but is usually thought more useful in suppository form.

Digitalis. The leaves of foxgloves contain substances with a powerful action on the heart. Its main action is on the Bundle of His, which it depresses, and its most important use is for atrial fibrillation. It slows and strengthens the heart beat, enabling the heart to fill better and thus increase its output. This improved performance in patients with heart failure results in better kidney circulation, so that the output of urine rises and œdema is diminished.

In large doses toxic effects are seen, and to avoid these the nurse should take these precautions:

1. The pulse should be taken before each dose is given, and if the rate is below 60 the doctor should be consulted before the drug is given. Should the temperature be raised (e.g. after thyroidectomy) a rate of 80 is low enough for the same precaution to be used.
2. Urine should be measured.
3. Coupling of the pulse, headache, nausea, vomiting and a fall in the urine output are the toxic signs to be noted and reported.

The most commonly used preparations are prepared digitalis, 30–100 mgms. by mouth; tincture of digitalis, 5 to 15 minims; digoxin 0·25 to 1 mg. Digoxin may be given intravenously, and so is valuable for urgent cases. At the outset of treatment much larger doses may be given than are used for maintenance doses.

A drug with a similar action on auricular fibrillation is *quinidine*, less often used than digitalis because it is reputed to be more dangerous. It is usually only prescribed for fibrillation of recent onset, and patients should be at rest in bed during the course. The pulse should be taken before each dose, and if a return to normal rhythm has occurred, the physician should be asked if he wishes the dose to be given or varied. Embolus is a complication to be feared if there is blood clot in the auricles.

Diuretics promote the output of urine, and so help to reduce œdema in suitable patients. The most widely used is *chlorothiazide* and its related drugs (hydrochlorothiazide, hydroflumethiazide) which can be taken by mouth. They all decrease the reabsorption of salt and water in the kidney tubules, and are liable to increase the excretion of potassium. Patients with ascites are especially susceptible to potassium loss, and nurses should look for such signs as muscular weakness. Potassium is sometimes added to these oral diuretics, and the letter " K " after the name is an indication of this. *Frusemide* (Lasix) is an oral diuretic with a much quicker action than the thiazide group and is especially useful for those who do not respond to other diuretics. *Spironolactone* promotes excretion of sodium and retention of potassium, and is used in special cases with other diuretics. *Mersalyl* is a mercury diuretic given by intramuscular injection.

Caffeine and *theophylline* are alkaloids that increase the output of urine.

Hormones, either natural or synthetic, are used when their secretion is deficient, e.g. *thyroid* extract for myxœdema, and insulin for diabetes. Many are of more general application, e.g. *adrenalin,* which because of its effects on the sympathetic system can be used in asthma, to relax bronchial spasm ; in hypoglycæmia, to raise the blood sugar ; with local anæsthetics, to secure a bloodless field ; and in heart block, to raise the pulse rate. *Cortisone* is a suprarenal cortical hormone the introduction of which threw a great deal of light on disease processes and the body's responses to them. It limits tissue reactions in inflammation, and has, therefore, been used in a great variety of complaints. In rheumatoid arthritis it causes a remarkable increase in the mobility of affected joints, but hopes that it was the cure for this condition have not been realized, since continued use causes undesirable side-effects, while withdrawing it allows the arthritis to return. Though less used than formerly, it may still be given for certain cases, and is also prescribed for inflammatory eye conditions, ulcerative colitis and many skin conditions. In ointment form it is an effective treatment for pruritus (itching) of vulva or anus, and for some cases of eczema.

Hypnotics produce sleep resembling the natural variety ; *narcotics* produce deep sleep. The nurse is well aware that these are not the only means of helping a patient to sleep. External conditions must be suitable—darkness, quiet and a suitable ward temperature are necessary. Bedclothes must be sufficiently warm but not heavy. Cold feet or a full bladder will prevent sleep, and pain must, of course, be relieved. A hot milk drink or, for elderly people, a little alcohol is often effective.

The biggest class of hypnotics is the *barbiturates.* From this large group a drug can be selected and dosage arranged to produce light or heavy sedation, narcosis or general anæsthesia. They range from short-acting ones like *quinalbarbitone sodium* (" seconal sodium ") to long ones like the very useful *phenobarbitone.* None has any pain-relieving action, and all are dangerous if taken with alcohol, a combination that may produce coma. Outpatients must be warned about this, and also against keeping their tablets beside the bed, since a further dose may be taken in a moment of confusion in the night.

Barbiturate poisoning, accidental or suicidal, is a common occurrence, and most hospitals have a routine for dealing with this emergency. The stomach should be washed out and if the patient is unconscious it is wise to pass a cuffed endotracheal tube, which will prevent fluid gaining entry to the airway, and will also enable a respirator to be used if breathing fails. The unconscious patient should be turned regularly to prevent hypostatic pneumonia, and penicillin is given to avert lung infection. If coma is deep, forced diuresis by intravenous mannitol and fluids is usually required. Nasal feeds, mouth toilet and catheterization if urinary retention is present are nursing procedures that will be necessary. When the patient has recovered, the circumstances that led to the incident must be investigated and the help of the medico-social worker and the psychiatrist may be enlisted.

Glutethimide is a useful alternative drug to the barbiturates. Its effects last about six hours. *Nitrazepam* (" Mogadon ") has a rapid action, and is rather longer lasting in effect.

Chloral hydrate is safe and effective, but has an unpleasant taste and is usually dispensed in a flavoured mixture. Chloral Elixir Pædiatric is made specially for children.

Paraldehyde is another useful drug, with the disadvantage that it has an unpleasant smell that lingers in the breath. It may be given by mouth or per rectum, and is excellent for alcoholics. By intramuscular injection it is valuable for confused and agitated patients. The B.P.C. dose is 2–8 ml., and in spite of its safety, some accidents have occurred with paraldehyde, from giving the wrong volume.

Hypotensives are drugs that lower the blood pressure and they have a place both in medicine and surgery. The surgeon uses them in order to reduce bleeding at operation, and the physician for patients with hypertension. Those receiving these drugs should have a daily reading of the blood pressure while lying down. These people are apt to feel faint if they get up too quickly from a recumbent position, and should be warned about it. *Serpasil, pempidine tartrate, mecamylamine* and *Guanethidine* are among those in common use.

Stimulants. In many acute conditions such as shock, post-operative anæsthetic collapse and acute heart failure there are drugs to stimulate the circulation or respiration or both. The method of action of these varies considerably. *Nikethamide* is one of the most commonly used in ward emergencies in doses of 1 to 4 ml. by hypodermic intramuscular or intravenous injection. *Methedrine* is often used as a circulatory stimulant in shock, and so is *noradrenaline* in intravenous saline. *Nalorphine* counters the depressing effects of morphine and its related drugs.

The **sulphonamides** are a group of chemically related substances capable of preventing the growth of bacteria in the body. They do not display the same specific action that the antibiotics do, and fall into two main groups—the soluble ones that are readily absorbed from the intestine and the insoluble ones that remain in the gut and exert their action there.

Of the insoluble ones, *phthalylsulphathiazole* is widely used to sterilize the intestinal contents before operations on the colon. *Succinylsulphathiazole* and *sulphaguanidine* are used in the treatment of bacillary dysentery.

Among the soluble ones, *sulphadimidine* and *sulphadiazine* are perhaps the most useful, and the ones least liable to toxic effects. In general they are given by mouth, and need to be given at four or six hourly intervals in order to keep up the level in the blood. Sulphafurazole and sulphamethizole (Urolucosil) are rapidly excreted in the urine, and so are active against urinary infections.

Patients having a course of a sulphonamide should have their fluid intake kept high, since the chief danger of these drugs lies in their relative insolubility in the urine, in which they are excreted. Crystals may form in the pelvis of the kidney or the ureters and cause anuria. Blood in the urine or a fall in the urinary output are warning signs. If the urine is kept alkaline while the sulphonamide is being given, complications are less likely.

Tranquillizers. The name of this group has taken hold of the imagination of the lay public, and since in modern life there are many suffering from anxiety of varying degrees they are much in demand. Many proprietary medicines are marketed ; most are only obtainable on prescription, and all should be.

Chlorpromazine hydrochloride has many actions, since it is a ganglion-blocking agent, affecting the whole of the autonomic system and having a sedative effect on the cerebrum. It is extensively used for agitated and anxious patients in mental hospitals, and has many uses in general hospitals for checking vomiting and for pre- and post-operative patients. It can produce severe reactions in sensitized people, and nurses should wear gloves while preparing injections. In hospitals where it is extensively used a more stringent routine may be devised for the protection of the staff, for whom sensitization to this drug may be an occupational hazard. *Chlordiazepoxide* (" Librium ") and *diazepam* (" Valium") are tranquillizers that do not cause sleepiness, and are widely used for mild anxiety states.

Antimitotic drugs. Cells are able to grow and reproduce themselves by means of the nucleus and the complicated structures within it, and since cancer cells grow faster than most of the body cells, they are sensitive to the action of drugs that interfere with cell-division.

These drugs, called cytotoxic or antimitotic, form a comparatively recent group. They are less effective, even in high dosage, than radiotherapy, and the amount that can be given is limited by the ability of the red bone marrow cells to survive their action. Such drugs can only usefully be ordered if the cancer cells are more sensitive to the drug-effect than the marrow cells from which blood cells develop.

Nitrogen mustard preparations include Mustine, given intravenously, and Melphalan, which can be taken by mouth. Cyclophosphamide (Endoxan) has been used with success in treating lymphadenoma. Busulphan (Myleran) may bring relief for some time in chronic myeloid leukæmia, while for acute leukæmia 6-mercaptopurine is often used. Thiotepa may be prescribed for patients with secondary or inoperable growth, and is said to have a larger margin of safety than most cytotoxic drugs.

In order to ensure that maximum concentration of these drugs reaches the growth, they may be given by intra-arterial infusion. If they are allowed to run into the artery that supplies the part affected, the blood stream will carry the drug directly to the growth.

An infusion running into an artery must overcome a pressure of about 120 mms. of mercury, and to do this the bottle must hang at least 6 feet above the level of the patient, so a special stand will be required, and a pulley to raise the bottle to the necessary level. The tubing should be wired to the glass connections or it may be forced off by the pressure in the artery. Care should also be taken in lowering the bottle for refilling, or again blood may rise into the apparatus.

This brief account of some of the groups of drugs indicates the scope of this subject today. New medicines are constantly being introduced and nurses are fortunate who work in hospitals where the pharmacist is able to issue periodic bulletins or produce displays of these recent innovations. Several books for nurses on pharmacology exist, and one of these should be read by all who want to know more of a subject so important to patients and nurses.

CHAPTER 8

INJECTIONS

A LARGE and increasing number of drugs is given directly into the tissue by a syringe and a hollow needle. Many of the drugs so given are dangerous, not only in the legal but in the literal sense, and the fact that injections are so commonly given should not make the nurse forget that there are many perils involved unless a scrupulous and intelligent technique is learnt and always followed. To be proficient in giving an injection implies not merely to have learnt the way to insert the needle, but to know how to sterilize and select the equipment ; to read the prescription and understand its implications ; to calculate the amount needed ; to give it painlessly and without harm to nerves or blood-vessels ; to know the effects expected and to watch for untoward reactions ; to cleanse and resterilize the equipment.

The routes by which injections are given are as follows :

1. **Intradermal.** Fluid is given into the skin, in which it raises a wheal. Such an injection is made at the beginning of local anæsthesia, and in many sensitivity tests. Quantities used are small.

2. **Hypodermic or Subcutaneous.** The fluid is injected into the connective tissue beneath the skin, and quantities up to 2 ml. can be given.

3. **Intramuscular.** The needle point penetrates muscle, which can accommodate amounts up to 20 ml., though quantities between 1 and 5 ml. are more usual.

4. **Intravenous.** Injection is made directly into a vein.

5. **Intrathecal.** After lumbar puncture has been performed drugs may be given into the cerebro-spinal fluid.

Injection has many advantages over giving medicines by mouth.

1. It is more speedy in action ; intravenous injection is notable in this respect.

2. It is a certain method of administration, whereas drugs given by mouth might be vomited. For unconscious patients it may be the only practical method.

3. Small doses of powerful drugs can be efficiently administered.

4. Some drugs, such as insulin, are inactive by mouth.

5. Drugs which do not readily pass from the blood into the cerebro-spinal fluid must be given by intrathecal injection.

6. It is an impressive method. Many patients think more highly of an injection than of a capsule.

There are, of course, drawbacks to this technique, of which these are the most important :

1. Drugs given by this means may be difficult to neutralize if any undesirable effect occurs.

2. An aseptic technique is needed, and there are many reports in the literature of sepsis, sometimes severe or even fatal, resulting from an injection.

3. Intramuscular injections may result in nerve injuries if the site is not carefully selected. Intravenous injections have similar complications: for instance, intra-arterial instead of intravenous injection of thiopentone has resulted in gangrene of the arm. In Britain, however, it is not usual for a nurse to give intravenous injections.

4. Sterilization of syringes costs money; the same is true of the supply of disposable syringes and needles.

SYRINGES AND NEEDLES

A syringe consists of a barrel, made of glass or plastic, with a nozzle to which the needle is attached. The barrel is etched with the graduations for the dose. Syringes may hold from 1 to 100 ml., and the smallest sizes are marked into 0·1 ml. divisions. Insulin syringes are graduated in "marks", 20 to each millilitre, to facilitate the measurement of different strengths of insulin.

Glass syringes usually have a metal nozzle, but plastic syringes are all of the same material. Nozzles are of a standard diameter (Luer fitting) and so can take needles of any size. Within the barrel is the piston, which can be drawn up to aspirate fluid into the syringe through the needle, or depressed to expel its contents.

Hypodermic needles are made in sizes 22 (the smallest) to 1. They have a hollow shaft and at the penetrating end are cut at an angle to give the sharpest possible point. The shaft is joined to a mount, that is fitted on to the nozzle of the syringe. Single-use disposable needles avoid problems of sterilization and sharpening.

STERILIZATION

Plastic disposable syringes and needles are supplied sterilized and packeted by the manufacturers. If glass and metal ones are used, they are sterilized by one of these means:

1. Baking in an electric oven at 160° C. for 1 hour.
2. Exposure to a temperature up to 190° C. for a shorter time in a chamber heated by infra-red lamps, through which the syringes pass on a conveyor-belt.
3. Autoclaving at a pressure of 15 lbs. for twenty minutes. The syringe must not be packed in a sealed container into which steam cannot penetrate.

Boiling for three minutes, disassembled will kill all bacteria other than spores.

Boiling in 2% sod. carbonate for five minutes has practical difficulties connected with maintaining the correct strength, and in getting rid of the alkali from the syringe, but can be used if syringes are infected in circumstances where none of the other methods of "absolute" sterilization is available. Syringes of glass and metal cannot be sterilized by chemical means, and immersion in any kind of fluid must not be relied on. Syringes and needles should be stored in a sterile container sealed where they are needed at intervals only.

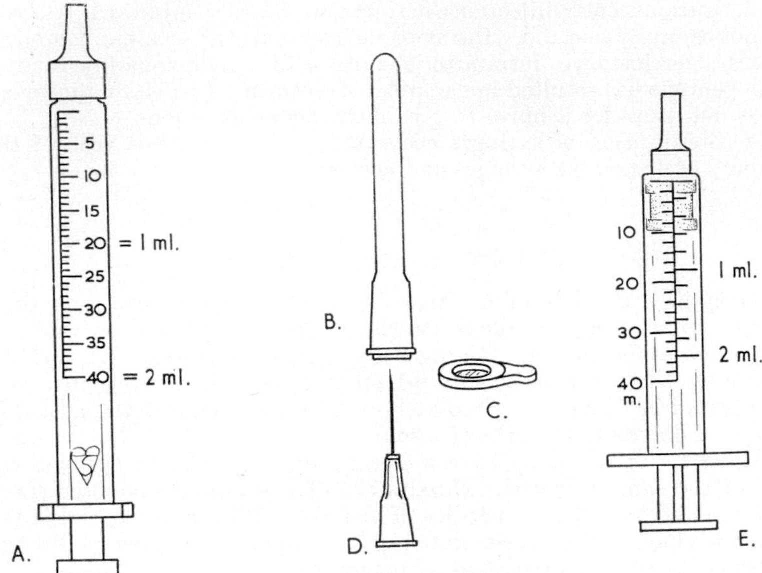

FIG. 17. Syringes and needles. (A) an insulin syringe, graduated in marks. On the right is a disposable plastic syringe (E). The disposable hypodermic needle (D) is supplied sterile in a case (B) with a cover (C).

GIVING A HYPODERMIC INJECTION

Equipment

Receiver or tray with a syringe bridge.
2 swabs or tissues.
Files for glass ampoules.
Small bottle of ether, or spray, with spirit.
Receiver for used swabs and empty ampoules.

The procedure to be described is the administration of morphine gr. $\frac{1}{6}$ (10 mg.) to a patient after operation. Every hospital has its own rules for giving dangerous drugs, and it usually involves the checking of each step in the preparing and giving by a second nurse, preferably a trained one.

A sterile 1-ml. syringe with a No. 19 needle is selected and laid on the bridge. Two sterile swabs are required, and a little ether is poured on each. The order for the drug is read—" Hyp. inj. morphine 10 mg. post-operatively "—by both nurses, the poison cupboard unlocked and the drug selected. In a ward it may be a multi-dose glass container with a rubber cover protected by a screw cap. The label (e.g. morphine 10 mg. in 5 minims) is read by both nurses and the screw cap removed and the rubber cleaned with an ether swab, which is discarded. To prevent the formation of a vacuum in the bottle, the piston of the syringe is withdrawn to the 5-minim mark and the needle inserted at a right angle through the rubber cap. The bottle is inverted and the

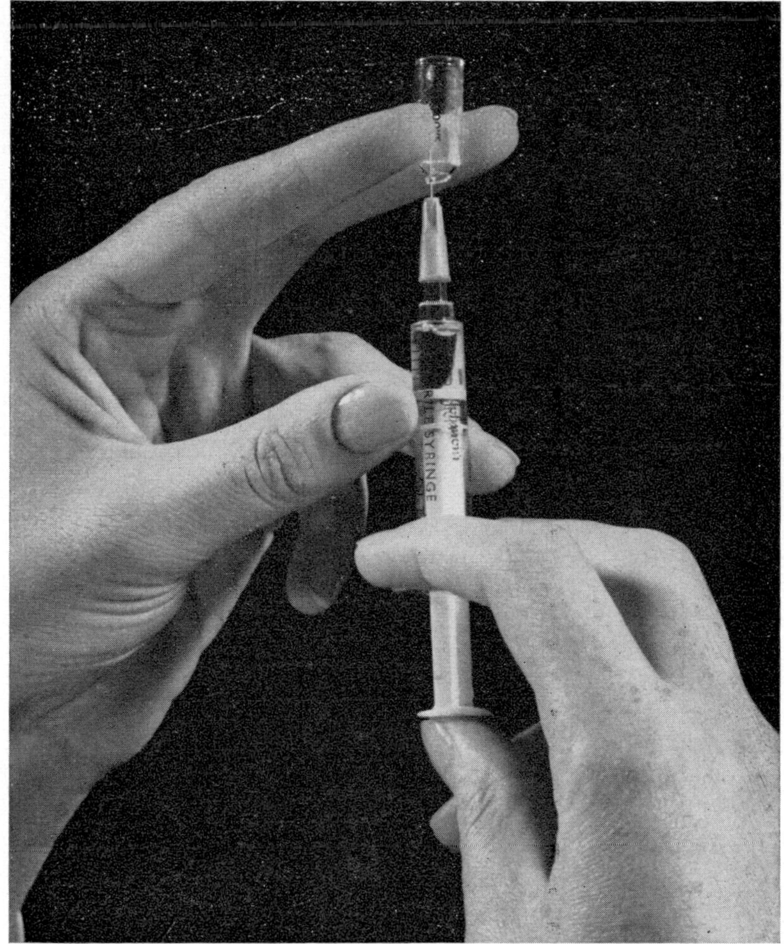

FIG. 18. Filling a syringe. Notice that the fingers do not touch the part of the piston that goes into the barrel.

air injected into the bottle. The piston is then withdrawn until 5 minims of fluid are in the syringe, when the needle mount is supported by the forefinger while the needle point is withdrawn. The loaded syringe is laid on the bridge, the dose once more checked with the order and the bottle, and the morphine bottle locked up again in the poison cupboard.

Both nurses take the tray to the patient's bedside, since the duty of the checking nurse is to see that the injection is given to the right person. A usual site in adults is the outer surface of the upper arm, which is easily accessible, not unduly sensitive, and not crossed by superficial veins. If the patient is conscious, while the arm is being exposed and the selected spot cleaned with the ether swab, she is told

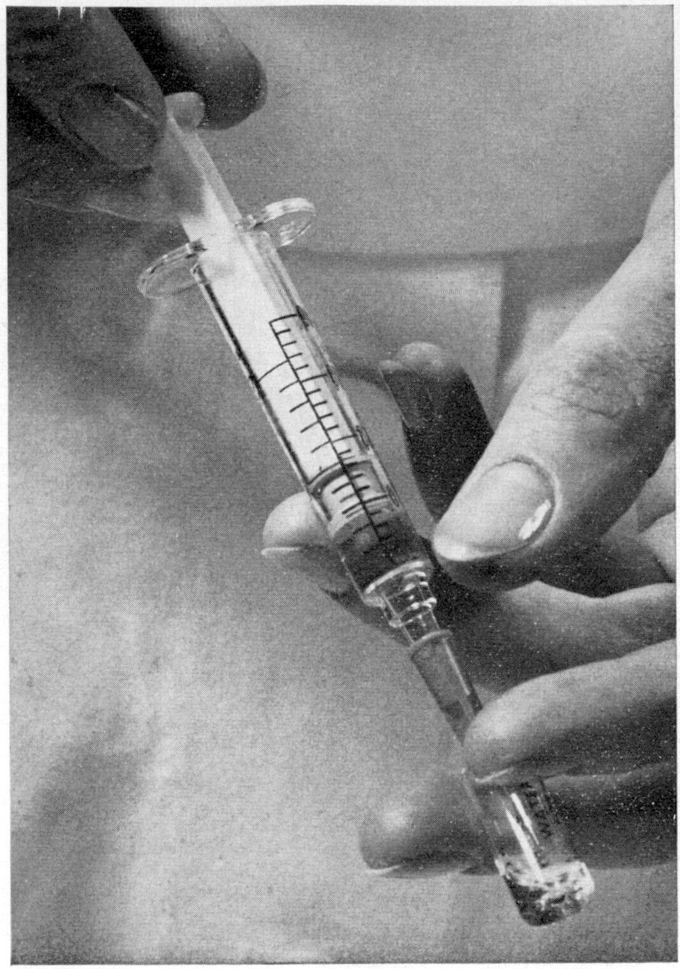

FIG. 19. A method of holding a syringe when drawing up an injection from an ampoule.

that the injection will keep her free from pain. The skin is made taut with the left hand, while with the bevel of the needle upward, the point is introduced at an angle of 45 degrees to the skin and allowed to penetrate about a $\frac{1}{4}$ in. into the subcutaneous tissues. The left hand is transferred to the piston of the syringe and slight traction is made to make sure that the needle point does not lie in a blood-vessel. If it were, blood would be drawn back into the syringe. If all is well the piston is pressed gently home and its contents expelled and the swab is held over the point while the needle is withdrawn. This pressure enables the needle to be withdrawn painlessly and prevents escape of the drug along the needle track. The site is massaged briefly with the swab to aid dispersal and give a minor comfort to the patient, whose gown is readjusted before leaving her to sleep.

Both nurses return to the office or desk, and sign in the ward drug book the date, time, patient's name, drug and both their own names. The syringe is rinsed, assembled, under running water with special attention to the patency of the needle, then taken to pieces and rinsed again, dried and put aside for resterilization. The hypodermic tray is left clean and in order for the next user.

If a glass ampoule is used, it will contain a single dose, and the amount will be etched on the glass. These are preferable to multi-dose containers, and their use is becoming general. Any drug in the neck of the ampoule is shaken down, and a swab held behind it while it is broken to prevent cutting a finger. Some ampoules have a mark filed on the neck ready for breaking, some will need a few strokes with a file at the base of the neck. The top is broken off, and the entire contents drawn into the syringe.

Drugs for injection are sometimes dispensed as tablets, and although this is a convenient method of storing and checking drugs it is not quite so easy to give. A spirit lamp, a spoon and a bottle of distilled water will be needed. The interior of the spoon is flamed over the lamp and the tablet dropped in. A convenient amount of distilled water (e.g. 1 ml.) is drawn into the syringe and squirted into the warm spoon on to the tablet. This is better technically than pouring distilled water into the spoon, since the lip of the bottle may be contaminated. The tablet will dissolve easily, and all the fluid in the spoon is drawn up into the syringe.

Fractional Dosage

Sometimes the dose to be given does not correspond to the dose in stock, and then a simple calculation will be required. Where the stock of drugs carried is small and such calculation is often needed, drugs should be dispensed in a volume that will make arithmetic easy.

Example. How to give morphine 10 mg. from a bottle containing 15 mg. morphine in 1 ml.

There is morphine 15 mg. in 1 ml.

Therefore there is 1 mg. in $\frac{1}{15}$ ml., and 10 mg. in $\frac{1}{15} \times 10 = \frac{2}{3}$ ml.

The dose given is to the nearest 0·7 ml. so 0·1 ml. is given.

INTRAMUSCULAR INJECTIONS

Drugs are given by intramuscular injection for one of three reasons:

1. Fluids which are too irritant to be given under the skin can safely be injected into muscle.
2. Bigger volumes can be given into muscle.
3. Action of a drug is faster by this route.

Sites. Since these injections are given more deeply and may be bigger in volume than hypodermic ones, the possibility of injuring nerves with such injections is of great importance, and must constantly be guarded against when giving them. Blood-vessels too are more readily entered, and the precaution of withdrawing the piston before giving the drug must never be omitted.

The gluteal muscles in the buttock are the first choice of most nurses for intramuscular injections, although the sciatic nerve runs beneath the inner and lower parts of the buttock. There are several ways of determining a safe site, but the simplest to a nurse is to consider the buttock, with the iliac crest as its upper boundary, to be roughly circular, and to give the injection in the upper outer quadrant of that circle, avoiding the outer part close to the iliac crest.

The muscles of the thigh are often used. The outer aspect of the

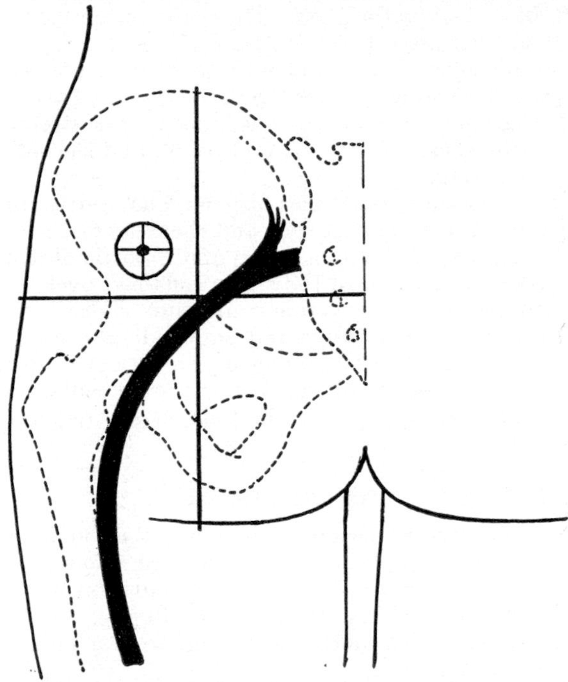

Fig. 20. Intramuscular injections. If these are given in the buttock, the upper outer quadrant must be used, to avoid the sciatic nerve and the ischial tuberosity.

thigh, a hand's span below the great trochanter in an adult, is safe, but injections in this area often seem to be painful, perhaps because of fascia in the region preventing dispersal of the fluid. The front of the thigh is also liked, injection being made into quadriceps extensor half-way between the groin and the knee, but it is just possible that the femoral canal may be entered if the injection is given too near the groin. The deltoid muscle may be used if the patient has a big enough muscle, and the region of the shoulder joint is avoided.

Many physicians and surgeons have strong preferences about intra-muscular injection sites, and the nurse must follow the wishes of her chief. In some cases, however, the choice of sites is severely limited, e.g. a patient may be in a plaster hip spica, and then injections will have to be made into the muscles of his upper parts.

Giving Intramuscular Injections

The syringe must be of a size adequate to hold the volume needed and the needle should be a 2 in. (4 cm.) one to ensure entering muscle. The site is selected with care, and the skin cleaned. The syringe is most conveniently held in the manner of a pen, with the middle finger tip resting on the needle mount. The skin is made taut with the left hand, and the needle introduced smartly but not too violently into the tissues at a right angle to the skin. It must never penetrate to its full length in case it breaks at its junction with the mount, and while the syringe is held firmly it must not be held so rigidly that an involuntary contraction of the muscle being pierced snaps the needle. The skilled operator holds the syringe so that the ulnar border of the hand meets the patient's skin at the same time that the needle penetrates. This contact seems to mask the prick, which should be scarcely felt.

The piston is withdrawn, and should blood enter the syringe another puncture site must be chosen. The fluid is expelled quite slowly, especially if the volume is large, and firm counter pressure is made with a swab while the needle is withdrawn to prevent escape of fluid into the surface tissues where it may do harm if irritating. The site is then very gently massaged with a swab.

Some Special Considerations

If antibiotics like penicillin or streptomycin are being given by this route, the possibility of sensitization to the drug arising in the nurse must be prevented. Repeated contamination of the fingers, and of the face by spray, not infrequently leads to severe dermatitis, very difficult to cure but easy to prevent if these precautions are taken :

1. Gloves should be worn while the syringe is filled, the drug given and the syringe and needle washed.

2. The same needle should be used for filling the syringe and giving the injections. Needles are not blunted by puncturing rubber, but by careless contact with hard surfaces.

3. The dose should be adjusted with the needle point still in the phial.

If multiple injections have to be given, as in bacterial endocarditis, the site should be regularly changed ; constant injections in the same place may lead to necrosis. Patients having such long courses need handling with tact and sympathy and the best possible technique, since they become apprehensive and not unnaturally critical about a procedure they know so well.

Very thin patients also need especial care, since if the available muscle is small, less latitude in avoiding nerves and blood-vessels is given. Children are a similar risk, and two people should always give such an injection, one making the injection and the other controlling the part selected. Very fat patients have their muscle deeper below the skin than normal, and a long enough needle to reach it must be chosen. Œdematous patients should have the œdema fluid pressed away from the site selected, or in these too the injection may be made too superficially and necrosis of the skin may occur.

Should the needle break during an injection, it usually does so at the mount and if it has not been too deeply introduced it can be removed without difficulty. An injection must never be given to a restless patient or child until movement in the part selected has been absolutely controlled.

Oily solutions and suspensions are more painful after injection than watery ones, and are probably best given in the buttock if this is possible. If suspensions are being given from a multi-dose container, they must be very well shaken until all sediment has gone, or the patient will not be receiving the proper dose.

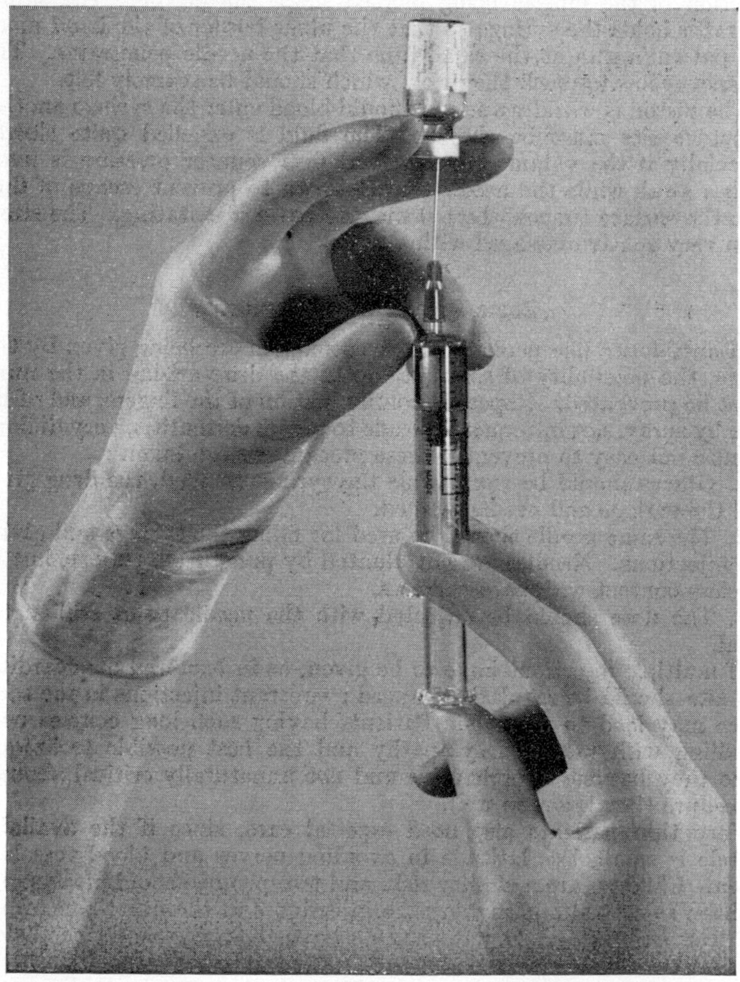

FIG. 21. Sensitization to drugs. Certain injections, especially penicillin, streptomycin and chlorpromazine, cause dermatitis in those sensitized to them. Gloves should always be worn; the same needle is used for drawing up and giving the drug; and the level is adjusted with the needle tip in the bottle.

INTRAVENOUS INJECTION

These are normally given by the doctor. Drugs are given in this way when a rapid effect is wanted, e.g. thiopentone as an induction to anæsthesia, glucose to terminate hypoglycæmia, nikethamide as a cardiac or respiratory stimulant. "Absolute" sterilization of the syringe needle by baking or autoclaving is necessary. A vein in the bend of the elbow is usually selected, and the elbow extended. The vein may be made more prominent by constricting the upper arm either by a piece of rubber tubing or by the hand of the assistant. Once the vein has been entered the pressure is released and the injection made. Firm pressure by a swab over the puncture site for a few seconds is made, and a dressing is not needed.

CHAPTER 9

Examination and Investigations

EVERY patient admitted to hospital normally has the heart, lungs and abdomen examined and the urine tested, and other investigations suggested by his complaints. Ideally the out-patient should be examined in the same way, but life is short and in some cases of trivial complaints and injuries it is not necessary. The nurse must, however, present her patient dressed in a way that makes examination easy and saves time for the patient and doctor. For instance, a lump or tumour calls for an examination of the lymphatic fields into which spread may have taken place if the swelling is malignant. If a woman has a lump in the breast, the doctor will want to examine the other breast, the axilla, the supraclavicular hollow, and the abdomen. Below are some of the examples of the way in which patients are got ready for examination in out-patient departments.

Heart and lungs. Nothing should be worn under the dressing gown above the waist.

Breast. Dressing gown and knickers.

Hernia. Dressing gown and decency towel, since it may be necessary to examine the patient standing.

Spine or hip. Dressing gown and decency towel.

Limbs. The opposite limb must be available for comparison.

Out-patients sometimes need encouragement and reassurance in getting undressed, and assert that they have not prepared themselves for an extensive examination. No such difficulties exist when they are examined in the wards.

General Examination

Requirements. Stethoscope.
Tendon hammer.
Sphygmomanometer.
Torch.
Spatula and receiver.
Treatment blanket and bedjacket.

It is generally necessary to examine the mucous membranes for signs of pallor ; the state of the teeth and tonsils; the heart and lungs.

The nurse screens the bed and closes the windows beside it. All pillows but two are removed, unless the patient finds it difficult to breathe lying down, and the nightdress is taken off. The bedclothes are folded singly down to the level of the symphisis pubis and the upper parts covered with a blanket. The nurse tells the doctor his patient is ready, and stands at the lefthand side of the bed to help him. The blanket is turned down and the heart and lungs examined, the patient's face being directed away from the doctor if he asks her to cough. She sits forward, with her arms around her knees, while he examines the back of the chest. For the abdominal examination, she lies down and will have the chest covered with the blanket. If the feet are to be examined, the upper clothes are returned to position, and the foot of the bed loosened and the ends folded back singly. Afterwards the nightdress is put on again and the bed remade. The nurse assures herself that the patient does not feel cold.

Rectal Examination

Requirements. Tray with receiver with disposable glove or caped finger stall, and finger stalls.
Receiver with proctoscope.
Lubricant jelly, or soft paraffin.
Plastic sheet and towel.
4 in. (10 cm.) swabs.
Cover.

Rectal examination will reveal if constipation is present, if there is tenderness in the Pouch of Douglas ; whether a growth is present in the rectum, or swellings can be felt in the reproductive organs, while hæmorrhoids can be seen through the proctoscope. It is used instead of vaginal examination in young girls.

Not more than two pillows are used, and the patient lies on her left side with the buttocks right at the edge of the bed and the nightdress rolled up. The spine, hips and knees are flexed in order to relax the abdominal and pelvic muscles and make discomfort minimal. The bedclothes are folded on to the hips and a blanket put over the shoulders.

If a finger stall is used, a large swab is held between the index finger and thumb in order to protect the hand from contamination from the perianal skin. In many cases a digital examination is sufficient, and a proctoscope need not be used. After it has been concluded, the anus should be cleared of lubricant with a swab.

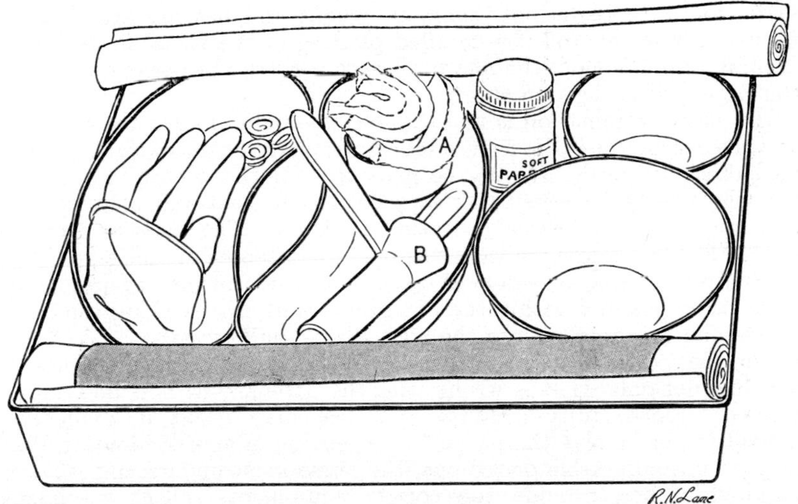

Fig. 22. Tray for rectal examination. Notice especially the 4-in. swabs (A) and the proctoscope (B).

Neurological Examination

Purpose. To investigate the efficiency of the nervous system, sensory, motor and reflex. New growths, infections or degeneration within the cord or brain will affect the peripheral nerves, and so may metabolic states like Vitamin B deficiency or diabetes. Hysterical complaints of paralyses and anæsthesia can be distinguished from organic complaints.

The special senses (sight, hearing, taste and smell) are located to limited areas or organs ; common sensation—sensitivity to touch, pain, heat and cold—is felt all over the body to varying degrees.

Requirements. Ophthalmoscope.
- Small bottles with distinctive smelling liquids, e.g. peppermint, lavender.
- Salt, sugar, vinegar, watch glasses and pipettes or glass rods.
- Tongue cloths.
- Spatula and torch.
- Pins.
- Wisp of wool, or camel-hair brush.
- One test tube of hot and one of cold water in separate stands.
- Tape measure.
- Skin pencil.
- Tendon hammer.
- Receiver.
- Treatment blanket and decency towel.
- Dressing gown and slippers if the patient is required to stand or walk.

Not all these will be needed for all patients ; testing the sensation of taste, for instance, is not common. Sight and hearing are roughly assessed clinically, and if a detailed plotting of the visual fields, or an accurate knowledge of the hearing loss is needed, the patient will visit the appropriate department.

If a total examination is to be made, the night clothes are removed and the decency towel put on, a blanket is put over the patient and the bedclothes stripped. It may be necessary for the doctor to examine the whole body for sensitivity to pain, touch, heat and cold, and to map any areas of loss of sensation he finds. The tape measure is needed for determining muscle wasting or shortening on one side. The ophthalmoscope is an essential part of the neurologist's equipment, since rising pressure within the cranium is transmitted along the optic nerves and causes œdema of the optic disc (*papillœdema*).

The diagnostic tests in which the nurse takes part will assist in deciding not only what is wrong with the patient, but how he is to be treated. Since faulty conduct of a test may result in diagnostic difficulties, or involve the patient in repetition of an examination that may be uncomfortable or tedious, the nurse must understand what is required of her, provide the correct equipment, collect specimens punctually where indicated, and label and dispatch them correctly. The co-operation of the patient is essential in many of them, and is

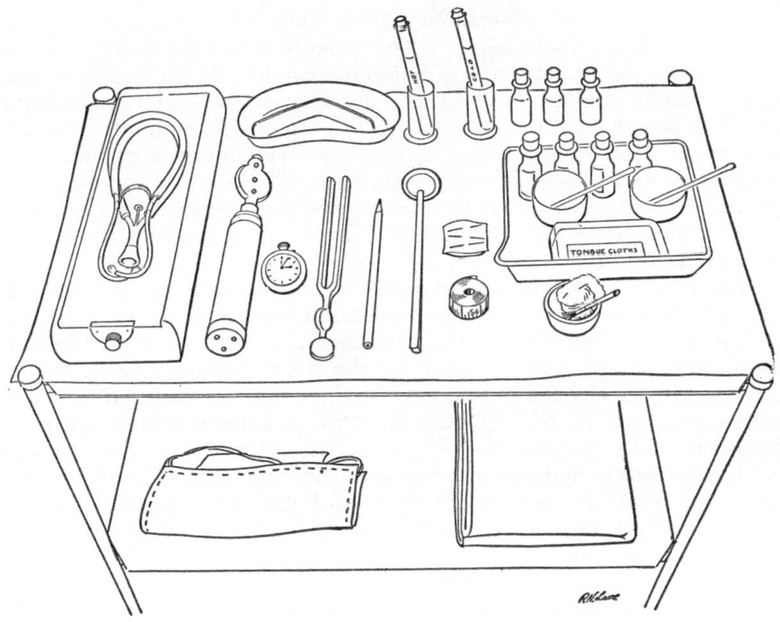

FIG. 23. **Neurological** examination.

gained by explanation in terms that he can understand, and when it is suitable the doctor will tell him of the result.

Erythrocyte Sedimentation Rate

Definition. The rate at which red blood cells sink in citrated blood, measured in millimetres in one hour. The normal rate is less than 10 mm.

Purpose. This rate (E.S.R.) is raised in many infections, and its chief value is to assess the progress of chronic conditions like tuberculosis and rheumatoid arthritis. A series of weekly readings may indicate whether activity of the disease is declining or not. It is not reliable in the presence of anæmia.

Equipment. Sterile 2 ml. syringe and No. 1 needle.
3·8 % sodium citrate solution, sterile.
Dry gallipot.
Westergren tube (or desired pattern) and stand.
Ether and swabs.

Method. 0·4 ml. of sodium citrate is drawn into the syringe, which is then filled with blood from a vein up to 2 ml. The mixture is squirted into the gallipot to mix it, and is sucked up the tube as far as the upper or " 0 " mark. It is stood in its rack and the time noted. Exactly an hour later the width of clear fluid showing at the top of the column is read on the graduated scale to give the result.

Basal Metabolic Rate

Purpose. Basal metabolism is the amount of metabolism going on in a person lying at rest, having fasted overnight. It is affected by the height, weight and sex, and by the activity of the endocrine glands, especially the thyroid and the pituitary. It can be estimated from a knowledge of the oxygen taken in and the carbon dioxide expired, and is expressed as a plus or minus percentage. The commonest cause of a rise in the basal metabolic rate is fever, and the temperature should be normal when the test is conducted. Thyrotoxicosis causes a rise, and myxœdema a fall.

Method. The patient's height and weight are ascertained overnight, and he is told that it is a simple breathing test, causing no more discomfort than having nothing to eat from supper time till after the test. Reassurance is especially needed for the toxic patient. Early in the morning the screens are drawn, the bladder may be emptied, and the patient is asked to rest quietly till the technician comes with his apparatus. An oxygen supply must be available. The patient simply breathes in and out of a bag for a few minutes. The results are calculated from the figures obtained and the data supplied by the nurse. Changes of less than 10% are not considered of much significance. Some physicians now prefer to estimate the level of the protein-bound iodine (for which only a blood sample is required) or to perform a radioactive iodine uptake test to give information on the metabolic rate.

Urine Concentration and Dilution Test

Purpose. To test the ability of the kidney to vary the specific gravity of the urine. This important function enables the body to deal with changes in the fluid intake, with the needs of the skin in changing temperatures, and with other emergencies in the fluid balance. The loss of ability to concentrate the urine indicates a late stage of renal failure, as in chronic nephritis.

Method. Many modifications of this test are in use ; this is a typical one, not too rigorous. Nothing to eat or drink is allowed from 6 p.m. on the evening before the test. At 6 a.m. and 7 a.m. the bladder is emptied. The specific gravity of at least one of these specimens should reach 1·022.

The dilution part of the test follows; it is not ordered for patients who have œdema. 1,000 ml. of water is drunk in the next half hour, and specimens are collected hourly for the next four hours. Normally most of this litre of water will have been excreted during this period, and a specific gravity of 1·003 or less is attained. If there is severe impairment of kidney function, the specific gravity of the urine usually remains fixed at about 1·010.

Urea Concentration

Purpose. The output of urea in the urine should rise if the amount of urea in the blood increases, and this test investigates the ability of the kidney to do this.

Method. Nothing is given after 9 p.m. until the test is complete on the following morning. At 6 a.m. the bladder is emptied, and 15 G. of urea is given dissolved in 100 ml. of water. At 7, 8 and 9 a.m. specimens 1, 2 and 3 are collected and sent to the laboratory. The amount of urea should exceed 2% in two of these if urea concentration is to be considered satisfactory.

Urea Clearance

Purpose. This is a test of glomerular function, and depends on the fact that urea is cleared from the blood into the urine at a steady rate, so that if the blood urea is known, and also the amount of urea per hour excreted into the urine, a satisfactory estimate of the filtration power of the kidneys can be made.

Method. No coffee or tea (which are diuretics) should be given on the morning of the test. At 10 a.m. the bladder is emptied and the specimen discarded. At 11 a.m. specimen 1 is collected, and at noon specimen 2. The blood urea is estimated at 11 a.m. Specimens 1 and 2 are sent for examination, and the whole amount passed must be included.

For an accurate result, specimens must be obtained with strict punctuality. If there is any delay (e.g. if the patient is unable to micturate) the exact time when the urine was passed should be put on the label.

Creatinine Clearance

Purpose. This is another and more reliable test of glomerular function.

Method. No preparation is required. A 24-hour specimen of urine is collected, and a sample of this and a note of the total volume is sent to the laboratory. 10 ml. of blood are collected on the same day. Sometimes the pathologist may ask for two 24-hour specimens: this is because collection for 24 hours is subject to fallacy because of loss of a specimen, especially if the patient is spending time out of the ward in connection with other examinations.

Renal Biopsy

Microscopic examination of small portions of kidney tissue obtained by needle biopsy may be a great help in diagnosis. An intravenous pyelogram is performed beforehand, unless the biopsy is to be done under X-ray control, to establish the position of the kidneys. The patient's blood group is ascertained, and a bottle of blood cross-matched and kept ready for emergency use. The prothrombin time and platelet count must be estimated, because abnormal findings indicate a risk of undue bleeding. If a local anæsthetic is used, adequate sedation must be given beforehand. The following equipment is needed.

2 gallipots.
Gauze and wool swabs.
2 pairs of dressing forceps.
French's or handling forceps.
Paper towels.
5 ml. syringe.

Needles size 1 and 20.
Vim-Silverman or Menghini biopsy needle.
Exploring needle (e.g. lumbar puncture needle).
Masks, gowns, gloves.
Cleaning lotion (e.g. chlorhexidine 1 in 200 in spirit).
(All the above are sterile)
Adhesives.
Preservative for biopsy specimen.

The patient lies face downwards on a firm surface for the puncture. The right kidney is a little lower than the left, and so easier to reach but the liver is close by, and may be punctured in error. The skin is cleaned and anæsthetized, and then the exploring needle is passed to find the depth at which the kidney lies; when the needle is in the right place it will move with each breath. It is then withdrawn, and the biopsy needle is passed along the same track. Cores of renal tissue are obtained and put into the preservative, and an adhesive dressing is applied.

Bleeding down the ureter is common, and brisk bleeding is often seen. The patient is kept at rest in bed, and encouraged to drink freely to keep the urine diluted. If bleeding is free, clotting will occur, and the patient will suffer from colic as the clots pass down the ureter and an analgesic must be given. The pulse and blood pressure must be taken hourly, and each urine specimen is saved separately to see if bleeding is getting less. Profuse hæmaturia or colic, falling blood pressure, rising pulse rate or sweating must be reported at once. Bleeding usually ceases spontaneously, and surgery is rarely necessary.

Glucose Tolerance Test

Purpose. To investigate the ability to metabolize sugar. Normally the fasting blood sugar, estimated before breakfast, is about 80 mg. per cent, and if sugar is taken there is a steep rise, followed by a gradual fall to normal in two hours as insulin action causes its removal to the liver. If the blood sugar rises above 180 mg. per cent, sugar will appear in the urine. In diabetes mellitus, the fasting blood sugar is often high, and taking sugar causes a rise without the steady return to normal. This test is used to distinguish diabetes from other causes of glycosuria.

Method. If the patient is ambulant, it may be more convenient for him to go to the laboratory. He fasts overnight, and at 9 a.m. a specimen of blood for fasting blood sugar is taken, and the bladder is emptied. He then drinks 50 G. of glucose in a glass of water flavoured with lemon juice. The blood sugar is estimated after ½ hour, 1 hour, 1½ hours and 2 hours, and specimens of urine are collected at 10 a.m., 11 a m. and noon and sent for examination. It is unusual for the blood sugar to exceed the renal threshold level of 180 mg. per cent.

Tuberculin Skin Tests

People who have had an overt or sub-clinical infection with the tubercle bacillus become sensitized to tuberculin, and will respond with a reaction if it is injected into or applied to the skin. A negative reaction indicates that the subject has never been exposed to such infection and is therefore susceptible. Most adults in urban communities show a positive reaction, but with the decline in tuberculosis now taking place, there are increasing numbers who are negative. A proportion of students taking up nursing or medicine will be negative reactors, and in view of their occupational risk it is common practice to immunize them with B.C.G. (Bacille Calmette-Guérin), a weak strain of the tubercle bacillus.

Mantoux Test. This is the commonest and most reliable skin test. The doctor will bring his own sterile glass syringes, tuberculin, and normal saline. He should be supplied with swabs and ether. He injects 0·2 ml. of tuberculin, 1 in 1,000, intradermally into the skin of the forearm, and a corresponding amount of control solution into the other. A positive reaction is the development of a red reaction with a central zone of œdema at least 1·5 cm. across on the tuberculin side.

Patch Test. A piece of strapping containing tuberculin is applied to the back, usually of a baby, and the result read after forty-eight hours. It is not very reliable.

Fractional Test Meals

Purpose. To investigate the quality of the gastric juice, and usually to assess the response of the stomach to food intake. The principle is to pass a Ryle's tube into the stomach of a fasting patient, and then to give some kind of "meal" and by serial withdrawals discover its effect on gastric secretion. The meal can consist of a pint of thin strained cereal, or 50 ml. of 7% alcohol. Some procedures still called "meals" are also used in which serial samples are collected after the injection of insulin, or of histamine, which usually provokes secretion of acid juice. Difficulty is sometimes experienced in collecting sufficient juice in these circumstances.

The information that may be gained is :

1. The amount of *resting juice*, i.e. the secretion in the stomach after a twelve-hour fast. It may be excessive in pyloric stenosis.

2. The amount of free and total hydrochloric acid in the stomach. Excessive acid (*hyperchlorhydria*) is characteristic of duodenal ulcer. Absence of acid (*achlorhydria*) is found in pernicious and some iron-deficiency anæmias, and usually in cancer of the stomach.

3. The response of the stomach to food. Normally there is a rise in the acid secretion, followed by a steady return to normal. In duodenal ulcer there is a steep rise and excessive free HCl is present throughout the test.

4. The response of the stomach to subcutaneous injection of histamine, if no acid is found at first. A histamine-fast achlorhydria is found in pernicious anæmia. Not all physicians like histamine.

5. The speed with which the stomach empties ; the hyperchlorhydria of peptic ulcer is usually associated with quick emptying.

6. The amount of *residual fluid*, i.e. the amount left after two hours. In pyloric stenosis some of the meal may still be left in the stomach.

7. The presence of excessive mucus or blood, as in gastric ulcer or cancer of the stomach.

Preparation of the Patient. The patient is told of the test, and of the valuable information to be gained, to secure his co-operation. He must fast overnight.

Equipment. Rack of six test tubes. Pathologist's request card.
Instrument dish with Ryle's tube ; 50 ml. syringe.
Two gallipots, one with swabs.
Measure for resting juice.
Alcohol, 50 ml. of 7%.
Liquid paraffin.
Litmus paper, blue and red.
Plastic cape and towel.
Receiver.
Vomit bowl.
Mouth wash.
Strapping and spigot.

Sometimes needed. Cup and saucer on tray for gruel.
Histamine 0·5 mg. in syringe if ordered.

Method. The Ryle's tube should be sterilized, or a disposable one. Some occupation, such as a book, should be provided for the patient.

The trolley is brought to the right side of the bed, and the patient sat up comfortably supported with pillows. The cape is adjusted round the shoulders, and the vomit bowl may be at hand, but is not given undue prominence. The end of the Ryle's tube is dipped in liquid paraffin, and it is now usual to pass it through the nose. Since the test is only performed on active patients, a preliminary cleansing of the nostril is not normally needed. The patient is asked to breathe steadily and regularly through the mouth, and to swallow when asked. The end of the tube is passed about 2 cm. upwards, then horizontally backwards along the floor of the nose. It will presently be felt to be passing into the pharynx, and the patient should then be asked to swallow, and usually the end enters the post-cricoid space and the œsophagus without incident.

If the septum is very crooked it will be necessary to pass the tube through the mouth. This method requires a little more skill from the nurse, is morely likely to cause nausea, but avoids the initial discomfort to the sensitive nasal mucosa. The patient is asked to swallow when told, and if he feels inclined to retch, to breathe steadily and deeply till the feeling passes, since retching involves holding the breath.

The tube is marked with one ring at 38 cm., the average distance to the cardiac orifice of the stomach ; two at 54 cm. for the pyloric sphincter, and three at 72 cm., the distance to the entry of the bile duct. It should be passed as far as the double ring, and then is strapped to the cheek firmly. The syringe is attached to the end and the piston withdrawn. Gastric juice should enter the barrel, and all that can be obtained should be aspirated and put in the jar, labelled "Resting juice." The feed is now given ; if alcohol is used it can be put into the tube by syringe. while gruel should be brought in a cup and saucer on a tray like any other feed, and drunk. The open end of the tube is closed with a spigot, and the patient settled comfortably with a book or some occupation until it is time to take the next specimen. The curtains may be drawn back if he prefers it.

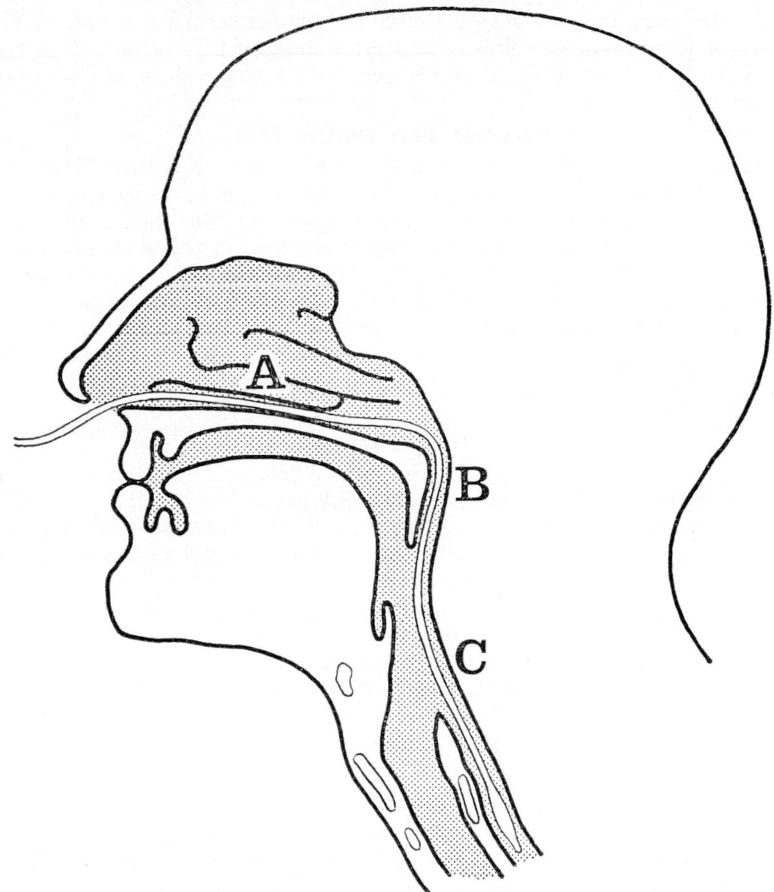

Fig. 24. Passing a Ryle's Tube. Care must be taken when the tube reaches (A) less the mucosa be injured, at (B), lest the end come forward into the mouth (C) or into the larynx.

The interval at which specimens are taken depends somewhat on local custom. Six specimens, withdrawn at twenty-minute intervals, is a usual number, and not more than 5 ml. should be taken at each aspiration, or the supply will be exhausted before the required number has been obtained. Each is put into a test tube, labelled with the time, and tested with litmus paper for acidity. Ifnone is found in the first two specimens, the nurse may be asked to give histamine 0·5 mg. by hypodermic injection. This sometimes causes uncomfortable flushing and headache, and if this is severe it may have to be relieved by giving one of the anti-histamine drugs.

When all the specimens have been obtained, the strapping is detached, and the tube pinched and withdrawn gently but briskly. The patient will welcome a mouth wash, and a late breakfast.

In the augmented histamine test, an antihistamine is given before the test is performed. This blocks all actions of histamine except the acid-secreting one, and permits a very much larger dose of histamine to be given.

Diagnex Blue Gastric Test

This is a tubeless form of test meal. The " meal " consists of Diagnex Blue, which is an ion-exchange resin. When it is immersed in dilute hydrochloric acid (as in normal gastric juice), the blue part of the resin is exchanged with the acid ions, and so set free in the stomach. The released dye is absorbed into the bloodstream, and eventually is excreted into the urine by the kidneys. Blue urine indicates that acid is present in the stomach, and the strength of the colour shows the degree of acidity. If the urine shows no colour change, no ion exchange has taken place in the stomach, which means that no free acid was present (achlorhydria).

Jejunal Biopsy

In order to take a biopsy of the jejunal mucous membrane (e.g. in malabsorption states), the patient swallows a tube with a Crosby capsule at the end. Applying suction to the tube draws a little mucous membrane into the capsule, and this is severed. Nothing is taken by mouth from 10 p.m. the previous evening, and an hour before the test sedation is given (e.g. metoclopramide and diazepam 10 mg. of each intramuscularly). The tube is passed, and the patient taken to the X-ray department to ensure by screening that the capsule is in the jejunum. Once the biopsy is taken and the tube removed, the patient may eat and drink.

SCHILLING TEST

This test is used to distinguish between types of anæmia, especially when pernicious anæmia is suspected, to find out if vitamin B_{12} (cyanocobalamine) is being absorbed, a measured dose of the vitamin labelled with radioactive cobalt (Co^{58}) is given to the patient. This substance can be traced, and its fate ascertained; the test is as follows:

1. The patient can have a cup of tea at 6 a.m., but no breakfast.
2. At 10 a.m. the isotope is given by mouth, and collection of all urine passed in the next 24 hours begins. This collection must be complete, or misleading results will be given.
3. At noon, an intramuscular injection of 1,000 microgrammes of vitamin B_{12} is given, which will flush the isotope from the liver, if it has been absorbed.

Normally more than 7% of it is excreted in the urine, within 24 hours. Less than 3% suggests pernicious anæmia. In cases of doubt, a similar test, with the addition of intrinsic factor, can be used a week later to confirm results.

Marrow Puncture

Purpose. To obtain a specimen of red bone marrow, in which the red cells and 75% of the white cells are made. Examination of this marrow helps in the diagnosis of obscure blood conditions, especially the aplastic anæmias in which erythrocyte formation is deficient. The bones usually selected in adults are the sternum (most frequently), the iliac crest or the body of a lumbar vertebra. The tibial crest may be used in babies.

Preparation. If the sternum is to be used in a man, the area should first be shaved. This procedure is not a pleasant one ; the puncture is made with some pressure, and the aspiration also produces a distressing sensation. Children will have some premedication (such as pethidine), and so will nervous adults, though the doctor may feel it is easier to gain the confidence and co-operation of an alert patient. Although the sternum is the easiest bone to puncture successfully, the iliac crest is perhaps better for an apprehensive patient, being less exposed to his view. Sterile technique is most important, since the penalties of bone infection are heavy, and the puncture needle and aspirating syringe must be autoclaved.

Equipment. Instrument tray with :

All sterile:
- 2 pairs of dissecting forceps.
- 3 gallipots.
- 2 ml. syringe ; No. 18 and No. 14 needles.
- Narrow-bladed sharp scalpel.
- Salah (or similar) marrow puncture needle and aspirating syringe.
- Towels and swabs.
- Small dressing.

Platinum loop, spirit lamp, watch glass, slides.
Iodine, ether, collodion and procaine 2%.
Receiver for swabs.
Receiver for instruments.
Strapping.

Method. The patient should lie flat for sternal puncture, with the chest exposed, and is encouraged to co-operate. The doctor may wear a mask, and should scrub his hands and dry them with a sterile towel. The site is cleaned, an injection of local anæsthetic made, and the sterile towels laid around. A small nick is made in the skin with a scalpel, so that skin resistance shall not hold up the passage of the needle. The needle possesses a stop to prevent too deep penetration, and this is adjusted according to the amount of tissue lying over the bone. The needle is pressed vertically into the sternum, the trocar taken out, and the syringe attached and the marrow withdrawn. The needle is taken out and the puncture covered with a small sterile dressing moistened with collodion and a dry swab and strapping put on top. Smears are made at once by the doctor from the marrow.

Patients often feel shaky and distressed afterwards, and should be covered up and given appropriate comfort, like a hot drink. The dressing is inspected occasionally to see that there is no leakage, and should not be removed or allowed to become wet for two days. Any rise of temperature or unusual symptoms following marrow puncture must be reported at once.

LIVER TESTS

Information about the efficiency of liver function can be gained from examination of the urine, the stools, the blood, or of a biopsy specimen. The *urine* may contain bile; the *stools* may show undigested fat, or absence of the bile pigments that are normally excreted by the colon. The physician may examine the *blood* to find if the levels of substances made by the liver are normal (e.g. serum albumin and prothrombin), or if substances which the liver excretes or alters have undergone any changes (e.g. serum bilirubin; blood urea).

Examination of liver tissue obtained by puncture is an important aid to diagnosis of hepatic disease. Specimens are secured by passing a needle through the side of the chest into the liver. The Vim-Silverman instrument is a trocar and cannula ; after introduction the trocar is removed and a split needle pushed through the cannula to cut out a minute slice of liver. The cannula is advanced to the same depth as the needle, and both are withdrawn together. Aspiration of specimens through a hollow needle is more liable to cause bleeding.

Bleeding is the main risk, but peritonitis from rupture of a bile duct, and pneumothorax from inadvertently piercing the lung are possible. Vitamin K is given to jaundiced patients by intramuscular injection. A bottle of blood is cross-matched ready for an emergency, and the prothrombin, clotting and bleeding times are estimated.

After the biopsy, pressure should be made over the site for 15 minutes. The pulse and respiration rate should be taken every quarter of an hour, and the blood pressure hourly for four hours. Intelligent observation should be kept up for 24 hours ; pallor, sweating, restlessness, dyspnœa, a rising pulse rate, abdominal pain or vomiting should be quickly reported.

ENDOSCOPY

Endoscopy is the examination of a cavity or organ by means of a lighted instrument passed into it. Fragments of tissue may be removed with special forceps to aid diagnosis. Bronchoscopy (inspection of the bronchi), thoracoscopy (inspection of the pleural cavity) and cystoscopy (examination of the urinary bladder) are described in the chapters on thoracic and urological nursing.

All the instruments used (except some proctoscopes) carry an electric light. The small bulbs used fuse readily, and must be handled with care. They should be tested before use. The terminals of the flex must be connected to the battery with the switch in the " off " position, and it is turned on steadily until illumination is sufficient.

Proctoscopy

Proctoscopy is inspection of the rectum, and it may form part of a rectal examination or may be the prelude to the injection of hæmorrhoids. The rectum should be empty.

Requirements. Proctoscope in receiver.
7 in. forceps and small swabs.
Battery and flex.
Lubricant.
4 in. swabs.
Waterproof and paper towel.
Treatment blanket.

The patient lies on the mackintosh and towel, with the buttocks at the edge of the bed. The proctoscope is lubricated and introduced through the anal sphincter, while the nurse connects the light to the battery and turns it on. The obturator is removed, and the light put in place. When the procedure is over and the proctoscope is taken out, the anal area should be thoroughly cleansed of lubricant. The proctoscope is scrubbed with soap and water and boiled for three minutes before being put away.

Sigmoidoscopy

The sigmoidoscope is a longer, narrower instrument which can be passed into the sigmoid colon, and although it is a common investigation, and can be undertaken without an anæsthetic except in very apprehensive patients, it is not without danger. It is possible to perforate the colon, especially if it is diseased.

Preparation for sigmoidoscopy varies considerably from one surgeon to another. The worst fault that can be made is to leave fluid in the sigmoid colon, so that it runs down the instrument to the eye-piece and obscures the view. An enema or washout should not be given on the day of examination, and an aperient should not be given less than thirty-six hours before. Some surgeons use no preparation; some use a "Dulcolax" suppository.

Requirements. Sigmoidoscope, complete, and battery.
Long forceps.
Lubricant.
Swabs.
Tall jar, or trough to receive instrument after use.

Sigmoidoscopy may be performed on a patient in the left lateral position, and the knee-chest is also a useful one. The sigmoidoscope is lubricated and introduced about 4 or 5 cm. through the anal canal. The obturator is then withdrawn, the light and the eye-piece are attached. The instrument is then advanced under direct vision, using the bellows to distend the bowel. In favourable conditions the whole sigmoid colon can be inspected. A biopsy may be taken with long forceps if appearances suggest a growth.

Gastroscopy

The interior of the stomach may be inspected with a gastroscope in the course of investigation of peptic ulcer, pernicious anæmia, and especially to aid in the differentiation of cancer of the stomach from simple ulcer. The gastroscope has a light-carrying tip which is screwed into a flexible metal middle portion in which are the lenses. This section is enclosed in a rubber sheath. The upper portion carries the handle, the eye-piece and a bellows for inflating the stomach. It is best performed with local anæsthesia. When cocaine was the anæsthetic used, severe reactions were sometimes met, and a sensitivity test to cocaine was necessary beforehand. With modern synthetic preparations, reactions are rare and are said to be unknown if a barbiturate is given the night before.

Some doctors like the stomach emptied by Ryle's tube beforehand, while if there is pyloric stenosis with retention of gastric contents, a

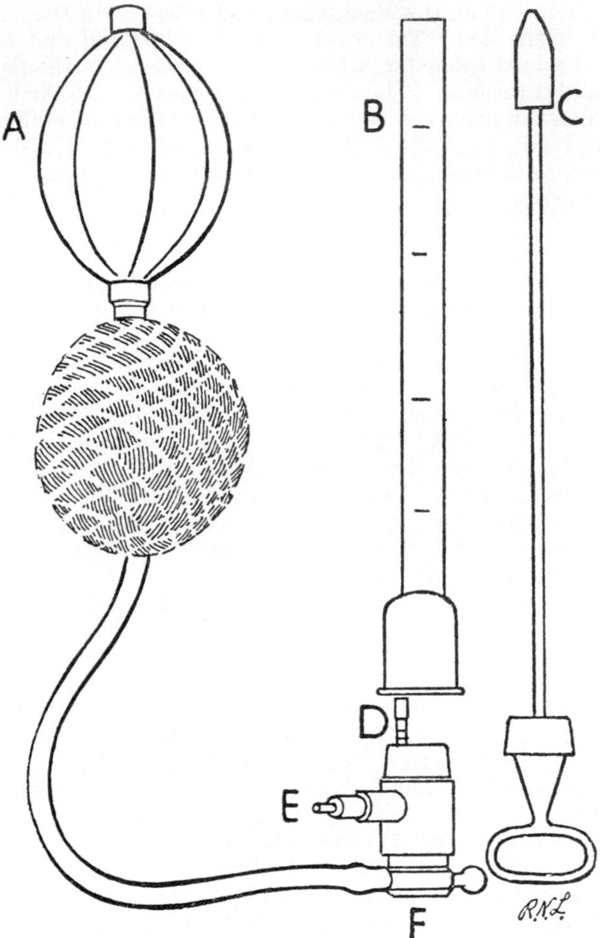

FIG. 25. Sigmoidoscope.

A. Bellows.
B. Sheath.
C. Obturator, used in the sheath during insertion.
D. Light carrier being inserted in sheath.
E. Point for battery connection.
F. Glass eye-piece.

stomach washout will be requested. Atropine is frequently ordered to diminish the secretions and morphine or a barbiturate may be added as premedication.

The procedure is conducted in the theatre and 2 ml. of amethocaine or lignocaine is used as local anæsthetic. It is dripped on to the lips and then into the mouth from a hypodermic syringe, and the patient is asked to move it around the mouth and then swallow it.

No food or drink should be given for three hours afterwards when

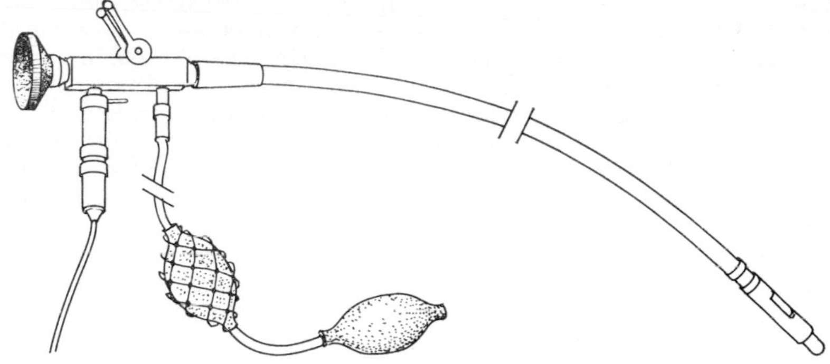

Fig. 26. Gastroscope. Hermon Taylor pattern.

sensation will have returned to the mouth and pharynx, and swallowing can be undertaken without risk of fluid entering the airway. A complication that is rare but not unknown is perforation of the œsophagus, which will lead to mediastinitis. If damage is known or feared to have occurred, feeding should be undertaken with a sterile indwelling œsophageal catheter. The temperature should be taken four-hourly for twenty-four hours after gastroscopy, and aspirin mucilage is usually ordered if the throat is sore.

Œsophagoscopy

It might be thought this examination was a less severe one than gastroscopy, since the instrument is not so long and the route is the same, but the œsophagoscope is a rigid, not a flexible tube, and œsophagoscopy is usually undertaken under a general anæsthetic. The preparation is the usual one for such an anæsthetic, and if there is difficulty in swallowing, as is found with a growth, the doctor may ask the nurse to pass a Ryle's tube down to the obstruction and aspirate any secretions or food débris that might otherwise be inhaled when anæsthesia was induced.

The patient lies on his back, and the anæsthetic is an endotracheal one. When relaxation is complete, the head and neck are extended over the end of the table in order to straighten the œsophagus, and a theatre nurse will support the head. The purpose is to examine the œsophagus ; perhaps to take a biopsy ; or to remove foreign bodies. A variety of foreign bodies may be swallowed and become impacted in the œsophagus, one of the commoner in adults being a dental plate. This often has to be broken up before it can be extracted.

After œsophagoscopy no food or drink should be given for three hours, and aspirin mucilage is usually needed for the sore throat.

PREPARATION FOR X-RAYS

X-rays will darken a photographic film on which they fall, and if the body is interposed, the X-rays are held back in varying degrees, so that lighter areas appear on the film. Bone is the most radio-opaque substance in the body, and shows up lightest, but still allows some rays to pass so that the pattern of cancellous bone may be seen. Muscle and solid tissue is fairly readily penetrated, allowing the film behind it to darken, while gas and air are the most transparent of all, and a film behind a hollow gas-filled organ darkens considerably. If a film of the abdomen is taken, the vertebral column and pelvis will appear nearly clear, with darker areas of muscle around, while if the colon is distended with flatus, its pattern will stand out darker still, and may considerably obstruct the view of the structures behind it.

Patients for X-rays sometimes need careful preparation, therefore, if a successful picture is to be obtained. A poor result may mean that the X-ray has to be repeated, involving hardship to a patient who may have gone without food in readiness for it, interference with the programme of the department and expenditure of public money.

X-ray departments have an ever-increasing load of work. They serve not only in-patients, but out-patients seen by appointment, and casualty work of which the amount cannot be foreseen. An X-ray involves not only the taking of a picture, but developing, fixing, washing and drying it ; presenting it to the radiologist for a report ; typing his findings, and delivering it to the ward or filing it. The nurse should not only prepare her patients carefully, but should take great care of films delivered to the ward, and should return them to the department promptly, protecting them from damage by contact or dust. When asking for the previous X-rays of a newly admitted patient, she should supply the Christian names as well as the surname, and diagnosis.

Increase in our knowledge of radio-activity shows that X-rays are not entirely devoid of risk ; for instance, repeated X-rays of the abdomen in pregnancy is associated with an increased liability for the baby of leukæmia in childhood. For all these reasons a successful picture the first time is highly desirable.

Plain and Contrast X-rays

Although gas in the colon may be a handicap to the radiologist, it may be helpful elsewhere in showing the shape of a cavity ; for instance, if it is injected into the ventricles of the brain, these will show as dark areas in the X-ray. Hollow structures may also be filled with substances opaque to X-rays, e.g. barium sulphate, and the stomach and colon may be visualized in this way. Iodine is radio-opaque, and preparations of it can be used to show up the outlines of the bronchi, or by different techniques the pelvis or the kidney or the gall-bladder. An X-ray may, therefore, be a plain one or may include the use of one of these contrast media.

The structures of the body can be seen on an X-ray screen in a darkened room. The bones are readily visible, as everyone knows who has seen the machines operating in shoe shops. The physician sometimes uses the screen in the regular examination of tuberculous patients, but its chief use is in the course of the contrast X-rays. For instance, during the course of a barium X-ray of the stomach, the radiologist may watch the action of the stomach on the screen, direct the radiographer to take the pictures at the best times, and notice if any unusual appearances are constant, or only the result of peristalsis.

Going to the Department

The garment worn while the trunk is being X-rayed must be of cotton, fastened with tapes—no rayon, strapping, buttons or mackintosh must be used. Dressing gown and slippers are worn, and in winter socks and enough blankets are added. The notes and previous X-rays are sent, and if serial X-rays are being taken a newspaper or book is an advantage.

Preparation

For *bones* of the limbs, *skull, chest.* No preparation is needed.

Abdomen, lumbar spine or *pelvis.* Bismuth medicines must be omitted for three days before examination. Intestinal flatulence must be prevented by such measures as an aperient twenty-four hours beforehand, restriction of fluids on the day of the X-ray, and encouraging the patient to walk about. Activity is most important. If the patient is confined to bed, charcoal biscuits may be a help.

Alimentary Tract

The intestinal canal is investigated by means of barium, which is not only radio-opaque, but non-toxic and not absorbed. The œsophagus is seen by means of a *barium swallow*, the stomach and small intestine by *barium meal*, and *follow-through*, the colon and rectum by a *barium enema.* Medicines, e.g. stomach mixtures, must be omitted before all these X-rays.

Barium Swallow. Omit the meal before.

Barium meal for stomach and duodenum. Medicines are omitted, and an aperient given twenty-four hours before. Nothing is given by mouth for six hours before.

Barium follow-through for small intestine and appendix. If the stomach is not to be X-rayed the barium may be given in the ward. The Department will give instructions as to the times of visits, and when meals may be taken.

Barium Enema. An aperient is given twenty-four to thirty-six hours before, unless diarrhœa is present. All medicines are omitted. A 2-pint enema or " Dulcolax " suppository is given not less than four hours before X-ray. The patient lies on the table in the department in a darkened room, and 2 pints or more of barium suspension are run into the colon, and will pass round as far as the ileo-cæcal valve. New growths, diverticulitis and organic changes due to ulcerative colitis are important among the conditions that may be seen.

Cholecystography

Certain iodine compounds are absorbed from the intestine, pass into the liver, and are passed back into the intestine with the bile. Since bile is concentrated and stored in the gall-bladder, a normal gall-bladder will also concentrate and store the dye, and will expel its contents readily when a meal containing fat enters the duodenum. The substance used is telepaque, and it can be given in tablet or granule form. The patient's weight must be known to calculate the dose.

A dye examination is normally preceded by a plain X-ray, which may show opaque gall-stones and render further X-rays unnecessary. Low residue meals are taken on the day before the X-ray, the last at 7 p.m. At 8 p.m. the tablets or granules are given with water, and nothing more is taken except sips of water until the investigation is over. The first X-rays should show the dye well concentrated in the gall bladder, which should empty after a fatty meal. If good concentration is not obtained, Biligrafin can be given intravenously not less than two days later and may enable a good view to be obtained. Stones not opaque to X-rays may be seen in outline, or in cases of chronic cholecystitis the gall-bladder may not be functioning at all. Since these patients are prone to flatulent dyspepsia, every effort must be made to see that there is no gas in the colon.

A *cholangiogram* is a picture of the bile ducts, and may be made at operation after injection into the common bile-duct, or into a T-tube if one has been inserted.

Pyelography

A number of commercial forms of iodized poppy-seed oil are made which if injected intravenously are excreted by the kidney, and examination at the appropriate times will show if the kidney is functioning, an outline of the pelvis and the ureter, and finally of the bladder when the dye has reached it. It is a test of function, and will also reveal anatomical peculiarities such as double ureter, fused kidneys or hydronephrosis (enlargement of the pelvis and calyces).

Medicines are omitted, except for an aperient thirty-six hours before. The diet should be low residue on the day before, and no fluids should be given for six hours before the appointment. Measures to dispel flatus are important, and the bladder should be empty before going to the department. The injection is made by the radiologist, and pictures are taken at intervals. Apart from the conditions mentioned above, stones in the pelvis, the ureter, or the bladder may be shown. A *cystogram* or X-ray of the bladder is obtained by injecting the dye through a urethral catheter.

If the kidney is not functioning, investigation will have to be undertaken by *retrograde pyelography*. The preparation is as for the intravenous kind, with the additional measures needed for cystoscopy (p. 351). An anæsthetic is used for nervous patients, but it is an advantage to have a conscious patient who can co-operate, and sometimes an injection of morphine is better than a general anæsthetic. A catheterizing cystoscope is passed, and a ureteric catheter passed into one or both ureters. Sodium iodide is injected along the catheter 10 ml. at a time until the patient can feel discomfort in the loin as the kidney pelvis is stretched. Not more than 20 ml. is normally used if the patient is unconscious. Sometimes the patient returns with the ureteric catheters in place in order that a specimen of urine may be secured from each kidney. It is usual, for instance, in renal tuberculosis, and it is important to see that post-anæsthetic restlessness does not disturb the catheters.

Some discomfort or pain in the loins is usual after retrograde pyelography, and analgesis will be needed. The temperature is taken four-hourly in case the instrumentation has aroused latent infection in a diseased kidney.

Bronchography

A bronchogram shows the bronchial tree outlined by iodine preparations. The introduction of the oil into the airway is not pleasant, and children will need a general anæsthetic, but for adults a local one is adequate. Iodine sensitivity was sometimes troublesome in connection with bronchography, but is very rare with modern preparations.

This X-ray is used for patients with new growths of the lung and with bronchiectasis. The bronchial tree should be as free as possible from secretion beforehand, and those with bronchiectasis should be treated by postural drainage and clapping of the chest. The patient sucks an anæsthetic lozenge before going to the department. The oil is introduced into the airway, usually through a catheter passed by the mouth.

Following the introduction of the oil, the patient is moved into positions that will allow all parts of the bronchi to fill before the X-ray is taken. On return to the ward the patient is encouraged by postural drainage to cough up the oil, and no food or drink is given until the effects of the local anæsthetic have worn off.

Cardiac Catheterization

A fine plastic catheter introduced into the heart enables the physician to obtain samples of blood from different parts of the heart and great vessels, and to measure pressure. Children usually need a general anaesthetic to prevent restlessness during the long examination, but adults only require a sedative. Antibiotic cover is sometimes necessary. Full aseptic precautions are taken during the introduction of the catheter.

The right heart can be reached by inserting the catheter into an arm vein, whence it can usually be manœuvred without difficulty into the superior vena cava, the right atrium and the right ventricle, and thence into the pulmonary artery. The progress of the catheter is checked on a screen.

Many of the more common conditions affect the left side of the heart and the aorta, and examination of this side is more difficult. The catheter can be introduced into the femoral artery by puncturing this vessel in the groin with a large bore needle, threading a guide wire through this into the artery, and passing the catheter over it. The catheter is then guided up the aorta, valve into the left atrium and the left ventricle. After the examination, the catheter is withdrawn, and firm pressure applied over the puncture site for ten minutes. An alternative method is to pass a long needle up the catheter when it is lying in the right atrium, puncture the septum, and pass the catheter over the needle into the left atrium.

Complications are not common after right heart examination, but catheterization of the left heart is more dangerous. The benefit to the patient of accurate assessment of his condition must be considered by the physician as greater than the risk involved. Disorders of cardiac rhythm, especially ventricular fibrillation or cardiac arrest, must be continually watched for, and the means available to deal with them. When the patient returns to the ward, the pulse rate and rhythm are observed every half hour, and the temperature is taken four hourly. The puncture site should be inspected regularly for signs of hæmatoma formation.

Among the facts that can be learned from cardiac catheterization are the presence, site and size of septal defects; lesions of the heart valves; the cardiac output; and the pulmonary resistance. In addition, angiocardiography may be performed by injecting hypaque 85% through the catheter and taking films.

Angiography

The blood-vessels may be visualized by the injection into them of a suitable medium, and efficient radiographic routine is needed to secure the X-rays with the necessary speed. A carotid angiogram may be of great help to the neurosurgeon in making a diagnosis of intracranial conditions.

Aortography is increasingly used as surgery of the blood-vessels advances. Blocks of the aorta or its main branches to the legs may be relieved by grafts, and an accurate estimate of the position and extent of the block and the state of the collateral circulation is most helpful. A catheter is introduced into the aorta by puncturing the femoral artery, as described in the foregoing paragraph, and advancing the catheter to the desired level before injecting the dye.

Salpingography

The Fallopian tubes must be patent if pregnancy is to occur, and a common investigation in cases of infertility is the insufflation of carbon dioxide into the uterus to determine whether the gas will escape along the tubes into the peritoneal cavity. If the tubes are not patent, the position of the block may be found by injecting iodized oil through a syringe and cannula through the cervix. The oil passes through the body of the uterus into the tubes as far as the obstruction, and an X-ray is taken. It may enable the surgeon to decide if there is any possibility of a surgical relief of the condition. A block occurring at the fimbrial end of the tube is the most hopeful in this respect.

Myelography

Introduction of iodized oil into the spinal canal permits a myelogram to be made that may show tumours or lesions connected with the spinal cord. The injection is made after lumbar puncture (p. 144) and a 5-ml. syringe may be autoclaved along with the lumbar puncture needles for introducing the oil. The injection is made in the ward and the patient is later taken to the department.

Ventriculography

The contrast medium used in a ventriculogram is oxygen. It is introduced through burr-holes in the skull into the lateral ventricles. It is an examination that is sometimes severe in its effects, and a consent form should be signed by the patient, and his relatives should understand that further treatment may be needed afterwards.

The head must be shaved, and although a local anæsthetic is used, food must be withheld beforehand, as tapping the ventricle may induce vomiting. Disturbances of consciousness may follow ventriculography, and it is usually done in the morning, so that if craniotomy is necessary because of deterioration in the patient's condition, it can be undertaken the same day. On return from the X-ray theatre, the patient should be nursed with the head of the bed on blocks, and regular observations made of the pulse and respiration and of the state of consciousness.

An *air encephalogram* is made by introducing oxygen after withdrawing 100 ml. of cerebro-spinal fluid by lumbar or cisternal puncture.

CHAPTER 10

COLLECTION OF SPECIMENS

Examination by the pathologist of specimens submitted to him will often provide the diagnosis, and in many cases decide the treatment of the patient concerned. It is, therefore, of the greatest importance that material sent to the laboratory is of the kind wanted, in suitable quantity, and as fresh as possible. The doctor will request the examination he wants and sometimes collects the specimen ; the nurse's duties include providing his equipment, or the collection of material, and the labelling and despatch of the specimen to the laboratory. The containers used should be suitable for the purpose, firmly closed, and labelled clearly with the name of the ward and patient ; the nature of the material ; the examination requested, and the date. Contamination of the outside of the container must be avoided in the interests of those who have to handle it. Specimens must be sent as soon as possible after collection, with the signed request card.

SPECIMENS OF URINE

Ward Specimen. The urine is passed into a clean, dry receptacle and a specimen glass filled from it. The bottom of this glass is conical so that small amounts of sediment are easily seen. It is covered with a glass slide (or it will become ammoniacal with standing) and the bed number is attached. Self-adhesive labels of the type used in shops as price tickets are inexpensive, do not need moistening, and can be peeled off after use without leaving a mark.

Clean Specimen. Urine is passed into a sterile container, after cleansing the urethral meatus. Examinations of the centrifuged deposit and for bacteria may be made on a clean specimen. Though used mainly for men useful information can be gained from women.

Catheter Specimen. These are used much less often than clean specimens, because of the risk of setting up urinary infection.

Twenty-four-hourly Specimen. A Winchester is labelled with the name of the ward and patient, and the date and times of collection. Nursing staff and the patient must be told that all urine is being collected. The patient empties the bladder early in the morning (e.g. 6 a.m.) and the urine is discarded. All urine passed up to and including the 6 a.m. specimen on the following morning is measured and put into the Winchester. The pathologist may want the whole amount, or a specimen from it together with a record of the amount passed.

One of the commoner reasons for collecting a 24 hour specimen of urine is for estimation of excretion of 17-ketosteroids. These substances are derived from the steroid hormones, mostly those of the suprarenal gland in women, while in men a good proportion are from the male hormone, testosterone. Undersecretion of the suprarenal glands (as in Addison's disease), causes a marked fall in 17-ketosteroid excretion, while suprarenal tumours, especially malignant ones, produce a rise.

Aschheim-Zondek Test. Four to six ounces of an early-morning specimen (which is the most concentrated) is sent to the laboratory. This test is used in the diagnosis of early pregnancy, and of certain malignant growths of the reproductive system.

SPECIMENS OF STOOL

Examination for Occult Blood. Amounts of blood in the stools indistinguishable to the naked eye may be detected chemically. Specimens of three consecutive stools are collected, and small amounts are sufficient. Bleeding gums or piles render the test valueless.

Organisms. A small representative sample, including any abnormality like pus or blood, should be sent if the bacteriology of the stool is being determined.

If examination is being made for amœbæ a fresh, warm stool is required, and it should be sent as soon as possible, preferably in the bedpan.

SPECIMENS OF SPUTUM

The patient must understand that the material required is phlegm from the chest ; saliva is not only useless, but a waste of the valuable time of the bacteriologist. If examination is to be made for tubercle bacilli, three consecutive specimens, or more if indicated, should be sent.

A patient with an early suspected lesion, for whom this examination is most useful, sometimes is unable to provide sputum. In such a case the nurse may be asked to send gastric juice, which may contain swallowed bacteria. Early in the morning a Ryle's tube is passed through the nose or mouth into the stomach, 5 or 10 ml. of normal saline is injected with a syringe, and all the fluid in the stomach withdrawn.

Specimens of sputum are best expectorated directly into a carton. If a specimen is taken from a sputum container, it must be one with no disinfectant in it.

SPECIMENS OF BLOOD

Capillary Blood. Blood obtained by puncturing a finger pad or ear lobe is used to estimate the hæmoglobin level and the red and white blood cell counts. The blood is drawn into a special pipette, and the technician will bring his own equipment.

It is also used for blood-sugar estimation, and the nurse may be asked to collect it, since the fasting blood-sugar level is an important one and must be taken early before technicians are normally at work.

Requirements. Blood-sugar tubes containing fluoride.
Hagedorn needle.
Dish with sterile swabs and ether.
Fine rubber tubing.

The patient is told that the procedure only involves a prick, and a finger pad is cleaned with ether and allowed to dry. Rubber tubing may be used as a tourniquet, or the sides of the finger tip may be pressed by the nurse's left hand to produce superficial congestion. The needle point is stabbed briskly into the finger tip, and the resulting blood collected in the fluoride tube. About 0·2 ml. will suffice. The patient is given a swab to press on the puncture site for a few minutes. The label should give the time of collection as well as the usual data.

Whole Blood. Venous blood is used for many investigations. Usually 5–10 ml. is taken.

Requirements. 5–10 ml. syringe and No. 14 Record or 20 Luer needle.
Dish with gallipot or ether and sterile swabs.
Sphygmomanometer, or tubing, as a tourniquet.
Paper towel.

The syringe and needle must be kept for this purpose : syringes or needles used for aspiration must never be used for venepuncture. They are best dry sterilized (e.g. hot air at 160° C.) ; if they have been boiled they must be well rinsed with normal saline, or hæmolysis (breakup of blood cells) will occur and spoil the result.

A vein in the bend of the elbow is the usual site. The arm is bared, and must rest comfortably on a mackintosh and towel with the elbow extended. The sphygmomanometer cuff is adjusted, and the pressure raised to 60 mm. Hg. If the veins are not prominent the patient is asked to open and close the fist a few times.

The skin is cleaned and allowed to dry. When the vein is successfully entered the sphygmomanometer cuff is released, and the syringe filled. A swab is pressed over the site as the needle is withdrawn, and may be kept in place for a few minutes by flexing the elbow. A dressing is not necessary.

The blood is squirted gently into a tube, which is closed with a cork, not a swab. A dry tube is used by most laboratories for the majority of investigations, such as blood calcium, chlorides, grouping (including the Rhesus group), potassium, sodium, urea ; van den Bergh, Wassermann and Kahn reactions. Some like to use a tube containing oxalate (to prevent clotting) for blood urea, uric acid and a few others. Blood for estimation of the alkali reserve is collected with a needle and tubing into a tube under a layer of liquid paraffin. Blood for the erythrocyte sedimentation rate (described on p. 113) is citrated.

Estimation of the blood sugar may also be made by a paper dip-and-read test such as Dextrostix. A large drop of capillary or venous blood is spread over the end of the test-strip. After one minute the blood is rinsed off, and the colour of the test compared with a colour chart. Such a quickly-performed test is of great value in the speedy diagnosis of causes of unconsciousness, and in diabetic clinics.

SPECIMENS OF PUS

A throat swab may be dipped in pus from a wound, returned to its tube, and sent at once to the laboratory. Such swabs dry quickly and become useless, so it is important that the swab is well charged with pus if possible, and despatched without delay. If pus is abundant, it may be transferred to a plain sterile tube with a pipette ; it should never be scooped up with a tube. This soils the outside of the tube with organisms dangerous to the nurse and the technicians who will handle it, and to the patients to whom they may spread the infection.

SPECIMENS OF TISSUE

Biopsy means the removal of tissue for examination. The amounts are often small if taken during sigmoidoscopy or bronchoscopy, and such fragments should be put into normal saline in a test tube, closed with a cork, not a swab.

Larger specimens (e.g. organs removed at operation) may be sent at once to the pathologist in a covered bowl, or enclosed in a polythene bag to prevent drying. Accurate labelling and careful handling of such specimens is vital, since in many cases the surgeon wants to know whether or no the condition is a malignant one.

CHAPTER 11

ENEMATA AND SUPPOSITORIES

THE large intestine has two functions. Firstly, it absorbs water, so that the intestinal contents, which are fluid when they enter the cæcum, are semi-solid when they reach the rectum. Salts dissolved in this water are also absorbed, though not nearly as efficiently as from the small intestine, where the villi are specially adapted for absorption. There are no enzymes in the colon, so no digestion takes place.

Secondly, the unwanted residue from the food is discharged once or twice a day from the sigmoid colon into the rectum, and the distension of the rectum arouses the desire to empty it. This desire can be stimulated by distending the lower colon with fluid; reflex peristalsis is excited, and the fluid is expelled, along with the bowel contents.

An enema is an injection of fluid into the rectum, and it is given for one of these reasons.

1. To empty the bowel. It may be used in some cases of constipation, and unless the colon is loaded will effect rapid relief, whereas an aperient might cause intestinal colic and several bowel actions. Before operations on the colon, or on pelvic organs like the bladder and uterus it is necessary for the surgeon that the rectum is empty. Distension of the colon by flatus post-operatively is sometimes an indication for an enema. Old people and paraplegics may accumulate large quantities of faeces in the colon, unless the possibility is guarded against, and repeated enemata may be ordered to relieve this. The amount given must be enough to distend the lower bowel in order to stimulate contraction, and 600 to 1,000 ml. is a usual amount.

2. To supply water or to give drugs in solution. For this purpose, the amount given at any one time must not be large enough to stimulate contraction, and 300 ml. is usually the largest amount that can be retained and absorbed.

3. To inject a radio-opaque solution, which is retained long enough for an X-ray to be taken that will allow visualization of the colon. Barium sulphate is used; the enema is given in the X-ray department. The nurse's duties in preparing the patient for a barium X-ray are on page 127.

Cleansing Enemata

The fluid used for an evacuant enema can be plain water, normal saline, or soap solution. Soap has some effect in breaking up hard faeces.

The soap enema (enema saponis) is probably still the most common kind, and is used to produce a bowel action, especially in cases of constipation suitable for such treatment, and in order to empty the colon before an abdominal or pelvic operation. Its administration is described in detail because it is the type of all enemata consisting of a fairly large quantity of fluid meant to be returned almost immediately.

The amount of solution is from 600–1,000 ml. for an adult and it is usually given with a funnel, about half a metre of tubing, a glass connection and a catheter size 20 F. A Higginson's syringe may be used, provided the bone nozzle is protected by a catheter. The solution is made from soft soap, a piece of the size of a walnut being dissolved in a pint of water. It is most convenient to melt it in a little boiling water and add cold water to bring the amount up to a pint at a temperature of 100° F. (or 38° C.). Soap solution can be dispensed ready-made, and this is a saving of the nurse's time.

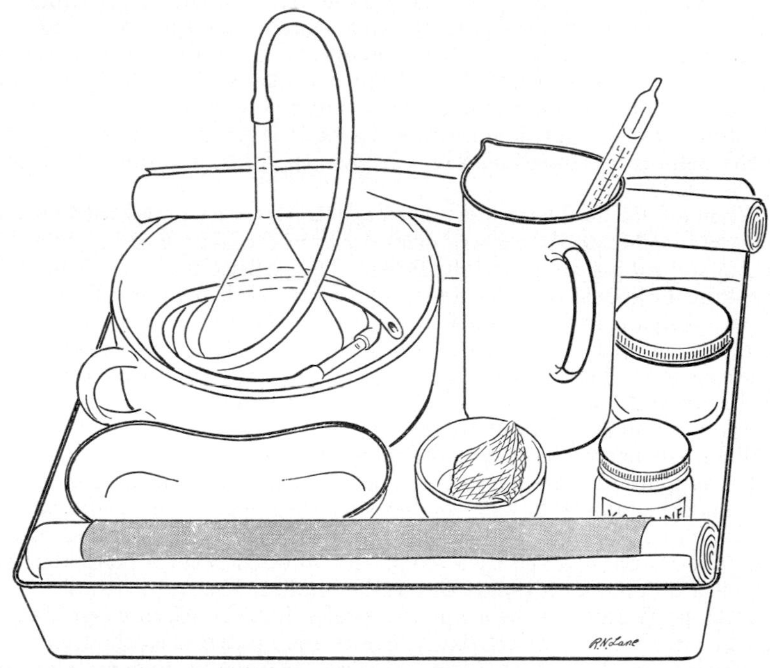

FIG. 27. Enema tray.

The following equipment is assembled on a tray:

Funnel, tubing and catheter in a bowl.
Jug of solution, 600–1,000 ml. at 100° F. (or 38° C.).
KY jelly.
Swab in a gallipot.
Kidney dish.
Mackintosh and towel.
Cover.
Warm dry bedpan.

The patient is told of her treatment, and if she is unfamiliar with it is reassured. Her bed is screened and the equipment brought to the right side of the bed. Enough pillows are removed to allow the patient to lie comfortably on her left side, and the bedclothes are folded singly down to mid-thigh level. The patient's upper parts must be adequately covered with a bedjacket or a small blanket. The buttocks are brought out to the edge of the bed and the mackintosh and towel slipped beneath them. If the patient is comfortable and relaxed, with hips and knees flexed, the treatment is easier for her and the nurse.

The last 3 in. of the catheter are lubricated with KY jelly, the funnel and catheter held in the left hand, and solution poured in until the apparatus is filled and all air excluded. The catheter, pinched to prevent the solution escaping, is taken in the right hand, and passed gently about 10 cm. into the anal canal. The solution is now allowed to flow in with the funnel held about half a metre above the level of the bed. As the level falls, it is replenished from the jug. The aim is to administer it at such a speed that the patient can accommodate the whole amount without discomfort, but briskly enough to produce a strong reflex peristalsis in the colon. If the patient complains of discomfort before the full amount has been given, the catheter should be pinched to stop the flow for a few moments, since the pain is probably due to spasm at the pelvi-rectal junction, and will pass off, when administration can be resumed.

When all fluid has been given the catheter is pinched and withdrawn. It is detached from the apparatus and put in the kidney dish, while the funnel and tubing are put in the bowl. The patient may be encouraged to retain the enema for a few moments, and then is comfortably settled on the bedpan, and the nurse takes away her equipment. An ill or highly strung patient should be visited occasionally as faintness sometimes occurs. The catheter is rinsed under running water, scrubbed with soap and hot water, and boiled for two minutes. The funnel and tubing are washed and put to dry.

When the enema has been returned, the bedpan is taken away and water supplied for the patient to wash her hands. The bed is tidied and made comfortable and the screens removed. The result of the enema should be noted—whether the fluid has been returned clear, coloured or accompanied by a stool, and whether relief from distention has been obtained. A report should be made to the ward sister.

Some physicians dislike soap, and prefer to order plain warm water, but hypotonic solutions are dangerous to such patients as children with megacolon or those with head injuries. Normal saline is safer for general use, and fluid return should always be measured. The signs of water intoxication due to over-absorption are restlessness, muscle twitching, and even convulsions.

Olive Oil Enema. Severe constipation may be treated by giving five or six ounces of olive oil with a narrow funnel and a 14 F catheter. It will take about ten minutes to give, and should be retained long enough to soften the rectal contents. A brown wool pad beneath the buttocks may help to give the patient the necessary confidence. If the enema is given in the evening, it should be followed by a soap enema next morning if a bowel action has not resulted.

Suppositories

Suppositories can be used to produce a bowel action, and because they are inexpensive and easy to give they are frequently used instead of enemata.

Bisacodyl suppositories (" *Dulcolax* ") are commonly ordered. They stimulate the rectum and lubricate its contents, and unless these contents are very hard are normally effective in about fifteen minutes. They are often used in the elderly, and by securing a regular bowel action are useful in the control of fæcal incontinence.

Glycerine suppositories are hygroscopic, and when they melt provide good lubrication. They contain 2 or 4 G. of glycerine, and when giving one the nurse collects the following articles on a tray:

Suppository.
Finger stall or caped finger stall.
Small gallipot with water.
Swabs.

The suppository is inserted with the patient in the left lateral position. A finger stall is put on the right index finger and a swab of adequate size put between the thumb and forefinger. The extreme tip of the suppository is moistened, and it is passed into the anal canal and pushed upwards the length of the index finger. The gelatine melts and allows the glycerine to exert its effect. A bowel action can be expected in about half an hour. A similar method is used in giving all suppositories.

DISPOSABLE ENEMA PACKS

Assembling the apparatus for giving an enema, and dealing with this apparatus afterwards, is time-consuming. The use of a disposable enema pack will save this time, and such a pack requires less skill in

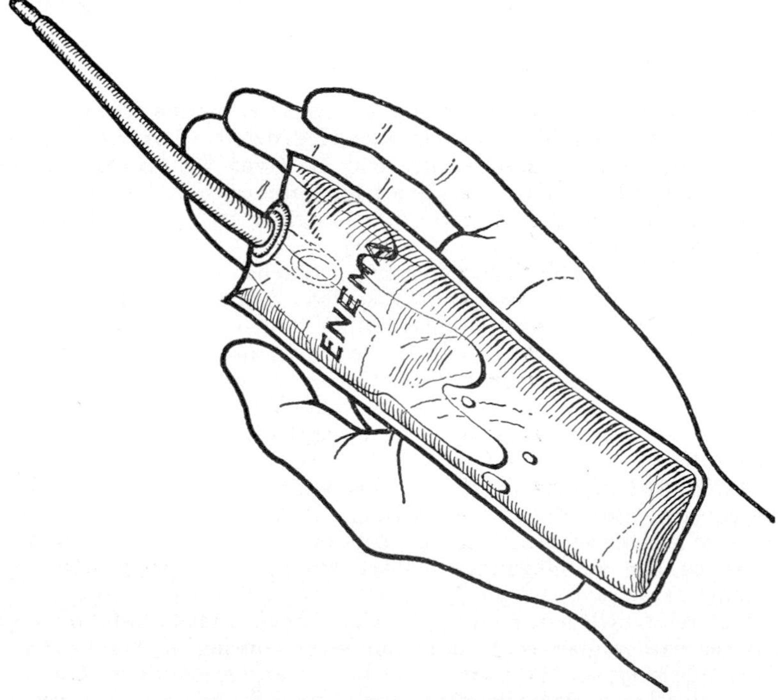

FIG. 28. Disposable enema apparatus.

use. More important, the patient feels no discomfort in administration, since these packs do not usually contain more than 150 ml. of solution. The chief obstacle to their wider use is the cost.

The substance used is sodium phosphate, or sodium acid phosphate, and it is contained in a small plastic envelope, either as crystals to which water is added, or in solution. From this leads a tube and nozzle. In use, the cap is removed from the nozzle, which is inserted into the anus, and the envelope is rolled up to expel the contents through the tube. The empty pack is then thrown away. The discomfort associated with the distension of the colon by a large volume of fluid is not experienced, and there is usually no difficulty in retaining the sodium phosphate for a few minutes until the bowel action is stimulated. Some people find the solution causes local irritation.

People who are attending the Outpatient Department for X-rays which require a clear colon, may be given such a pack with instructions as to the time it is to be given, since there is no difficulty about self-administration.

Magnesium Sulphate Enema. 60 G. of magnesium sulphate in 200 ml. of water is occasionally ordered for patients with raised intracranial pressure. This is another hygroscopic solution, and the amount returned should be greater than that given. This enema is sometimes retained by an unconscious patient, and if it is not returned in half an hour it should be siphoned back by running a little water into the rectum, then inverting the funnel over a bedpan below the bed level, and allowing the enema fluid to run out. The amount returned should be measured.

ENEMATA TO BE RETAINED

Some drugs are quite well absorbed from the rectum, though twice the amount given by mouth is usually ordered. Paraldehyde and Lugol's iodine are examples, and may be given with a small funnel and tubing and a 14 F catheter in a little water or saline. Alternatively, drugs may be added to a rectal infusion given by the drip technique described below.

Caffeine is also absorbed, and black coffee has enjoyed a reputation as a stimulant in cases of opium poisoning. 6 or 8 fl. oz. (180–250 ml.) of freshly made coffee is administered.

Patients with ulcerative colitis are occasionally ordered retention enemata such as sulphaguanidine in mucilage, or prednisolone. They must be given very slowly, as the inflamed rectum in such cases is very intolerant, and are best used at night when colonic activity is at its lowest.

Starch and Opium Enema. This enema is intended to check diarrhœa in cases of rectal irritation. It is obviously not suited to cases of extensive enteritis, but patients with ulcerative colitis, or tenesmus due to infiltration of the rectum by new growth, may benefit.

A starch mucilage is made by mixing a heaped teaspoonful of starch powder with a little cold water and then pouring on boiling water, stirring briskly, till the mixture becomes translucent (about 250 ml.). When this has cooled, the consistency should be adjusted if necessary with more water till it will run easily, though still tacky. 150–200 ml. of this mucilage is used, and the usual dose of tincture of opium is 2 or 4 ml. Half of the mucilage is poured into a funnel with not more than 12 in. of tubing and a 14 F catheter, and allowed to run into the rectum slowly until the level in the funnel has sunk nearly to the bottom. The whole of the tincture of opium is poured in, and then enough starch is added to carry the opium through. The mucilage is thought to form a protective coating to the mucous membrane, while the opium has a well-known anti-peristaltic action. In fact, opium acts through the nervous system, and not locally, and might quite as well be given by mouth.

RECTAL INFUSION

The use of rectal injection to supply fluid to a dehydrated patient is much less common than formerly in hospital practice, since intravenous fluid can be given so simply with better control than by the older method. It is still a very useful way of supplying fluid in situations where medical help is not readily available. Plain tap water is better absorbed than anything else, and should be preferred unless the patient is thought to need salt as well. In that case dilute saline, perhaps one-fifth of normal strength, will be tolerated. Normal saline is absorbed with rather more difficulty, while if dextrose saline is used the patient

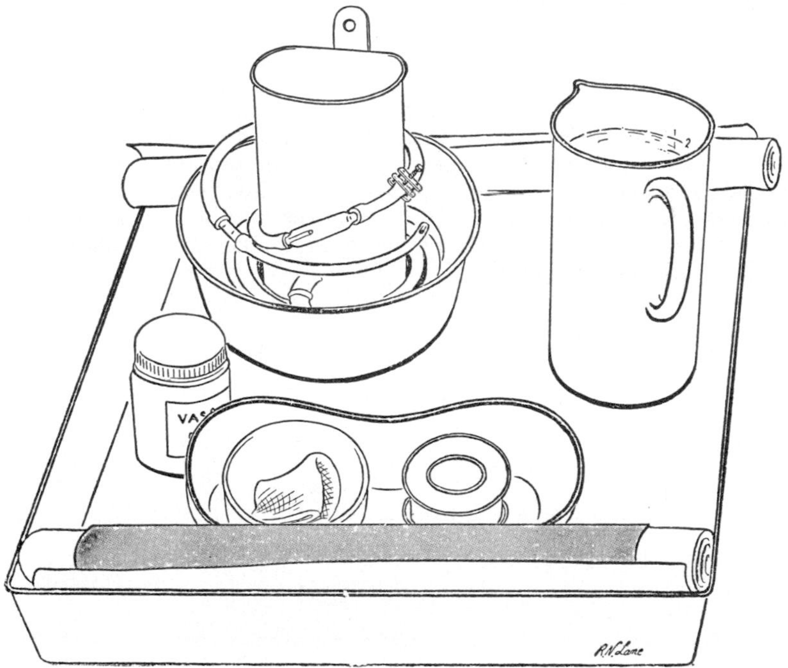

FIG. 29. Tray for a rectal infusion.

not infrequently fails to absorb it and it may be returned. If it is felt that dextrose is needed, probably an intravenous rather than a rectal infusion should be ordered.

If a small amount of fluid is needed, up to 300 ml. may be administered with a funnel and tubing and a No. 8 catheter. The left lateral position is convenient, but it may quite well be given with the patient on her back if that is more comfortable. In that case the bedclothes must be folded singly on to the thighs, and the upper parts warmly covered.

The nurse should sit while giving the infusion, lest she be tempted to give it hastily. 300 ml. of water or saline will take twenty minutes to give. The bladder should be empty, since micturition later may stimulate a desire to void the rectal fluid as well. If the patient is conscious and anxious, a brown wool pad may be put beneath the buttocks. 300 ml. infusions may be given at four-hourly intervals, but it is undoubtedly more comfortable for the patient, if some quantity is needed, to use the next method.

Continuous Rectal Infusion

The apparatus needed is a reservoir, 3 ft (1 metre) of tubing with a drip connection in the middle and a clip below it, a glass connection and a 14 F catheter. The can hangs at a height of about 1 metre above the bed. It is taken to the bedside with a jug of solution or water at 100° F. (38° C.), lubricant, a receiver and narrow strapping. The can is filled, solution is run through the apparatus and the clip tightened. The catheter is lubricated and passed 6 in. (15 cm.) into the rectum. It is most comfortable to have the tubing passing beneath the leg in the fold of the buttock, and a piece of strapping attaches it to the inside of the thigh. The clip is opened to allow a drip rate of 40 drops a minute and the patient comfortably settled. At intervals the apparatus and the level in the can should be inspected, and if the patient is feeling distended the rate of flow can be slowed or even halted temporarily. There is no need to adopt any means of keeping the fluid warm ; at the slow rate at which it is given it will not need to be warmer than room temperature once it is running.

CHAPTER 12

LAVAGE

THE stomach, colon and rectum may be irrigated in order to remove their contents ; the bladder may be washed out in order to apply a therapeutic lotion or to check hæmorrhage. Except for the stomach washout, which is used extensively for people suffering from poisoning, and as a pre-operative measure, all these washouts are less commonly used than formerly.

Certain nursing considerations apply to all of them. They involve the introduction of a catheter or tube, never pleasant and sometimes actively uncomfortable, and all precautions to avoid unnecessary discomfort must be taken. Where the cavity irrigated should be sterile (like the bladder) the lotion, equipment and technique must be sterile. The temperature of the lotion introduced must be known accurately, and therefore a thermometer must be used. The organ to be washed out must not be unduly distended, so that the quantities used must be watched. All the fluid used must be regained, unless there is a therapeutic purpose in leaving some behind.

GASTRIC LAVAGE

The stomach may be washed out in cases of non-corrosive poisoning, the majority of which today are barbiturate poisoning. It is used extensively for patients with pyloric stenosis to remove the retained gastric contents, and may be given daily in the medical preparation of such people for operation. Gastric lavage is not a routine procedure before stomach operations unless stenosis is present.

Equipment. Funnel, rubber tubing, glass connection and œsophageal tube, boiled, in a bowl.
Clip.
Lotion thermometer.
Irrigating lotion in a 6-pint (3 litre) jug.
Empty 2-pint (litre) jug.
Instrument tray with gallipot of liquid paraffin or glycerine, and one of swabs.
Senoran's evacuator if liked.
Jar for stomach contents in cases of poisoning.
Mouth gag and spatula for an unconscious patient.
Waterproof and towel.
Receiver for swabs.
Vomit bowl and tissues.
Bucket and floor rug.
Mouth wash.

The method of giving this treatment to a conscious and co-operative patient about to undergo a stomach operation for pyloric stenosis will be described. The patient is sat up against sufficient pillows and the bed screened and the trolley brought to the right-hand side of the bed. If the patient has not received this treatment before, he will be regarding these preparations with apprehension, and it cannot be denied that the procedure is unpleasant. He must be asked to co-operate in the passage of the tube, which is the disagreeable part, and to try to follow instructions. The floor rug is spread beside the bed, and the bucket stood on it. The small jug is filled with lotion from the big one, and the temperature ascertained to be 98° to 100° F. (or 37° to 38° C.). The vomit bowl should be at hand. The funnel, tubing and connection are joined, but the tube is kept separate until it has been passed. Glycerine is a slightly more pleasant lubricant than liquid paraffin. The patient is now told that he should breathe steadily and deeply in and out all the time until asked to swallow, and that the lips should be closed over the tube, but the teeth must not be clenched. He is asked to open his mouth and keep his head back. The lubricated tip is passed over the tongue and directed downwards towards the œsophagus. As it enters, he is asked to swallow, and the tube is then carried down a few inches. He is reminded to keep breathing steadily, as this will prevent retching and nausea. When he is breathing quietly he is asked once more to swallow, and the tube is pushed onwards at the same time. Haste is to be deprecated; it will only result in retching, and perhaps vomiting of the tube.

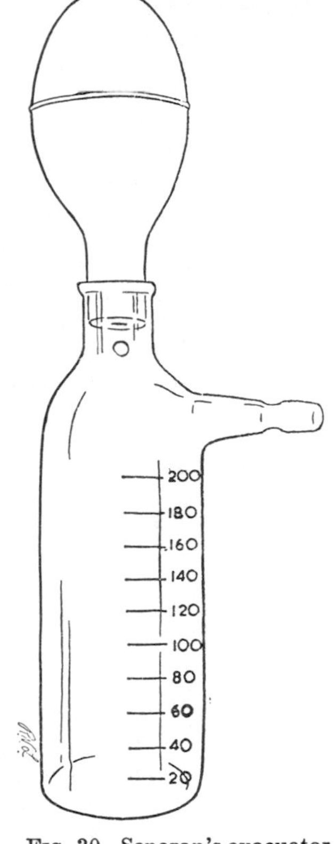

Fig. 30. Senoran's evacuator for aspiration of stomach contents.

Before starting the washout, the position of the tube in the stomach must be checked in one of these ways :

1. Senoran's evacuator is attached to the tube, the bulb is squeezed and the hole covered with the thumb. When the bulb is released, stomach contents should flow into the container.

2. The end of the tube may be put into a gallipot of water.

Bubbles coinciding with expiration would indicate that the tube was in the airway. In fact, it is unlikely that an œsophageal tube will pass in a conscious patient in the wrong direction.

The clip is applied, the funnel and tubing filled with lotion and attached to the tube. When the clip is opened, the fluid runs in. About 300 ml. is allowed to flow in, then the funnel is lowered until the level in it begins to rise, then inverted over the bucket, when the stomach contents will be siphoned out. This should be repeated until the lotion is returned clear. The tube is then pinched and withdrawn, and the patient will welcome a mouth wash.

The lotion used may be sodium bicarbonate, 1 teaspoonful in 500 ml., or normal saline. Plain water is best for cases of poisoning. If washouts are to be repeated, the doctor should be consulted as to the lotion used, since chloride is lost in the gastric contents which are removed.

A patient who is unconscious should be laid prone, with the head turned to one side, since no anxiety need be felt about the airway if he lies face downwards. A gag will be needed to open the mouth. Senoran's evacuator should be used to empty the stomach, and the residue should be put into a jar and labelled. The washout may be continued with this apparatus ; the bulb is removed and lotion poured into the flask which is used in the same way as the funnel and tubing.

A form of gastric lavage suitable for endeavouring to recover tubercle bacilli from the stomach is described on p. 133.

WASHING OUT THE BOWEL

Some confusion exists about terms in connection with treatment of the large intestine, and doctors should be sure that nurses understand the sense in which they are being used.

An enema is a pint or two of fluid which distends the rectum and sigmoid colon and produces a contraction which evacuates the solid contents and the enema solution. It is suitable for rectal constipation (dyschezia), in which the intestinal function is normal except in the atonic rectum.

A rectal washout implies that fluid is run into the rectum and siphoned back again. It is used as a final cleansing process before rectal operations, to remove mucus, blood or debris. It is quite unsuitable for treatment of a loaded rectum ; to try to irrigate away hard masses through the eye of a catheter is obviously uneconomic. Not more than a pint is normally used.

A colonic washout is especially used when obstruction (e.g. carcinoma) in the rectum or sigmoid has allowed chronic distention of the colon and the accumulation of fæces above the obstruction. In these cases fluid is run in through a large-sized catheter at a gentle pressure until the patient feels distention, and then siphoned back. If the process of giving a barium enema is watched on a screen it will be seen that the barium passes without difficulty along the whole colon back as far as the ileo-cæcal valve, so that a colonic washout efficiently administered should remove all the contents of the large intestine.

A colostomy washout is badly named, since it is in fact an enema given through the colostomy.

Rectal Washout

Equipment. Funnel, tubing, glass connection and 20 F catheter in a bowl.
500–1,000 ml. of normal saline at 100° F. (or 38° C.)
KY jelly and swabs.
Receiver for catheter.
Waterproof and cover.
Blanket.
Pail and floor rug.

A comfortable position for the patient is essential. He lies on his left side, with the buttocks on the waterproof and cover at the edge of the bed. His upper parts should be covered and only two pillows are needed under the head. The pail stands on the floor rug beside the bed. The catheter is lubricated, the apparatus is filled with saline, and the catheter introduced about 6 in. within the anus. About 4 oz. of fluid is run in, then the funnel is lowered and the solution siphoned out into the bucket. This is continued until all the solution has been used, when the efflux should be clear. If it is not, a further pint should be used. The amount returned should be measured to ensure that none has been retained, since it is a serious inconvenience to the surgeon at operation.

Colonic Washout

1. The Dierker apparatus for colonic lavage is used in hospitals or clinics specializing in diseases of the large intestine. It is connected to the mains water supply, and has a thermometer so that the incoming fluid can be adjusted to 100° F. (38° C.). The outflow is by plastic tubing which is connected to a 4-in. wide-bore rectal tube with a flange which rests against the anus. When the " on " switch is turned, water flows into the colon at a steady but brisk rate, and the pressure within the colon is read from a mercury manometer. When this shows an additional ½ lb. pressure (or earlier if the patient feels pain) the switch is reversed and the fluid siphoned out through tubing containing a glass segment through which the contents can be observed, and empties into the main drain. The process is repeated until the operator is satisfied that the colon has been cleared, and it may take 10 litres to do this. It is an efficient apparatus that leaves no water in the colon at the end of treatment. The patients receiving such a washout are often ill people, and their condition should be assessed constantly while the treatment is in progress.

2. Colonic lavage may be undertaken with the same apparatus as was used for rectal washout, except that a greater quantity of fluid will be needed, and an additional small jug to replenish the funnel. The catheter should be a large one, and the glass connection a straight-sided one.

Some like to raise the end of the bed in order to facilitate the flow of water into the colon, and as it is a fairly lengthy procedure the patient must be in a comfortable lateral position, covered, and with well-placed pillows. The most important points are to run the solution in gently enough to allow the fluid to run in quantity into the colon, and to see that it is all siphoned out again.

3. Operators in clinic or private practice sometimes use a modification of Dukes' apparatus (p. 361). The Y-tube and the tubing leading to the rectal catheter must be wide bore. The clip on the bottom section of the tubing is closed while lotion runs in, and opened to allow it to siphon into the bucket while the clip below the reservoir is closed.

COLOSTOMY WASHOUT

After removal of the rectum and anus for malignant disease, the divided end of the sigmoid colon is brought onto the surface of the abdomen in the left iliac region, and stitched to the skin. This opening is a colostomy, from which the fæces will be permanently discharged. Daily washouts of the bowel through this opening were once an integral part of colostomy management, but are now very rarely used like this. Washouts may be ordered (1) to encourage an action in a recently established colostomy, (2) to relieve constipation for a patient who finds difficulty in managing his colostomy.

Occasionally a terminal colostomy is performed on the sigmoid colon to relieve obstruction, but the rectum is too involved in growth for removal. The upper end of this portion is closed and returned to the abdomen. This blind rectal pouch will require a washout from time to time to remove mucus and débris.

Colostomy Washout

Equipment. Douche can, tubing, clip, glass connection and 20 F catheter, in bowl.
Stand or hook.
One or two pints of water, normal saline, or enema solution at 105° F. (or 40° C)
Two kidney dishes.
Tray with two pairs of dissecting forceps, swabs, cut gauze and wool.
KY jelly.
Skin ointment if necessary.
Binder and pins.
Pedal bin.
Waterproof.
Bucket and floor rug.

A washout is best given immediately after breakfast, to establish a morning routine of action. The patient must be arranged comfortably sitting up, with the abdomen exposed, and a waterproof covering the folded bedclothes. His shoulders are warmly covered. The can is filled and hung about 0·5 metre above the bed, the pail is stood on the floor rug beside the bed and a kidney dish placed below the colostomy. The catheter is lubricated and passed about 6 in. (15 cm.) into the colon, and the fluid allowed to run gently in. It will be found necessary to hold the catheter in place, which is why it is better to use a can than a funnel and tubing.

When all the fluid has run in, the catheter is removed and the outflow runs into the kidney dish carrying with it the fæcal contents of the colon. If it is emitted from the colostomy at an awkward angle, the second kidney dish may be used to direct it into the lower dish. This is emptied at intervals into the bucket. All the fluid given must be returned before the dressing is done.

When the washout has been completed, the abdomen is well washed with soap and water and dried. The skin around the colostomy may be lubricated with ointment, such as vaseline or a water-repellent barrier cream, but the colonic contents are not irritating, and trouble is not common. The colostomy itself is dressed with gauze moistened with vaseline, and a dressing added, the size of which depends on the confidence felt in the regularity of the colostomy. In hospital a many-tailed bandage is usual to retain the dressing. Types of appliance suitable for everyday use will be mentioned in discussing the management of a colostomy without a washout (p. 274).

BLADDER WASHOUT

Bladder washouts used to be extensively used in cystitis, to wash away infected material with an antiseptic lotion. Such infection is much better treated by sulphonamides or antibiotics, which do not involve the trauma, however slight, involved in catheterizing the bladder. The only occasion on which washouts are at all frequently used is in the treatment of hæmorrhage, reactionary or secondary, following prostatectomy. If the bleeding is reactionary a urethral or suprapubic catheter will already be *in situ*. Secondary hæmorrhage is most usual after the first week, when the catheter is not likely to be in position. It will have to be passed before a washout can be given.

Equipment. Bladder syringe, sterile.
Two sterile kidney dishes.
Lotion thermometer.
Jug of lotion (e.g. silver nitrate 1–1,500) at 115° F. (46° C)
Sterile glass connection (wide bore) and tubing for open drainage.
Blanket.
Waterproof and towel.

The patient will be alarmed and in pain, and morphine is commonly ordered. He should have only two pillows and be warmly covered. The waterproof and towel are placed between the legs, where the patient cannot see the result of the irrigation, and one of the sterile kidney dishes put under the end of the catheter. The syringe is filled with lotion, and held upright while air is expelled completely. It is connected to the catheter, and an ounce or two of solution gently directed into the bladder. The nozzle is disconnected, and the fluid should run out into the dish. Small quantities are used at first in case a clot is lodged valve-fashion over the catheter eye, allowing lotion to go in but not out. If this is so, the empty syringe is attached to the catheter, and suction exerted to try to withdraw the clot. Should this be unsuccessful, the house surgeon must be told ; it is useless and dangerous to distend the bladder with lotion that cannot escape, and treatment in the theatre is usually needed. If, however, the fluid runs freely out, the washout may be continued. Afterwards the catheter should drain by a glass connection and tubing into a jar, so that the course of the bleeding, if any, may be observed. More discussion on this subject will be found in the chapter on urosurgery.

Washouts of the female bladder are not common. They may be performed with a sterile funnel, rubber tubing and glass connection into a kidney dish, running the lotion in and siphoning it out. While a syringe is traditionally used for men, and a funnel and tubing for women, there is no necessity to observe the distinction.

CHAPTER 13

THERAPEUTIC AND DIAGNOSTIC PROCEDURES

THE measures that were described in the chapter on diagnostic methods are designed to give information that lead to effective treatment. Some of the ones in this chapter may be used for this purpose too, but all are used as therapeutic measures that will improve the patient's condition. In connection with all of them the nurse must consider the equipment needed, and how sterilization, if it is needed, can be best effected ; how the patient is prepared and how to tell him what is being done ; what complications can occur and how they may be averted ; the after-care that is required and the observations that should be made.

Apparatus used naturally varies in different hospitals, though a tendency to standardization is noticeable. Equipment becomes simplified, and unwieldy and complicated apparatus that is difficult to sterilize gradually becomes obsolescent. Sterile equipment may be provided ready packed and sterilized by a Central Supply Department. Where such a service is not available, equipment is most conveniently dished up in sterile trays with lids, or in the container in which it was sterilized, on a dry clean trolley.

Lumbar Puncture

The spinal cord ends at the level of the first lumbar vertebra, but the arachnoid and dura mater are prolonged below it, so that a sac filled with cerebro-spinal fluid lies below the termination of the cord, and may be tapped by passing a needle and stilette between the second and third, or third and fourth lumbar vertebræ. This process (*lumbar puncture*) may be performed for these reasons :

1. *To Examine the Cerebro-spinal Fluid.* It should be crystal-clear and turbulence indicates infection, i.e. meningitis, while blood may be found in subarachnoid or cerebral hæmorrhage. Alterations in the protein and sugar content can occur, and the Wassermann reaction for syphilis is often performed. The normal pressure is 80–120 mm. of water, and it may be much raised in intracranial new growth, and hydrocephalus (*inter alia*).

2. *To Relieve Raised Intracranial Pressure.* A rare complication of this use is impaction of the medulla oblongata in the foramen magnum by the downflow of fluid, causing sudden death from cardiac arrest.

3. *To inject substances*, e.g. streptomycin for tuberculous meningitis ; spinal anæsthetics ; radio-opaque oil for a myelogram (p. 130).

Lumbar puncture needles are about 5 in. long for an adult, with a stilette to facilitate introduction, and are made in Record or Luer fitting. Many have a sidearm and tap to permit taking the cerebro-spinal pressure. They must be perfectly sharp, and are carefully inspected and felt after use in case they need sharpening. Sterilization must be by autoclaving since boiling cannot be relied on to destroy spores. The manometer is of glass, graduated in millimetres up to 200, with a bulb near the top to prevent overflowing in cases of high pressure. This also should be autoclaved ; boiling will dull the interior, and if a meniscus of water remains inside, it is awkward when reading pressures. A convenient method is to autoclave together in a pack the manometer, two lumbar puncture needles and the syringe and needles for the local anæsthesia if these are not supplied in separate sterilized containers. If a myelogram is to be performed a 5-ml. syringe should be included.

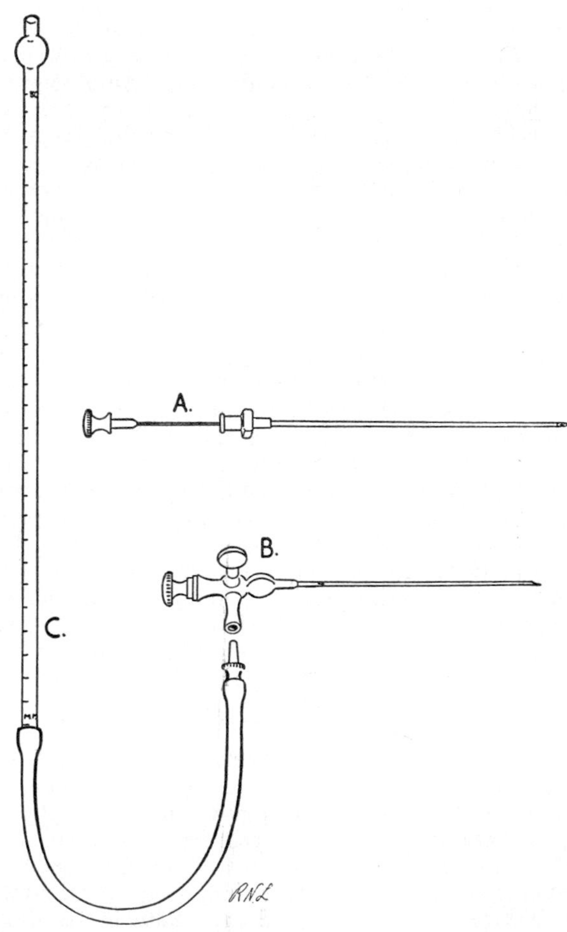

FIG. 31. Lumbar puncture needles and manometer.

A. Needle with stilette partly withdrawn.

B. Needle with two-way tap for connection with manometer C

Equipment. 2 lumbar puncture needles. ⎫
Manometer. ⎪
2-ml. syringe. ⎬ sterile
2 No. 19 and 2 No. 14 needles. ⎪
2 pairs of French's forceps ⎭
Sterile covered tray with 3 gallipots.
2 pairs dissecting forceps.
Sterile packet of 2 towels.
Swabs.
Small sterile dressing for puncture.
2% procaine.
Skin lotions (ether, spirit, iodine, cetavlon) and collodion.
3 specimen tubes.
Plastic sheet.
½-in. strapping.
Receiver or bin for swabs.

Sterile gloves are often used by the doctor. If he is giving an intrathecal injection a sterile mask and gown should be provided.

Preparation of the Patient. The patient is told that a needle is to be put into his back to obtain a specimen to help the doctor treat him correctly, or is given a similar simple explanation. He is asked to help by lying still in the desired position.

The pyjama trousers are taken off, and a light blanket used to cover the upper parts. All pillows are removed but one, and the bedclothes folded to mid-thigh level. The buttocks are brought to the edge of the right side of the bed with a waterproof and towel put beneath them. The spine, hips and knees must now be fully flexed, in order to separate the lumbar spinous processes, but there must be no lateral flexion of the spine at all. The pillow is adjusted under the cheek. If the patient is not fully conscious and co-operative an assistant should stand on the left side helping the patient to maintain his position by steadying him behind the neck and knees. An alternative position, often used for spinal anæsthesia, is to have the patient sitting up, and flexing his spine by bending his head towards his knees.

The doctor scrubs, dries his hands on a sterile towel, and puts on his gloves if he uses them. He drapes the area with sterile towels, cleans the skin, injects the local anæsthetic and passes the lumbar puncture needle into the theca, between the second and third, or third and fourth lumbar vertebræ, and on withdrawal of the stilette cerebro-spinal fluid should begin to drip out. The manometer is attached and the pressure read. Sometimes the nurse is asked to compress the jugular veins first on one side, then on the other, a manœuvre which should cause a rise in the cerebro-spinal fluid pressure and is called *Queckenstedt's test*. Two specimens are taken, or three if many investigations are required, the needle removed and the puncture hole sealed with a collodion dressing. It is not a procedure likely to be followed by any complication (provided that adequate sterilization has removed the risk of meningitis) except headache. The patient should lie quietly afterwards with only one pillow ; many physicians believe that raising the foot of the bed on blocks for twelve hours is helpful in preventing headache.

A child who is to have a lumbar puncture should have enough premedication to ensure co-operation if it is not old enough to accord it without. Pethidine is suitable. It is best performed on a firm couch, and two assistants should always be available, one of whom is solely concerned with maintaining the child's position. Large amounts of fluid will not be obtained for specimens, and a fluoride tube is often needed for sugar estimation. Small children cannot be induced to lie flat if they do not want to, but older ones should be encouraged to do so.

Cisternal Puncture

In places around the base of the brain, the arachnoid is widely separated from the pia mater, and spaces filled with cerebro-spinal fluid are formed, called the subarachnoid cisternæ. The largest of these lies in the angle between the cerebellum and the medulla, and it can be reached by passing a needle between the first cervical vertebra and the skull. This is the procedure of cisternal puncture, and it is similar in technique to lumbar puncture. It is performed generally with the patient sitting up with the neck flexed, and the cisternal needle used is a fine one graduated in centimetres, to inform the neuro-surgeon of the depth to which he has penetrated.

Paracentesis Abdominis

Free fluid within the peritoneal cavity is called *ascites*, and it may accumulate in many different conditions. It may be an item in generalized œdema, e.g. in subacute nephritis, when fluid may be present in the limbs, serous cavities and face. Extensive œdema is often found in congestive heart failure, especially in the legs, sacral area and often in the abdomen as well. Ascites may occur in inflammatory conditions, such as tuberculous peritonitis. Finally, if there is obstruction to the portal circulation by cirrhosis of the liver, or peritoneal metastases from carcinoma of the digestive tract or ovary, ascites may be considerable. In the latter group of cases, relief of the distension by tapping the fluid (*paracentesis abdominis*) is often undertaken to diminish the discomfort and respiratory embarrassment. It may also be used, though less generally, in some of the other cases.

Trolley.

- 2 gallipots. (sterile)
- Scalpel. (sterile)
- 2-ml. syringe and No. 19 and No. 14 needles. (sterile)
- 2 pairs dissecting forceps. (sterile)
- Southey's tube, with shield, stilette and rubber tubing, or trocar and cannula. (sterile)
- Packet of sterile towels and swabs.
- Small sterile dressing.
- Sterile gloves, if the doctor wishes.
- Cleaning lotion.
- 2% procaine.
- Large abdominal binder.

Trolley. (cont.)

Winchester on a small tray.
$\frac{1}{2}$-in. strapping.
Specimen tubes if needed.
Stimulants tray.
Clip.
Pedal bin or disposable bag.

If Southey's tube is used, a suitable size should be selected and the shield screwed into place. Four feet of narrow tubing is needed, with $\frac{1}{2}$ in. of wider tubing threaded over it near one end. This end is drawn on to the mount of the Southey's tube, and the needle and stilette are boiled or autoclaved.

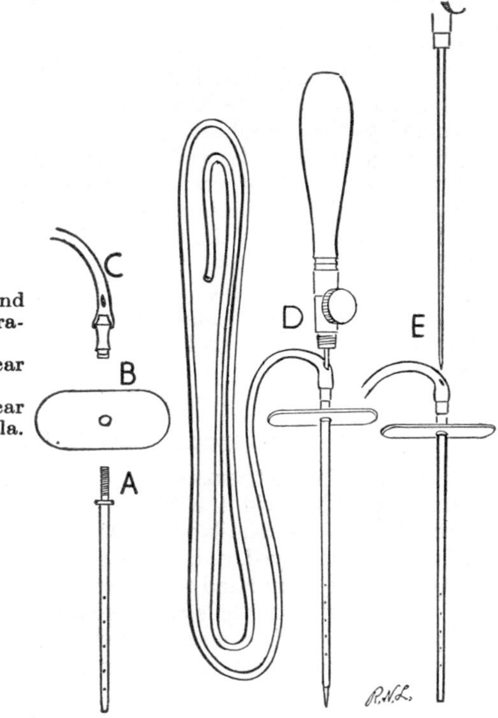

FIG. 32. Southey's tube.
A. Cannula.
B. Shield used between A and C when abdominal paracentesis is being formed.
D. Cannula, tubing and trocar assembled ready for use.
E. Method of inserting trocar through tubing into cannula.

Preparation of the Patient. If the patient has not experienced paracentesis before, he is told how much relieved he will be by this painless procedure. The patient must empty the bladder immediately beforehand; puncture of a distended bladded is the main hazard in the performance of paracentesis.

The skin of the abdomen must be clean, and it is sometimes necessary in men to shave the abdomen between the umbilicus and the symphysis pubis. The patient sits well up, so that the fluid may drain downwards and forwards to an accessible position. The pyjama jacket is opened, the chest covered, and the binder slipped behind the back. The bedclothes are folded on to the thighs and covered with a waterproof. The Winchester stands or hangs beside the bed.

When the doctor has scrubbed, he cleans the skin and inserts local anæsthetic halfway between the umbilicus and the symphisis to one side or other of the midline. He passes the stilette through the rubber and into the tube, adjusting it until the point is in the correct position. It is usual to nick the skin with a scalpel to facilitate the introduction of the tube, which will then pass easily into the abdomen. The end of the tubing is dropped into the Winchester and when the stilette is withdrawn fluid should flow out. When it does the cuff of tubing is slipped down to cover the puncture hole, a small dressing may be put over the shield, and strapping used to keep it in position. The binder is adjusted as firmly as possible, and the rate of flow regulated. If this is the first time paracentesis has been used, the rate must be moderate, or distress and faintness due to the falling intra-abdominal pressure may be experienced, but if the patient is accustomed to it, the fluid may be allowed to run as fast as the tube allows. A safety pin secures the tubing to the drawsheet.

Subsequently the pulse and appearance should be observed, and the binder tightened at intervals. Collapse is unusual, but nikethamide should be available in case it occurs. A hot drink is more generally useful. If no clip is on the tubing, the flow will cease in a few hours, but if the flow is modified, the process may continue for twenty-four hours or more. The level in the jar should be watched, and when necessary it is emptied and measured. When the flow has ceased, the tube is withdrawn and the puncture hole sealed with a sterile dressing.

Tapping Fluid in the Legs

Excess fluid in the tissues may be dispelled in one of two ways. The natural method is via the kidneys ; the other way is to drain it externally, in a way similar to that described for ascites. In practice both may be employed, and in heart failure and some other states the kidneys may be stimulated to excrete more, and at the same time fluid may be removed from the legs, where it tends to accumulate by gravity. This procedure used to be attended by the risk of cellulitis, but now this need no longer be feared, since prophylactic penicillin can be used.

The patient should be prepared beforehand by spending forty-eight hours sitting in a heart bed with the legs dependent to allow the œdema to intensify. Southey's tubes are convenient and if they are used the following equipment is needed :

Trolley.

2 gallipots.
2-ml. syringe and No. 19 and No. 14 needles.
2 pairs dissecting forceps.
2 Southey's tubes, prepared as before, but without shields
} sterile

Packet of sterile towels and swabs.

Trolley. Small sterile dressings.
Cleaning lotions.
2% procaine.
Containers for fluid, e.g. two Winchesters.
Waterproof and towel.
Bed cradle.

The tubes are inserted into the outer aspect of the lower leg just above the ankle, parallel with the skin in the subcutaneous tissues, and the tubing is brought over the end of the bed into the jars. The bedclothes are made up over a cradle, with the end divided to allow the tubing to pass through.

Acupuncture

An alternative method of draining œdema fluid is by means of superficial incisions or punctures on the outer aspect of the legs. It is a quick and effective method, but rarely needed now diuretics are so much used.

Trolley.

2 gallipots. } sterile
Scalpel, or triangular needle, or No. 1 intravenous needle. } sterile
Packet of sterile towels and swabs.
Lassar's paste and spreader.
Cetrimide 1%.
Long waterproof, carbolized.
Bed cradle.
Small bath.

The legs are arranged on towels on the waterproof, the end of which passes over the foot of the mattress into the bath, while the edges are rolled inwards to direct the fluid. The skin of the calves is thoroughly cleaned with cetrimide and spirit, and then is covered with a layer of Lassar's paste from below the knees to the heels, leaving a narrow strip down the outside into which the punctures will be made. These may be very superficial incisions with a scalpel, or needle punctures, and from them the œdema fluid will begin to trickle. The bedclothes are arranged over a cradle, and if the legs feel cold a lamp with a 40-watt bulb may be tied to the inside of the cradle.

The rate of flow can be controlled by raising or lowering the foot of the bed, and the legs must be inspected at intervals. The chief danger of acupuncture is that if flow is rapid the patient may suffer from sodium depletion, with a low blood pressure, muscular weakness and vomiting. When the desired effect has been secured (and it is not usual to continue for more than twenty-four hours) the end of the bed should be raised and sterile tulle gras dressings applied until the incisions are dry. This procedure and the preceding one are not frequently needed now that diuretics are so effective.

Aspiration of Chest

Pleural effusion can be caused by inflammation (pneumonia or tuberculosis) ; by trauma (chest operations, rib fractures) or by new

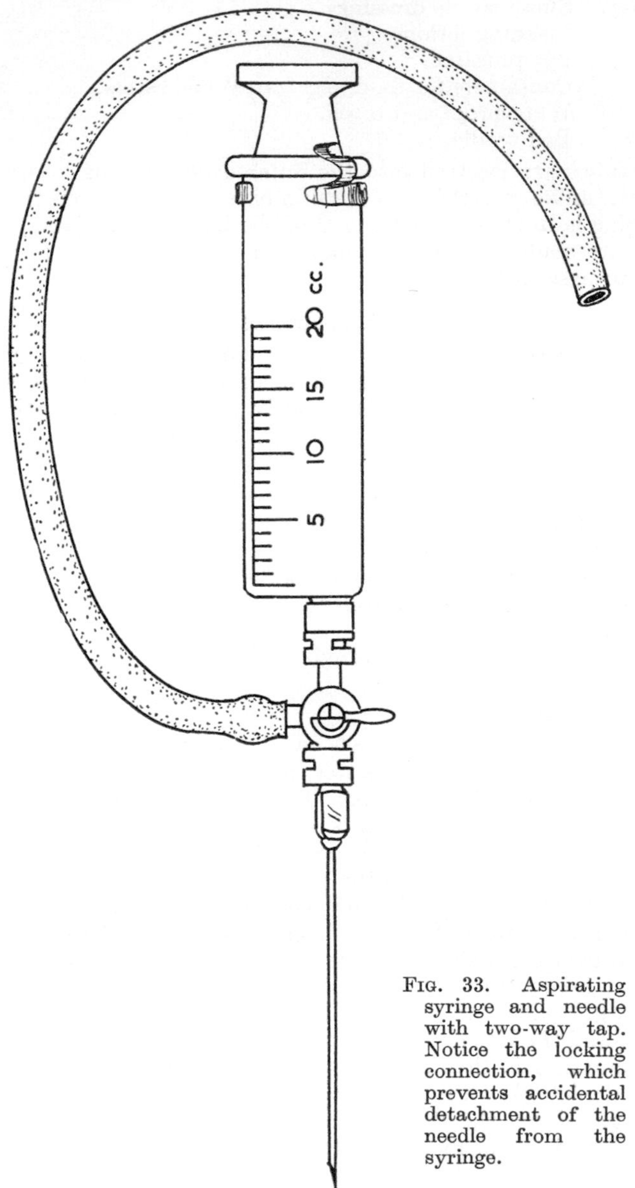

Fig. 33. Aspirating syringe and needle with two-way tap. Notice the locking connection, which prevents accidental detachment of the needle from the syringe.

growth (carcinoma of breast, lung metastases). It can also be part of a general œdema, as described above. Not all effusions need aspiration, but generally those that are large enough to embarrass breathing are aspirated, and so are those that follow pneumonia, since they often give rise to *empyema*, or pus in the pleural cavity. Although the removal of a large effusion can give great relief, it is a procedure that sometimes causes the patient to faint, and more severe collapses, said to be due to *pleural shock* when that membrane is punctured, are also seen. Onlookers such as young nurses and students not uncommonly feel faint when first watching a chest aspiration, and the sister in charge is not only alert to the needs of her patient and doctor, but also spares a glance from time to time at her assistants.

The fluid in the chest cannot simply be allowed to run out through a trocar, as described for ascites, because air would enter through the needle and cause a pneumothorax. The simplest apparatus is a syringe connected with an aspirating needle by a two-way tap (see Fig. 31). When the needle is in the effusion, suction on the syringe with the tap parallel to the needle will fill the syringe with fluid. The tap is turned through a right angle, and as the piston is pressed in the fluid, is expelled by a side arm and tubing into a jug.

Trolley. Pack or tray with :

- 3 gallipots.
- Luer-Lok syringe with two-way tap and assorted aspirating needles.
- 2-ml. syringe, and needles size 19, 14 and 1.
- 2 pairs dissecting forceps. All sterile.
- Packet of sterile towels and swabs.
- Sterile jug (1 or 2 pint).
- Sterile gloves.
- Specimen tubes if required.
- Small sterile dressing.
- Cleaning lotions and collodion.
- 2% procaine.
- Receiver for swabs.
- ½-in. cellotape.
- Waterproof sheet.
- Small blanket.
- Stimulant tray.

Preparation of the Patient. The patient is told that there is fluid in the chest, and that he will feel easier when it has been withdrawn. Repeated aspirations can try the nerves of the most co-operative, and sometimes premedication will be indicated. The most useful position for the patient is sitting up, as the puncture is made towards the base of the lung at about the ninth intercostal space. He may lean forward on to pillows on a heart table, or if this is uncomfortable for his legs, may sit on the edge of the bed with the heart table parallel to it, and his feet on a stool. A position recommended in books for the ill patient is to lie on the sound side with the arm above the head, but in practice few are comfortable lying down on the side which is mainly responsible for respiration. The doctor will examine the X-rays and the chest, and indicate where he expects to make the puncture.

The patient is asked not to cough without warning while aspiration is taking place, and may be given a lozenge to suck if he finds it comforting. He is settled into an easy position, with the back exposed and a waterproof sheet behind him. The skin is cleaned and anæsthetized and puncture of the pleural cavity is made ; if fluid is drawn into the syringe, the jug is placed under the outlet and the effusion aspirated. Finally the puncture hole may be sealed with a collodion dressing or a dry dressing and cellotape. The fluid is measured, the patient is comfortably settled, and his temperature, pulse and respiration rate are recorded. His colour is noted, and his pulse taken again at the intervals his condition suggests.

If an effusion becomes infected it is usual to aspirate as much fluid as possible at daily or two-daily intervals, and to inject penicillin at the end of the procedure. If this is to be done a three-way tap to the syringe should be provided. It is hoped by this means to clear the infection without resorting to surgery, but in a small proportion of cases it will be found necessary when the pus is thick and well localized to open the chest (with or without rib resection), remove the fibrin that has accumulated, and drain the cavity.

Exploration of the chest is a term sometimes used by physicians about the withdrawal of small quantities of fluid for diagnostic purposes. A 10-ml. syringe and a suitable needle are used. It is not undertaken unless X-rays give evidence of effusion, since puncture of an inflamed lung may give rise to pleurisy.

Venesection

Withdrawal of blood in small quantities for diagnostic purposes is *venepuncture* (p. 134). Larger amounts can be taken for therapeutic reasons (in right heart failure with venous engorgement) or when obtaining blood from a donor, and in either case the usual amount taken is 600 ml.

For a therapeutic venesection, the following equipment is used, though it is possible and sometimes convenient to use the routine donor apparatus.

Trolley.

- Sterile covered tray with:
  - 2 gallipots.
  - Needle and 6 in. of tubing.
  - 2 pairs dissecting forceps.
  - 1-ml. syringe and No. 14 needle
- Sterile 600 ml. jug.
- Packet of sterile towels and swabs.
- Sterile intravenous dressing.
- Cleaning lotions.
- 2% procaine.
- Sphygmomanometer.
- Jaconet-covered pillow.
- Strapping.
- Receiver for swabs.

The patient will be sitting up, and is usually breathless and cyanosed with distended systemis veins. The pyjama sleeve is rolled up so that the sphygomanometer cuff can be smoothly applied to the upper arm, with the tubes uppermost so that the veins in the bend of the elbow are accessible. The arm rests on the jaconet-covered pillow with the elbow extended. When the doctor is ready the pressure in the sphygmomanometer is raised to about 60 mm. Hg. and the patient can be assured that the procedure will bring him great relief. The doctor cleans the skin and covers the forearm with a sterile towel. Although a local anæsthetic should be provided, it is not always deemed necessary. The needle used can be any hollow one with a short bevel ; French's needle, once very popular, is now usually thought unnecessarily large. The nurse holds the jug at a convenient level, and releases the sphygmomanometer pressure when the needle is inserted and the blood flows out. Pressure by a swab is sufficient to stop the bleeding when the required amount has been withdrawn, and a small sterile dressing is strapped into place.

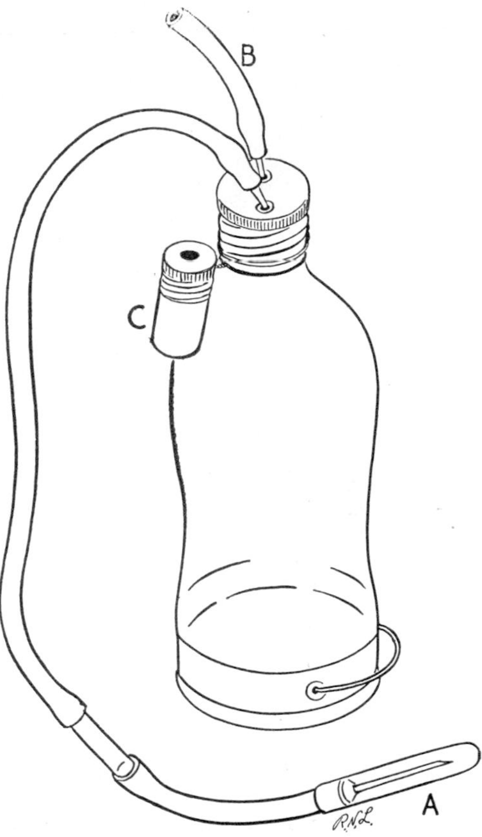

Fig. 34. Apparatus for collecting blood.

A. Needle which enters vein.
B. Air outlet.
C. Small bottle in which a little of donor's blood is put for crossmatching.

Taking Blood from a Donor

Two factors or *agglutinogens* named A and B are found in red blood cells. Some people possess both A and B, some either A or B, and some neither. On this basis there are four blood groups, called by international classification AB, A, B and O. Similarly, plasma contains substances named *agglutinins* which are capable of clumping together cells of a different group. This means that blood cannot be transferred from a donor to a recipient unless their blood groups are known to be compatible, or agglutination of the incoming donor cells may occur, causing a reaction often severe enough to be fatal.

People of group AB can receive blood from any other group, while group O can act as donors to anyone. Groups A and B can receive

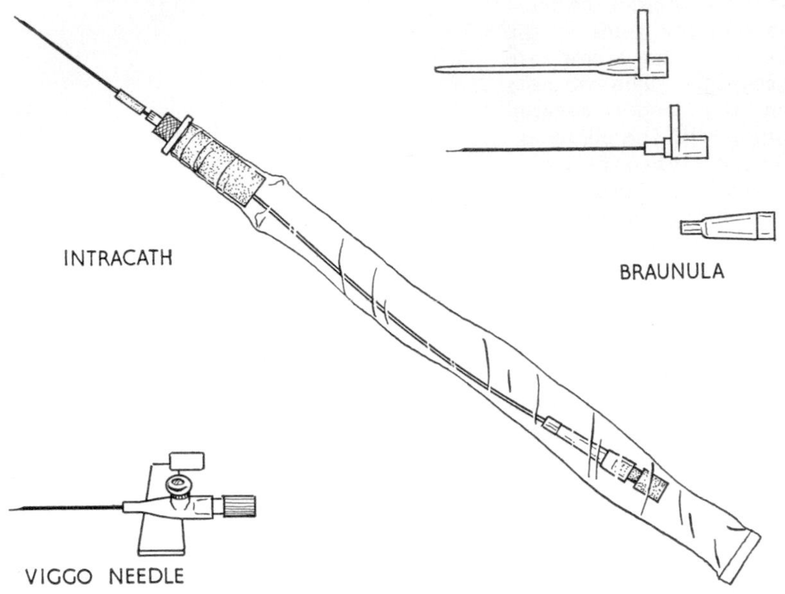

Fig. 35. Intravenous therapy. The Braunula is a disposable trocar and cannula. The viggo needle has a diaphragm, through which intravenous drugs can be given. The Intracath allows a fine plastic catheter to be introduced into a vein through an intravenous needle.

blood from their own groups, or from group O. In transfusion, the main effect to be considered is the action of the recipient's serum on the donor's cells. The donor's serum is so diluted during intake that the effect of his serum on the recipient's cells is not noticeable in small transfusions. In repeated or massive transfusion, however, this action may obviously be important, and it is best to use blood of the same group.

Group	*Red Blood Cells Agglutinogens*	*Serum Agglutinins*
1	AB	None
2	A	B
3	B	α
4	O (none)	αB

In addition to these agglutinogens, the Rhesus factor is present in 85% of people in the British Isles. These are said to be Rh+ve, while those who do not have it are Rh−ve. Rh−ve people should never be transfused with Rh+ve blood, since they will make immune substances which will cause hæmolysis of further incoming Rh+ve cells. The most important clinical effect of this Rhesus factor is that a Rh−ve woman, married to a Rh+ve man, may have Rh+ve children. During the first pregnancy she may make anti-Rh immune substances in her blood, and these may be potent enough in subsequent pregnancies to cause hæmolysis of the Rh+ve cells of the fœtus. This hæmolytic disease can be severe enough to cause pre-natal death. Young women find this knowledge alarming, but should remember that the hæmolytic effect may not become obvious until after several pregnancies, and that treatment such as exchange-transfusion at birth for affected babies has much improved their prognosis.

The blood group is ascertained by testing a drop of the patient's blood with two sera, A and B. Agglutination can be seen as a cayenne-pepper appearance with the naked eye.

If serum A agglutinates it, the group is B.

If serum B agglutinates it, the group is A.

If sera A and B agglutinate it, the group is AB.

If there is no agglutination, the group is O.

Rhesus grouping is done as a tube test, after two hours incubation, and is done microscopically.

A donor who comes to a transfusion centre to give blood first has his group and his Rhesus type ascertained, and is given a card with these inscribed on it. Donors may normally give blood every six months, and many do so. Since the only way to obtain blood for transfusions that may be life-saving is from donors, it is obvious that a great debt of gratitude is owed to their selflessness, and the nurse working among them must never forget to thank them for it.

On arrival he is greeted, his coat is hung up, and he takes off his shoes and lies on a couch with his arm extended on a jaconet-covered pillow. These requirements are brought on a trolley :

Trolley.

- 2 gallipots. } sterile
- 2 pairs dissecting forceps. } sterile
- Packet of sterile towels and swabs.
- Sterile donor set.
- Blood bottle with 100 ml. of sodium citrate.
- Small sterile dressing.
- Cleaning lotions.
- Sphygmomanometer.
- Waterproof.
- Receiver for used swabs.

The "taking" set which is standard in most hospitals consists of a needle, protected in a glass tube, attached to tubing with a glass window in the middle, and a needle at the other end which transfixes the rubber cap of the receiving bottle. The needle and short tubing packed with it are to provide an air outlet from the bottle. The set is packed in two layers of cellophane and a tin sealed with adhesive tape. The sets are packed and sterilized at the blood banks of the Department of Health and Social Science and are supplied to the transfusion depots which collect blood from donors.

The method of taking the blood is the same as for venesection, except for the management of the apparatus. The nurse removes the protective cap from the top of the bottle, and exposes the metal cover which has two holes in it. She opens the tin, takes out the set, and unfolds the outer layer of cellophane. The doctor takes it and removes the inner protective layer. The air inlet needle is inserted into one hole, and the distal needle of the "taking" set into the other. The nurse stands the bottle at a convenient level slightly below the donor's arm, and the doctor removes the glass tube that protects the intravenous needle and inserts it into the vein. It will take about fifteen minutes to fill the bottle, and during this time the donor must be watched for signs of faintness. Sweating, pallor or nausea are signs that the bleeding

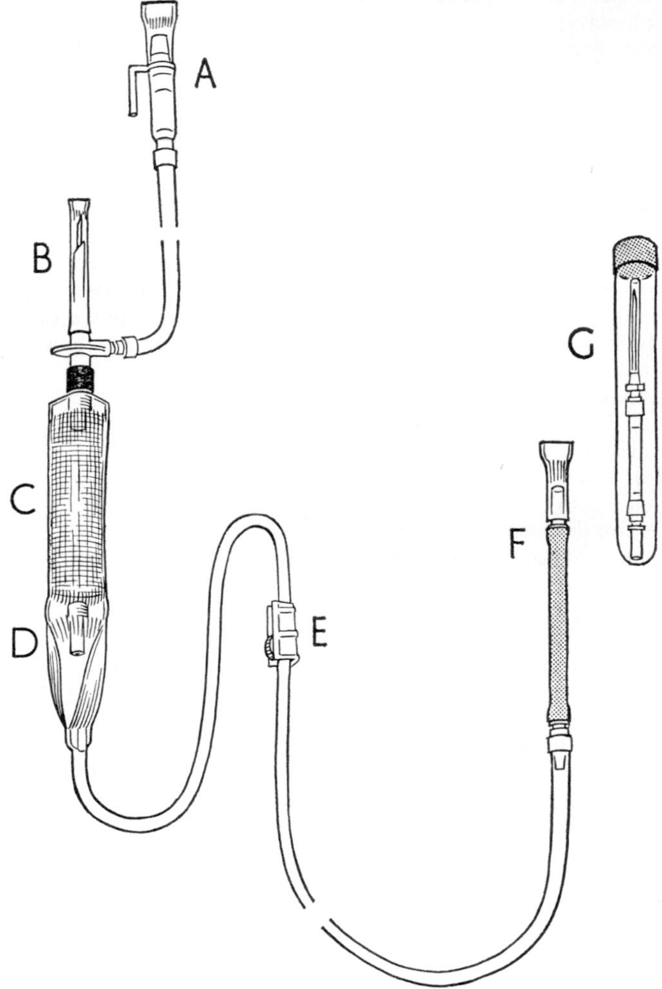

FIG. 36. Disposable transfusion or intravenous set.

A. Air inlet.
B. Needle for piercing cap of flask.
C. Filter
D. Drip chamber.
E. Clip.
F. Section of rubber tubing through which drugs may be injected.
G. Intravenous needle.

must be stopped. Marked collapse is rare, but stimulants such as methedrine should be at hand to raise the blood pressure.

When the bottle has been filled, the needle is withdrawn and the small amount of blood remaining in the tubing is put into the small tube attached to the bottle. This is subsequently used for cross matching with the recipient, and avoids the necessity for opening the bottle (with its attendant risk of contamination) until it is used. A dressing is applied and the donor rests on the couch for twenty minutes before leaving, and receives a cup of hot tea or coffee. The nurse assures herself that he is quite fit before he goes and he is thanked for his service. Labels of different colours for the different blood groups exist, and the correct one is selected, the donor's name is added, and it is attached to the bottle before it is stored in the refrigerator.

FLUID REQUIREMENTS

Every day about 5 pints of fluid is lost from the body in the following ways.

Urine	1,500 ml.
Insensible loss from skin	600 ml.
Insensible loss from lungs	400 ml.
Fæces	100 ml.
	2,600 ml.

If this loss (which in round figures we will call 3,000 ml.) is not made good, there will be first a fall in the amount of urine secreted, then fluid will be withdrawn from the intercellular spaces into the blood vessels, and finally the intracellular fluid will be called upon, and life cannot continue, unless the loss is replaced.

In health, this 3,000 ml. is taken by mouth either as liquid or as water contained in food, and will contain also the other substances, especially salt, which are lost in the urine and sweat. If a patient is unable to take anything by mouth (e.g. after an operation on the stomach) it may be possible to supply this fluid by rectal infusion (p. 142). The salt (sodium chloride) needed is 5 G. a day, and since normal saline contains 0·9% sodium chloride, 1,000 ml. contains 9 G., and the necessary 5 G. would be contained in 600 ml.; 600 ml. of normal saline and 2,400 ml. of water would, therefore, contain the necessary allowance of water and salt, and if mixed together would yield 3,000 ml. of fifth-strength (N/5) normal saline. Giving fluid by the alimentary tract is known as *enteral* feeding ; if neither the oral or rectal methods is possible, fluids must be given *parenterally* either into the tissues (subcutaneous infusion) or into a vein (*intravenous infusion*), or if the fluid is blood, *transfusion.*

Intravenous infusion has problems and difficulties not met with in rectal infusion, of which these are the most important :

1. The procedure must be sterile, or septicæmia will occur.
2. The speed of infusion must be carefully regulated, or overloading of the venous system may cause right heart failure.
3. The fluid must be of the same electrolyte concentration as the

plasma, or breakdown (hæmolysis) of the red blood cells will occur. We cannot, however, give 3,000 ml. of normal saline, as that would give five times too much salt ; neither can 3,000 ml. N/5 saline be used, as that would not be isotonic with the blood. A much-used solution is dextrose saline, which contains 4% dextrose and 0·15 sodium chloride. Dextrose saline has the additional advantage of providing calories.

In practice, the problem is rarely as simple as this. Additional loss of fluid and salts may occur by vomiting or gastric aspiration or diarrhœa. This loss must be measured accurately (in the case of the first two) and made good as normal saline. If hæmorrhage has occurred, blood must be used in making up the deficit, while if shock is severe but there has been no bleeding, a fluid like plasma or dextran which will raise the osmotic pressure of the blood will be used.

A fluid balance chart should be kept of all patients having intravenous fluids, showing the amount lost by the kidneys and from the stomach and on the other the amount and nature of the fluid given. Other observations which will help the doctor to decide what fluids the patient needs are the temperature, pulse, respiration, blood pressure, bowel actions and whether sweating has been severe. It may also be helpful to test the urine for chloride (p. 47).

If intravenous infusion has to be continued for more than three days, potassium must be supplied. Although important, this substance has dangers. Not more than 4 G. is given in twenty-four hours, and it is not used if the patient is excreting less than 1,000 ml. of urine, in that time. The potassium is added to the bottle of fluid so that it is well diluted, and the rate of flow should be lowered while it is being given, or stopping of the heart (cardiac arrest) may occur.

Patients who cannot take food for some days require calories to keep up their metabolic activities. Fat is the most valuable source of calories, but if given into a vein must be emulsified into very fine particles, or fat embolism will result. Such patients break down their own body proteins, and this loss must be made good, or wasting will occur. Protein can be supplied in the form of essential amino acids. The water soluble vitamins (B and C) are usually added to the fluid.

Very careful assessment is required of the patient's needs when using these complicated solutions, and the nurse must check the label most carefully to see it is what the doctor has prescribed. The contents are a good medium for bacterial growth, and every aseptic precaution must be taken in setting up the infusion. The speed of flow must be carefully regulated to give the rate desired.

When the amount of fluid needed has been estimated, the rate in drops per minute can be found by multiplying by 12 the number of litres needed for the day, e.g. if 5,000 ml. (5 litres) is to be given, the rate in drops per minute is $5 \times 12 = 60$.

Intravenous Infusion

Trolley.

2-ml. syringe and No. 19 needle. 2 pairs dissecting forceps. 2 pairs mosquito forceps. 1 pair Spencer Wells forceps.	} sterile, if cut-down is necessary.

Trolley (*cont.*)

1 pair fine-stitch scissors.
Scalpel.
Aneurysm needle.
Small curved cutting-edge needle.
Small straight cutting-edge needle.
White and black linen thread.
Intravenous cannula, or Frankis Evans needle, or similar.
2 sterile gallipots.
} sterile, if cut-down is necessary.

Sterile intravenous recipient's set.
Small sterile dressing.
Packet of sterile towels and swabs.
Sterile bottle of fluid (e.g. normal saline).

Cleaning lotions.
2% procaine.
Sphygmomanometer.
½-in. strapping.
Straight splint, padded, or back splint for leg.
2-in. bandage.
Plastic sheet.
Receiver for swabs.
Stand or hook for the bottle.

The site is usually the forearm. A simple explanation is given to the patient and the arm selected is removed from the shirt. If there is no contra-indication, the left arm is the most sensible one to use in a right-handed patient. It is extended on a pillow with a mackintosh or jaconet cover with the sphygmomanometer-cuff in position, and should be covered up if the procedure is not to begin at once, since cold pre-disposes to spasm of the vein. The trolley is conveniently disposed, with plenty of room for the doctor to work.

While he scrubs his hands, the nurse prepares the lotions and exposes the sterile towels. The set illustrated is a disposable one of which the interior and the parts enclosed in plastic caps are sterile. The piercing needle B is unsheathed, and pushed into the rubber cap of the intravenous bottle; the clamp is closed, the bottle suspended, and the air inlet filter A hooked up and its sheath removed. The doctor squeezes the filter chamber C a few times until it is full, and then the drip chamber is similarly treated until it is a quarter full. The clamp E is opened, all air expelled from the tubing, and the clamp shut. The intravenous needle G is inserted into the vein, the sheath removed from the connection F, and junction made. The nurse lowers the sphygomomanometer pressure, and the clamp is opened to allow the fluid to drip in at the required rate. When satisfied that all is well, the doctor adjusts the clip until the drip rate is satisfactory. A dressing is put over the needle, and strips of strapping keep the tubing in place, and a light forearm splint is bandaged into position.

Subsequently, the nurse must inspect the apparatus at frequent intervals to see that the flow is regular. Slowing or stopping may be due to:

1. Spasm of the vein. Stroking the vein above the needle, or clamping the tubing and squeezing the filter chamber a few times may help. The doctor may inject a millilitre of nikethamide into the rubber tubing section above the needle.

2. The needle is displaced, and fluid is running into the tissues, as shown by local swelling. The flow must be stopped, and the procedure started again, elsewhere.

3. A minor displacement of the needle has occurred within the vein. If the doctor is available, it is best to summon him at once, while making sure that there is no external pressure or kinking of the tube. If he is not, the nurse may try lifting the needle mount, but should not try to move the needle in the vein.

The bottle will have to be changed for a full one as it empties, and vigilance is needed to see that the infusion is not allowed to run through. It would be most dangerous to put up a new bottle on empty tubing, since air would be forced into the vein as an air embolus, and if the quantity were large enough to impede the heart's action, it might be fatal.

When it is time to begin a new bottle, the nurse should ascertain what is needed, and *read the label* on the bottle. She clamps the tubing, unhooks the old bottle, removes the protective cap on the new one and hangs it up. The piercing needle is extracted from the old one and inserted into the new; the air filter is put into place and the clamp reopened.

Cutting Down Onto a Vein

If the veins are collapsed it may be impossible to start an infusion simply by inserting a needle, and the vein will have to be exposed and opened and a cannula tied in. This method is also used when it is important to keep the infusion going for several days. A blunt metal cannula, or a disposable plastic one, or a piece of fine polythene tubing can be used. Under local anæsthesia an incision is made across the vein which is exposed and isolated. The aneurysm needle is passed under it, threaded and drawn back. The loop is cut and forms two strands under the vein, one of which is used to tie the vein, and the other to tie the needle in place in the vein.

While infusion is in progress, the temperature, pulse and respiration rate should be recorded four-hourly. A rise of temperature may indicate inflammation in the vein (phlebitis). This is most common if dextrose saline, which is rather irritating, has been used.

Blood Transfusion

The technique of transfusion is exactly the same as for intravenous infusion, and indeed many doctors like to start a transfusion with a bottle of saline, which is replaced by one of blood when all is running smoothly.

A meticulous routine is adopted for all patients having transfusion to ensure that they receive blood of the correct group. A sample of blood is taken for grouping and for Rhesus type, the patient being carefully identified by christian and surname. A bottle, or bottles, of the appropriate group is ordered, and should be cross-matched with the patient's own blood. The doctor performing the test writes the patient's name on the bottle, and each bottle used should be verified by two people as the correct one.

Blood is not warmed before use, as this increases the incidence of transfusion reactions. It should not be taken from the refrigerator until the transfusion is about to begin.

Mis-matched or incompatible blood gives rise to severe symptoms very quickly. The patient feels pain in the arm, begins to shiver and may soon complain of pain in the back, because products of the hæmolysed cells begin to block the tubules of the kidneys. Hæmaturia or anuria may follow, and the patient may die of uræmia. A bottle of normal saline should be put up in place of the bottle of blood, which is kept for examination.

Small rises of temperature are quite common, and need cause no alarm. Patients with blood diseases may have a more marked pyrexia with headache, and the use of an anti-histamine drug may abolish such reactions.

Subcutaneous Infusion

Fluid is absorbed quite readily from the subcutaneous tissues, especially if it is accompanied by hyalase, a tissue enzyme that hastens absorption. It used to be used almost entirely for children, but today it is frequently prescribed for adults. Its advantage for the adult who needs a litre of fluid but for whom the rectal route is contra-indicated, is that a subcutaneous infusion can be readily set up by a nurse, and that the needle never blocks. For small children, it is most important to know exactly how much fluid is to be given.

The sites used are :

1. The outer aspect of the thigh in its middle third. This is the most suitable site for adults.
2. The chest wall lateral to the border of pectoralis major.
3. The abdominal wall, halfway between the umbilicus and the flank.

Trolley.

2 gallipots. ⎫
2 pairs of dissecting forceps. ⎪
1 ml. syringe with No. 14 needle. ⎬ sterile
No. 14 or No. 1 needle. ⎪
Packet of sterile towels and swabs. ⎪
Recipient's infusion set. ⎭
Ampoule of hyalase.
Ampoule of distilled water and files.
Intravenous dressing.
Cleaning lotions.
Bottle of normal saline.
Receiver of used swabs.
Mackintosh.

The site is exposed and carefully cleaned. The ampoule of hyalase is opened and a millilitre of distilled water is squirted into it, and when the powder is dissolved the solution is drawn back into the syringe and placed on one side with the needle on a sterile swab. The "giving" set is opened, and is filled with saline as described for intravenous infusion. The intravenous needle in its glass shield will not be used. A fold of skin is pinched up, and the No. 14 or No. 1 needle is inserted into it, with the point towards the patient's head. The needle should lie in the subcutaneous tissues more or less parallel to the skin.

The hyalase syringe may now be attached to the subcutaneous needle and its contents injected. The adapter of the saline-filled intravenous set is joined to the needle mount and the clip opened to begin the flow. Alternatively the hyalase may be injected into the tubing. A swab is placed beneath the needle mount, so that if the needle moves its point shall not come out through the skin. It is covered with a small dressing lightly strapped into place, and the tubing is appropriately tethered with strapping.

The infusion site must be frequently inspected, for the rate of flow must not exceed the rate of absorption. If any swelling occurs, the clip must be closed until it has disappeared. It is possible to give a bottle of saline in about two hours, but if it is wished to give more it is better to start another infusion on the opposite side. Saline is the fluid usually given ; dextrose saline is apt to be as irritating subcutaneously as it is elsewhere.

CHAPTER 14

OXYGEN AND INHALATION THERAPY

Oxygen is needed by all cells for their metabolic activities, and is brought to them in combination with the hæmoglobin in the red blood cells. This combination is oxyhæmoglobin, which is bright red in colour, and is responsible for the normal colour of the skin. Once oxyhæmoglobin has given up its oxygen to the tissues, it becomes reduced hæmoglobin, darker in colour, and if this substance is present in any quantity in the tissues, a noticeable change towards blueness or *cyanosis* takes place. This is first seen in the fingers and toes, lips, tip of the nose and ears.

The commonest causes of oxygen lack are:

1. Interference with the airway.
2. Interference with the oxygenation process in the lungs, e.g. by pneumonia and chronic bronchitis with emphysema.
3. Inefficient cardiac action, as in heart failure.
4. Severe anæmia. Cyanosis is not seen in such a case, because the hæmoglobin is fully oxygenated.
5. Shock, causing stagnation of the blood flow.

Since oxygen lack, or anoxia, harms all tissues, especially those of the brain, it should be corrected as soon as possible. The doctor will seek to restore an adequate airway and normal lung ventilation, remove fluid that may be embarrassing the lung, deal with lung infection, improve the heart's action, and in addition will frequently order the administration of oxygen. It is in the second and third cases listed that it is most effective.

In large institutions, oxygen may be stored in tanks, and piped to the wards and thence to outlets by the patient's bed. Rather more commonly, it is supplied in cylinders, which by international agreement are coloured black with a white top. The name is stencilled on, and a printed label attached by the supply company. All oxygen is supplied from such cylinders and where wards and operating theatres can obtain oxygen from taps on the wall, these cylinders are kept in the basement. At the top is a socket into which is secured the cylinder head with the indicators and control devices, and at right angles to this is the main tap (with arrows pointing to the "on" and "off" positions) which is opened by means of a key which should be kept with the cylinder. A supply should be kept in every ward and the staff nurse should check daily that the cylinder is not empty. When a new one is needed, a porter brings one from the store, and outside the ward opens the main tap momentarily to blow any grit out of the valve. The cylinder head is then screwed firmly home. No grease must be used on the thread for fear of fire.

The cylinder head should consist of these parts :

1. A wing bolt by which the screw can be tightened.
2. A pressure gauge. When the main tap is opened, the needle

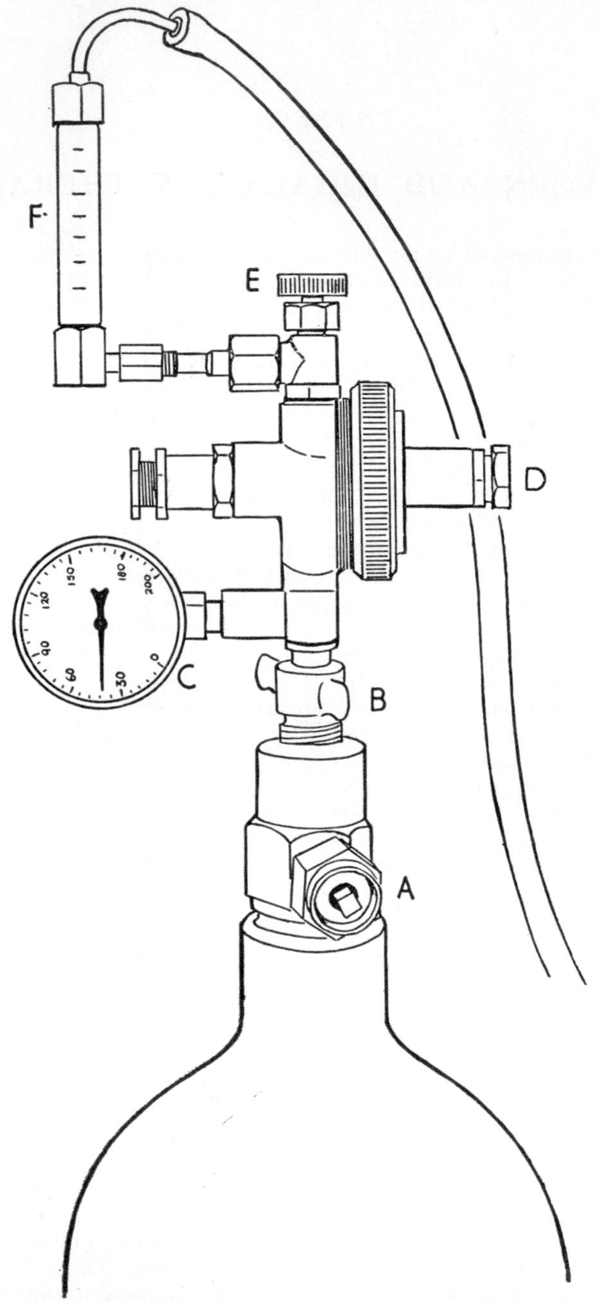

FIG. 37. Oxygen cylinder and fittings.

A. Main tap.
B. Wing bolt for attaching head to cylinder.
C. Pressure gauge.
D. Reducing valve.
E. Fine adjustment valve or regulator.
F. Dry flow meter.

on the dial should move to " full ", and will continue to register until the cylinder is empty or the main tap turned off.

3. A reducing valve. This is a safety device for reducing the pressure of the escaping oxygen, and needs no adjustment.

4. A regulator or fine adjustment valve. This must be shut when the main tap is turned on. It is a knurled disc big enough to be turned readily by finger pressure.

5. A flowmeter, described below, is often incorporated.

6. A side opening allows the oxygen to pass out.

Flow Meters

Oxygen flow is measured in litres per minute, and an apparatus to measure the rate is a flow meter. Dial type flow meters are attached to oxygen tents and to some ward apparatus. The most common type is

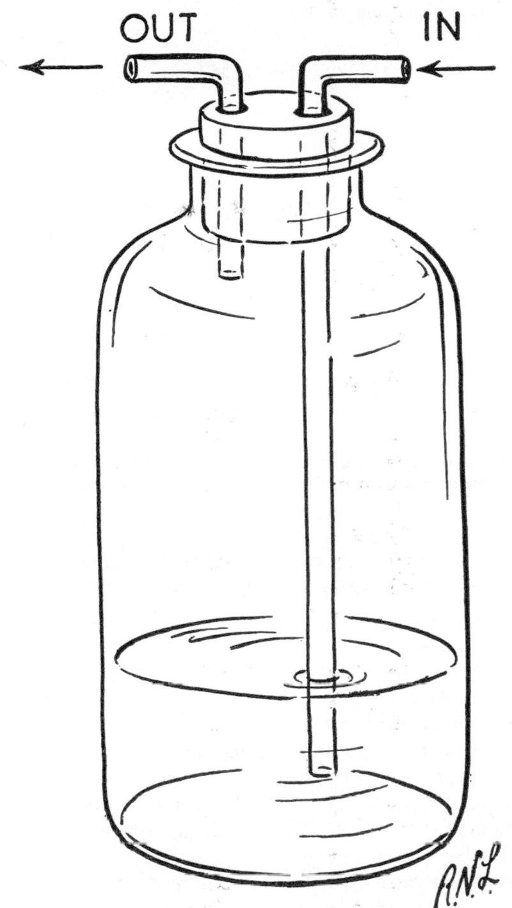

FIG. 38. Woulfe's bottle.

the one in which a bobbin lies in a graduated glass tube. It is raised by the current of oxygen, and rides at a level which indicates the rate.

Methods of Giving Oxygen

There are two categories of patients needing oxygen, those who need it in strictly controlled quantities, and those who need it in high concentration. The apparatus used for these two purposes is different, and if the wrong kind is used, the therapy may be ineffective in some cases, and dangerous in others.

Those needing controlled oxygen therapy. The majority of patients in this group are chronic bronchitics. They have had increasing respiratory failure, sometimes for a long period, and the stimulus to the respiratory centre which maintains breathing is lack of oxygen. If the oxygen level in the blood is raised too high, this stimulus is abolished, and the patient's breathing becomes increasingly shallow, carbon dioxide accumulates and will cause coma.

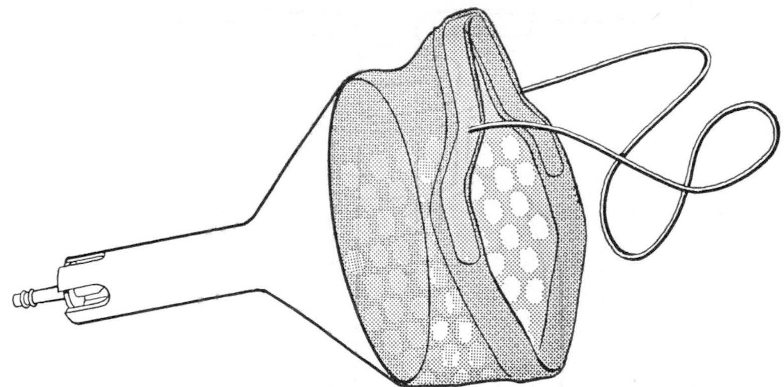

Fig. 39. Disposable mask suitable for the administration of oxygen in moderate amounts to a patient with chronic bronchitis.

The amount of oxygen given to such patients must not exceed 24–28%; this amount will raise the oxygen in the blood to an acceptable level without stopping respiration. A special mask, such as the Venti-mask, is required. This is a disposable mask, which will deliver the percentage of oxygen indicated on each mask (24%, 28% or 35%), when the flowrate indicated on the mask is employed. Oxygen tents and intranasal methods should not be used.

Those needing a high percentage of oxygen. This is a large group, who have a low level of arterial oxygen which is not due to respiratory failure. It includes people with heart failure, post-operative patients, and those with a low blood pressure. The amount of oxygen required is from 30% to 60%, but provided it is high enough to relieve the symptoms, the exact percentage does not matter. The oxygen may be given by masks of various types, by intranasal methods, or by oxygen tents.

Masks for high oxygen concentration therapy include:

(*a*) The Harris mask, which gives a concentration of 30–40% at a flow of 2–4 litres per minute.

(*b*) The M.C. mask, which delivers an inspired concentration of 40–60% oxygen at a flow of 6–8 litres per minute.

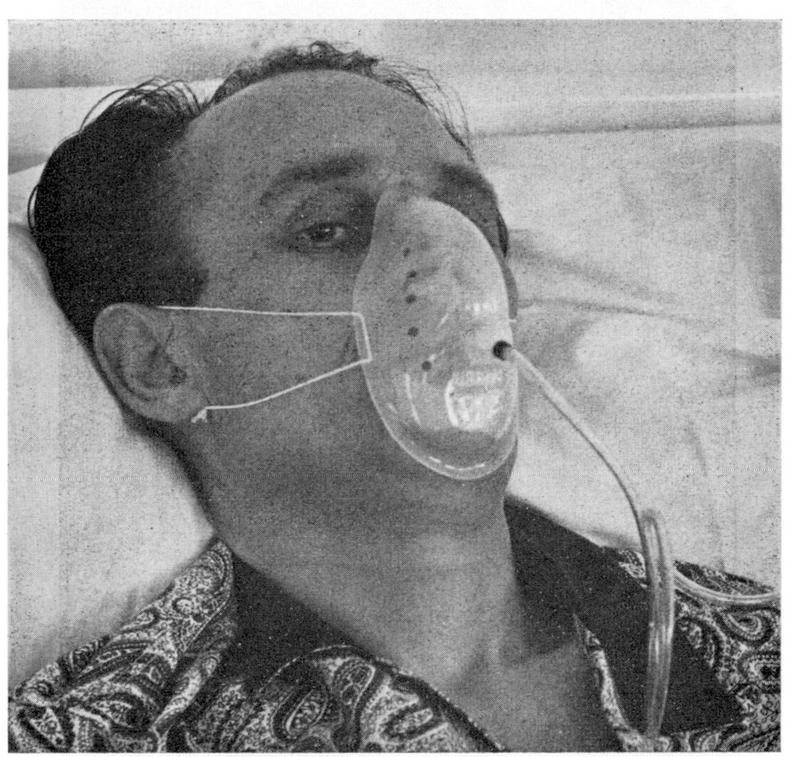

Fig. 40. Harris Disposable Mask.

(*c*) Non-rigid plastic masks. It will be seen from the illustrations that the amount of dead space in such masks is larger than that in the rigid Harris and M.C. masks. Even with a flow of 10 litres per minute carbon dioxide may accumulate in such a bag.

All the masks described are disposable.

Intranasal methods include:

(*a*) Nasal catheters, lubricated with xylocaine and inserted about 2 cms. into the nostril. These may be carried on a spectacle frame e.g. in Tudor Edwards spectacles. This method is satisfactory, provided that the patient can keep the mouth closed.

(*b*) Nasal cannulae inserted 7 to 10 cms. (i.e. into the nasopharynx) can give a higher concentration of oxygen, but are not very comfortable.

Babies who require oxygen are best nursed in heated humidified incubators. The amount of oxygen given to newborn babies must not rise above 40%, since giving high concentrations of oxygen is believed to cause formation of fibrous tissue behind the lens of the eye (retrolental fibroplasia) which may lead to blindness.

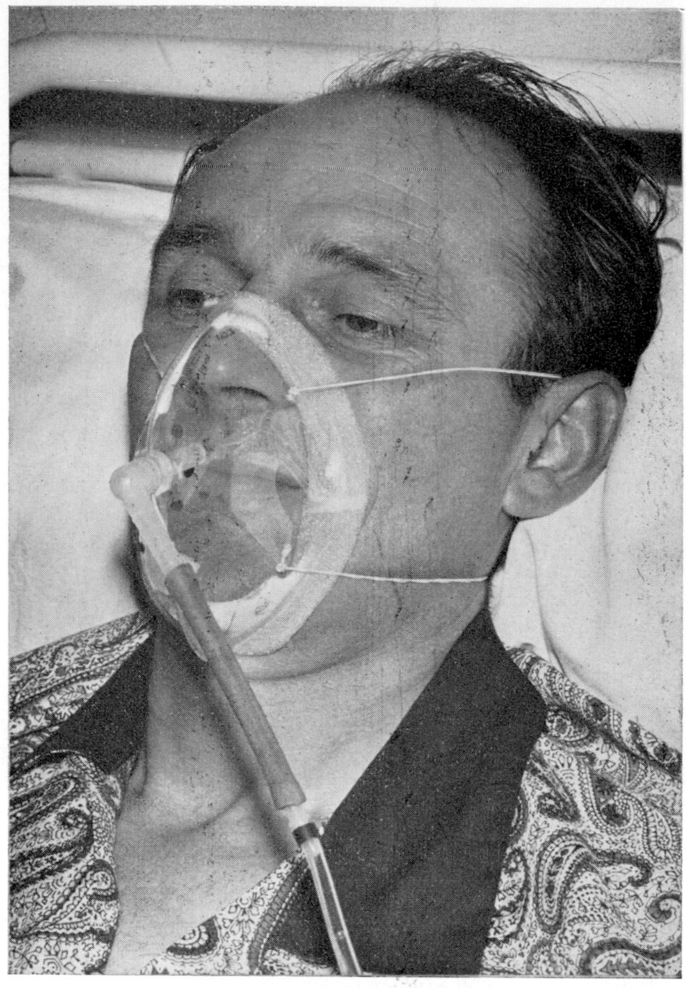

FIG. 41. M.C. disposable mask.

A very small number of patients (e.g. those with carbon monoxide poisoning) will benefit from very high oxygen concentrations, approaching 100%. Such concentrations have always been thought irritating, and they are only given for short periods, with careful attention to moistening.

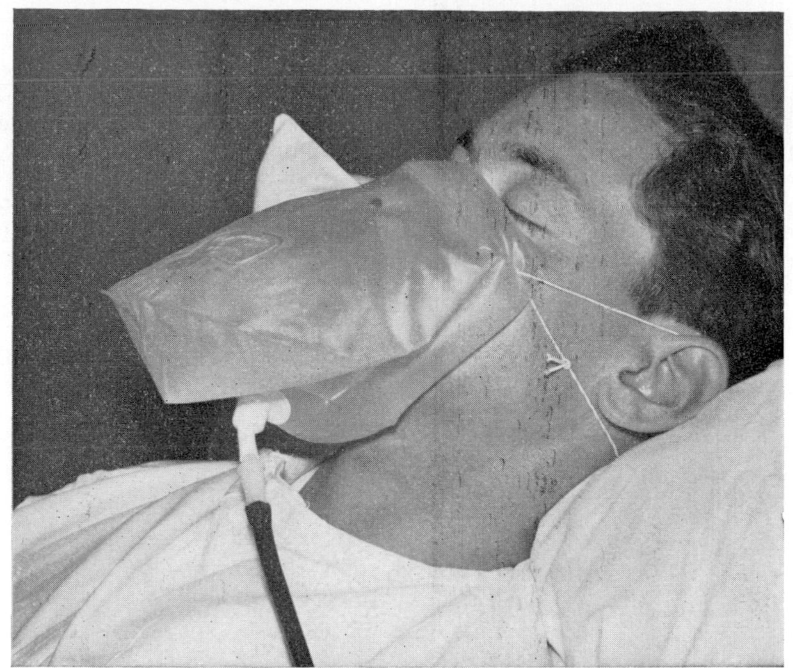

FIG. 42. Non-rigid disposable mask. Notice that the amount of dead space is greater than in the two preceding types.

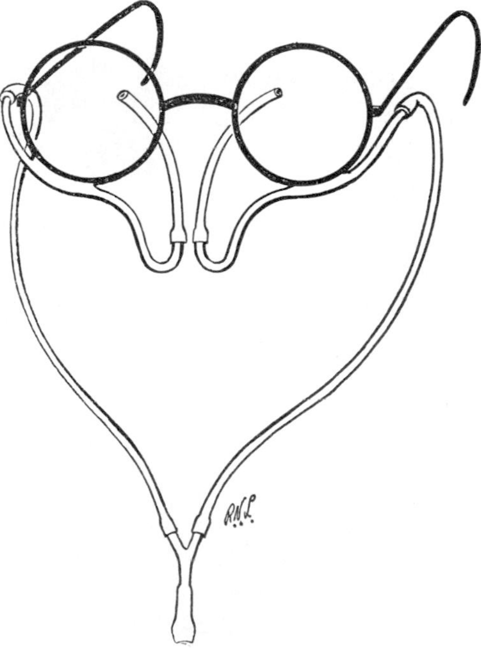

FIG. 43. Tudor Edward's oxygen spectacles.

Hyperbaric oxygen. By raising the pressure of the oxygen which the patient breathes to 2 or 3 atmospheres, the blood may be supersaturated with a high tension of dissolved oxygen. Special hyperbaric tanks or chambers are used, which may accommodate only the patient, or his attendants as well. Hyperbaric oxygen was first introduced as a preliminary to radiotherapy, the effect of which it is thought to enhance. It has since been used effectively for carbon monoxide poisoning, gas gangrene and following operations involving large skin flaps.

Moistening Oxygen

High concentrations of dry oxygen irritate the lining membranes of the bronchi and alveoli. If a plastic mask is used, the moisture from

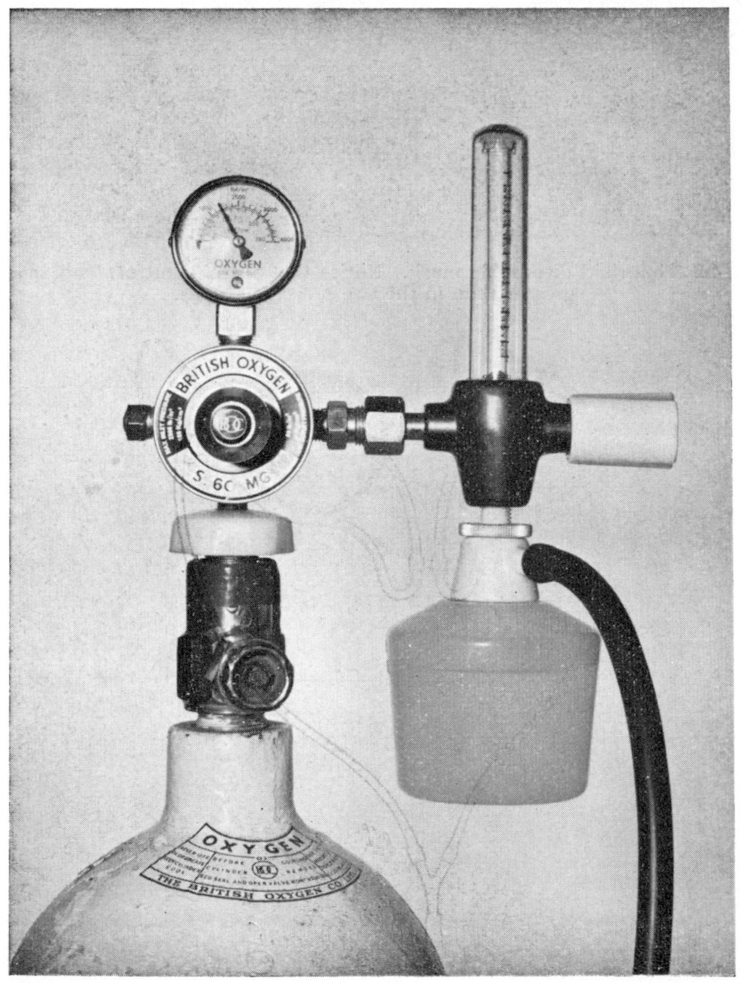

Fig. 44. Cold nebulizer for moistening oxygen. The water container is below the flow meter.

the patient's breath in the mask may provide sufficient humidification. If nasal catheters are used, moistening is absolutely necessary. The means that are available are:

1. *Woulfe's bottle.* This is the oldest method. The bottle has a rubber bung pierced by two tubes. One is long, and reaches below the surface of the water in the bottle; the other is short. The oxygen enters through the long tube, bubbles through the water, and emerges through the short tube. Care must always be taken to attach the oxygen to the right tube, or water may be forced out of the bottle, and even into the

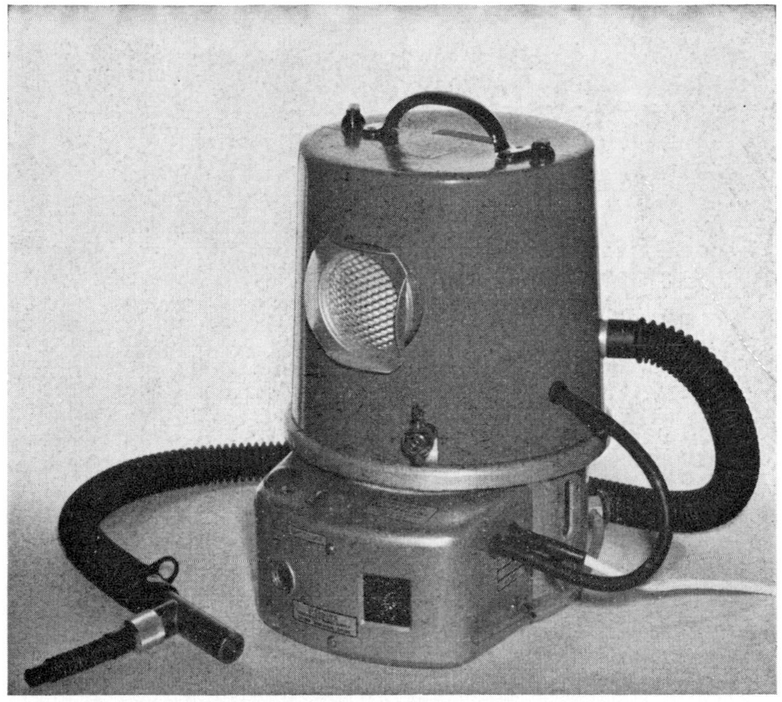

Fig. 45. Heated water-vapour humidifier. The fan is in the upper part, and the water, kept at a temperature of 50° C, in the lower.

patient's airway. If high concentrations are used, the bung may be blown out. The most that can be said for Woulfe's bottle is that it is better than nothing.

2. *Cold nebulizers.* The oxygen passes over the surface of water in a container attached to the oxygen source (see illustration). The principle is the same as that in a scent spray.

3. *Heated water vapour humidifiers* (see illustration). In the lower part the water is kept at a thermostatically controlled temperature of 50° C. In the upper part is a fan which blows air over the water, and oxygen is led in to enrich the mixture.

4. *Ultrasonic cold water* ("*cold steam*") *nebulizers.* A fine and penetrating mist is produced in this type, said to penetrate most effectively to the alveoli.

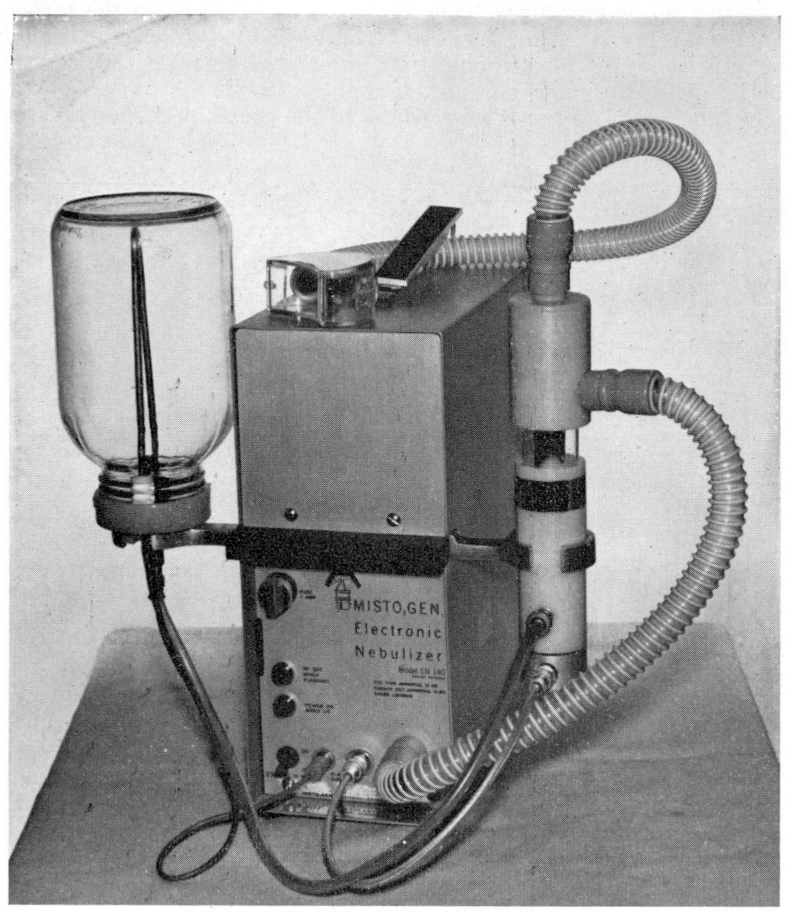

FIG. 46. Cold water ultrasonic nebulizer.

5. *Heat exchange humidifiers.* The one illustrated is attached to a cuffed tracheostomy tube, and is often used in this way. Within the apparatus is a wire mesh screen, one of which is shown separately. The patient's breath condenses on this and provides humidification.

Setting Up the Apparatus

When all is assembled, the oxygen is turned out to the required rate. If a mask is used, it is held to the patient's face, and he is told of the help it will be to his breathing, and it is fastened in place. The nurse

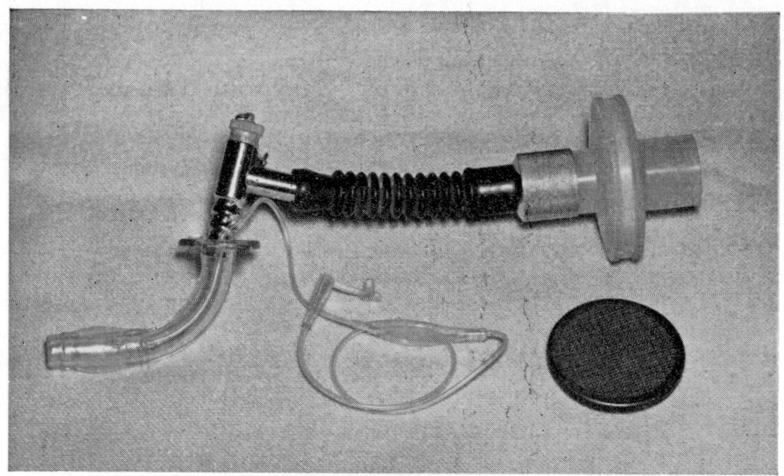

FIG. 47. The parts shown, from left to right, are:
1. Cuffed Portex tracheostomy tube.
2. Cobb's suction union.
3. Catheter mount.
4. Condenser-humidifier.

Below is the wire gauze insert of the humidifier.

remains with him making sure that he will co-operate with the treatment. The colour, respiration and pulse should be noticed.

Oxygen Tents

The basic idea of an oxygen tent is to enclose the patient in a plastic tent or canopy, and to fill this with oxygen so that the patient is surrounded by a high-oxygen atmosphere. The chief difficulty is to keep down the temperature inside the tent, and some device for securing this must be incorporated in the design. This is usually an electric refrigeration unit.

Tents are used for adults only if they cannot tolerate a mask or nasal catheters, but tents and incubators are extensively used for children.

The most modern ones consist of a refrigeration unit to which the oxygen is led through a moistening device. This part can be pushed under the bed. From it rises a metal frame from which is suspended a plastic canopy which is large enough to be tucked in all round the bed to enclose the patient. Zip fasteners allow access to all parts of the patient, and there are holes through which tubes and leads can pass. There are hooks for suspending intravenous bottles.

When the tent is in use it is brought to the bedside, and plugged into an electric supply. The water-bottle through which the oxygen passes is filled with distilled water, which must be renewed daily. The patient must be assured of the benefit he will feel from the use of the tent. A thermometer is fastened to the bed, the canopy is drawn over the bed and flushed with oxygen. The temperature within is regulated by a control on the outer panel, and should not rise above 65° F. The transparent canopy allows the patient to be observed from all angles, which lessens his sense of isolation. He should not be left alone at first ; the nurse will need to observe his mental reactions to the tent, as well as the effect on his colour, respiration and pulse.

There is a very real risk of fire when an oxygen tent is in use, and no electric fires, naked lights or smoking should be allowed in its vicinity. Visitors and fellow patients should be warned about this. Static electricity may also start a fire, and children should not have metal toys in a tent, especially those which wind up. Friction of blankets on mackintoshes may also generate electricity in a dry atmosphere, and bedmaking should be gentle. Should a fire occur, the oxygen must at once be turned off.

Steam Inhalations

The inhalation of steam is beneficial in inflammation of the air passages and the accessory nasal sinuses. During the early acute stages it lessens the pain and in the later stages it loosens the secretions and helps in their expulsion. Sometimes the patient is best helped by being nursed in an atmosphere impregnated with steam ; those with bronchitis and patients after tracheotomy (when air passes directly into the trachea without being warmed and moistened in the nose) are instances. For these, a steam tent may be used; for those with head colds, sinusitis, laryngitis or bronchitis, inhalation of steam from a receptacle of hot water is practised.

Proprietary forms of inhaler such as the Maw and Nelson are made, but have no special advantage over a jug. Steam is inhaled from them through a glass spout fitted in a cork, and this mouthpiece is easily broken. Moreover, the steam is inhaled through the mouth, so that colds and sinusitis cannot be well treated in this way.

Steam from boiling water is unpleasant and affords opportunity for scalds. It should never be used. A pint of hot water made of 15 oz. of boiling water and 5 of cold will afford steam of a comfortable temperature, and if the container is wrapped in a wool cover, it will continue to do so for the ten minutes that the inhalation should last.

Other safety precautions include supervision of patients not well enough to be left alone with the inhaler, and standing the jug in a flat-bottomed bowl to prevent spilling. Children should never be left alone.

Equipment Two-pint earthenware jug.
Flannel or wool cover.
Flat-bottomed bowl, with handle.
Small hand towel.
Pint measure.
Poison measure.
Boiling and cold water.
Inhalant (Friar's balsam, pine or menthol as prescribed).

At bedside. Bedjacket.
Sputum carton.
Heart table or locker.

The patient should be sitting up, supported with pillows and with the upper parts warmly covered. Fifteen ounces of boiling water and 5 oz. of cold are put into the jug. The inhalant is measured and added ; in the absence of other instructions from the prescriber, the dose is 1 dr. The towel is folded round the mouth of the jug, and the inhaler firmly placed where the patient can comfortably breathe the vapour, and the nurse assures herself that she can manage it safely and efficiently. The nose and mouth are put into the opening made by the towel, so that the steam only reaches the air passages. A dry bath towel may be put over the head and inhaler if the patient cannot lean forward, but this is not a very comfortable method especially for women, whose hair is ruffled, and who dislike the sweating and flushing of the face that follows enclosure of the head in a towel. Such an enclosure should never be used with a menthol inhaler, as the vapour irritates the eyes. After the inhaler has been used for ten minutes, it is taken away, the face is dried, and the patient comfortably settled. Ambulant patients being treated with inhalers should remain in a room at an even temperature, and not expose themselves to cold air while the blood vessels in the nasal mucosa are dilated.

If Maw's inhaler is ordered for laryngitis and bronchitis, it is used in exactly the same way. A single fold of gauze is wrapped around the glass mouthpiece, and while the inhaler is in use the outlet must be directed away from the patient's chest, or steam will saturate her night clothes.

Friar's balsam forms a deposit on the container which cannot be removed by soap and water. Immediately after use stains should be rubbed off with a rag dipped in spirit.

Steam Tents

A steam tent is most conveniently made by erecting a canopy on screens over the head of the bed or cot. An electric kettle is highly desirable, for a spirit lamp beneath a kettle adds the danger of fire to the hazards described later. If such a lamp is used, a bucket of sand should be near by and the patient is not left alone.

Requirements. 1 sheet.
1 or 2 screens.
Bronchitis kettle of boiling water.
Wall thermometer.
Safety pins.

The screen (or screens if small) is arranged around the head of the bed to form three sides of a rectangle, and the feet steadied with sand-bags or weights. The sheet is put over the top, with about 12 in. overlapping in front, and the ends at each side of equal length. The corners are folded square and secured with pins, so that the final result is neat and symmetrical. The thermometer is fastened to the inside. The kettle is placed on a suitable stand, plugged in, and the spout directed into the tent along its side wall.

The dangers of this form of treatment are :

1. The kettle may be overturned by a restless patient. It must be well out of reach.

2. The patient may be scalded by steam. This cannot happen if the spout is correctly placed.

3. The kettle may be overfilled and may spurt boiling water. Common sense precautions will prevent this.

4. The kettle may boil dry. Again, the remedy is obvious.

While the tent is in use, the temperature within it should be watched, and should not be allowed to rise above 75° F. or 24° C. The kettle is replenished at regular intervals with boiling water. The temperature, pulse and respiration of the patient are regularly noted, and the amount of relief obtained from the steam. Though a steam tent can be erected in a general ward, a separate room for the patient is a great convenience.

Cold water humidifiers, if available, are efficient and safe, and will be preferred for children's use.

CHAPTER 15

ARTIFICIAL FEEDS

ARTIFICIAL feeds are given into the stomach (or occasionally the small intestine) by a catheter and do not have to be swallowed by the patient. The catheter may be passed via the nose or mouth or through an artificial opening into the alimentary tract. They may be :

1. **Œsophageal.** The catheter by which the feed is given may be passed by the *nasal* or the *oral route.*
2. **Gastrostomy.** The meal is given through an in-dwelling catheter fixed in the stomach through the abdominal wall at operation. An ileostomy may be similarly used.

SOME PRINCIPLES OF ARTIFICIAL FEEDS

1. In all patients who are not eating in the normal way the *care of the mouth* is of the greatest importance.
2. Food swallowed is warmed during the passage down the œsophagus. An artificial feed must have the *temperature* adjusted to 100° F. (38° C.) before being given.
3. The *calorie value* and *constituents* of the meal must be considered if artificial feeding is to be continued. Milk, eggs and sugar form the basis of most fluid feeds ; extra protein can be added in the form of casilan, and vitamins must not be forgotten. If feeds are supplied in bulk by the diet kitchen, the fluid must be well stirred before the feed is measured out. A recipe for a fluid feed is given on p. 82.
4. Patients who are conscious and alert (e.g. those with carcinoma of œsophagus having gastrostomy feeds) will be interested in their feeds. Appetite can be felt and the thought of food enjoyed even though it is not swallowed, and the aroma of coffee or soup may make them want some, and fluids that the patient fancies can be given.
5. Precautions must be taken to prevent fluid entering the airway of those who are unconscious. It is best to pass tubes far enough to reach the stomach, since regurgitation of fluid is less likely to occur. Once the tube has been passed, one of these methods should be used to ensure that the tube has not entered the trachea.

1. A syringe and Tubbs' adaptor is attached to the tube, and a few drops of stomach contents withdrawn. These can be tested with litmus paper for acidity.
2. The funnel and tubing through which the feed is to be given can be connected to the tube, and the mouth of the funnel inverted under water. An odd bubble may escape even if the tube is in the stomach, but a stream of bubbles indicates that it is in the airway.

Artificial feeds to the unconscious should always be given with the patient lying on his side, or with the head turned to one side to guard against possible inhalation of regurgitated fluid.

Nasal Feeds

These are widely used for the unconscious and for those who have had laryngeal operations.

Requirements. Feed, at 100° F. (38° C.) in a measure in a bowl of warm water.
Food thermometer.
Fine œsophageal catheter.
Narrow funnel, 12 in. (30 cm.) of tubing and glass connection, in receiver.
Instrument tray with gallipots with swabs, liquid paraffin and blue litmus paper.
10 ml. syringe and Tubbs' adaptor.
Dissecting forceps.
2 oz. of warm water.
Waterproof and napkin.
Mouth tray, with spatula and gag.
Strapping and spigot.
Receiver.

Method. The patient is adjusted to a suitable position, and if there is any crusting of the nostrils, these should be cleaned with liquid paraffin and forceps. The mackintosh and towel are placed in position. The tube is lubricated and introduced into one nostril, and passed along the floor of the nose into the pharynx. As it passes down, the patient may swallow if not too deeply unconscious, and this will confirm that it is passing into the œsophagus. The length needed to reach the stomach is about the distance between the bridge of the nose and the xipisternum, and when this amount has been passed it should be fastened to the cheek with strapping, and its position in the stomach checked. The commonest wrong direction it can take is not into the airway, but forward into the mouth, and the spatula should be used to ensure that this has not happened.

An ounce of water is introduced into the funnel and tubing, which is connected to the tube. If it runs in uneventfully the feed is now poured into the funnel and allowed to run slowly in. When it is finished, the rest of the water is added to rinse the tube. If it is to be removed, it is pinched to prevent any fluid entering the larynx during removal and gently withdrawn. If it is to be left in, a spigot is inserted and the strapping made secure. Feeds can be given through the indwelling tube, which must be taken out, cleaned, boiled and repassed every twenty-four hours.

Continuous Milk Feeds ("Drip" Method)

Milk run continuously into the stomach from a reservoir, drip chamber and indwelling transnasal tube, is occasionally used in the treatment of acute peptic ulcer to relieve severe pain. The gastric hyperacidity is controlled, and pain usually disappears in twenty-four hours. From 2 to 3 litres are given a day, usually citrated, and there is no contra-indication to the patient taking small meals as well if his physician permits it.

Requirements. Jug of milk.
Glass reservoir with cover, two 12-in. (30-cm.) pieces of tubing and drip and plain connections.

Requirements. (cont.)
Fine œsophageal catheter.
Instrument tray with gallipots of swabs and liquid paraffin, 10-ml. syringe and litmus paper.
Waterproof and towel.
Receiver.
Stand.

The patient should sit up and the tube is passed with the precautions described above. The reservoir is filled with milk, which is allowed to run as far as the glass connection, clipped off, and joined to the in-dwelling tube. The rate of flow is adjusted to 40 drops a minute.

If the drip stops, or the drip connection becomes full of milk, the glass connection should be disconnected from the tube. Milk will probably flow from the connection, showing that the block is in the œsophageal catheter. If it is, the tube should be syringed through with 10 ml. of water, and this will always clear it. The reservoir must be kept covered, and replenished as required with a measured amount of milk.

Œsophageal Feeds

Œsophageal feeds are most used in general hospitals for small babies who are too ill or weak to suck. They may also be used for psychiatric patients.

Requirements for a baby.
Feed, in its sterile bottle, or measure, standing in a bowl of water at 105° F. (or 40° C.)
Thermometer.
Narrow funnel, tubing glass connection, and fine catheter (10 F). Small clip.
Swabs.
Glycerine.
Waterproof and bib.

The baby is turned on to its side, and the mackintosh and bib put in place. The tip of the catheter is lubricated in glycerine, and when put on to the back of the tongue is usually sucked and so swallowed with no difficulty. The correct position of the tube should not be checked by stomach aspiration, but by connecting the funnel and tubing and putting the funnel into water. Water can be run through the catheter before the milk, as described for nasal feeds, but is usually omitted for small babies who cannot accommodate large quantities of fluid. The rate of flow must be slow if regurgitation is to be prevented. After the catheter has been pinched and gently removed the baby's wind must be brought up in the usual way.

Gastrostomy Feeds

A gastrostomy is an opening into the stomach through the abdominal wall into which a catheter is secured. It is most often performed to maintain the nutrition of patients with a cancer occluding the œsophagus, but may also be done as a prelude to œsophageal surgery, or for an innocent stricture. In either case, the catheter remains in position, closed by a spigot, and does not have to be passed for each

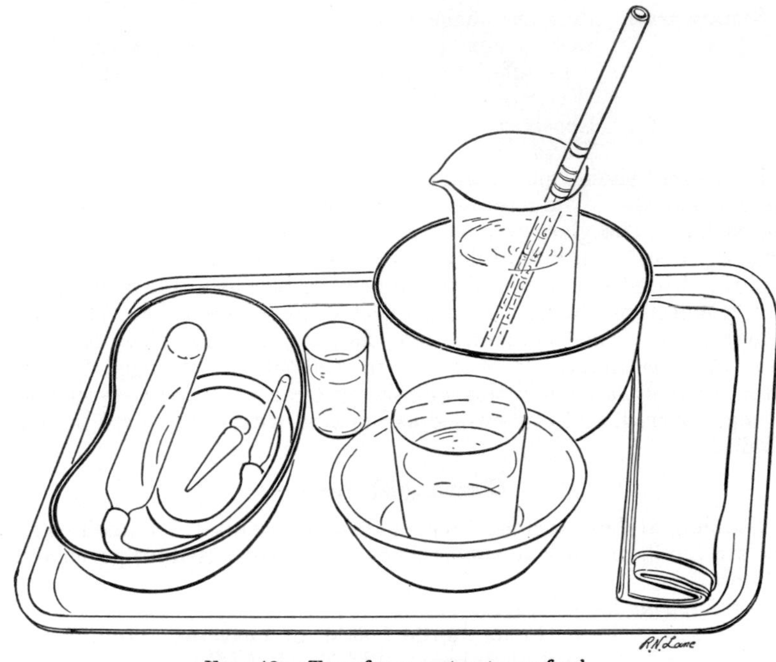

FIG. 48. Tray for a gastrostomy feed.

feed. These people, it must be remembered, are not unconscious. What is a " feed " to the nurse is a meal to them, and the tray should be arranged neatly.

Requirements. Narrow funnel, 12 in. (30 cm.) of tubing, glass connection.
Feed at 100° F. (38° C.), in a bowl of warm water.
30 ml. of warm water.
Waterproof and cover.

The feed is given with the patient sitting up, and the bedclothes folded down. The catheter is exposed and unspigotted, and the protective and cover arranged. Some of the water is put into the funnel and tubing, which is joined to the catheter, and as the water runs in the feed, is added to the funnel. If the patient is to return home with a gastrostomy, he may gradually be introduced to the process of feeding himself by helping to hold the funnel or the jug, and finally both.

Toilet of the abdominal wall is performed daily, and the strapping renewed. Leakage of gastric juice, causing soreness of the skin, is not usual because the stomach wall is turned in around the catheter at operation, but if it occurs, a protective application such as aluminium paint should be made at once before excoriation can take place.

CHAPTER 16

MEDICAL NURSING

The discussions of some common conditions that make up this chapter are not intended to be full medical accounts ; for these a textbook of medicine must be consulted. The subjects selected are those which present nursing problems to be solved, or opportunities for health education, or which are linked to other conditions.

Patients in medical wards generally stay longer than those on the surgical side, so that there is more time in which to establish a helpful relation, but also the problems of rehabilitation are more difficult. Many of them are suffering from chronic diseases, and recovery can be only partial. Many have to be taught while in hospital how to adjust themselves to life with some permanent condition, like diabetes or pernicious anæmia.

HEART FAILURE

Failure of the heart means failure of the cardiac muscle efficiently to perform its functions. The kinds of causes that can produce failure are these :

(*a*) *Toxic.* The muscle can be poisoned by substances in the blood.

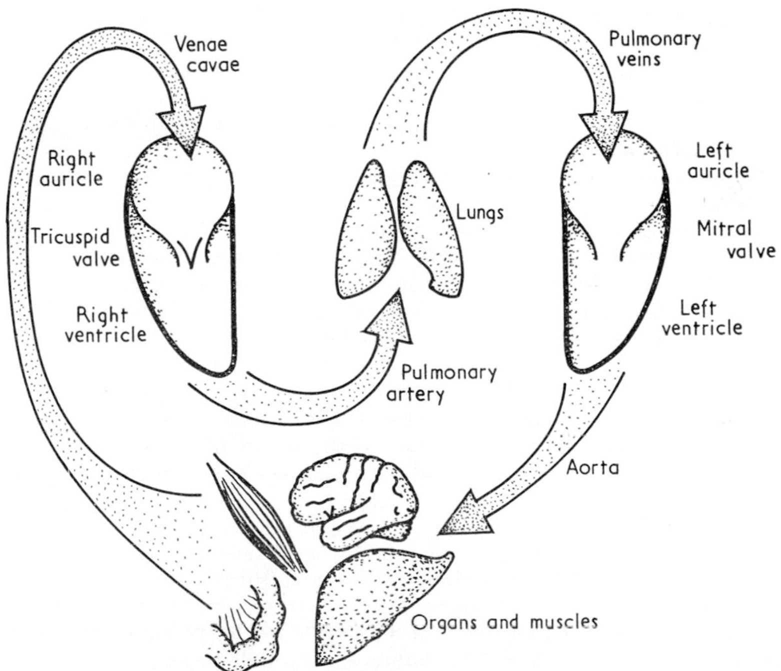

Fig. 49. The pathway of the blood.

Diphtheria is a disease in which toxic heart failure is a feared complication.

(*b*) *Mechanical.* If the conditions of work of heart muscle are unfavourable the heart may by overwork compensate for the handicap, but in time failure supervenes. Examples of such handicaps are hypertension, when the heart has to force blood out against raised arterial pressure ; congenital cardiac deformities ; narrowing (stenosis) or incompetence of heart valves ; overloading of the circulation by injudicious transfusion.

(*c*) *Ischæmia.* Interference with the blood supply from the coronary arteries is a common cause of failure.

The signs and symptoms of congestive heart failure vary because one side of the heart is usually affected before the other. The accompanying diagram may make this clear. The blood may be thought of as following a continuous path around the body, and if obstruction to the onward flow occurs at any point, there will be congestion behind it. For instance, if a patient has hypertension the left ventricle may eventually dilate and become inefficient, when blood will collect in the lungs, so that the patient with left heart failure has pulmonary œdema, and acute attacks of breathlessness at night. If the right ventricle fails, blood tends to stagnate in the systemic veins, causing venous engorgement of the liver and the superficial veins. In clinical practice, failure of one side of the heart is followed by failure of the other within a comparatively short time.

Since the heart supplies blood to all organs, the signs and symptoms may relate to any system in the body :

Circulatory—decreased pulse volume and irregularities in rhythm ; œdema of dependent parts, coldness of extremities, palpitation, cardiac pain, venous engorgement.

Respiratory—cyanosis, dyspnœa, orthopnœa, cough, hæmoptysis, cardiac asthma.

Digestive—anorexia, constipation.

Renal—oliguria, albuminuria.

The aims of the medical and nursing staff are :

(*a*) *To improve the heart's efficiency* by absolute rest, oxygen for cyanosis, and such drugs as digitalis preparations (see p. 96).

(*b*) *To relieve the œdema* by a low salt diet (p. 72); diuretics such as chlorothiazide, ethacrynic acid or frusemide.

(*c*) *To forestall complications by vigilance.* An accurate intake and output chart is essential; the pulse is recorded four hourly, and if there is atrial fibrillation, the pulse deficit is ascertained. The drugs used in treatment may cause upset of the blood potassium level, and such signs as thirst, confusion and muscular weakness must be watched for.

(*d*) *To relieve discomforts* by all available nursing measures. A heart bed which allows the foot end to be lowered is very useful for the œdematous breathless patient, as it allows fluid to drain downwards. A sorbo ring will relieve pressure on the buttocks, the feet should have a support to prevent foot drop, and a cradle to carry the weight of the bedclothes. Pillows should be numerous enough to support him in a sitting position, and a heart table may help the really breathless patient by enabling him to fix his shoulder girdle. The pressure areas must be frequently and adequately treated, which is not easy if the patient is heavy and breathless. Sleeplessness is common because of the many discomforts, and anxiety is understandable. Both can be relieved by drugs.

Acute attacks of congestive failure can often be surmounted, and if the cause can be treated the prognosis is much improved. If it cannot, the patient may be discharged to a life of limited activity within his cardiac reserve. He must be warned against putting on excess weight. Treatment by diuretics may be continued at home by the doctor or district nurse.

PACEMAKERS

Damage to the conducting system of the heart may result in heart block, in which the ventricles receive less than the normal number of impulses from the atria, or may even be cut off completely. Patients such as these may have abnormally slow pulse rates, and are prone to attacks of dizziness and less of consciousness, and also to cardiac arrest. For the severely disabled, the implantation of an electrical artificial pacemaker may be considered. A wire is passed along the internal jugular vein into the right ventricle, and along this are passed impulses from a small unit which is implanted beneath the skin of the axilla. The batteries in the unit must be replaced every two or three years. Although the mechanical reliability of pacemakers improves continually, there is always a risk of the system failing or a wire breaking, and only people who are severely handicapped are given this form of treatment.

SOME DISEASES OF ARTERIES

Degeneration of the walls of the arteries is a common accompaniment of increasing age, and as the age of the population rises more patients with arterial disease and its complications appear in medical wards. The pathology of these conditions is difficult and the naming confused, and the account given here is only of the main clinical effects of these arterial changes.

HYPERTENSION

The blood pressure is maintained and varied mostly by the tone of the muscular walls of the arterioles. In elderly patients thickening and hardening may occur widely in these muscular walls, leading to a rise in the blood pressure. This rise may be secondary to kidney disease and a few endocrine disorders, but appears often to be primary, when it is known as *essential hypertension.* The effects are felt first by the heart, which has to put out the blood against increased resistance ; by the cerebrum, where a vascular accident like hæmorrhage or thrombosis may occur ; by the retina, shown by limitation of sight ; and by the kidney, which may show albuminuria leading to uræmia.

Mild hypertension is compatible with many years of comfortable life, and treatment consists of giving phenobarbitone in small doses, and advocating a quiet life on a simple non-fattening diet. Severe hypertension, especially arising rapidly in comparatively young patients, requires active treatment if sight is to be saved, and heart failure, cerebro-vascular accident or uræmia averted.

The patient is admitted to a medical ward and his clinical condition carefully assessed; accurate observations on the pulse, urine and blood pressure are especially important. New drugs to treat hypertension are regularly introduced; the two most commonly ordered today are methyldopa and guanethidine. Methyldopa reduces the constricting effects on blood vessels of the sympathetic system, and can cause big falls in the blood pressure. Such a fall may occur suddenly when the patient gets up from bed, and gastric upsets, nasal congestion, dry mouth and drowsiness are unwanted side effects. Diuretics like chlorothiazide enhance the action of methyldopa. Guanethidine reduces sympathetic activity and is a long-acting drug which may only have to be given once a day. Dizziness can arise quite suddenly and patients must be warned of this hazard.

The most striking clinical impression made on nurses by these drugs is the disappointing fact that though they may lower the blood pressure effectively, this fall usually makes the patient feel worse for a considerable time. He must be warned not to get up suddenly from bed or the drain of blood from the brain can cause fainting. Constipation and difficulty in micturition are common complications, and the patient must be helped through the initial discouraging phase by assurance that once his blood pressure is stabilized at a lower level he will feel better, and complications will be averted.

Atherosclerosis

Narrowing and hardening of the arteries is quite a common accompaninent of advancing age, especially in men with diabetes. The narrowing occurs most often in the arteries to the legs, and the first symptom is pain in the calves on walking.

This pain is ischæmic, because the narrowed arteries cannot provide the extra blood the muscles need when active. If the patient stands still, the pain disappears. Such patients run the risk of gangrene of the feet, and should take special precautions to avoid it. Socks should be clean, dry and free from bulky darns; shoes should be well-fitting; chiropody and toe-nail trimming should if possible be done professionally, since minor injuries to the feet are often the starting point of gangrene.

In nursing patients threatened with gangrene of the leg, it must be remembered that the needs of the tissues for oxygen and foodstuffs rises as the temperature rises, so the threatened limb should be kept cool by exposing it to room temperature. The head of the bed can be raised on blocks so that the blood supply to the leg is increased by gravity. Pressure must be completely removed from the heel by placing a small pillow under the Achilles' tendon, and the same care must be given to the other heel, the blood supply of which is usually little better than on the affected side. Smoking should be forbidden, since nicotine is a vaso-constrictor in action, but alcohol, which dilates superficial vessels, may be permitted. Vaso-dilator drugs like tolazoline may be ordered, and if the vessels are still capable of dilating, a lumbar sympathectomy may be helpful by removing the constricting effect of the sympathetic nerve fibres.

Often after successful medical care and skilful nursing it will be found that the amount of tissue that actually becomes gangrenous is little, if any, and very small operations may be needed. There are other cases, however, in which treatment is unsuccessful, and amputation has to be undertaken at a level where the blood supply is adequate to allow healing, and this may be as high as the mid-thigh.

Atheroma

In atheroma, changes in the lining of arteries produces raised ulcerative plaques. These slowly diminish the volume of the blood flow through the arteries, and also encourage the formation of blood clots on the rough areas, which may cut off suddenly the blood flow to the part affected. The commonest conditions due to atheroma are:

(*a*) Cardiac ischæmia, causing the painful and alarming *angina pectoris*, and predisposing to thrombosis in the coronary arteries.

(*b*) Cerebral thrombosis if it is the vessels of the brain that are affected.

(*c*) Uræmia due to atheroma of the renal arteries.

Coronary Thrombosis

A very large number of patients, mainly middle-aged men, suffer thrombosis of a coronary artery every day. A number of them die suddenly, but for those who reach hospital alive the prognosis is fairly good. They are admitted pale and sweating, with a low temperature and blood pressure, irregular and sometimes imperceptible pulse, and severe pain in the centre of the chest.

The patient is admitted to a warm bed with a few pillows to maintain him in a comfortable semi-recumbent position. Morphine is usually ordered at once to reduce the pain and anxiety, and oxygen is given with a mask at 6 litres per minute. The pulse is recorded every fifteen minutes, and the blood pressure hourly until stable.

In a severe case like the one described, anti-coagulant drugs are usually given to prevent extension of the clot in the coronary artery. Until the condition is under control, the patient is nursed at complete rest. The stages of activity will be decided by the physician after studying the pulse, blood pressure and electrocardiogram. It is usual to allow the patient to use a commode at the bedside after the first twenty-four hours, since it appears less strain than being lifted on to a bedpan. Convalescence should be leisurely, and a good proportion of patients can return to a life of medium activity, but it must be remembered that the atheroma that caused the clot is still present.

Cardiac arrest is more likely to occur in connection with coronary thrombosis than with any other medical condition. Arrest may be due to an upset of rhythm, and if this temporary difficulty can be overcome, the heart may be started again. The cardiac oscilloscope (cardioscope) if attached by leads to the limbs, will give a continual picture of the heart's action and the more complex machines will print on tape a

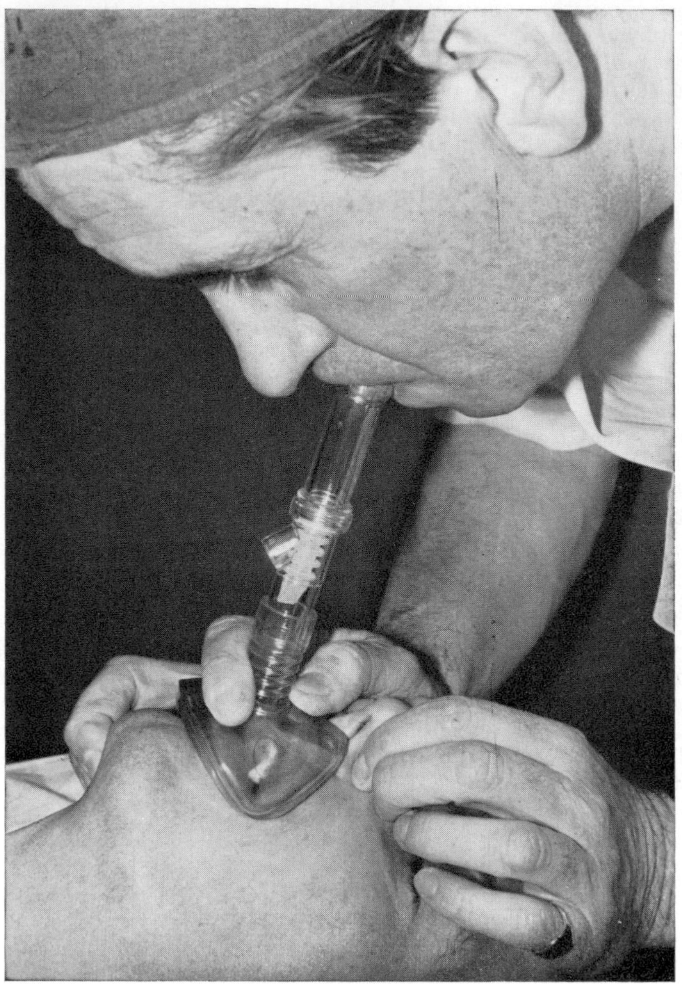

Fig. 50. The Brooke airway in use.

continual recording. The machine may also sound an alarm if the heart rate rises above or falls below a preset level. It is therefore possible to receive warning of impending trouble, and for the doctor to see on the cardioscope whether the ventricles have ceased to beat (asystole) or if they are beating ineffectively (ventricular fibrillation).

In cardiac arrest, no pulse can be felt in the carotid artery; breathing ceases; the pupils dilate, and the skin is pale or cyanosed. Treatment must be prompt, or irreversible brain damage will occur.

If enough help is available the patient is lifted onto the floor; if not, the board which should be kept for this purpose in every ward is put on the bed, and the patient rolled onto it. A firm thump on the sternum may restore the heartbeat in some cases.

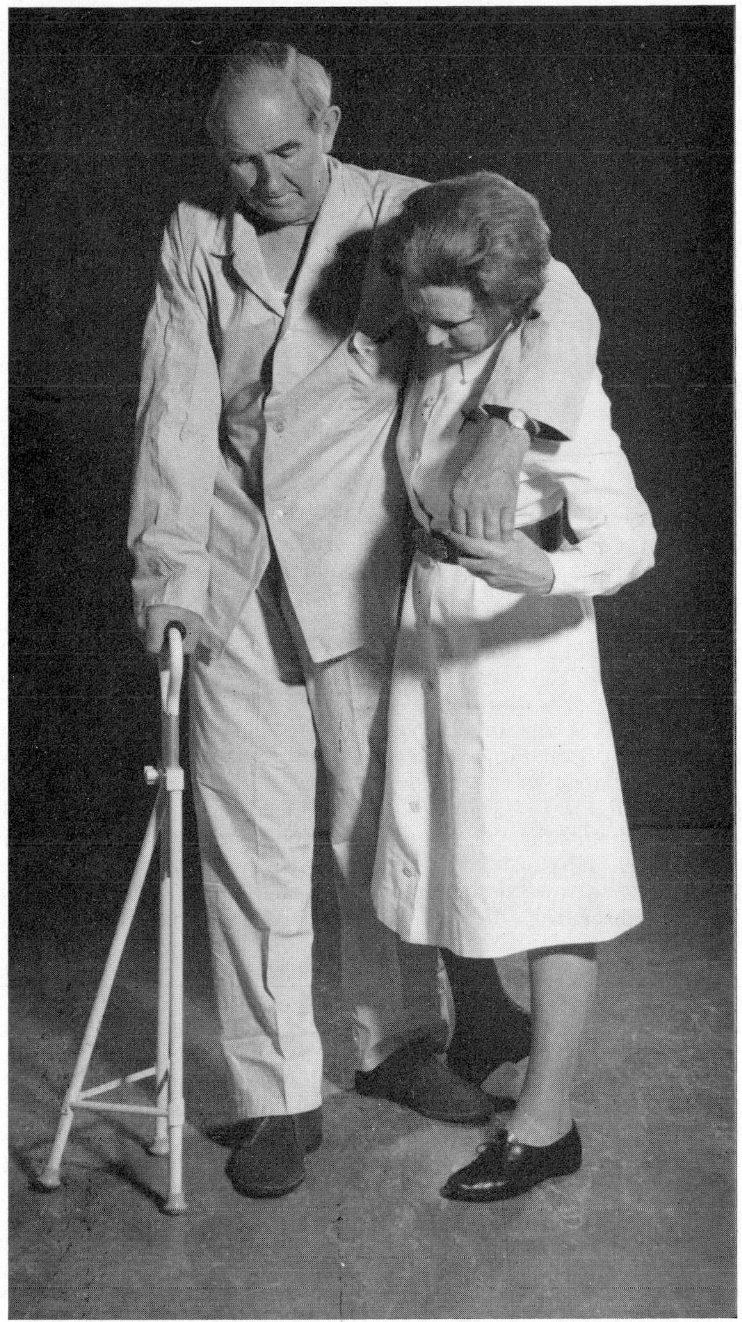

Fig. 51. Physiotherapy for the hemiplegic.

The designated resuscitation officer is summoned, and closed chest cardiac massage is begun, as described on p. 516. Artificial respiration is begun either with an Ambu bag or a Brooke airway. If the bag is used, the mask is applied to the face, with one hand, while the chin is supported by the ulnar border of the same hand. The bag is compressed at a rate of about 12 a minute, which allows time for the bag to refill completely. The illustration shows the method of use of the Brooke airway; the valve in the centre prevents aspiration of the patient's secretions by the operator.

When the doctor arrives, he will intubate the trachea and continue ventilation. An intravenous drip is set up, and sodium bicarbonate is given to neutralize the acid that has been accumulating as a result of respiratory failure. If the cause of arrest is ventricular fibrillation, an electric defibrillator is used. Cardiac massage is continued until the beat is restored, or further efforts are useless.

Such a dramatic episode causes much alarm to other patients, especially those with a similar condition, and the nurse must calm and comfort them.

Cerebral Thrombosis

Clotting of blood in a cerebral artery produces nervous effects related to the size of vessel affected, varying from mild difficulties with speech, or transient weakness of a few muscles, to *hemiplegia*, or complete paralysis of one side of the body. Only the more severe cases arrive in hospital, and on the success of treatment there depends the kind of life that the patient will be able to lead afterwards. Many people who formerly would have been confined to bed or a chair for the rest of their lives are now restored to considerable activity with the help of the physiotherapist, and a field of preventive medicine of great importance is open to the nursing staff who look after these patients.

On admission with hemiplegia following a stroke the pulse is slow and full, the breathing stertorous and the colour congested. Consciousness is not generally lost, but since the patient may not be able to speak or turn his head towards his attendants, this fact may not be realized by the less observant. It is possible to treat such a patient physically with great efficiency, but with lack of insight by handling him as if he were unconscious. Incontinence, for instance, is frequently a result of the patient's inability to make himself understood.

He should be nursed with the head and shoulders raised on pillows or with blocks at the upper end of the bed, and the usual records made. He is turned four-hourly to avoid pneumonia and pressure sores, and the mouth kept moist. It is usually possible to give fluids orally after the first twelve hours, so there should be no hurry to institute nasal feeds. When feeding such patients, care must be taken not to put food into the paralysed cheek. Restlessness may indicate a full bladder, and the timely offer of a urinal may prevent incontinence.

Once a patient has survived twenty-four hours, it can be assumed that he will recover, and the aims of the nurse and physiotherapist will be to mobilize him before he has forgotten his walking reflexes and become obsessed by the idea that he is paralysed. To ensure this it is also necessary to see that no contractures of the paralysed parts take place. Frequently some movement returns rapidly, as the spasm of cerebral vessels in the neighbourhood of the thrombus relaxes ; usually the leg recovers first, speech is frequently regained, while fine movements of the hand are the last to return.

A walking stick is not a very safe support for a handicapped patient, and the introduction of the tripod has been an advance that increases confidence. The wrist may need support to prevent flexion, and very light plastic splints can be made to fit. Even if the residual paralysis is extensive a patient can usually be taught to sit down and get up from a chair or lavatory unaided, and thus to attend to his own basic physical needs.

Acute Rheumatic Fever

Acute rheumatic fever or rheumatism is a disease believed to be caused by a streptococcal toxin, and it mainly affects the young people who are most likely to have streptococcal sore throats. It is less frequent now than formerly in this country, there are many parts of the Far East and South America where it is still a disease which carries a high mortality and affects the heart severely.

The patient, who is usually a child, has a fever of 101° or 102° F., and inflammation of one or two of the medium-sized joints of the limbs, such as the knees, ankles, elbows and shoulders. The joint is swollen, red and tender, and any movement is painful. In the course of a day or two, the inflammation subsides in one joint, but appears in another. In spite of the fever there is often well-marked sweating. The great danger of this disease is not, however, to the joints at all, but to the heart. Myocarditis, endocarditis and pericarditis may all occur in the acute stage, and lead to chronic disease that can eventually lead to heart failure.

The aim of medical and nursing care must, therefore, be absolute rest to avert the risk of heart complications and relief of fever and joint inflammation. Most physicians have abandoned the practice of nursing patients between blankets, but if sweating is marked a cotton blanket next to the patient will increase comfort. Only one pillow is given, a cradle takes the weight of the bedclothes from the tender joints.

Penicillin is given for at least ten days. Salicylates are always prescribed, either as soluble aspirin or as sodium salicylate. Patients who do not show a good response may be ordered a steroid drug such as prednisolone. During the time that the joints are inflamed they must be rested with small pillows and gamgee pads, and while the temperature and pulse are above normal the child must be nursed flat, fed and washed and rolled for bedmaking and pressure area treatment. A blanket bath is given daily and the fluid intake kept high. As the child begins to feel better, amusements must be found to relieve the tedium of lying flat. Activity is gradually resumed, but in most cases it will be three months before the child is up again, and it may be much longer if there is any sign of cardiac affection.

Observations to enable early diagnosis are of great importance. The pulse should be taken as frequently as its condition suggests. A rising pulse rate (especially if the temperature is normal), irregularities of rhythm, decreasing volume ; breathlessness or cyanosis should always be reported at once. Vomiting or ringing in the ears are signs of salicylate intolerance.

A holiday in a convalescent home is beneficial before return to school, and the parents are advised that sore throats must be taken seriously. Phenoxymethyl penicillin by mouth over long periods as a prophylactic is often prescribed after severe attacks; in such a case the patient and his parents will need encouragement and support by their doctor and health visitor. Effective treatment of tonsillitis reduces the incidence of acute rheumatism and its sequels of chronic valvular disease and heart failure, and also of the condition described next.

Bacterial Endocarditis

Endocarditis is inflammation of the heart lining and of the valves, which are made of endocardium. Rheumatic fever, described in the last section, may cause endocarditis. The bacterial form is that in which there is infection of the heart valves, which become crusted with layers of fibrin and clot which contain bacteria.

Bacteria gain entry to the blood stream occasionally—for instance after dental extraction—and normal people can usually deal with these without trouble. Those have existing valvular disease, or congenital heart lesions, may be unable to do so, and bacterial endocarditis develops.

The signs and symptoms in the acute case fall into 3 groups:

1. Those related to the septicæmia—swinging fever, tachycardia, anæmia and toxæmia.
2. Those resulting from emboli from the vegetations on the valves ; these emboli may lodge in the brain, kidney, spleen, lungs, or indeed in almost any organ.
3. Those of heart failure may appear.

The infection is usually streptococcal, but a variety of organisms may be responsible. The treatment is massive doses of the appropriate antibiotic, either by intramuscular or intravenous injection. Large intramuscular injections six hourly for long periods are very trying for the patient, and also for the staff who have to give them. The usual safe sites should be used in strict rotation. Intravenous injection through an indwelling plastic catheter may be preferred.

This is a disease with a high mortality, and people with pre-existing heart lesions should be given antibiotic cover to protect them from possible infection in these circumstances.

1. Before dental extraction or scaling.
2. Before cystoscopy or pelvic surgery.
3. Before tonsillectomy.
4. After abortion; some physicians would give antibiotics before a normal delivery.

The varied signs that may arise suddenly from embolism mean that the nurses must be alert in observation and reporting. The prognosis depends on how early the diagnosis is made, how severely the heart is affected before the infection can be controlled, and the skill with which the nursing is performed in this long and weary illness.

ANÆMIA

Anæmia is a reduction in the oxygen-carrying powers of the blood, either as a result of a fall in the number of red blood cells, or the hæmoglobin they contain, or both. It is a subject of fundamental importance in surgical as well as medical wards. The signs and symptoms of anæmia, whatever its cause, are pallor of skin and mucosæ, headache, lassitude, palpitation, tachycardia, breathlessness on exertion, and swelling of the ankles. In addition to these, there are special signs associated with the specific anæmias, and a medical textbook must be consulted with regard to these.

In the normal person taking a good diet, red cells are made at a rate which exactly balances the rate at which old cells are broken down (hæmolysed) in the spleen, and the colouring material resulting from hæmolysis is excreted by the liver in the bile, which owes its colour to these pigments.

Anæmia can be classified under these headings :

A. Anæmia due to Blood Loss, Acute or Chronic. This variety is most commonly seen in surgical wards, either as a result of operative loss, or because of such conditions as bleeding piles, or excessive menstrual loss. Such anæmia, even if not very severe, leads to indolent healing of wounds and must be corrected, usually by transfusion if rapid results are required.

B. Anæmia due to Deficient Blood Formation.

1. *Iron Deficiency.* Red meat is the chief iron-containing food and since this is expensive a simple dietetic anæmia is not uncommon in poorer patients, especially women, who have the usual monthly loss to make good. Those with dyspepsia or hypochrondria, or domestic difficulties often construct home-made diets which are lacking in iron, and need advice on food. An iron-deficiency anæmia due to faulty iron absorption is not uncommon in middle-aged women with achlorhydria and menorrhagia.

While diet is important, many people in this group must take iron. It may be given by mouth as ferrous sulphate, citrate or gluconate. Women who are given iron pills must be warned that they are poisonous to children, who will eat them for the sake of the sugar covering, and such pills must be locked up out of their reach.

Intramuscular iron is valuable for those who find difficulty in absorbing iron by mouth. When giving such an injection, the skin must be drawn to one side before inserting the needle, so that when it is withdrawn the needle track is angled, not straight. A swab is used to maintain firm counter-pressure round the needle as it is withdrawn, since if any of the solution leaks into the subcutaneous tissues it will cause an ugly and long-lasting discoloration of the skin.

2. *Vitamin B_{12} Deficiency.* This vitamin is present in food and is absorbed in the stomach in the presence of the intrinsic factor in the gastric juice. If the gastric juice is abnormal, the vitamin is not absorbed and pernicious anæmia results. It is a disease of adults, all of whom have achlorhydria, and may show motor and sensory changes due to an associated nervous condition, subacute combined degeneration of the cord.

The name is a relic of the time when this was a fatal disease ; today patients can be maintained in normal health by administration of the vitamin, either in liver extract, or more usually by giving the vitamin itself by intramuscular injection. Nurses must impress on their patients on discharge that as long as they attend regularly for their injections they will never suffer again from the symptoms of this condition.

C. Anæmia due to Excessive Hæmolysis. If breakdown of red blood cells occurs at a rate greater than their manufacture, anæmia will result, and the patient will suffer from jaundice because of the inability of the liver to clear the excess bilirubin from the blood.

The cause of the hæmolysis must be sought and found. Malaria, streptococcal septicæmia and neonatal jaundice in babies due to Rhesus incompatibility are examples of conditions in which hæmolysis causes anæmia.

Anæmia occurs as a secondary condition in many conditions such as cancer, chronic nephritis, rheumatoid arthritis, and leukæmia. It may be a cause of many of the patient's complaints, and if it can be relieved may greatly increase the sense of well-being, even if the primary condition is incurable.

JAUNDICE

Jaundice means yellowness, and it results from retention of bilirubin in the blood. It may be nothing more than a yellow tinge to the conjunctivæ, or may be enough to colour the whole skin dark brown. The kind which is easiest to understand is obstructive jaundice, in which the outflow of bile from the liver is prevented by such causes as a stone in the common bile duct, a carcinoma of the head of the pancreas, or malignant lymphatic glands. The common feature in each type is that the stools are pale because bile is failing to reach the intestine.

Another cause of jaundice is the excessive hæmolysis referred to in the last section. The jaundice is not commonly very pronounced, the stools are normal in colour, and it is always accompanied by anæmia.

The third group of cases have toxic or hepatic jaundice. The bile ducts are normal, but the liver cells are inflamed or degenerate and cannot excrete the bilirubin. Such jaundice is instanced by infective hepatitis, poisoning by arsenic, chloroform, chlorpromazine, etc., and cirrhosis or fibrous degeneration of the liver.

Obstructive and toxic jaundice produces symptoms such as depression, anorexia, nausea, skin irritation, and a tendency to bleed due to a fall in the prothrombin level of the blood. These symptoms may be treated, even if the cause itself is not amenable to cure. Bile salts may be given in capsules by mouth, and in obstructive jaundice may do much to relieve the nausea and vomiting. The diet should contain plenty of sugar, while any articles ill-tolerated should be omitted. Calamine lotion with phenol is useful for skin irritation, and vitamin K by intramuscular injection will raise the level of the prothrombin, of which it is a precursor.

Cirrhosis of the Liver

Cirrhosis is a fibrous degeneration of the liver which sometimes follows acute hepatitis, prolonged malnutrition, or chronic poisoning by toxins known (such as alcohol) and unknown. Dyspepsia, anorexia, and jaundice may occur early ; ascites is a later and serious sign, while bleeding from dilated veins in the œsophagus or rectum is a troublesome and dangerous complication. Coma is due to accumulation of the breakdown products of protein, which are normally dealt with in the liver.

The diet should be low in fat and high in glucose, and when coma threatens, the protein should be reduced as far as possible. In this connection, it must be remembered that bleeding into the stomach constitutes a high protein meal, and that hæmatemesis, therefore, is a double problem, threatening the life both because of loss of blood and from hepatic coma. A dextrose saline infusion is used if the patient is drowsy, and there is some indication that bacterial invasion of the small intestine is important, and that antibiotics may be of great value.

In a proportion of cases in which liver failure is not too advanced, the surgeon may anastomose the portal vein to the inferior vena cava, shunting the blood from the digestive area into the systemic circulation instead of into the liver.

ENDOCRINE DISORDERS

The hormones secreted by the endocrine glands influence not only the bodily structure and physiological activity but also the emotional reactions. All the ductless glands may show states of disordered activity marked by over or under secretion of their hormones. In general, under activity of a gland is treated by supplying the lacking hormone, while over secretion is treated by removal of part of the gland or the administration of a drug suppressing the hormone secretion of the gland affected. Two endocrine disorders will be described here ; thyrotoxicosis, in which the thyroid gland produces excess thyroxin, and diabetes mellitus, in which insufficient insulin for the physical needs is available in the blood.

Thyrotoxicosis

The typical thyrotoxic patient is a young woman complaining of nervousness, loss of weight, and protrusion of the eyeballs (*exophthalmos*). The pulse is rapid, the thyroid gland usually enlarged, the hands show a fine tremor, the appetite is good in spite of the loss of weight, and there is such restlessness that it is often possible to locate the thyrotoxic patient in a medical ward by the disorder of her bedclothes. There is another group of patients with overactive thyroids who are in their forties and have less florid toxic signs, but in whom the effects fall on the heart, so that atrial fibrillation is common and heart failure occurs early. In all cases the basal metabolic rate is raised.

Such a patient is admitted to a bed in a quiet part of the ward, if possible not within sight of cases that might distress her. She will have enough pillows to enable her to sit up, and light bedclothes, since she feels the heat. Her temperature and respiration rates are recorded four-hourly, and the pulse should also be taken while she is asleep to see if the tachycardia is still maintained. The rate should be taken at the apex as well as at the wrist if there is any irregularity, and the pulse deficit charted. An attitude of kindly calm must be maintained in nursing her, as she is easily upset. The diet should be high in calorie value, but excess protein must be avoided, because of its stimulating effect on metabolism, and extra carbohydrate as sugar, honey, jam or chocolate is useful. A high fluid intake is encouraged. A daily bed bath is given, and the pressure points of this thin, restless patient must be regularly treated, not forgetting the elbows which she often uses a great deal in changing her position. No difficulty is encountered in securing a bowel action.

The drugs prescribed will include phenobarbitone two or three times a day to allay restlessness, and if the thyrotoxicosis is to be treated medically an anti-thyroid drug such as propyl thiouracil or carbimazole (neo-mercazole) is given. Skin rashes, drug fever, and leucopenia sometimes attend their use, and relevant symptoms should be reported at once. If atrial fibrillation is present digitalis is indicated. If medical treatment is being undertaken preparatory to partial thyroidectomy Lugol's iodine is given for the three weeks preceding the operation.

The patient's emotional state has sometimes disturbed her relations with her family, who have not realized that she is ill rather than difficult, and relatives can be reassured that as her physical condition improves she will benefit mentally.

DIABETES MELLITUS

This disease is characterized by inability to metabolize carbohydrate, owing to a relative or absolute shortage of insulin secretion by the islets of Langerhans in the pancreas. The glucose which should be stored as glycogen in the liver accumulates in the blood, and when a level of 180 mg. per cent. has been exceeded, sugar begins to appear in the urine. Fat metabolism is affected, so that such substances as *ketones* (which are acids) and acetone begin to appear in the blood.

Two groups of diabetics are seen in the wards and clinics of hospitals :

(*a*) Obese middle-aged people, mainly women, with mild diabetes. They secrete insulin, but not in sufficient amounts to provide for their surplus weight and calorie intake. The treatment is dietetic ; once the weight has been reduced to normal, sugar will disappear from the urine. A diet of 1,000 C. is suitable, and the nurse should encourage the patient to persevere with it.

(*b*) Patients whose insulin secretion is not sufficient for normal needs. This group includes all the young people with diabetes.

The symptoms include *polyuria, thirst, loss of weight*. The urine contains sugar and usually acetone. *Skin irritation* and *boils* frequently accompany diabetes. The acute complication is *diabetic coma,* due to acidosis, but this is not now commonly seen, and does not carry the high mortality once associated with it. The chronic complications have assumed greater importance as diabetics are better treated and live longer. They are *arteriosclerosis*, with a tendency to cause ischæmic gangrene in the legs; infections such as *tuberculosis* and *cystitis*; *diabetic nephritis*; *cataract* and *retinitis*.

The treatment of diabetes falls under three headings:

(*a*) *Dietetic.* A diet containing a known amount of carbohydrate is ordered, and one containing 150 G. of carbohydrate is often used. The principles of constructing a diabetic diet are given on p. 77.

(*b*) *Insulin injection,* to supply the missing factor. All diabetic children and all severely affected patients need insulin, which unfortunately is destroyed in the stomach and must be given by injection.

(*c*) *Education.*

Types of Insulin

Insulin injection (*B.P.*) (*soluble insulin*) is a clear solution, which begins acting soon after administration, and is effective for about eight hours. It was the earliest type of insulin marketed, and though it has many uses when a rapid effect is needed, it is not generally suitable by itself for control of diabetes because it may have to be given three times a day to keep the blood sugar normal. It is made in strengths of 20, 40 and 80 units per ml.

Globin zinc insulin injection, B.P. (*Globin insulin*) is a solution containing globin and zinc chloride, with a somewhat larger action than soluble insulin. Its strength is 40 or 80 units per ml.

Protamine zinc insulin injection, B.P. is a suspension preparation, slowly absorbed and, therefore, effective over twenty-four hours. One morning injection may suffice. It is available in strengths of 40 or 80 units per ml.

Insulin zinc suspension B.P. (amorphous) = insulin novo semilente.
Insulin zinc suspension B.P. (crystalline) = insulin novo ultralente.
Insulin zinc suspension B.P. = insulin novo lente.
Isophane insulin = NPH insulin.

These are the latest introductions in insulin therapy, and their names indicate their relative speed of action. It will be seen that there are approved names as well as others in these varieties, and the greatest care must be taken to see that the correct sort is being used. Every word of the name must be read, as well as the number of units per ml. The most used forms of insulin are the soluble insulin injection, and insulin zinc suspension (lente).

Giving Insulin. An insulin syringe is used specially calibrated for measurement in units. The word unit does not appear on the syringe, so that no anomalies arise in using single, double or quadruple strength. It is divided into "marks"; 20 marks make up 1 ml.

If single strength (20 unit) soluble insulin is being given, the number of marks to which the syringe is filled is the same as the number of units prescribed, e.g. if 10 units of insulin injection, B.P. (soluble insulin) 20 units per ml. is to be given, 10 "marks" will be given.

If the strength of insulin is 40 units per ml., the volume given will be half that of 20 units per ml. insulin, and the number of "marks" drawn up is half the number of units prescribed, e.g. if 40 units of insulin injection B.P. (soluble insulin) 40 units per ml. is to be given, the syringe is filled to the 20 mark.

If the strength is 80 units per ml., the "mark" to which the syringe is filled is one quarter of the number of units prescribed, e.g. 40 units of insulin of this strength will correspond to 10 " marks " on the syringe. Nurses who give or check insulin must be quite sure they understand the simple arithmetical principle involved.

Insulins of different kinds are put up in packets of differing colours and bands. There are now so many of these that the colours are not helpful to a nurse using several varieties and strengths, and she should rely entirely on reading the names and strengths. They are, however, of assistance to patients, who know the pattern of their brand, and can

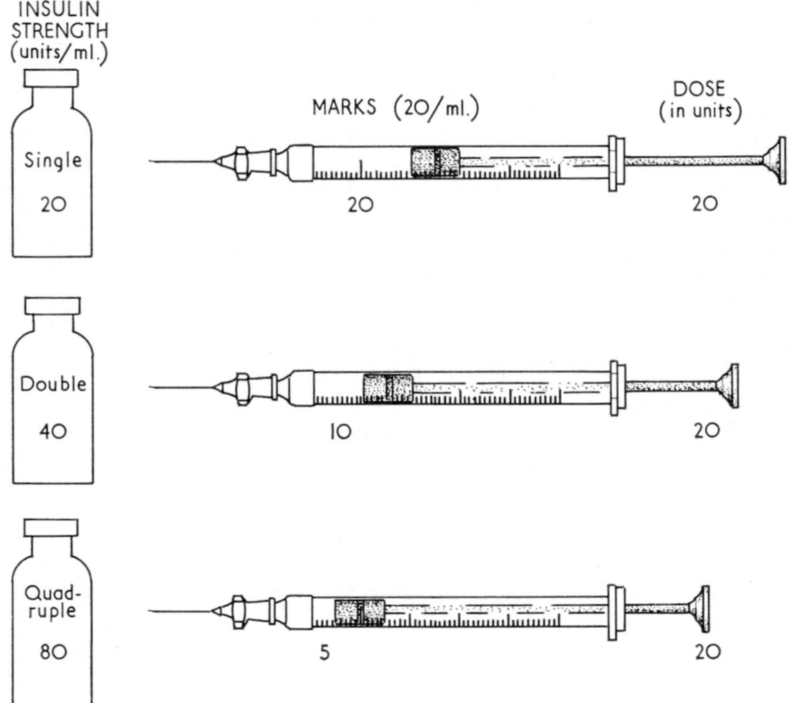

Fig. 52. Measuring insulin. The volume of the dose depends on the strength selected. Each of the syringes photographed above contains 20 units.

feel assured that the volume they use is the one familiar to them as long as they are using the same kind of insulin.

Education of the Diabetic

A newly diagnosed young diabetic is usually admitted to hospital for stabilization of his regimen. He is frequently alarmed and despondent, and a full and careful explanation should be given by the physician, while the dietitian and the nurse have a big part to play in raising his morale. The main points on which he will want instruction, or may ask advice, are these :

1. **Insulin.** He must know the type, amount and the time of giving ; how to sterilize the needle and syringe at home, how to fill the syringe, choose the site and give the injection. Detailed instruction must be given and opportunity allowed for practice under supervision. The most important point is that insulin must *never* be omitted ; if illness prevents him taking his diet he must go to bed and send for the doctor at once. Infections increase the need of the body for insulin.

2. **Diet.** He is told the importance of regular meals ; how to exchange items ; what foods to weigh and how often. Many ask about diabetic patent foods and the answer is that none should be taken unless the carbohydrate content is on the label, and that the dietitian can be consulted about the others.

3. **Hypoglycæmia.** If the blood sugar falls too low, symptoms will appear that the patient should recognize. They are weakness, hunger, fainting and sweating ; in addition, signs such as mood changes, prominence of the eyes, full rapid pulse and unconsciousness with muscle twitching may be observed by the nurse. Patients should carry sugar lumps with them to ward off such attacks, and a card stating their complaint and giving the name of their doctor, in case they become unconscious in the street.

Hypoglycæmia can be relieved by these means :

(*a*) Sugar, glucose or sweetened fruit juice by mouth.

(*b*) Glucose (20 G.) in solution by nasal tube into the stomach.

(*c*) Adrenalin 5 minims by hypodermic injection. This mobilizes the liver glycogen.

(*d*) Intravenous dextrose.

4. **Urine Testing.** The urine should be tested for sugar at regular intervals, and at such times as the everyday routine is at all upset. The use of reagent strips has made this a simple procedure to perform and to read. The results should always be recorded and taken to the clinic when attending there.

5. **Social Problems.** While the diabetic may pursue almost any occupation in which regular meals are possible, the risk of hypoglycæmia would preclude him from piloting an aeroplane or driving a train. The question of car driving is more difficult and a court case has indicated that someone with hypoglycæmia can be charged with driving under the influence of drugs.

Younger people often ask about marriage. The diabetic tendency is a recessive gene, and a diabetic marrying a normal person has no increased risk of having diabetic children, but two diabetics are likely to pass diabetes to their offspring. There is little risk in pregnancy to a diabetic woman with good antenatal supervision, but the infant mortality rate is much above normal still.

Diabetics of a suitable type may be told about the Diabetic Society which has a good welfare programme.

Because insulin is destroyed in the stomach, and therefore must be given by injection, search for a substance that could be given orally to control diabetes has been going on for many years. The first success came as a result of observing that some sulphonamide drugs lowered the blood sugar, and investigation of related substances produced tolbutamide and chlorpropamide. Phenformin and metformin belong to another chemical group. These oral drugs are at present only suitable for mild cases in which ketosis does not occur.

It is believed that there are 300,000 undiscovered diabetics in Great Britain, and search for these might avoid some of the later degenerative complications of diabetes, such as gangrene and retinitis. The introduction of Dextrostix, a strip paper test for blood sugar, seems likely to make the search for these undiscovered diabetics simpler.

SOME DISEASES OF THE KIDNEY

Pyelitis

Pyelitis is a bacterial infection of the pelvis of the kidney, commonly by bacterium coli, streptococci or staphylococci. It produces general signs—rigors, anæmia, and local ones—pain in the loin, pyuria and cystitis.

Such patients are nursed with two or three pillows until they feel well enough to sit up, and the amount of bedclothes depends on the temperature. If sweating occurs, the nurse must be alert to notice when dry clothes are needed, and when warm sponging and drying with a warm towel will promote comfort.

As soon as possible after admission a clean specimen of urine is sent to the bacteriologist and until his report names the organism and the antibiotics to which it is sensitive, a course of sulphadimidine is frequently begun, and if it proves effective may be continued. The urinary output and frequency is recorded, and a high fluid intake encouraged. Alkalis are often ordered and have the effect of decreasing the frequency. Nitrofurantoin is another very useful antibacterial drug. A specimen of urine is saved daily for examination, and though ward tests for pus are not informative, estimation of the amount of deposit in the glass may show improvement. The chosen should be continued until the bacteriologist pronounces the urine sterile. Relapse is quite common, so thorough treatment of the first attack is important, and on discharge the patient is advised to maintain a good fluid intake.

Nephritis

Nephritis is an inflammation of the kidney, but not an infection, so that the anti-infective treatment that is so effective in pyelitis is of no avail. Though the pathology of this condition is difficult and the naming rather confused, the nurse will meet in clinical practice three main types :

(*a*) **Acute nephritis** (acute diffuse glomerulo-nephritis).

(*b*) **Subacute nephritis,** a condition of insidious onset, with little clinical resemblance to the acute form.

(*c*) **Chronic nephritis.**

Acute Nephritis

This usually occurs in the third week after a streptococcal infection (often tonsillitis) to which it appears to be an allergic response, and since such infections are commonest in children, the patient is usually young, and boys predominate in number. The inflammation interferes seriously with renal function, so that the constituents of the urine are retained in the body, as can be seen from the raised blood urea, and there is a compensatory rise of blood pressure. The patient will have diminished urinary output (even anuria), albuminuria, hæmaturia, œdema, fever, headache, nausea, backache and hypertension. No drugs affect the kidney condition, so that nursing under the best conditions is of prime importance in aiding recovery.

Chilling of the skin causes spasm of the renal vessels, and this must be avoided, so the patient must be warmly clad. Although it is not now general to nurse these people in a blanket bed, many physicians believe it to be of value. If blankets are ordered, it is for the reason given above, and not to induce sweating. Physical activity retards recovery, and the raised blood pressure may strain the heart, so absolute rest is ordered until improvement is well established.

The nurse's records are important in assessing progress. The urine is meticulously measured, and a specimen put up daily to demonstrate the amount of hæmaturia. Esbach's test should also be performed daily, filtration of the specimen being necessary if blood is present. The fluid intake is measured and the blood pressure taken daily, while a four-hourly temperature, pulse and respiration chart is kept. The occurrence of severe headache, twitching of muscles, changes in the pulse rate and dryness of the tongue must be reported at once.

The diet is of great importance, since water, salt and excess protein taken by mouth must be excreted by the kidney or retained in the tissues. A salt-free, low protein diet with restricted fluids is usually recommended. In the early days appetite is absent, and sweetened fruit juices are usually sufficient ; as recovery begins, fruit purée, mashed potato, and butter are given, then protein is gradually added as milk, then a little egg, fish and finally meat. During the stage of restricted intake, mouth care will be necessary.

It is impossible to keep a young child lying down as soon as he feels better, but bed rest is maintained until the blood pressure is normal and albumin has disappeared from the urine, or until it appears that bed rest is no longer helpful. The big majority of cases recover completely, but in a few a trace of albumin or of hypertension indicates that recovery is not complete, and in a longer or shorter time chronic nephritis will supervene. Adequate convalescence is necessary, and the child's mother is warned that sore throats must be taken seriously and must receive early medical attention.

Subacute Nephritis

Patients with subacute nephritis have massive albuminuria, and the drain of plasma proteins into the urine lowers the osmotic pressure of the blood and allows generalized œdema (*anasarca*), often of an extensive degree. Anæmia is often marked, but the normal blood urea and blood pressure show that there is no impairment as yet of kidney function. Very few patients, however, recover, though it may be years before the rising blood pressure heralds the onset of the last chronic stage.

Treatment aims at restoring the level of the plasma proteins and so diminishing the œdema. A high-protein, low-salt diet can help considerably, but it is not an easy one to tolerate for the long periods necessary, and patients need much encouragement. Since the kidney function is adequate, diuretics are ordered by some physicians. While these patients are being nursed in bed, regular attention must be given to the pressure areas on which so much weight is put owing to the œdema.

Cortisone is sometimes ordered for these people, and though its effect may be marked, it is only temporary, as in so many other conditions for which it has been tried.

Chronic Nephritis

Long-standing and progressive kidney disease results in renal failure and a rise of blood pressure, both indicative of the last stages of nephritis. Typically the patient has hypertension, with severe headache and giddiness and a raised blood urea, the urine contains a trace of albumin and is of fixed specific gravity day and night, showing that the kidney is no longer able to vary it in accordance with the changing needs of the body. The hypertension may lead to heart failure, or the kidney disease may cause uræmia ; in any case the outcome will be unfavourable so that treatment is merely designed to promote comfort. Restrictions on the diet are rarely justified, since they cannot influence the course of the disease, and symptoms should be alleviated as far as possible as they arise.

Uræmia

Failure of kidney function if unrelieved, will lead to a toxic state called uræmia. Such failure can be caused by nephritis ; chronic pyelitis ; prostatic enlargement ; involvement of the ureters in new growth ; by severe shock or bleeding causing prolonged hypotension ; by incompatible transfusion ; by upset of the chemical balance of the tissue fluids by prolonged vomiting or by ketosis.

The symptoms can be grouped under three headings :

Cerebral. Drowsiness, headache, muscular twitchings, disorientation, stupor.

Respiratory. Cheyne-Stokes breathing is common because of the increasing amount of acid in the blood.

Gastro-intestinal. Hiccough ; vomiting ; diarrhœa ; dry, brown. offensive tongue, and a bitter taste in the mouth due to urea in the saliva.

In uræmia due to chronic nephritis the treatment is symptomatic, since recovery cannot be expected. Venesection or lumbar puncture may help the cerebral signs by lowering the intra-cranial pressure. Treatment of the mouth should be frequent and meticulous, since its offensiveness is a great source of discomfort to the patient. Chlorpromazine is often tried in the treatment of vomiting, and is sometimes most effective, while an occasional stomach washout may be helpful, provided the patient does not feel the remedy to be worse than the disease. A daily warm blanket bath is given to remove the acid sweat, and will help to check skin irritation, which is often troublesome.

Paraldehyde 5 to 10 ml. by intramuscular injection can be given for restlessness, but the nurse will notice that this restlessness is often terminal, and means that life will not be long. Morphine is effective in checking hiccough and restlessness, but by depressing respiration shortens life, so is only given by those physicians who value its effects in the last stages.

MANAGEMENT OF CHRONIC RENAL FAILURE

In some patients with renal failure, the cause of this failure may be fatal in itself (e.g. extensive pelvic carcinoma). Patients with chronic nephritis, however, are often in a different category; if renal function could be restored, or artificially imitated, they might be capable of something like normal life.

The work of the kidney is to control the volume constituents and reaction of the blood, and to excrete soluble waste products; unless this is done life cannot be maintained. When the kidneys have ceased to function, however, their tasks may be performed artificially by *dialysis*, which is the separation of the crystalloid constituents of a fluid from its colloid part. The peritoneum may be used as a dialysing membrane (peritoneal dialysis), or the blood may be led into a kidney machine where it is only separated from the dialysing fluid by a thin membrane before returning to the body. This process is hæmodialysis. When circumstances are favourable and the facilities are available, the management of the chronic nephritic will therefore fall into these stages.

(*a*) Medical and dietetic management, perhaps with intermittent peritoneal dialysis.
(*b*) Hæmodialysis, in hospital or at home.
(*c*) Renal transplant.

Medical Management

The symptoms of uræmia, such as nausea and vomiting are due to the accumulation in the blood of products of protein metabolism. The diet in chronic nephritis must therefore be low in protein to reduce the amount of urea to be excreted, and high enough in calories to avoid the breakdown of body protein to provide energy. The caloric value of the diet can be raised by carbohydrate foods such as honey, jam and sugar, or concentrates such as Hycal. Most low protein diets are deficient in vitamin B, and this must be added. A diet containing as little as 18 grammes of protein a day may be required, and this is a very unpleasant one, but a patient in uræmia who loses his gastro-intestinal symptoms will usually tolerate it because he feels so much better.

Other problems that may present as time passes include:

(*a*) *Hypertension.* The usual drugs are given but must be very carefully regulated because of lack of excretion in the urine.

(*b*) *Electrolyte imbalance.* The regulation of the sodium, potassium and calcium in the blood is very difficult, and for details of its management the student is advised to consult a medical textbook.

(*c*) *Anœmia* is usually present, because the red cells are shortlived. Transfusion is usually avoided if at all possible, because the donor cells are rapidly broken down, and because of the risk of serum hepatitis, which may prejudice the patient's chances of obtaining hæmodialysis later.

(*d*) *Itching* may seem a minor problem, but can cause great distress. Frequent hot baths and small doses of chlorpromazine may be helpful.

(*e*) *Gout* can occur because the failing kidneys cannot excrete uric acid.

(*f*) *Calcium* may be deposited in the eyes, arteries or joints.

If complications become severe, or if kidney function is so reduced that dietary restriction is of no avail, peritoneal dialysis is used, in the hope that a kidney machine will become available for this patient.

Peritoneal dialysis. The principle of the procedure is to run fluid into the peritoneal cavity, leave it there to absorb urea, fluid and excess electrolytes, and then allow it to run out. This is repeated hourly, using 2 litres of fluid at a time, and a total of 40–60 l. Keeping regular accurate records is of the utmost importance, since undesirable effects and complications are not unusual. Before dialysis the physician ascertains the hæmoglobin, blood urea, plasma proteins and electrolytes (sodium, chloride, calcium and potassium). An electrocardiogram is usually necessary, and the weight must be known.

Requirements. Intravenous stand.
Dialysing fluid in plastic bags.
Water bath at 40° C.
Ampoules of potassium chloride.
Tetracycline.
Heparin.
Abdominal catheter set.
Peritoneal administration set.
Tray of sterile equipment; 2 ml. and 5 ml. syringes; no. 20 and no. 12 needles; scalpel or steralet; trocar and cannula; towels and swabs.
Local anaesthetic.
Gentian violet.
Sterile plastic bags (e.g. uribags) for receiving outflow.

Procedure.

The patient should be relaxed and pain-free throughout, and an analgesic like pethidine will be necessary, and perhaps a sedative. The bladder must be emptied immediately beforehand, or it may be accidentally punctured. The patient lies flat, the skin of the abdomen is cleaned, and local anaesthetic injected about 5 cm. below the umbilicus. Two bags of dialysing fluid are put to warm in the water bath. A small incision is made into the skin, and the trocar and cannula introduced into the peritoneal cavity; the trocar is withdrawn, and the plastic catheter introduced through the cannula, and passed down towards the left iliac fossa. Two bags of warm dialysing fluid are hung on the stand, connected to the catheter by the giving set, and run rapidly into the peritoneal cavity. When it has all run (usually in about ten minutes) the tubes are clamped, and the solution allowed to remain in the abdomen for an hour. The clamps to the drainage bags are then opened and the fluid allowed to run out. The amount is measured, and recorded against the input; the whole amount may not be recovered on each occasion but if retention continues the physician

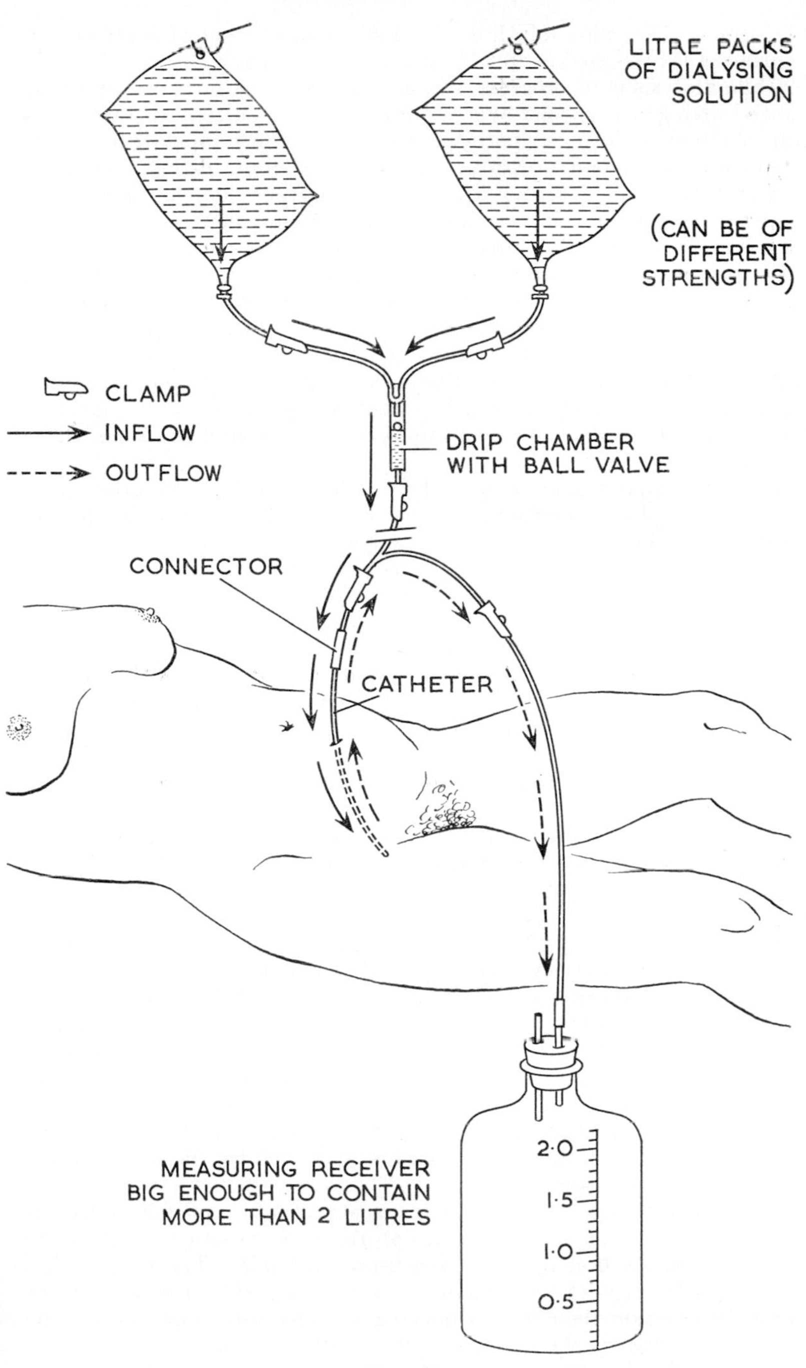
LITRE PACKS
OF DIALYSING
SOLUTION
(CAN BE OF
DIFFERENT
STRENGTHS)
CLAMP
INFLOW
OUTFLOW
DRIP CHAMBER
WITH BALL VALVE
CONNECTOR
CATHETER
MEASURING RECEIVER
BIG ENOUGH TO CONTAIN
MORE THAN 2 LITRES
2·0
1·5
1·0
0·5

Fig. 53.

is informed. Dialysing solution with a stronger content of dextrose can be ordered if increased excretion of fluid is wanted.

While dialysis is in progress, the area around the incision should be painted with gention violet every four hours, to avoid entry of infection from the wound into the peritoneal cavity. The temperature, pulse, respiration and blood pressure are estimated four hourly. Fever is usually treated with tetracycline; a fall in the blood pressure may indicate the need for intravenous fluids. Pain must be relieved by pethidine, or a drug of comparable strength. The patient is weighed, and a specimen of the outflow sent daily to the bacteriology Laboratory.

Hæmodialysis. The artificial kidney in current use is the Kiil dialyser. In this, a thin film of blood is separated only by a permeable membrane from the dialysing solution, which is automatically blended by the machine from soft water and a concentrated solution of electrolytes, and runs to waste after it has passed once through the machine. Patients at a dialysis centre commonly spend two nights a week there for a period of 14 or 15 hours.

In order to take the blood into the machine and back into the body, easy access to the circulation must be possible. This is provided in one of two ways. The first is by means of a Scribner shunt, which consists of a shunt made of two Teflon-silastic tubes introduced into a peripheral artery and a nearby vein. These tubes are joined by a connector except during dialysis. When the shunt is in good state there is no tenderness around it, and there is a continuous column of blood in the tube, which feels warm and pulsates. Naturally the patient feels concerned about the shunt, which is a kind of lifeline. Hæmorrhage from accidental separation of the ends is rare, but can be most alarming. Infection is quite common, but it is clotting (especially on the venous side) which is the most troublesome complication, and may be a source of pulmonary emboli.

The second method is to create surgically an arterio-venous fistula, which produces a dilated superficial vein into which a double puncture is made at each dialysis. This does not sound pleasant but many patients prefer it to the rather awkward external shunt.

If the patient's domestic circumstances are suitable, a dialyser may be established in his home, and this will free a place at the centre for someone else. Patients on home dialysis usually prefer three ten-hour periods a week, which keeps them rather fitter than those on less frequent dialysis. It must not be thought however that dialysis involves only technical problems. He has a very restricted diet and fluid intake, cannot take a holiday, and must guard against many complications. In addition, the family of such a patient may feel the strain very severely. The long-term solution to his problems will lie in the possibility of a renal transplant.

Dialysis centres now maintain a group of patients kept in good health by regular treatment, tissue typed, and ready to submit themselves to operation when a donor kidney becomes available. The cooperation of hospitals where such kidneys may become available, and of relatives willing to sanction their use, is necessary. The better the tissue-type match, the better is the chance of the grafted kidney surviving, and the lower is the dose of drugs necessary to prevent its rejection.

SOME DISEASES OF THE CHEST

Bronchitis

Acute bronchitis is not very commonly seen in hospital wards because it is not a serious disease except in the old or the very young. It frequently begins as a cold in the head, which descends to the chest, causing fever with its usual accompanying signs and a cough at first dry but soon becoming productive, frequently with quite large amounts of muco-purulent sputum. A moderate attack is over in about a week, but the course can be shortened and made more comfortable by treatment.

The first requisite is to remain in a room with a warm, even temperature, adequate humidity ; the typical British bedroom unheated in the depth of winter is not suitable. The temperature should not fall below 60°, and moisture should be provided by a steam kettle or four-hourly steam inhalations. Enough pillows are provided to keep the patient sitting comfortably, and the shoulders are kept warm in a bed jacket. Fluid intake should be high, but there is no need to press solid food for a day or two until the appetite improves. If the fever is slight and breathing not impeded antibiotic therapy is not always prescribed, but if the attack is a sharp one, or the patient is frail or subject to recurrent attacks, it will be ordered. A broad-spectrum antibiotic like tetracycline is popular.

While a single attack of bronchitis is not normally serious, repeated attacks during the winter months will lead to chronic bronchitis. Infection leads to excess production of mucus with diminished air entry, expiratory difficulty and eventually to break up of the alveoli, into cyst-like spaces, i.e. emphysema. Chronic bronchitis and emphysema with resultant heart failure is the third commonest cause of death in this country, only being exceeded by arterial disease and cancer. The patient is most likely to be a middle-aged man with a rounded, barrel-shaped chest and prominent sterno mastoid muscles. He relies mainly on his diaphragm for breathing ; his chest movement is slight. He is short of breath, often while at rest, and is troubled by a chronic productive cough. The lines of treatment are :

1. *Advice.* The patient must try to avoid exposure to inclement weather and fogs, and if residence in an industrial town can be avoided, it should be. He should take care not to let the sedentary life imposed on him by breathlessness be the cause of weight increase, and smoking should be prohibited.

2. *Breathing exercises.* The physiotherapist can often improve his respiratory excursion.

3. *Drugs.* Antibiotics may lessen infection ; expectorants may help expulsion of sputum ; broncho-spasm can be helped by ephedrine or aminophylline. Prednisone is often prescribed with benefit.

In its early stages chronic bronchitis is not spectacular, but if progressive, heart failure will eventually follow, while the appearance of a bronchitic patient in a surgical ward is viewed with misgiving since he is a very likely candidate for post-operative broncho-pneumonia.

Pneumonia

Pneumonia, or inflammation of the lung, is not only an important primary disease, but is a secondary and always serious complication of many conditions. The chief varieties and the situations in which they may be encountered are as follows :

(*a*) *Broncho-pneumonia.* The inflammation is usually at the bases, with patchy consolidation around the bronchi. The infection enters through the air passages, and is usually secondary to some other conditions, e.g. surgical operations, especially those involving the upper abdomen ; specific fevers, such as scarlet fever, measles or typhoid ; cachexia as in the later stages of cancer ; stagnation of lung circulation through lying still (*hypostatic pneumonia*) or congestive heart failure.

An account of broncho-pneumonia in the post-operative phase is to be found on p. 245. Whatever the cause it runs an irregular course with a fluctuating temperature for about a fortnight. The organisms found in the muco-purulent sputum are mixed, and pain is not a prominent symptom because pleurisy is not present.

Broncho-pneumonia complicates so many serious illnesses that it is often a terminal event, but there are many precautions that may be taken to prevent it in susceptible patients, e.g. by treating fevers with severe naso-pharyngeal inflammation, with sulphonamides or antibiotics ; by deep breathing and coughing exercises before surgical operations ; by frequent turning of the helpless. The treatment of surgical broncho-pneumonia is described on p. 245.

(*b*) *Lobar pneumonia.* This disease is now rarely seen to run its classical course. It is an infection, usually pneumococcal, though streptococci and staphylococci are sometimes responsible, which reaches one or more lobes of the lung via the bloodstream and causes consolidation. The onset is sudden with a rigor, fever and a marked rise in the respiratory rate with pain in the chest over the inflamed lobe. In the absence of effective treatment the disease lasts about ten days with continuous pyrexiam herpes on the lips, cyanosis, marked toxæmia and sometimes delirium until in favourable cases the temperature falls by crisis and a long and trying convalescent period follows. Heart failure is always to be feared, while empyema and lung abscess are complications.

Many cases are nursed at home, since a response to antibiotics can be expected in twenty-four hours. At the onset, the patient is put into bed lightly covered, with enough well-placed pillows to make breathing comfortable. A specimen of sputum must be obtained at once for identification of the organism and its sensitivity to organisms. The temperature, pulse and respiration rate are recorded four-hourly, or more often if it seems indicated. There is no need to press the patient to take food for the first forty-eight hours, but a high fluid intake must be encouraged ; this needs skill and persuasion from the nurse as the breathlessness and chest pain makes swallowing laborious. The mouth is regularly treated, and if herpes appears on the lips the blisters are kept dry with powder. Cyanosis indicates the need for oxygen with a polythene mask, or the use of an oxygen tent. The sputum, usually scanty and viscid at first, and stained orange from red blood cells, should be measured. A kaolin poultice over the chest may be comforting, but feverish patients sometimes resent it, and few doctors would then insist on its being used.

Penicillin is usually begun at once, and if when the bacteriologist's report is available the organism is penicillin-resistant, a broad-spectrum antibiotic is used, of which today the choice would be tetracycline. In the ill or the old, it might be thought desirable to begin with tetracycline. Although the temperature soon falls, lung consolidation must clear by natural means, and this clearance is checked by X-rays.

Failure to resolve sometimes indicates an obstruction to a bronchus, and carcinoma is the commonest and most important cause. A fair proportion of patients with cancer of the lung have pneumonia as an early sign. If feasible, resection is the treatment.

Pneumonia due to a virus such as that of influenza or psittacosis (ornithosis) appears to be increasingly common. The temperature rises to about 102° F. (38·9° C.), and settles slowly over three weeks. The number of white cells in the blood is lowered (leucopenia), in contrast to the rise (lencocytosis) usual in lobar pneumonia. In general, there is no antibiotic at the moment that influences virus infections, but super-added bacterial infection may be prevented or treated by tetracycline.

PEPTIC ULCER

Peptic ulcers occur in those parts of the digestive tract exposed to gastric juice, and are especially found on the lesser curvature of the stomach, and the first part of the duodenum. Though increasingly common in all industrial communities, the cause is quite unknown, though many factors are commonly associated with such ulcers. The sufferers are predominantly men, though women are by no means immune, and they are usually adults from 35 to 50 years old. They complain of pain (related in some way to meals), heartburn, and sometimes vomiting. Irregular meal times, heavily seasoned indigestible food, excessive cigarette smoking or drinking, and worry have all been blamed, but in fact it will be seen that most of these are part of a single behaviour pattern ; highly strung volatile men who are anxious (with or without cause) about their affairs are likely to smoke heavily and bolt their meals. The only common physical finding is that excess hydrochloric acid is found in the stomach if a duodenal ulcer is present, but this is not always true of gastric ulcers.

Nurses sometimes do not realize that the people whom they see in the wards with ulcers are only a small proportion of the whole ; most are treated in out-patient clinics or doctors' surgeries. Diagnosis is made by barium meal (p. 127) or a fractional test meal may also be used. The chief elements in the treatment is *rest* for the mind, the body and the stomach.

If admitted to a medical ward, the patient should be weighed and put to bed, where he must spend most of his time. If he is in acute pain, a continuous drip feed of milk (p. 184) is usually effective in relieving it in twenty-four hours. His diet is adjusted to his condition

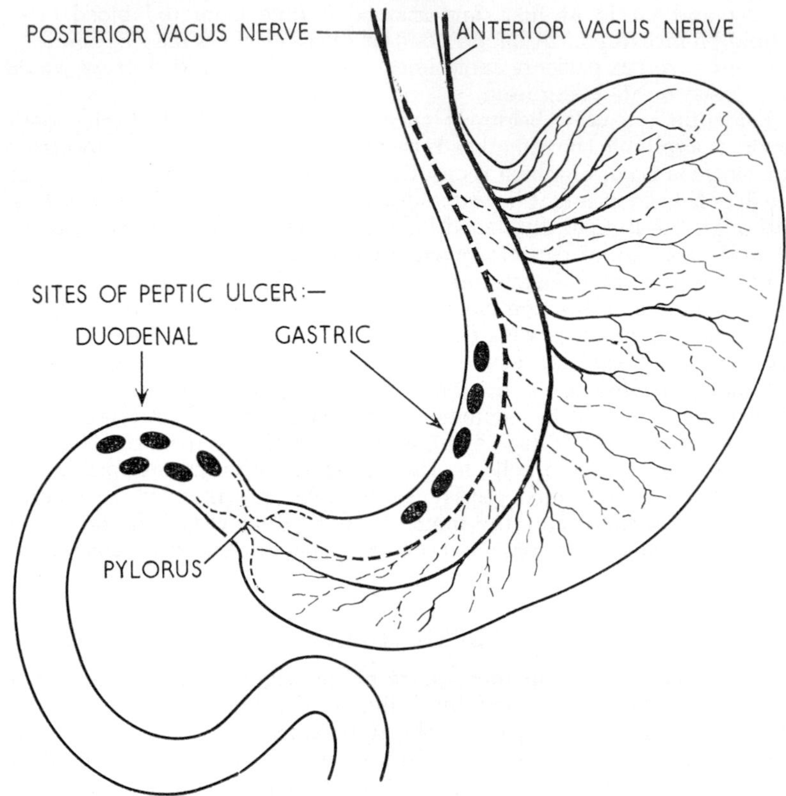

Fig. 54. Peptic ulcer sites.

and needs. A talk with the almoner may be helpful in resolving difficulties that prevent him from relaxing. Among the most useful drugs are :

1. **Phenobarbitone, to reduce tension.**
2. **Tincture of belladonna before meals to relax the stomach.**
3. **Alkalis or antacids.** An alkali like sodium bicarbonate neutralizes the gastric acid, with evolution of carbon dioxide, but stimulates more acid production. The neutral antacids like magnesium trisilicate or aluminium hydroxide are preferable, and should be given after meals and last thing at night. Many proprietary preparations exist.
4. Other remedies. Carbenoxolone (Biogastrone) is the drug in current use. Probanthine, a ganglion-blocking agent which reduces acid secretion and stomach activity, is another. Since ulcers are liable to remission and relapse, the effect of drug therapy is difficult to estimate, and many drugs of which high hopes were entertained once, have now fallen into disuse.

On discharge, the patient should be gaining weight and free from pain. He has received advice on his mode of life and his attitude to his complaint, and he and his wife have had an interview with the dietitian.

The complications of peptic ulcer are :

1. *Perforation.* The ulcer erodes the stomach wall completely, so that stomach contents escape into the peritoneal cavity.

2. *Hæmorrhage.* A blood vessel is opened by extension of the ulcer, and blood is vomited (hæmatemesis) or passed altered per anum (melæna).

3. *Stenosis.* Chronic ulcers may cause fibrous contractions either at the pylorus, or in mid-stomach.

4. *Penetration.* The ulcer bores its way into the pancreas.

5. *Malignancy.* An uncertain proportion of peptic ulcers of long standing become malignant.

All these complications are treated surgically, except hæmorrhage, which calls for emergency admission to a medical ward, though the surgeon may sometimes endeavour to save a life when repeated hæmorrhages have occurred.

Hæmorrhage from a Peptic Ulcer

Whether such bleeding is revealed as hæmatemesis or melæna does not influence prognosis or treatment. On hearing that a patient is to be admitted following a gastro-intestinal hæmorrhage, the nurse should see that a bed is ready with one pillow covered by a towel and mackintosh, admission blankets, and blocks ready to elevate the foot. On the locker is a vomit bowl and paper towels, a mouth tray, and a board for recording treatment and a sphygmomanometer. When the patient arrives he is lifted into bed, and if inspection reveals a pale, cold and collapsed man, he should be wrapped in the blankets, covered over, and allowed to rest before his clothes are removed.

The temperature, pulse, respiration and blood pressure are recorded at once, and repeated at the intervals indicated by the findings. The nurse while making these records also notices whether there is pallor, sweating, nausea, yawning, anxiety, or audible peristalsis that might indicate that further bleeding was taking place. Morphine is usually ordered at once, and transfusion is given if the hæmorrhage was big enough to produce general signs.

Physical and mental rest is obtained in this way, and all physicians would agree about it ; all would agree that rest for the stomach and duodenum is necessary, but would not be unanimous on the way it should be given. Some think that fluids should not be given by mouth until bleeding has ceased, and that small feeds of iced water should then be cautiously resumed. This conservative attitude was once universal, but most physicians now allow a more liberal intake. N/5 saline can be given as desired from the beginning, and milk drinks and soft purées can be added fairly soon. Supporters of this view believe that the stomach contracts most when empty and can point to the improving mortality figures in recent years as evidence in support of their régime.

This patient will be washed, given mouth toilet and nursed lying down until the danger of further bleeding is passed. The blocks should be removed as soon as the blood pressure is normal, and another pillow given in case hypostatic pneumonia develops. The bowels are kept confined for a few days and mild aperients are cautiously prescribed only when it is felt that the colon can be stimulated without risk of causing further bleeding. The first stool will always contain altered blood, and subsequently a stool should be saved daily for inspection.

Some physicians feel that after such a hæmorrhage the surgeon should be consulted about the advisability of partial gastrectomy, especially if the ulcer is a long-standing one.

Ulcerative Colitis

In the same way as peptic ulceration is associated with a personality-pattern, this condition of ulceration in the colon is usually thought of as psychologically determined. Patients at the time of the first onset are usually young people, but if the condition becomes chronic it can persist throughout life.

The symptoms are diarrhœa, with presence of mucus, blood and pus in the stools ; anæmia ; wasting and dehydration. In addition ulceration of the skin of the legs (*pyoderma*), arthritis and psoriasis may be associated with the chronic state. Two varieties are met : (1) the acute fulminating kind in which death from anæmia and dehydration can occur ; (2) the subacute variety with a less striking onset, but a tendency to become chronic with remissions and relapses. Once organic changes have taken place in the colon a complete cure cannot be expected.

Medical treatment consists of : (1) treatment of the anæmia, usually by transfusion; (2) a bland diet, to avoid colonic stimulation or irritation ; (3) antibiotics to deal with secondary infection ; (4) a course of cortisone, or a cortisone-like substance which often produces a remission though it cannot cure.

If the medical means of treatment are limited, the nursing care is exacting and offers great scope for thought and imagination. A bed should be chosen within easy reach of the service-rooms, so that bedpans can be fetched quickly and emptied easily. A comfortable mattress, well protected against spills, will give comfort to an emaciated patient.

The arrangements for dealing with the many bowel evacuations must be carefully made ; a commode by the bedside may give confidence, especially at night, when the nurses may be occupied with another patient and unable to answer an urgent request quickly enough. If the patient is emaciated a pad should be placed on the rim of the bedpan, and wool is kinder than paper for the local toilet. The stools are usually offensive, and a bottle of deodorant can be kept unobtrusively on a near-by windowsill. An accurate record is kept of the stools passed, and whether blood or pus is present in unusual amounts.

The diet is presented in an appetizing form, and it is usual to build it up gradually from simple bland foods, noticing any untoward effect on the bowel action of the addition of any new item. Sodium is lost in large quantities in diarrhœa and must be replaced. Hot drinks stimulate peristalsis and are best avoided, but if ice cream can be taken it is a good vehicle for extra protein and fat as casilan and cream. Abundant fluids are given.

The pressure points are regularly treated, and the anal area washed four-hourly and covered with a silicone barrier cream or a similar water-proofing substance. The incessant painful offensive stools often bring these young patients to the edge of despair, especially as they are often introspective by temperament and obsessively neat. They must never be given the least excuse to feel that the nursing duties involved are in any way irksome.

Among the acute complications that may occur are perforation of the colon and recto-vesical fistula ; these are treated surgically, and the surgeon today also sees a number of cases which medical measures have failed to control. He may bring the terminal ileum to discharge its contents on to the abdominal wall (ileostomy), and thus divert the fæces entirely from the colon. In a proportion of cases pus and blood will continue to discharge from the colon, and for these people total colectomy offers the only prospect of relief. Life with a permanent ileostomy sounds harsh, but there are many varieties of bag today that make the disability minimal. (See p. 271.)

The nurse who has looked after a patient with acute ulcerative colitis will realize that it is possible for the state of mind to influence the course of this disease, but it is difficult to believe that mental reasons alone could begin such an acute inflammatory state. Doubtless there are underlying physical as well as mental reasons that permit a patient to fall ill with ulcerative colitis.

ARTHRITIS

Inflammation of joints may be caused in many ways, but there are two kinds that can be seen commonly in medical wards, and in the general public. These are *rheumatoid* and *osteoarthritis*, two conditions linked in name, but differing in cause, onset, prognosis and treatment.

Rheumatoid Arthritis

Rheumatoid arthritis is not a disease confined to joints, but a systemic one having general effects throughout the body. Women of 20 to 45, mostly at the two extremes of this age group, are the principal sufferers. The disease can be of acute onset, usually with rapid involvement of many joints, or subacute repeated attacks can occur, sometimes resulting in damage just as severe. The joints first affected are those of the wrists, ankles and fingers, but eventually practically every joint can be involved. The joint swelling is symmetrical and tender, with wasting of the surrounding muscles that throws the swelling into prominence. The skin over the joint is waxy and shiny, and as time progresses movement becomes limited and typical deformities occur ; for instance the joints between hand and fingers are enlarged and flexed, while the fingers deviate towards the ulnar side. That the disease is a constitutional one is shown by fever, anæmia, a raised sedimentation rate, fatigue and sweating.

The aims of treatment which are limited by the fact that we do not yet know the cause of rheumatoid arthritis, are :

1. Rest during the acute inflammatory stage, with prevention of deformity.
2. Interruption of the inflammation by drug therapy.

3. Active rehabilitation once the acute painful stage is over.
4. Help, both orthopædic and social, for the chronically disabled.

The bed should contain enough pillows to allow a view of the surroundings, but not enough to cause acute hip flexion. A well-sprung firm mattress is usually to be preferred, but an air-ring may give comfort, and a cotton blanket above the patient will absorb the abundant sweat which is a feature of rheumatoid arthritis. A blanket bath must be given daily because of this symptom.

Having assessed the stage of the disease the doctor will decide the amount of activity that can be allowed or encouraged. He usually orders sodium salicylate, which relieves the joint pain and lowers the temperature. Cortisone and ACTH both have a marked but temporary effect on the joint reaction, and it is more usual now to prescribe prednisolone, a cortisone-like substance which represses inflammatory reactions without affecting the salt balance of the tissues. Acutely inflamed joints especially those of the hands, will be rested in featherweight plastic foam splints at night to prevent deformity. A normal temperature, falling sedimentation rate and decrease of pain are indications that more active therapy can be begun.

Once pain has been relieved enthusiastic physiotherapy is begun. Patients can be shown how much easier movement is under water (which supports the weight) and are encouraged to practise movements in a warm bath. Other forms of drug treatment may be tried now, e.g. intramuscular gold injections. Like all the metals, gold is poisonous, and when a patient comes up for an injection, a specimen of urine is tested for albumin, enquiries are made about any skin symptoms, and at intervals the white cell count is taken, since albuminuria, dermatitis and leucopenia are the chief complications of treatment.

Even when the disease has become chronic, there is much that can be done to help the patient imprisoned by the crippling of her joints. Orthopædic operations such as tenotomy may be helpful, or traction can straighten flexed joints. Special appliances may help the patient to undertake such activities as feeding herself, cleaning her teeth or doing her hair. For the less severely handicapped, there are many ingenious gadgets to help with household tasks and the Women's Voluntary Services should be consulted if a housewife needs help and may benefit from mechanical aids.

Osteoarthritis

Osteoarthritis is a degenerative process, commoner in men than in women, and since it is the result of the stresses of life on the joints, affects mainly the big weight-bearing joints of the elderly ; the knees, hips and spine are commonly involved. The articular cartilage becomes worn away, the bone beneath is eroded and roughened, leading to pain and progressive limitation of movement.

From the nature of the condition it is obvious that a cure cannot be expected, but advice and local treatment may help to alleviate pain and delay the advance of the arthritis. The most useful step is to encourage the loss of excess weight ; joints that found difficulty in carrying an obese person may prove adequate to sustaining a normal weight.

Unfortunately, pain and stiffness lead to a sedentary life that encourages weight gain, and some elderly lonely people feel that their meals are a great source of enjoyment.

Warm clothing is helpful, and the physiotherapist can often provide short-wave therapy or massage. Simple analgesis can be prescribed for the night-time, when pain may render sleep difficult. The chief point to remember is that the patient must learn to live with his arthritis, but that there is never any need to describe the condition as incurable or hopeless, since there are many minor forms of comfort that can be given. If osteoarthritis of the hip threatens to confine the patient to bed, the advice of the surgeon should be sought on the possibility of operative treatment.

DISEASE OF THE NERVOUS SYSTEM

Epilepsy

Epilepsy of some form is said to affect one person in two hundred in this country. It is a condition in which there are disturbances of movement, or of feeling, or consciousness, or all three (epileptic fits), which may occur seldom, or with severity and at short intervals. These fits are of three types; *grand mal*, or generalized convulsions in which consciousness is lost (see p. 524); *petit mal*, which are very short attacks often only lasting a second or two; and *focal* attacks originating in a definite part of the brain and following a certain pattern.

The patient who is thought to be epileptic is investigated by means of a careful history-taking: an account of an attack from an observer if possible; examination of the urine and blood chemistry, X-ray of the skull, and electroencephalogram.

Electroencephalography. The electroencephalogram is a record of the electrical activity of the brain, made through the intact tissues of the scalp and skull. This electrical output is very small, and must be amplified before it can be written out as a tracing on paper. It is used only for diagnosis, in the same way as the electrocardiogram, and is used in the following conditions.

1. *Suspected intranial lesions.* The presence of a tumour can be verified, where it is situated, and whether it is more likely to be innocent or malignant. It can distinguish between a tumour and cerebral thrombosis.

2. *Disturbances of function,* of which epilepsy is the most important. It can distinguish the type, sometimes the cause, and the response to drugs. In patients who have sustained severe brain injuries, and are being nursed on respirators, the electroencephalogram will show whether any brain activity is present.

3. *Diffuse cerebral disease,* e.g. dementia.

4. *Systemic illnesses* which affect brain function, such as liver or heart failure.

5. *Research* into the effects of physiological and pathological states on the brain.

This investigation can be done on outpatients, as preparation required is small. The most important is that the patient understands that no electric current is applied to him, as most people fear when they hear the name of this test. Preferably the hair should be washed, so that it is quite free from grease. The bladder is emptied immediately beforehand, so that the patient can rest and relax while the record is being made. Fasting is sometimes required, and if so instructions will be given. The doctor must know what drugs the patient is receiving.

Four pairs of electrodes are attached to the scalp, and since these must be accurately placed the head is first measured. Some electrodes are held by adhesive plastic discs, some by collodion. To make satisfactory contact, electrode jelly is injected into the middle of each electrode through a blunt-ended needle, which is rotated to scarify the skin slightly, and the slight tingling felt then is the only discomfort.

The patient lies on a couch, with the electrodes connected by wires to the machine behind him. He may be asked to open and close the eyes, to watch a flashing light, or to breathe rapidly. When the test is over, the electrodes are removed, and the collodion dissolved with a mixture of ether and spirit. It is difficult to remove, and thorough combing is needed. If on return to the ward a deposit of collodion reappears as the solvent dries, further treatment will be given with the same mixture and a little arachis oil to prevent undue drying. A fine tooth comb may be used if necessary.

The fits of most epileptics can be controlled by the correct combination and dose of anti-convulsant drugs. Once this has been found, the epileptic must be encouraged to regard his drugs as the diabetic does his insulin; they are the passport to a normal life. It is hard to continue such a regime for years when no fits occur, but to abandon it may mean a return of attacks which will damage the patient's confidence and his chances of employment.

The British Epilepsy Association, which is linked with the International Bureau for Epilepsy, issues a card for epileptics to carry, giving the name and address, and simple instructions as to what to do for someone who has a fit. It includes an appeal not to send the patient to hospital; the sight of someone in a fit is alarming to the lay public, but if the patient is protected from injury during the fit and allowed to rest afterwards he will soon recover.

The epileptic needs more help in the community than in hospital, to enable him to obtain suitable employment and to retain it, and to keep himself in good health. He should not only persevere with his drugs, but avoid the circumstances which precipitate fits—undue fatigue, hunger, drinking large volumes.

CHAPTER 17

NURSING PATIENTS WITH SKIN DISEASES

THE skin lies between the exterior and the deeper tissues, and so is exposed to influences from both sides. From without it may be affected by heat and cold; by chemicals; by mechanical irritation; and by infection from bacteria or skin parasites. The blood stream may carry to it from within toxins which may cause rashes, as in measles or scarlet fever; products of nutrition which can produce skin sensitivity; chemicals such as drugs which often cause eruptions. The skin is a very extensive organ, so that a widespread skin reaction can be a very big one.

The nurse will already be familiar with its structure and its many functions, but it is necessary to remind her of one very important fact. The epidermis is made from the same embryological structures as the nervous system and the retina, and can be regarded, not too fancifully, as an external part of the nervous system. Not only is it an important sense organ, but it is closely linked with the nervous system in that it has a psychic function. Many people express their emotions violently through the skin by flushing, paling and sweating, and it is now well known that these vascular changes can become fixed in skin rashes, so that emotional and psychological causes can operate very powerfully in irritating and maintaining skin conditions. Itching can be easily induced subjectively, as everyone knows who has listened to a lecture on pediculosis, and if scratching occurs, skin lesions follow very quickly. Dermatologists have long known of the effect of the patient's state of mind on the state of his skin, but today it is recognized as a major factor in the treatment of skin disease.

The converse is also true; the state of the patient's skin affects the state of his mind. One has only to think of severe pustular acne on the face of a girl in her 'teens, and the effect it must have on her social development and self-esteem.

This connection must at all times be considered in dealing with people with skin affections. In addition the lay public believes that all skin diseases are infectious, so that sufferers feel isolated and shunned. In fact, few are contagious and such precautions as wearing gloves when dealing with them are not only needless but cruel. A patient whose rash is conditioned by guilt may subconsciously feel that it is a punishment, and accept it as such, so that there is little incentive to healing.

There is a well-known saying that skin patients never die and never get well. This, of course, is not true; there are infective conditions that will never recur once they are efficiently treated, and many that occur acutely but never return. Unfortunately, there are many which are very chronic indeed, and who may attend skin clinics over long periods. The reasons for this are important to the nurse.

1. The cause of some skin conditions is imperfectly understood.
2. The skin is one of the main organs which express an allergic

reaction, and it is slow to forgive an injury. Sensitization to one substance may lead to intolerance of others. Modern life in an industrial community allows exposure to a large and increasing number of irritants.

3. Treatment of an extensive rash is very difficult for the patient to apply himself. It takes a lot of time, is messy, ruins the clothes, and is unpleasant to do in winter in a cold bedroom. If it is to be done properly at frequent intervals, it often means staying away from work, and this the patient is reluctant to do because the condition is not disabling.

4. Itching is a prominent feature of many rashes and leads to scratching which makes the skin hot and increases the itching. This circle must be broken before healing can start, and it is often impossible without bed treatment.

This allows easier and more thorough application to the skin, avoids heating and irritation from friction by the clothes, and the difficulty about staining underwear. Just like any other inflamed organ, the skin benefits from rest.

PRINCIPLES OF TREATING SKIN CONDITIONS

Patients admitted to a ward are nursed between special sheets to avoid the discoloration of linen caused by many ointments. The purpose of this must be carefully explained, and if the condition is not infectious, this must be stressed, or the patient will be depressed at the mere sight of his bed. Blankets must be few and light, and cradles may be used to keep them from the trunk or legs. Nightclothes should be of cotton, and are provided by the ward. Pyjamas are not good for generalized rashes ; they may cause friction between the legs. Hot-water bottles and all such forms of heating must be avoided.

The itching-scratching circle must be broken, and for this sound and uninterrupted sleep at night is invaluable. Phenobarbitone two or three times a day is useful in reducing tension, and extra sedation can be given at night. The nurse should notice and report if there is any scratching during sleep.

On general grounds, the bowels should be kept open, the fluid intake good, and the diet adequate in all essentials. Diet does not play as great a part in dermatology as in some other medical conditions, except where an allergy to a foodstuff is known to exist. Acne is a disease which can be made much worse by injudicious carbohydrate intake, and cocoa in all its forms as chocolate should be absolutely prohibited. Alcohol is a vaso-dilator and will increase irritation in an inflamed skin.

Many drugs once used by mouth in the treatment of skin complaints are not now prescribed ; the ones likely to be exhibited are :

1. Sedatives.
2. Anti-histamines for allergic conditions.
3. Hormones in a few cases. Cortisone is the most important, having a marked if temporary effect in reducing skin inflammation. The penetrating power and anti-inflammatory action of corticosteroids can be increased by sealing the area to which they have been applied

by a polythene occlusive dressing. Hands or feet can be enclosed in a polythene glove or bag; the air is expelled, and the edges sealed to normal skin with sellotape. Such dressings are not left on for more than twelve hours, or the skin will become macerated, and it is usually most convenient to apply them at night and remove them in the morning.

4. Antibiotics can be used by mouth or by injection for infected lesions.

Skin Applications

Powders increase the radiating surface and so are cooling to the skin.

Lotions can be solutions and when applied cause heat loss by evaporation. Suspensions are insoluble substances suspended in liquid, and calamine lotion is one of the best known. They have the cooling effect of solutions, and when dry leave a powder on the skin which continues the action.

Liniments are liquids with an oily base.

Creams are thin ointments, containing enough water to allow them to cool the skin by evaporation.

Pastes are preparations in which the solid ingredients and the base are present in equal parts. The ones used for skin conditions, such as zinc paste, are thick, somewhat porous and absorbent.

Ointments are greasy and are heavy applications which reduce the cooling power of the skin.

For erythema, powders and lotions are cooling ; lotions, liniments or creams are used on weeping surfaces ; crusts are removed with oils or starch poultices ; ointments are used mainly for scaly surfaces.

Baths

For widespread skin conditions, baths may be soothing if much irritation is present. Tar baths are of value in psoriasis. Sulphur, once popular in the treatment of scabies, is not now used, having been superseded by less irritating substances.

The temperature of baths for these patients should be 100°–103° F. (37·8°–39·5° C.) and prolonged soaking is not advised ; about fifteen minutes is usually sufficient. An average bath holds 25–30 gallons of water.

Oatmeal. Two breakfastcupsful of oatmeal are cooked with 2 pints of water for half an hour in a double saucepan. The result is put in a muslin bag, and well squeezed in the bath water. The nurse who tends the patient in the bath will be able to notice its softening and soothing effect on her own hands and forearms.

Bran. Three pounds of bran is put in a muslin bag and tied under the hot tap while the bath is running. When the bath is full the bag is detached and squeezed under the water for a few minutes. This is also a soothing bath. The bran must not be put loose into the bath, or it will block the outflow.

Soda. Half a pound of sodium carbonate or bicarbonate is dissolved in the bath. As bath salts, soda is very widely used in softening water.

Starch. One pound of starch is put in a large washing bowl, mixed to a paste with cold water, and stirred to a mucilage with boiling water.

This is then poured into a bath and well mixed. It may be prescribed for irritation with scaling.

Tar. Four to eight ounces of coal tar extract is used per bath, usually for psoriasis. The bath must be cleaned immediately after use if it is not to become badly stained. Spirit is used first to dissolve the tar, and small amounts left over from dressings should be saved for this. Finally a scouring powder is used.

Antiseptic. Sitz or hip baths are prescribed for, e.g., furunculosis of the vulva. Eusol 2 oz. per pint, or potassium permanganate 1 in 6,000 are effective antiseptics.

Skin Dressings

The cooling properties of skin applications are of great value, and these must not be wasted by putting heavy dressings over them. Wool has very little place in dermatology except as swabs for cleaning, or for dabbing on lotions.

If lesions are being treated by lotions, it may be convenient not to use any dressing, so that lotion can be constantly applied and allowed to cool the skin in drying. If pastes or creams are used, a dressing which is light and open, but capable of retaining the paste must be found. Gauze is suitable for many cases, but the threads detach very easily, and it should not be used where there is crusting. Skin muslin, which is firmer but still open in texture, is most useful. No other dressing is used.

Bandages cannot follow any regular pattern ; they must be open wove, and no more than is sufficient to retain the dressing in place. Reverses and figures of 8 which make the bandage thicker must be avoided. Tubegauz is useful in retaining dressings in awkward situations, and conforming cotton or Netelast bandages are useful.

Dressing a patient with extensive lesions must be performed with the utmost thoroughness. Had a cursory application been enough, the patient would not have needed hospital care. The requirements vary greatly, but the skin muslin, gauze, open-wove bandages, swabs, forceps, wooden spatulæ, pedal bin and the medicaments ordered are all needed.

The part to be treated must be fully exposed and seen in a good light. If the rash is at all extensive the bed-clothes should be entirely stripped and the patient left covered with a sheet. All dressings are removed, and the lesions carefully examined for activity, or signs of improvement. Dried pastes or lotions should be gently removed with swabs dipped in oil, but where the application is still moist it can be left. Vigorous toilet of the skin, which heats it and removes epithelium from healing areas, is to be deprecated. A nurse's natural instinct is to cut blisters, remove all traces of paste and tidy up meticulously, but this will delay healing. If it is possible to say that the lesions are progressing, or at least to point out places where this is true, it should be done. Application of lotions or creams must be adequate, and every part affected must be treated.

CHAPTER 18

APPLICATIONS TO THE SKIN

Applications of heat or cold can be made to the entire body, and hot, cold or chemical substances can be used locally on the skin in the expectation of affecting the tissues beneath it. The field of usefulness of such applications has greatly diminished in the last quarter of a century. Very much better alternatives exist to many of the treatments described in this chapter, and sometimes the purpose with which they were used is now not deemed a desirable one. Some of these the nurse will never see in use, but there are circumstances in which they may be required, and even in hospitals where all the most modern methods are available requests recur from time to time for some procedures that are usually considered outmoded.

GENERAL

Lowering the Temperature

Since the principal channel of heat loss is the skin, it is natural to use this function when it is desired to lower the temperature. Rise of temperature is in most cases a response to infection, and to deal with the cause by specific or antibiotic treatment is obviously more desirable than merely treating symptoms. There are still many occasions however when reducing fever is desirable or vital.

1. For hyperpyrexia in drug-resistant infections, e.g. pneumonia.
2. To lower the temperature after brain operations, when the heat-regulating centre is temporarily ineffective.
3. For useless fever, such as the hyperpyrexia that sometimes occurs with lymphadenoma.
4. In heat stroke.
5. To lower the temperature below the normal level as a means of reducing the metabolic needs of the brain, or the activity of the heart, as a means of medical treatment, or to assist surgery (i.e. hypothermia, p. 382).

The skin loses heat in four ways, and advantage can be taken of all of them.

1. *Conduction.* Cold packs or baths are means employed.
2. *Radiation.* Removal of the garments allows this.
3. *Convection.* Cradling permits air currents to pass over the skin and cool it, and an electric fan hastens loss in this way very effectively.
4. *Evaporation.* As water evaporates from the skin it takes from it the heat necessary for evaporation. Sponging the skin and leaving it moist will hasten heat loss.

Baths

Hot baths, between 100° and 105° F. (38 to 40° C.), are used by sick and well alike for cleansing purposes. They dilate the superficial skin vessels and induce a feeling of warmth and comfort that is especially welcome at bedtime. A warm bath is between 90° and 95° F. (32 to 35° C.), and those not able to take regular baths often prefer them warm rather than hot. Cold baths constrict the skin vessels temporarily, and are only suitable for the robust, except in cases of heat stroke, when it is vital to reduce the temperature quickly.

Mustard baths for infants are unlikely to be ordered today, though once popular in treating convulsions or collapse. One ounce of dry mustard is tied in cloth and squeezed in 3 gallons of water at 100° F. (38° C.). The baby is laid in it, with a cold compress on the forehead, and should be lifted out in three minutes, or earlier if the nurse feels tingling of the skin of the forearm supporting the baby. It is lifted on to a warm towel and most gently dried before being returned to its cot. (For medicated baths, see p. 223.)

Sponging

This word is loosely used for two quite different procedures. If a patient feels hot, or is sweating, " sponging " the limbs and trunk with warm or hot water is refreshing, raises the morale and encourages sleep. It only differs from a blanket bath in that it is not primarily cleansing, and that soap may only be used for the flexures that need it.

Sponging in its technical sense is a procedure for reducing pyrexia by allowing water to evaporate from the skin ; care should be taken by doctors and nurses that each understands what the other means when using this term.

Since hyperpyrexia is largely due to infections, it follows that efficient antibiotic therapy has reduced the indications for sponging. It may be used in these instances.

1. Hyperpyrexia resistant to antibiotics.
2. Hyperpyrexia in lymphadenoma, in which periodic crises of useless fever may recur (Pel-Ebstein fever).
3. In thyroid crisis.
4. Following disturbance of the heat-regulating mechanism after a brain operation.
5. In some tropical conditions characterized by high fevers.

Trolley. *Top.* Washing bowl of water at 100° F. (38° C.)
Bowl of ice cubes.
Bath thermometer.
Two lint compresses on ice.
Bowl of sponges (five if available).
Bath thermometer.
Talcum powder.
Backflannel and soap.

Bottom. Two cotton bath blankets.
Long mackintosh.
Face and back towels.
Warm bath towel.

Also : Bed cradle.
Clinical thermometer.

Method. Sponging must be performed without hurry and with careful attention to the patient's reactions to it if it is to be effective. The top clothes and nightclothes are removed, and the patient covered with a cotton blanket, while a cotton blanket and long mackintosh are rolled beneath her. Her face is sponged to refresh her, and dried, and an iced compress wrung out and applied to the forehead. The sponges are dropped in the water and a moist one placed in each axilla and groin. An arm is exposed, and sponged from shoulder to fingers with a sponge just wet enough to leave small beads of water on the skin. It may seem that water at a temperature of 100° F. (38° C.) is too warm to cool the skin very effectively, but it must be remembered that it is the evaporation that takes up the heat, and if the water is cold to begin with, the patient may start to shiver, and that this will raise the temperature faster than the nurse can lower it. As the sponging progresses, a little ice can be added if there is no untoward effect. The whole procedure should take about twenty minutes.

If the patient appreciates it, the bowl can be put on the bed, the hand placed in it, and water streamed over the forearm from the sponge. The second arm is treated like the first, and then the chest and abdomen. At intervals the iced compress and the sponges in the flexures are changed. The upper parts are covered, the legs sponged, and then the patient is turned on her side with her back to the nurse. At least five minutes should be taken over sponging the back, which presents a large evaporating surface. At the conclusion, the back should be dried, and the pressure areas powdered, since they would be uncomfortable to lie on if left moist. Without turning the patient the long mackintosh and blanket are rolled up, and the drawsheet freshened ; she is turned towards the nurse, and the mackintosh removed. The pillows are turned over, and the patient left with a clean nightdress and light coverings supported by a cradle. When the trolley has been cleared the temperature should be taken, and a fall of 2° F. or 1° C. is satisfactory, and quite often it will continue to fall slowly for the next few hours.

Untoward effects are not usual, but if the colour changes or the pulse becomes poor, sponging should be stopped, the patient is dried with the warm towel that has been kept in readiness, and covered with a blanket while her doctor is consulted. A little shivering is not an indication for stopping if the pulse is not affected, but usually shows that the procedure must be continued with more caution.

Cold Pack

A cold pack may be ordered to reduce the temperature in heat stroke.

Requirements. Cold compress on ice.
Small bath of cold water (50° F. (10° C.) or as ordered).
Bath thermometer.
Pail.
Bowl of ice.
Ten small towels.
Long mackintosh and sheet
Jaconet pillow case.
Clean gown and linen.
Bed cradle.
Stimulant tray.
Clinical thermometer.

Method. At the beginning of treatment the patient should have the sheet and long mackintosh beneath him, a jaconet cover over the pillow, a sheet to cover him, and a cold compress on his forehead. The towels are each folded into half lengthways and then in three in the other direction. They are dipped in the bath, excess water is pressed out, and they are unfolded and placed in position. One is put on to each arm, two on the trunk and two on each leg, and they are changed in rotation, the water being kept cold with ice. The procedure may be continued for twenty minutes or longer, but the temperature should be taken every five minutes, and a rectal thermometer is usually the most reliable. The pack is usually discontinued when the temperature has fallen to 101° F. (38·3° C.), as it will drop further afterwards.

Hot Packs

Hot packs may be used to induce sweating, but it is not now usually thought desirable to do so. In acute nephritis when there is fluid retention and diminished output of urine, it may seem that to encourage fluid loss through the skin would help the patient, but in fact it does not help the kidney.

Hot Wet Packs

Although hot wet packs to induce sweating have fallen into disuse, they may be needed in some parts of the world for painful spastic muscular conditions. Moist heat is soothing, and is applied in this way.

Pieces of old blanket are cut to the size of the limb on which they are to be used ; each must be big enough to wrap well round, and a piece of jaconet somewhat larger is needed to cover it. The pack is wrapped in a roller towel and boiling water is poured over it. Two nurses should wring it out unless it is a very small one, because it is important to wring it dry. It is tucked round the limb, pinned in position and covered with the jaconet. Each pack should be changed as soon as it begins to cool in about five minutes. A series is usually ordered, lasting perhaps for half an hour every three or four hours.

If a hot wet pack is to be applied to the entire patient, a long mackintosh between two blankets is rolled beneath him. An old blanket is folded in a sheet, put in a bath of water as hot as can be managed, and wrung thoroughly out by two nurses. It is applied carefully, and covered with a long mackintosh and two dry blankets. Hot-water bottles can be put around outside the blankets to maintain the heat. A towel is tucked under the chin, and can be used to dry the face at intervals. A cold compress on the forehead is desirable, and hot drinks can be given to increase the sweat-provoking properties of the pack. The pulse should be taken at the temporal artery at frequent intervals, and a nightgown blanket and towels are warming for use when the pack is removed. When it is over, the blanket and mackintosh beneath the patient are removed, leaving him lying on a blanket. The pack is taken off, the patient rubbed down and dressed in a dry shirt and covered with a warm blanket. Sweating will continue for some time and the nurse should be prepared to change the shirt at intervals.

Hot Dry Pack

Three blankets are rolled beneath the patient, and folded loosely over. Hot-water bottles or hot bricks are packed around. An electric blanket is a more efficient way of warming the patient, but it is not very likely to be available in the circumstances in which such a pack might be ordered. As in the wet pack, a towel should be put under the chin and a cold compress on the forehead. Dry garments should be ready to put on when the pack is discontinued, and watch is kept on the pulse in case it is necessary to interrupt the treatment.

POULTICES

Kaolin Poultice

Requirements. Small saucepan.
Tin of kaolin.
Poultice board.
Metal spatula.
Old linen or lint.
Gauze.
Scissors.
2 metal or enamel plates, warmed.
Wool pad or gamgee to cover.
Bandage or other means of securing.

Method. The cover of the tin is loosened, and the tin set in a saucepan of water, where it must boil for ten minutes in order to be thoroughly heated. While it is warming, the remaining articles needed are laid on a poultice board in the dressing room, and the linen or lint and the gauze cut to the size needed. The patient must then be prepared to receive the poultice, and the area is left readily accessible but covered.

The tin is lifted out on to the poultice board and its contents thoroughly stirred to amalgamate the contents and bring them to an even temperature. With the spatula the kaolin is rapidly and evenly spread to a thickness of 0.5 cm. on the smooth side of the lint, or on to linen. Old linen is the better choice for small poultices to septic fingers, and of course costs nothing, while lint is usually better for large poultices to the chest.

The gauze is spread over the kaolin and the edges of the poultice trimmed if necessary to neaten them. Folding the margins inwards is a common practice but has no advantages, and if the poultice is a small one the folded edges may prevent efficient contact with the skin. The poultice is put between two warm plates and taken at once to the patient. It is tested for temperature against the nurse's forearm, and if it is not too hot is applied, covered with wool and secured.

For medical purposes kaolin can be applied directly to the skin without the intervention of gauze, when it will retain its warmth longer. A little olive oil applied to the skin beforehand will prevent sticking. If it is being used on the chest for pneumonia, a chest many-tail bandage with shoulder straps or a crepe bandage can be used to secure it. If it is important not to disturb the patient, gate strapping is useful, especially for children. Applied without gauze, it may be left on for twelve hours ; for inflammatory lesions, four-hourly renewal by day is customary, with one change by night if the patient is awake.

Linseed Poultice

Linseed makes a comfortable supporting poultice for pain in the back or kidneys, but is rather bulky for the chest. Though not used frequently now in this country, there are others in which it is commonly ordered.

Requirements. Poultice board.
Linseed.
Bowl.
Kettle of boiling water.
Jug of hot water with spatula.
Old linen of required size.
Gauze of same size.
Scissors.
Wool or gamgee pad.
Two warm enamel plates.
Many-tail bandage.

The patient is prepared for the application, and the wool pad left covering the area while the poultice is being made. The bowl is warmed with a little boiling water and the work must be speedily completed once it is begun. Enough boiling water is poured into the bowl (and a little experience is needed to gauge this correctly) and then linseed is added rapidly with the left hand while stirring the mixture briskly with the spatula in the right hand. Linseed is added until the consistency is that of a Victoria sandwich mixture, and it comes away from the sides of the bowl, then it is turned on to the linen, spread quickly and evenly to within an inch of the edge. The gauze is laid over, and the edges must be turned in to help retain the poultice, which should be about ½ in. thick. It is folded or rolled and carried at once to the bedside between the hot plates, tested on the forearm for temperature, and put in position. It must be removed every four hours and if the skin is at all reddened a little olive oil should be applied.

Surgical Fomentation

A triple fold of white lint is folded into a towel or wringer and boiled for five minutes with the ends of the wringer well out of the water and fastened to the saucepan lid if gas is the method of heating lest they scorch. When the wound has been prepared, the fomentation is carried to the bedside in its wringer in a bowl, and must be thoroughly wrung out by an assistant who opens the wringer so that the dresser can extract the fomentation with forceps, shake it free from steam and apply it. It is covered with jaconet and a pad. The usual practice is to put on a series of fomentations—perhaps one every ten minutes for half an hour or so—every four hours. In between a dry dressing is used to prevent skin maceration.

Medical Fomentation

A triple fold of lint or flannel is put into a wringer in a bowl and boiling water poured over. The fomentation is wrung tightly out and applied under jaconet and a pad. It is not sterile, and is used for stiff and painful joints, or muscular aches and pains, and since it costs nothing may be useful in home nursing. It can also be used over the suprapubic area for acute retention of urine.

APPLICATIONS OF COLD

Cold applied to the skin constricts the superficial blood vessels, and so may check capillary bleeding, reduce extravasation of fluid, and relieve congestive pain. It is not suitable for inflammatory reaction due to infection, in which the hyperæmia is a desirable effect, and heat will be found much more comforting.

Evaporating Lotions

As noticed in connection with sponging, evaporation of liquid removes heat from the surface on which it takes place. Sprains of the ankle or knee are sometimes treated with such lotions as lead lotion. A double fold of lint is soaked in the lotion and applied with the least possible covering so that evaporation can take place readily. As the compress dries it is re-soaked in lotion.

Cold Compress

A double fold of lint is wrung out of iced water and applied to the suspected area, which is often an aching head. A spare compress should be cooling in the iced water, and should be changed at frequent intervals.

Ice Bag

The icebag is made of rubber with a wide stopper, since when filled with ice it is heavy for direct application; it is usually suspended over the part that it is desired to cool. Perhaps its most common use is on a bed cradle to help in lowering temperature.

Requirements. Poultice board.
Ice bag and lint cover.
Ice.
Stout pin.
Salt.
Teaspoon.
Cradle.
Open-wove bandage.

Method. A heavy pin will be found much more convenient than the conventional ice pick for breaking the ice into pieces about the size of a walnut, and the bag is two-thirds filled with these. A teaspoonful of salt is added to lower the temperature, and air is excluded before screwing in the stopper. A cover must be put on the bag, otherwise condensation may take place on the exterior and drip on to the bed. The bag must be refilled as soon as the ice melts.

COUNTER-IRRITANTS

A counter-irritant is a substance which dilates tbe superficial blood vessels when applied to the skin, and this produces a reflex constriction of deeper vessels. This reflex effect must be stressed ; the amount of blood brought to the surface is not an accurate measure of the relief afforded.

This interesting old branch of medicine is falling into disuse ; the times when a physician might be called a leech because of the frequency with which he ordered leeching are a long way off. Some of these procedures are tried in emergencies when other remedies have failed ; some are still used to a limited extent ; and some have fallen into merited disrepute. It is difficult to imagine circumstances in which their use might be revived. A few of the less uncommon are given below.

Turpentine Stupe

Requirements. Those for a medical fomentation.
Turpentine ½ fl. oz. (15 ml.) in a poison measure.

The turpentine is sprinkled on to the material used for the fomentation before putting it in the wringer and pouring on the boiling water. A turpentine stupe is usually applied to the abdomen, and is said to relieve distension. It should be looked at after five minutes and subsequently every two minutes and can be left on for ten minutes if there is no undue skin reddening earlier. It is sometimes useful for those with abdominal pain of functional origin, withdrawing their attention from the abdominal sensations to which they are abnormally sensitive. A little oil should be applied when the stupe is removed.

Mustard Leaf

A mustard leaf is a sheet of paper with a dry layer of flour and mustard on one side, and it is usually obtained ready made. It is dipped in water, applied to the skin, and removed when a good reddening effect is obtained, when the skin is dried, powdered and covered with a pad of hot wool. As a domestic remedy for stiff backs or joints, it is as successful as proprietary medicated wools sold for the same purpose, and is sometimes called a mustard plaster. Other " plasters " are little used ; belladonna plaster was once popular, but belladonna has no effect on the skin unless the patient is sensitive to it, when it can produce a severe reaction. The only comfort derived was from the supporting action of the plaster, but although doctors now think little of them, it will be noticed that the general public still has sufficient faith in them to buy them from the chemist.

Iodine

Iodine fortis (10% in alcohol) can be painted over painful joints. Two coats are applied, and the area must dry very thoroughly before it is covered. Before painting a large area, it is wise to make a small application to ensure that there is no adverse effect. Dentists often make use of iodine as a counter-irritant, painting it around an inflamed or tender tooth.

Counter-irritant Liniments

A variety of liniments are in use which redden the skin on rubbing in, and are bought as "embrocation" by the lay public, not only for their own joint pains, sprains and muscle stiffness, but for those of horses.

Methyl salicylate is absorbed through the skin, which it reddens, and is the main ingredient of a well-known liniment which also contains camphor, eucalyptus and menthol. Apart from its counter-irritant action, the massage with a warm hand that rubs it into the skin is most comforting for stiff joints.

CHAPTER 19

PRE- AND POST-OPERATIVE NURSING

NOT every patient who enters a surgical ward does so in order to have an operation, but a big number do, and it is important for the nurse to remember that no operation is a minor one to the person who is undergoing it. Improvements in surgical and anæsthetic technique have made operations safer, until comparatively big operations like partial gastrectomy may seem to the nurse a routine procedure with an unfavourable outcome almost unknown. To the patient, however, it is a formidable undertaking, arrived at often after much pain and anxiety and some disagreeable preparation, and is something that is going to influence the whole course of his life.

The surgical nurse has the pleasure of seeing many patients undergoing successful operations and being sent home quickly, well on the road to recovery. She sees sometimes, too, trouble and even disaster arising after some surgery. Such complications may arise with great suddenness, and she must constantly be alert, comparing her patient's condition now with what it was five minutes ago.

PREPARATION FOR OPERATION

The amount of pre-operative preparation and the time needed for it vary very widely. One patient may be elderly, anæmic, underweight, with a malignant growth necessitating a formidable operation, while another may be young and fit with some minor complaint. The following section indicates the scope of preparation that may be needed for surgery, while remembering that some operations are small enough to be performed in an out-patient department, with no more preparation than ensuring that the stomach and bladder are empty.

Patients undergoing an operation of moderate extent are admitted to a surgical ward about two days beforehand, for the following reasons :

1. **Investigation.** The temperature, pulse and respiration, and the weight are recorded, and the condition with regard to an anæsthetic assessed. A chest X-ray may be needed, the hæmoglobin level and the blood group may be ascertained, and the many tests relevant to special operations will be mentioned elsewhere. The nurse, meanwhile, is making an important observation of her own—how the patient is reacting to admission and the coming operation, what is the best attitude to adopt to reassure and help him.

2. **Preparation, Physical and Mental.** The patient must be made ready in these respects :

(*a*) *Confidence.* He must feel trust in his surgeon, and in the nurses whom he sees going competently and calmly about their work. His operation is explained to him in terms he can understand, and he gives his written consent. If he is a minor, his parents consent. His peace of mind is ensured by sound sleep, helped if necessary by a hypnotic.

(*b*) *Nutrition.* An underweight patient may need building up with a high calorie diet. If he has been living on a diet lacking fruit and vegetables he will need vitamin C and should be given ascorbic acid by mouth (50–150 mg.) or by intramuscular injection. If he has jaundice he must be given vitamin K (10–20 mg.) by intramuscular injection to prevent bleeding after operation. Plenty of fluids and glucose will help to prevent post-operative shock.

(*c*) *Digestive System.* The rectum should be empty before any major operation. If it is an abdominal one, an aperient is given thirty-six hours beforehand, and usually an enema the night before. The stomach must be empty, or vomiting may occur during anæsthesia and cause inhalation pneumonia. Food should be withheld for six hours, and fluid for four hours before operation.

(*d*) *Respiratory System.* Exercises in deep breathing and coughing taught before operation will help to avert post-operative chest complications. Just as important is the fact that free movement of the diaphragm encourages return of the blood to the heart from the inferior vena cava, averting the circulatory complications that will be described on p. 247.

(*e*) *Local Preparation.* The skin through which the incision is made must be as free as possible from organisms. Any hair must be shaved. A man undergoing an abdominal operation is shaved from the nipple line to the pubis by the hospital barber, while the nurse shaves the female patients. Small areas can usually be done most easily by the dry method, using powder and a new blade, but for the abdomen and vulva, a soap lather is the most comfortable way. Really hot water, and a lather stiff enough to keep the hair upright will facilitate the procedure. Preparation of the skin for an orthopædic operation is extensive, since joint cavities are susceptible to infection ; for instance, an operation on the knee is preceded by a shave from the groin to the toes. For large areas like the head an electric razor is recommended. The shave is followed by a bath, with careful attention to the umbilicus. Preparation of the skin in the ward by antiseptics is not now universally practised except by orthopædic surgeons. If it is required before an abdominal operation, the skin of the whole abdomen is painted, using sterile swabs held in sterile forceps. Ether, surgical spirit and 2% cetrimide are often used. Sterile towels are then bandaged in position using an open-wove bandage, and sewing or strapping the end. A great many surgeons now rely entirely on the toilet of the skin in the theatre and do not find any increased incidence of sepsis.

OPERATION DAY

Operation day in a surgical ward needs to be well organized if all is to go smoothly. The list is given to the ward sister the day before, and she sees that her staff know the order in which patients are going to the theatre, and the times of their last meal. Relatives will be told of the approaching operation, and the time at which they should telephone for news. It is not convenient to have visitors during operating sessions unless anxiety is felt about the outcome. They will be made uneasy by the sights and sounds of recovery from anæsthesia and gain nothing by seeing their relative unconscious. Telephone enquiries should, however, be answered as helpfully as possible and not in stereotyped phrases. "He is as well as can be expected," is a reply that dismays lay people, who do not know how well one can be expected to be after an operation.

Stock should be checked for possible deficiencies. *Linen* should be in good supply—operation gowns, socks, nightdresses, sheets and pillowcases. *Drugs* such as morphine, papaveretum, hyoscine and nikethamide will be needed. Sterile syringes, needles and dressings are available in adequate quantities. *Intravenous* equipment must be in order, and bottles of sterile *saline* available. *Oxygen* cylinders should be full, and equipment for its administration complete. If operations involving drainage are to be performed, *drainage jars*, rubber tubing and suitable glass connections must be ready.

SAFETY OF THE SURGICAL PATIENT

Unless adequate precautions are taken, there is a possibility that an operation may be performed on the wrong patient, or on the wrong side, limb or digit. The safeguards against such an accident by the Medical Defence Union and the Royal College of Nursing include the following:

1. All patients should be labelled on admission, whether they are going to medical or surgical wards.
2. The casualty sister or her deputy should be responsible for labelling all unconscious patients admitted through the casualty department. The lable should include the patient's registry number.
3. The surgeon or his houseman should see the patient before he is anaesthetized, and ensure that the notes are indeed those of the patient.
4. All patients going to the theatre should be labelled with their name, initials and number. The labelling should be the responsibility of the ward or casualty sister, or her deputy.
5. A copy of the operation list should be displayed in the anaesthetic room as well as the theatre, so that the anaesthetist can check his patient. The patient's name and not merely his operation should be given on the list. The ward sister should also have a list
6. Patients should be sent for by name and number, and if a porter is sent from the theatre for a patient, he should be given an order slip.
7. The ward sister is responsible for seeing that:

(*a*) the correct patient goes to the theatre.
(*b*) that he has signed a consent form
(*c*) the premedication has been given
(*d*) that where appropriate, the correct side or limb or digit for operation has been marked by the house surgeon. If this has not been done, the sister should inform the surgeon, but NOT undertake the marking herself.

Operations on the wrong limb may occur if:

(*a*) the description in the case papers is incorrect
(*b*) writing is illegible
(*c*) "right" and "left" are abbreviated to rt. and lt. and misread.
(*d*) The wrong notes accompany the patient to the theatre.
(*e*) The wrong limb or digit has been prepared by the ward nurse.
(*f*) The entry on the operation list is not checked with the patient's notes.

It will be seen that the nurse is responsible for seeing that the patient, correctly prepared and labelled, is sent with the correct records to the theatre. It is not her responsibility to mark a limb or organ that is to be operated on or removed, and she should never do this. Mistakes have occasionally been made because beds have been moved on busy operating or duty days.

IMMEDIATE PRE-OPERATIVE CARE

About an hour and a half before the operation is due, the nurse draws screens around the bed, and brings the patient a bowl of warm water to wash the face and hands, and mouthwash. She collects the following articles :

- 2 theatre blankets.
- 1 headshawl.
- 1 vomit bowl and towel.
- Set of anæsthetic instruments :
  - Tongue depressor.
  - Mouth gag.
  - Tongue forceps.
  - Sponge-holding forceps.
  - 6 gauze swabs.
- 1 open-backed theatre gown.
- 1 pair of operation stockings.

The patient is helped into the theatre gown, which must not be tied behind but folded well around. Long socks are put on. If the patient is a woman, all clips must be removed from the hair, which, if long, is made into two plaits fastened with open-wove bandage. Jewellery is removed and given into sister's keeping, but if a woman dislikes parting with her wedding ring it may be completely covered with elastoplast. False teeth are removed and put in a glass of mouthwash in the locker. The bladder is emptied and the amount passed recorded on the patient's notes. The pre-operative injection is given and recorded. It usually includes morphine or one of its allies to induce relaxation and drowsiness, and atropine or hyoscine to depress secretion from the respiratory tract. The patient is reassured, and settled down to sleep until the time arrives for her to go to the theatre. Beside her are the anæsthetic instruments in a bag, the vomit bowl and towel, her notes and the X-rays. The ward sister or staff nurse checks that the patient is correctly labelled.

The theatre trolley, which will be brought by the theatre orderlies for her, has a sorbo rubber mattress covered with a canvas stretcher by which she will later be lifted from the trolley to the theatre table. Like all theatre equipment, it has some anti-static device, and preferably a bag or rack to take notes and equipment. The patient is lifted on to the trolley with one of her feather pillows and the two operation blankets. If she is awake, the nurse speaks to her quietly and reassuringly by name and accompanies her to the anæsthetic room, where she remains till the patient enters the theatre.

OPERATION BEDS

As soon as the patient has gone her bed is made ready for her return. It should be made with clean linen, unless the operation is a very minor one, to provide clean surroundings for the operation site. For many years the traditional method of preparing it has been to warm it with hot bottles or an electric blanket for most patients. The number of patients for whom warmth is not indicated is, however, increasing and includes the following classes :

(a) The thyrotoxic patients.
(b) Those operated on in hot weather.
(c) Those whose surgeon believes that shock is best treated by the patient being kept cool (p. 242).

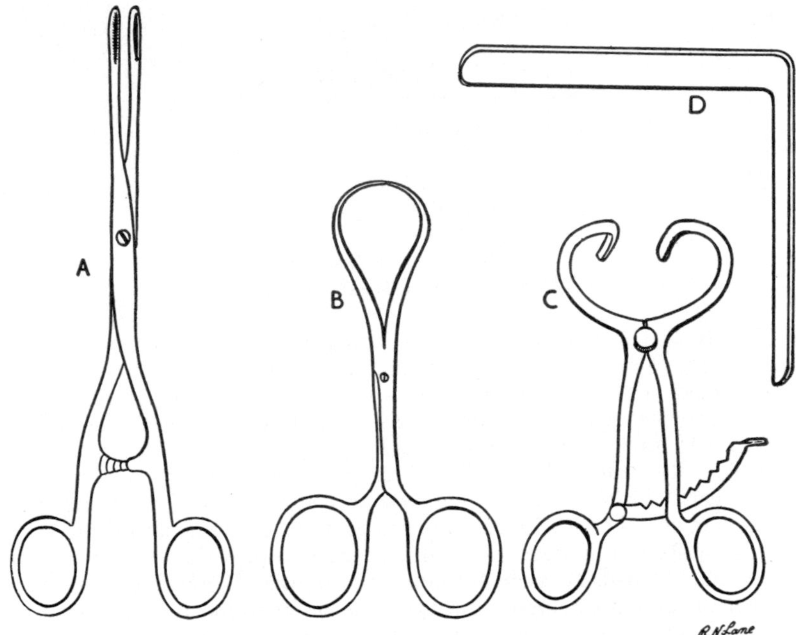

FIG. 55. Instruments for maintaining and clearing the airway of the unconscious patient.

A. Sponge-holding forceps. C. Doyen's gag.
B. Tongue forceps. D. Spatula.

A warm bed is, however, so widely used that it will be discussed here. The bottom of the bed is made up as usual, and on it is laid an electric blanket, or two hot-water bottles in distinctively coloured covers. On top a blanket is folded, and the top clothes are added. The sides must not be tucked in, so that they can easily be rolled either to the bottom of the bed or to one side to receive the patient. Pillows are not usually allowed until consciousness is regained, but one flat one may be permitted, especially after neck or head operations, when it should have a jaconet cover. A mackintosh and towel at the head of the bed is necessary for some cases (e.g. tonsillectomy), and may be liked by the ward sister for all patients. If the bed is going to the theatre, the sides of the clothes should be rolled up on to the bed to prevent them brushing against doorways. Blocks may be ready for the foot of the bed, either to help in the treatment of shock in the recovery phase, or to help prevent the patient slipping down the bed later.

Beside the bed are the pillows ready for insertion when consciousness is regained. On the locker are the following :

1. Vomit bowl and towel, or paper handkerchiefs.
2. Anæsthetic instruments.
3. Receiver for artificial airway and used instruments
4. Any of the following deemed necessary :
   (*a*) Thermometer.
   (*b*) Mouthwash and receiver. If the patient is to take no fluids by mouth, a mouth tray is substituted.
   (*c*) Treatment board.
   (*d*) Special equipment, such as sterile tubing and connections in a covered dish.

POST-OPERATIVE NURSING

Some hospitals have recovery rooms (p. 309) where patients are nursed for the first few hours following operations, but in many the patient returns at once to the ward. A ward nurse goes to the theatre for her, and receives a message about the operation and any relevant instructions from the house surgeon. An artificial airway of rubber will usually be in the mouth when the anæsthetist hands the patient over, and the colour and breathing will be satisfactory. No difficulty should occur on the brief journey back to the ward, since anæsthetists like the patient to be transferred either with the cough reflex restored, or sufficiently anæsthetized to remain quiet. The nurse walks closely beside the patient, keeping the head turned to one side and the angle of the jaw held forward to support the tongue if the patient is still deeply unconscious.

Screens or curtains should be drawn round the bed while the patient is settled. The electric blanket must be switched off, if it is in use, and the bedclothes folded to the bottom or one side. Any hot-water bottles must be removed. These are the circumstances in which many of the recorded cases of bottle burns occur—the unconscious person is laid on a bottle which is not noticed. The dressing is rapidly inspected for bleeding, and usually the socks can be removed before adjusting the top clothes. The policy as regards warmth or otherwise will be decided by the surgeon and is further discussed under shock (p. 242).

A thermometer is put under the axilla and the pulse and respirative rate taken and recorded. If all are satisfactory, there is no need to record these more frequently than four-hourly, but the pulse rate must be regularly checked. The colour of the skin is observed. A pink skin and normal temperature are reassuring, and if sweating is taking place it is a sign of overheating. If, however, a patient with a low temperature is sweating, it is an indication that the skin is too cold to evaporate the normal sweat, and the patient is suffering from shock that needs treatment.

During this phase the preservation of the patient's vital functions—respiration and circulation—are of paramount importance, and must be discussed in detail.

Maintenance of Respiration

No one should be left alone until the cough reflex has returned Once this level of consciousness has been regained the patient is safe if the nurse is within reach in case of vomiting or restlessness. During the dangerous period before the cough reflex returns, asphyxia may occur for one of these reasons :

1. **Obstruction of the Airway by the Tongue.** This cannot take place if the artificial airway is correctly in place, and it should, therefore, not be removed until the patient is making movements of the tongue and lips to reject it. If the airway is out, and the patient lying on the back, the relaxed tongue may obstruct the glottis. It can be prevented by keeping the patient on her side, or at least keeping the head turned to one side. It is much safer to keep a plump patient with a short neck on her side rather than to attempt to rotate the head on the neck. Keeping the angle of the jaw well forward helps to support the tongue.

The tongue forceps should not be used by the nurse unless she is alone and must keep the tongue forward while engaged on other restorative measures. Even when carefully used it must damage the tissues. It is applied with the blades parallel to the surface of the tongue, and is put on to the dorsum of the tongue, in the midline, so that its teeth pass through the fibrous central septum. The handles lie outside the mouth and can be used to steady the tongue in position.

2. **Obstruction of the Airway by Mucus.** Mucus may be freely secreted by the respiratory tract in response to anæsthesia and instrumentation, and if the breathing becomes rattling or the colour congested, this should be suspected. The jaws of the gag should be inserted at the side, and the mouth opened by pressure on the handles. If the tongue is not well forward in the mouth, it should be depressed with the spatula, but if the obstruction is mucus a gauze-covered swab held in a pair of sponge-holding forceps is used to clear it.

3. **Obstruction of the Airway by Vomit.** This cannot occur unless the patient is left lying on her back unattended. In intestinal obstructions reflux of stomach contents occurs easily, and the Ryle's tube, which will be left in the stomach after operation, should be aspirated before the patient leaves the theatre and at sufficient intervals on return to the ward to keep the stomach empty.

4. **Spasm of the Glottis.** This is more likely to occur during induction of anæsthesia than after operation, but occasionally follows lifting the patient from the trolley into bed. Breathing ceases, although the artificial airway is in position and no mechanical obstruction apparent. The nursing staff must summon the anæsthetist, lay the patient on the back with the head and neck extended, give oxygen at 8 litres per minute, raise the foot of the bed, and prepare a 5-ml. syringe, No. 1

needle and nikethamide for intravenous injection. If breathing is not quickly resumed, artificial respiration by rhythmic pressure over the sides of the thorax is begun.

In any case of difficulty with respiration after an operation the anæsthetist must be informed. It is better that he should arrive and find the emergency over rather than be called too late.

Maintenance of Circulation

Shock is a condition of which the underlying pathology is a fall in the blood pressure. For detailed theories as to its mechanism, a text-book of surgery should be consulted, but its signs and symptoms are important to the nurse, and she must know the contributing causes so that she can mitigate them as far as she is able.

Signs and Symptoms. The *blood pressure* is low (i.e. the systolic pressure is less than 100 mm. Hg.). The *pulse* is feeble, tending to be slow at the onset and becoming quicker in rate and thinner in volume as the condition progresses. The *temperature* is subnormal, and the *skin* cold and moist. The colour is "livid," i.e. pale with a tinge of cyanosis. *Vomiting* is common and *thirst* is complained of if the patient is conscious. The characteristic mood is *apathetic*.

Shock is produced by trauma, especially *crushing* injuries, *fractures*, *painful* injuries like burns, major *operations* involving resection of tissue, or traction on the mesentery or lung roots. It is made worse by *fluid loss*, as from hæmorrhage, vomiting, diarrhœa or profuse sweating, or leakage from raw areas ; by *pain* ; by *fear*. Until recently, exposure to cold would have been added to this list, but recent work makes this doubtful.

Knowledge of the physiology of shock is constantly growing and methods of treatment are constantly under review. The classical mainstays of treatment are these :

1. **Rest.** The patient must be moved as little as possible. The head low position allows the blood to reach the heart and brain where it is most needed.

2. **Relief of Pain.** Fractures must be temporarily splinted, and burns covered. Morphine has enjoyed a high reputation, and for patients with internal bleeding, pain or fear is excellent. Its chief danger is that when given to a patient with circulation impaired by shock, it may remain in the tissues and only be released as the condition improves.

3. **Fluids.** If shock is not severe, fluids by mouth can be freely given. If these are contra-indicated, tap water or N/5 saline per rectum is useful. If the condition is more than moderate, intravenous fluids will be needed. Blood is incomparably the best, but plasma or dextran may be life saving. Saline can only effect a temporary improvement. Large amounts of fluid are sometimes needed, and watch must be kept on the pulse, respiration and superficial veins lest right heart failure threaten from dilation of the right side of the heart by the incoming fluid.

4. **Oxygen.** Poor circulation results in lack of oxygen in the tissues, and for severe shock oxygen at 8 litres per minute is valuable.

5. **Warmth.** This is the most controversial of the means recommended for treating shock. A nurse's instinct is to warm a patient who looks and feels so cold, but it is becoming increasingly obvious that it may be unwise. Heating such patients with radiant heat cradles has long been abandoned, since warming the skin may draw blood from the vital centres where it is needed and increase fluid loss by sweating. For some time the guiding principle has been to prevent heat loss with warm coverings, but not to leave hot bottles or electric blankets in the bed. Now many surgeons think that a patient with a low blood pressure is better off with a low temperature, and allow no effort to raise the temperature. The nurse should see that she understands the wishes of her chief.

Post-operative Shock. The patient is returned to bed and the surgeon's wishes with regard to warmth and position followed. The *temperature* is taken, if necessary with a low-register thermometer, and if the skin temperature is below 96° F. (35·5° C.) it is taken every half-hour. A pulse record is made every fifteen minutes. The nurse is often asked to record the blood pressure every half-hour, and if this is done, she must ask at what level she may discontinue this rather disturbing procedure, or what fall should mean summoning the doctor. Records are useful only in so far as they influence treatment, and nurses must understand their purpose.

Hæmorrhage

Hæmorrhage may be *internal* when it takes place into the peritoneal or some other body cavity, or *external* when it is manifest on the surface. It can be classified according to the vessel from which it is taking place :

1. **Arterial.** The blood is bright red and appears in spurts corresponding to the heart beats. It may be seen (briefly!) in the theatre when small arteries are severed, before artery clamps are applied.

2. **Venous.** The blood is darker in colour, and wells out. Such loss may be very severe. If a large vein near the heart (e.g. internal jugular) is cut, the negative pressure in the vein may allow air to be sucked in and carried to the heart.

3. **Capillary.** The blood oozes out. If capillary bleeding is taking place from a large raw area, it can be troublesome, especially if it is maintained by a failure to clot, as in *jaundiced* patients, or those in whom the intestine has been sterilized by antibiotics ; both are short of vitamin K, and therefore have a low prothrombin level.

A classification of bleeding useful to the nurse depends on the time at which it occurs.

1. **Primary hæmorrhage** occurs at the time of injury. In surgical practice it takes place in the theatre and the surgeon sees that it is checked before the patient leaves.

2. **Reactionary hæmorrhage** occurs as the blood pressure rises following shock, and vessels begin to bleed that were unnoticed at operation. It, therefore, takes place within a few hours of operation. Patients who are suffering from shock must be watched closely for bleeding as their condition improves.

No patient is immune, but the operations most commonly followed by bleeding are *prostatectomy*, *tonsillectomy*, and operations on the *rectum*, *vagina* and *blood vessels*.

3. **Secondary hæmorrhage** is always due to sepsis, and, therefore, a few days normally elapses before it occurs. The classical day is the tenth, and the danger period is the second week. Infection erodes the clot that is sealing the severed vessels, and arterial bleeding is possible.

Such bleeding is not unheralded ; fever and signs of inflammation in the wound usually precede it. It is virtually unknown after most operations, and very common in some, e.g. *prostatectomy*, in which some infection of the cavity where the prostate gland was removed is very difficult to prevent.

The *signs* of internal hæmorrhage are as follows : low temperature and blood pressure, a pulse rising in rate and falling in volume (" thready "), pallor and sweating, sighing respiration, yawning (especially with bleeding into the stomach), fainting, and an air of anxious unease that is characteristic. If the patient is still unconscious, this picture will, of course, be somewhat modified, and a nurse may be undecided if her patient is suffering from shock or concealed bleeding. She should make regular observation of the temperature, pulse, respiration and blood pressure and watch the colour. A progressive deterioration in these, however small, will make her suspect hæmorrhage and inform the surgeon, since shock should become less when the operation is over and adequate anti-shock treatment instituted.

OTHER POST-OPERATIVE COMPLICATIONS AND DISCOMFORTS

Pain. Wound pain is normal, but can be effectively relieved. *Morphine* or one of its allies (e.g. *omnopon*) is necessary after major operations, and usually is repeated once or twice. It is used very cautiously after chest or head operations because of its depressing effects on the respiratory centre. *Pethidine* by mouth or intramuscular injection is less depressing, and very effective for gynæcological and thoracic patients. Once the first day or so is over one or two compound codeine tablets are effective. *Aspirin mucilage* is excellent for sore throats, as after tonsillectomy or thyroidectomy. Pain may be associated with many of the complications described below, and their effective treatment will relieve it.

Vomiting. This is a traditional accompaniment of anæsthetics, but is becoming less common. It may occur once or twice as consciousness is regained, and will not be remembered by the patient. A clean bowl should be given each time a patient vomits, and the mouth rinsed out, since if ether has been given its nauseating taste will still be apparent. No morphine should be given, since it often perpetuates the vomiting. An anti-emetic drug like perphenazine (" Fentazin ") is often prescribed.

If vomiting continues for more than twelve hours it is possible that nervous tension and anxiety are sustaining it, but more probable that it indicates some abdominal complication. A **Ryle's tube** is passed transnasally into the stomach and retained there by strapping the end to the cheek, and it is aspirated often enough to prevent vomiting. The character of the fluid and its amount is noted and the usual records of the temperature and pulse made frequently. Fluid is given intravenously.

Abdominal Distension. Flatulence after abdominal operations is due to wind collecting in the inactive gut. It is at its worst on the second and third days, and is not only distressing in itself but stretches the wound painfully and impedes the movement of the diaphragm. Early mobilization will help to prevent it ; drinks of peppermint water or the passage of a *flatus tube* may help. The tube is lubricated at the eye end, and the other is attached to a glass connection and a piece of rubber tubing which lies under a bowl of water. About 6 in. is passed into the rectum, and left for ten minutes, or longer if relief is experienced. Heat (e.g. an electric pad) to the abdomen is comforting.

An enema or glycerine suppository may be given on the third day if there are no contraindications; it is not usually effective earlier. Once the bowels are open no further trouble is experienced.

Urinary Complications

Retention of urine means inability to pass urine although the bladder is full. It is not uncommon if the patient must lie in an unusual position, or after operations on the rectum or vagina. It may be prevented sometimes by introducing the patient to the use of urinal or bedpan before the operation, and by seeing that the patient is comfortably settled in privacy when the first attempt is made to empty the bladder. A note should always be made as to when the patient first passes urine, and the amount recorded.

To allow a patient to sit on a commode is usually effective in curing nervous retention, and many who would once have been thought too ill may now be permitted to do so. No perturbation should be shown if difficulty is experienced, and simple methods of suggestion such as a sharp drink like lemonade, or the sound of a running tap may help. A woman may have a pint of warm water poured over the vulva while sitting on a bedpan. An injection of *carbachol* helps to increase the tone of the bladder and is often effective. Catheterization must not be delayed until the bladder is unduly distended, and urine measurements must be continued until the bladder is being satisfactorily emptied. If very small amounts of urine are being passed at frequent intervals it usually indicates that *retention with overflow* has been reached, and catheterization is needed. The re-establishment of micturition after the use of an indwelling catheter is discussed more fully in connection with gynæcology (p. 292).

Suppression of urine or *anuria* means that no urine is being secreted and the bladder remains empty. It is a serious condition, since if secretion is not re-established it must be fatal. Treatment depends on what the surgeon considers to be the cause.

Cystitis or inflammation of the bladder is signalized by frequent painful micturition and may occur if the operation causes trauma to the bladder or retention is allowed to go untreated, or catheter technique is faulty. Its incidence may be reduced by good operative methods, aseptic catheterization and guarding against bladder distension. A high fluid intake, and an alkaline mixture like potassium citrate with hyoscyamus are good prophylactic measures. If it occurs, the infecting organism is identified from a catheter specimen by the bacteriologist, and the appropriate antibiotic or sulpha drug begun. An intake of about 5 pints, or 3000 mls. a day is aimed at, to dilute the infection within the urinary system.

Respiratory Complications

Broncho-pneumonia. This is quite common after abdominal and thoracic operations, and may follow any type of anæsthetic. Contributory causes are :

1. Poor movement of the chest and abdomen allowing accumulation of bronchial secretion. Since men depend more on abdominal movement than women, they are more liable to broncho-pneumonia.
2. Immobility in bed permitting congestion of the lung bases.
3. Pre-existing bronchitis.
4. Heavy smoking. On this count, too, men outnumber women.
5. Irritating anæsthetics.
6. Heavy sedation with drugs depressing to the respiratory centre, e.g. morphine.

Signs and Symptoms. About twenty-four hours after operation there is a slight cough and mucus can be heard rattling in the bronchi. The temperature, pulse and respiration rate all rise slightly (e.g. T. 99·6° F. (37·5° C.); P. 90; R. 22). If not promptly and effectively treated, the temperature will fluctuate irregularly up to 101° or 102° F. (38·3 or 38·9° C.), and the pulse and respiration rate are correspondingly elevated. An undue rise in the pulse rate indicates that the myocardium is feeling the strain and beginning to fail. The course of bronchopneumonia is indeterminate with remissions and relapses as the infection spreads in one part of the lungs and clears in another.

Treatment. Prevention is better than cure. Before operation any bronchitis should be treated effectively, smoking should be cut down or forbidden, breathing exercises should be taught ; nurses should see that they are performed. After operation, deep breathing and coughing are encouraged ; supporting the wound may be a great help, and percussion over the chest by the physiotherapist will help to loosen secretions. Post-operative drugs should be judiciously prescribed and given to susceptible patients.

When pneumonia is first suspected, all these efforts at improving the chest movement should be redoubled. Steam inhalations are helpful if the sputum is tenacious, and fluids are freely given. A course of a broad-spectrum antibiotic, such as ampicillin, is begun. If improvement is not obvious in twelve hours a specimen of sputum is sent to the bacteriologist to find the antibiotic to which the infecting organism is sensitive. Although broncho-pneumonia is painful and prolongs convalescence, it is not as dangerous as formerly.

Lobar Collapse. If a bronchus is plugged with mucus, so that air entry is stopped, the air remaining in the lobe is absorbed and that portion of lung becomes solid. The onset is more dramatic than that of broncho-pneumonia, with a sudden and marked rise in temperature, pulse and respiration rate (e.g. T. 102·4° F. (39·1° C.); P. 120; R. 32) and the patient looks ill and anxious on examination; the chest is dull over the collapsed lobe.

It is vital that the mucus be coughed up at once to allow the lung to re-expand. The patient may be laid on the good side with the head low and vigorous clapping over the affected lobe and coughing undertaken. If the mucus is too thick to be expectorated, resort will have to be made to bronchoscopy. A good fluid intake (intravenous if necessary) must be kept up to make the bronchial secretions more fluid.

Pulmonary embolism. A pulmonary embolus begins as a blood clot, usually in a vein and the measures described in the next section on how to avoid such clotting will also help to prevent embolism.

Minor cases of embolism are treated by encouraging activity and giving anticoagulant drugs by mouth. In more severe cases, intravenous heparin is given to prevent extension of the clot. Some surgeons once the initial stage of shock is over, perform arteriography by intracardiac. catheterization, to see how much of the lung is affected, and if it is large, give intravenous streptokinase to attempt to dissolve the clot and restore function to the lung. Patients with a large embolus who might be expected otherwise to make a good recovery may be taken to the theatre, and have the clot removed after opening the pulmonary artery. This is a severe operation for a dangerously ill person, but is sometimes successful.

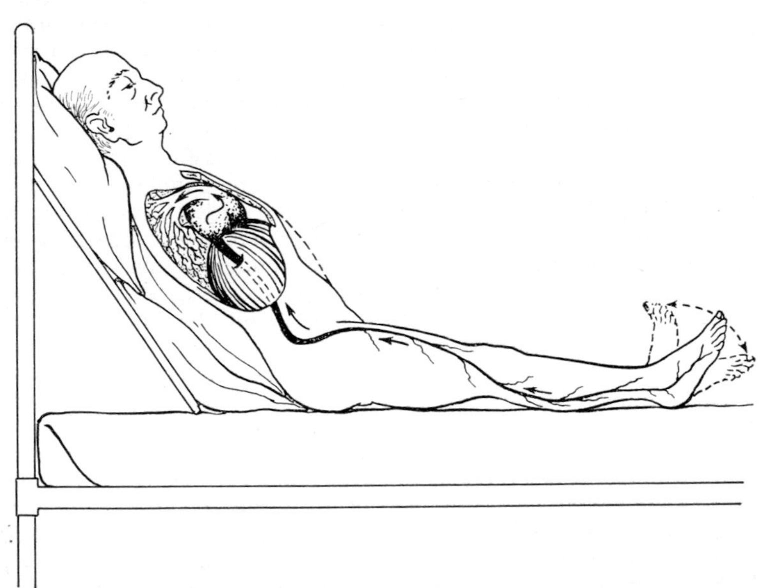

Fig. 56. Prevention of vascular complications.
1. The upright position allows free diaphragmatic movement.
2. Raising the foot of the bed helps venous return.
3. Foot and leg exercise involve the action of the muscle pump on the veins.

Intravascular Thrombosis

Clotting within blood vessels occurs in two different ways, and the cause, prognosis and treatment is quite distinct. (A) *Thrombophlebitis* is clotting within an inflamed vein, and in surgical practice is most often seen at the site of an intravenous infusion. Pain is invariably present, and the vein is tender and can be felt as solid with clot ; the temperature rises, usually to 99°–100° F. (37·2–37·8° C.), but sometimes higher. The clot is firmly adherent to the inflamed vein, and its detachment to form an embolus is unlikely. Warmth by kaolin poultices will relieve the pain, and the patient's progress is not delayed long. Intravenous dextrose is especially liable to cause thrombophlebitis, and infusions should not be continued longer than is strictly necessary. (B) Clotting within the *deep* veins of the calf appears to be caused by a combination of some of these factors:

1. Pressure on the calves on the theatre table or in bed.
2. A prolonged subnormal blood pressure, as in shock.
3. Anæmia.
4. Pelvic operations.

The vein wall is normal, the clot does not usually fill the lumen, and is only loosely adherent, so that the danger of pulmonary embolism is very great, and is what makes this condition so important. There may be a little fever, cramp or tenderness may be felt in the calves, and if the clotting becomes extensive there may be œdema of the leg.

This phlebothrombosis should be *prevented*. Pressure on the calves on the table can be relieved by a sandbag under the Achilles tendons. Shock should be adequately treated and anæmia relieved. Deep breathing exercises will improve the return of blood to the heart, and early rising after operations and mobility in bed are important. Nurses should feel the calves while giving a bed bath after abdominal or pelvic operations, and report tenderness at once.

If clotting occurs, an intravenous course of heparin (e.g. 10,000 units six-hourly on the first day) followed by dindevan (e.g. 50–100 mg. twice a day) is usual, to lower the clotting powers of the blood, unless hæmorrhage is feared. Surgeons' practices vary according to whether they believe mobilization will bring the risk of embolism nearer, or if they think confinement to bed will encourage the growth of the clot. Most would probably keep the patient in bed if there was any fever, but encourage mobility as soon as it disappeared. The prothrombin time is estimated daily as long as dindevan is being given, and not allowed to fall below 20% lest bleeding occur.

The importance of breathing exercises and of activity is apparent in several of the above sections. Good diaphragmatic movement lessens the risk of pneumonia, of thrombosis in the legs, and of pulmonary infarct and lobar collapse. It must not be thought however that post-operative patients need little care other than of their wounds. It is true that many of them benefit from performing their own toilet, but unless they are encouraged and helped with it in the early days, they may quite understandably do it with as little disturbance to themselves as possible, and not very efficiently. Activity should be

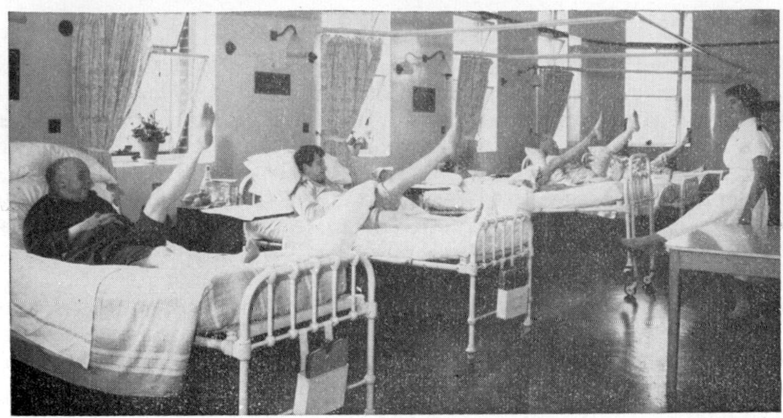

FIG. 57. A physiotherapist conducts ward exercises to avert venous thrombosis in the legs.

planned ; to hope that it will result from leaving the patient to fend for himself shows lack of nursing insight.

Infection

Infection has always been a problem in surgical wards and still is. We rarely see the gas-gangrene that used to be common in the eighteenth century, and streptococcal infections can be speedily and successfully treated. It is the staphylococcus, strains of which have acquired resistance to many antibiotics, that is still a major problem.

Staphylococci infect human tissues to produce boils, styes, osteomyelitis, pneumonia or pyelitis. But staphylococci may also be present on the skin and in the anterior part of the nose of people who are quite healthy, and who merely carry the organism. Patients, nurses, doctors and domestic or lay staff who work in surgical wards may thus be sources of infection to others. This is termed cross-infection.

In addition, staphylococci from such sources may be transferred to objects in the ward by direct contact or through the air, and bedclothes, curtains, dust, baths, screens and all kinds of ward equipment. These act as depots in which organisms can survive for long periods, and eventually may be transferred to patients. Staphylococcal infections may endanger life, and at least will prolong the patient's stay in hospital.

The measures that will reduce the incidence of infection include these:

1. Ward premises should be adequate and beds well spaced. Surfaces that can be easily cleaned are desirable.

2. Nursing staff should be plentiful enough to maintain a high standard of hygiene in their work.

3. Techniques for dressing should be aseptic, and carried out conscientiously.

4. Wound and other infections must be recognized early; precautions to prevent spread are taken, and the patient isolated.

5. Contamination of the articles in the ward must be avoided. Wounds are kept covered, discarded dressings are disposed of quickly. Hands must be washed after touching infected surfaces.

6. Possible depots of infection must be removed. Ward cleaning must be effective, and methods that disperse dust into the air are dangerous. Bedding, curtains and screen covers are changed regularly.

7. Methods of sterilization must be effective.

8. Susceptible people must be protected; small babies are an obvious example.

9. The guidance of a bacteriologist on acceptable techniques of ward hygiene should be available.

DRESSING MATERIALS

The materials most used in surgical dressings are these:

1. *Gauze.* This is made of cotton in a wide mesh, and is the most extensively used of all. It is put next to all surgical wounds, since it is absorbent yet allows the passage of air. It is supplied in rolls, and cut into sizes suitable for dressings and theatre swabs, or made into rolls for theatre use. Gauze is expensive and should not be used if a cheaper substitute is efficient, e.g. paper handkerchiefs rather than a pile of gauze swabs should be used during the phase of recovery from anæsthesia.

2. *Cotton Wool.* White wool absorbs fluid readily, and a layer over a wound provides protection and support if this is needed. It is sold in rolls and should be unrolled and warmed before cutting into dressings to thicken and fluff it up. Swabs used in ward dressings are of cut wool, but since fibres of wool detach fairly readily, they should not be used in situations where this may be dangerous. Mouth swabs for the unconscious patient, for instance, must be covered with gauze, and wool must never be packed into cavities or wounds.

Gamgee tissue is a commercial dressing of wool in two layers of gauze.

3. *Brown wool* is not used for wound dressings or any sterile purpose, but has many nursing uses, especially when made into pads with gauze. It is non-absorbent, and many references to it will be found in other chapters.

4. *Lint* is less used now than formerly. It is too close in texture to be a satisfactory wound dressing alone, but finely perforated polyester plastic may be bonded to lint to make a non-adherent smooth dressing. Boracic lint is coloured pink and is impregnated in boric acid, but has little advantage over the plain sort. Lint is another substance which is expensive, and for which cheaper substitutes may be available. Poultices for instance can be made on old linen as effectively as on lint.

5. *Tulle gras* is a cotton net material impregnated with petroleum jelly (soft paraffin or "Vaseline") and is extensively used for dressing burns and raw areas from which exudate must be allowed to escape. It does not stick to wounds and can be removed painlessly. Manufacturers supply it in tins in various sizes, interleaved with paper, and sterilized.

6. Oiled silk and plastic are used for their waterproof qualities, e.g. above poultices and fomentations. Since they prevent evaporation of sweat from the skin they should not be used for very lengthy periods.

Theatre Dressings

If a wound is clean and no drainage tube is used, the dressing applied in the theatre is often not changed till the sutures are removed. Such a dressing may consist of dry gauze soaked in Whitehead's varnish, mastisol, or Nobecutane. These dry to make a firm adherent dressing which is an effective barrier to infection. Wool is used if discharge is expected.

Bandages have been nearly replaced by strapping after most operations on the chest, and many on the abdomen. They are still used for retaining dressings on the perineum, and usually for the limbs.

DRESSING TECHNIQUE

The technique of surgical dressings must be influenced by the circumstances in which they are performed. The industrial nurse, working single-handed and dealing largely with injuries that are often contaminated, will use a method different from a ward sister with an assistant dressing operation incisions. Training schools should try to establish a common dressing technique in all surgical departments, for confidence and understanding by the students will avoid breakdowns in technique that may lead to infection. The types of instrument dish and receivers differ between one hospital and another, but it is possible to state certain principles that must be borne in mind, whatever technique is adopted.

1. Open wounds may be infected from the air. To avoid this a dressing room is available in some wards to which patients may be taken. In any case, sweeping and dusting should be finished an hour before the dressing round begins, and blankets should not be agitated needlessly while uncovering the wound. The technique of dressing should be one that leaves the wound exposed for the minimum period.

Respiratory infection is also a cause for anxiety. An increasing number of nurses carry staphylococci in the anterior part of the nose, and for dressing raw areas (like burns) and some similar cases, a mask covering the nose and mouth should be worn, thick enough to prevent organisms being transmitted to the wound.

The question of the use of masks is a controversial one. A few years ago they were used for dressings of all kinds ; now the best advice that can be given is that hospitals should regulate their practice by the latest research. Disposable masks are generally used for ward work. A used mask should be discarded; if it is put moist into the pocket or apron front and worn again later it may be a danger rather than a protection to the patient. Many wounds are cleanly stitched and dry when dressed, and not susceptible to respiratory infection. There is also some evidence that constant mask wearing increases the nasal staphylococcal carrier rate in nurses. These are the reasons advanced by those who limit mask-wearing to dressing raw areas and wounds with drainage tubes. Those who advocate masks for all dressings believe that meticulous anti-infective technique in all details should be used, and that it is difficult to teach discrimination between one type of dressing and another.

2. The wound may be infected from hands, instruments, lotions and dressings if these are contaminated. Such infection may be avoided thus :

(*a*) Hands. It is not possible at present to sterilize the hands, so these should not touch the wound or its neighbourhood or anything

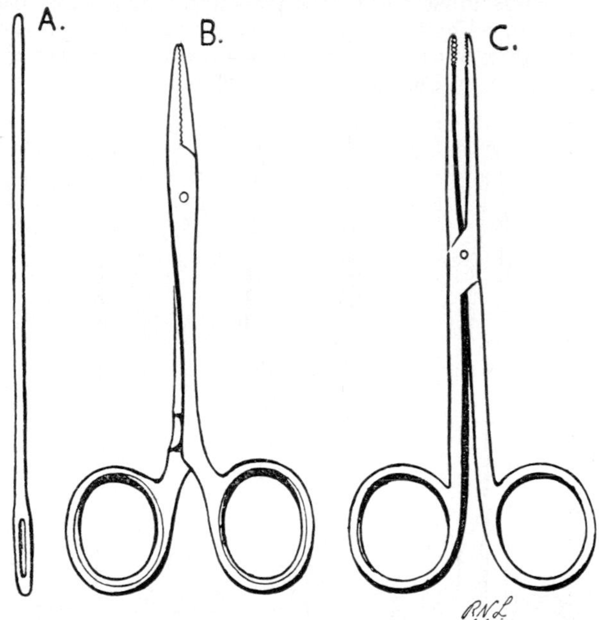

FIG. 58. Dressing instruments
A. Probe.
B. Spencer Wells' forceps
C. Sinus forceps.

else that will come into direct contact with it. The hands should be washed clean with soap and warm water, with attention to the nails, and dried on a clean towel. Disposable ones are satisfactory.

(*b*) Lotions which have been sterilized should be covered with metal caps; some of them (e.g. cetrimide) may become contaminated if fitted with corks.

(*c*) Instruments, bowls and gallipots must be sterile, and though boiling will destroy non-spore forming organisms, it cannot be relied on under usual ward conditions. Boilers may take a long time to reach the required temperature, and often do not possess a thermometer. Unless one nurse is in charge of it, more instruments may be added that send the water off the boil, and there is a risk of shortening the "sterilizing" time below an effective level. Autoclaving should be used whenever possible.

(*d*) Dressings. These should be made up in individual packets for each procedure. The practice of filling a drum with a variety of stock and extracting with Cheatle's forceps the amount required for a dressing cannot be justified, for contamination of the contents by recurrent opening is inevitable. Drums are expensive, noisy and heavy to handle, and easily damaged so that they do not close properly. They are also difficult to pack in a way that ensures efficient sterilization in the autoclave.

Soiled dressings must be at once placed in a disposable bag or in a covered bin operated by a foot pedal. At the end of the procedure they should not be taken out to the clean or sterilizing room, but disposed of in a covered bin or an incinerator in the sluice room.

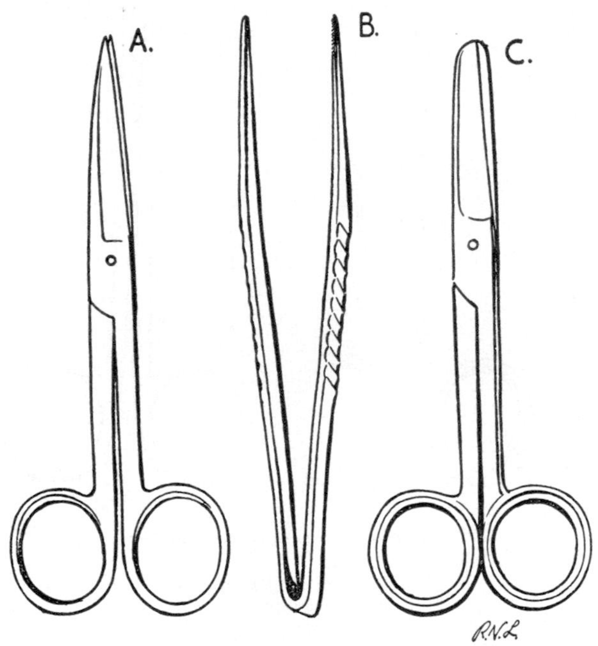

FIG. 59. Dressing instruments.

A. Stitch scissors.
B. Dissecting forceps.
C. Scissors.

4. Preparation of the patient efficiently makes the procedure easy for the dresser and comfortable for the patient. Nearby windows are shut, and screens or curtains drawn round the bed. If the wound is an abdominal one, the air ring is withdrawn and enough pillows removed to leave the patient semi-recumbent and relaxed. The bedclothes should be folded singly and smoothly to the level of the symphisis pubis. A nightdress should be rolled up and tucked in at the sides so that it cannot fall down while dressing is in progress. Bandages should be undone or strapping loosened from the skin so that forceps can be used to remove the soiled dressing.

STERILIZATION

To sterilize is to destroy all living organisms, including the spore-forms that some of them can assume, which are difficult to kill. The methods of sterilization are as follows:

Physical. Heat. Dry heat (hot air).
Moist heat (steam).
Irradiation. Gamma rays, beta particles.
Chemical. Liquids and gases.

Some of these methods are only suitable for large-scale use, by manufacturers or big institutions. These will be described separately from the ways that may be used in small units.

CENTRAL STERILIZATION OF SUPPLIES

Heat. *Dry heat* is widely used to sterilize syringes, which are passed on a conveyor belt through a heated tunnel. At a temperature of 190° C. sterilization is complete in 1½ minutes, and the process is controlled by a thermostat.

The only way in which *moist heat* is used in large-scale methods is in the autoclave. This is an appliance in which articles for sterilization are exposed to steam under pressure. A rise in pressure causes a rise in temperature. Textiles, lotions, instruments, rubber and some plastic goods can be autoclaved.

Before the sterilizing process begins, air must be removed from the autoclave, since a mixture of air and steam is less hot than pure steam at the same temperature. Modern autoclaves used in C.S.S. departments are high-vacuum, high-temperature machines ; that is, air can be efficiently and rapidly withdrawn, and sterilization-time is shortened because of the high temperature reached. The whole process is automatically controlled.

Articles from a central sterilizing unit are distributed to the departments or hospitals which use them, and so they must be wrapped. Plastic film or paper of an appropriate quality is usually employed, and as long as the outer layer is intact and dry, the contents will remain sterile almost indefinitely. Some hospitals like to issue a complete pack for every sterile procedure. This, however, means that large numbers of packs not in frequent use must be stored. Others design basic packs to which sterile items may be added.

Constant checking of the sterilizing process must be done, and Browne's tubes are often used. These little tubes contain red fluid, which changes through amber to green when exposed to a sterilizing temperature. Tape on which a pattern appears after sterilization can be used to fasten packages.

Considerable saving of stock is made when sterile packs are used ; trays for instruments and bowls for dressings are not required. The bag in which the equipment is packed can be used to receive soiled dressings, and if the pack is enclosed in a paper towel, this can be opened to form a sterile field.

Irradiation, either with gamma rays from a radio-active source (e.g. Cobalt 60) or beta-particles from a linear accelerator is a method best suited to commercial firms sterilizing very large amounts of stock.

The apparatus required is expensive, and skilled supervision is necessary.

Chemicals are little used in large-scale sterilizing ; fluids cannot be relied on to kill spores, and these " disinfectants " are most used in small units for purposes where destruction of spores is not important. Increasing use is being made, however, of the gas ethylene oxide, especially for plastics which are sensitive to heat. Ethylene is toxic and inflammable, and its use must be carefully controlled. Reference is made on page 464 to its use in sterilizing positive-pressure respirators.

Small-scale Sterilization

In small institutions, and in wards and theatres where centrally sterilized stock is not available, other methods are used. The smaller autoclaves found in such situations are commonly of a less advanced pattern than those previously described.

The air in the autoclave must be removed before textiles can be sterilized, and there are two ways in which this is generally done, and two corresponding types of autoclave. The air can either be withdrawn by a vacuum pump, or displaced by gravity by the incoming steam. If the vacuum method is used, an absolute pressure of the order of 15 mm. Hg. is required. Steam is then admitted and the length of time that sterilization takes depends on the materials being autoclaved and the temperature attained. The following *minimum* times and temperatures have been recommended by a working party on pressure-steam sterilizers for the Medical Research Council (1959).

3 minutes at 134° C. (30 lb. per sq. in.)
10 ,, ,, 126° C. (20 ,, ,, ,, ,,)
15 ,, ,, 121° C. (15 ,, ,, ,, ,,)

In downward-displacement sterilizers the steam enters at the top and the air, which is heavier, flows out at the bottom. Autoclaves of this type must be packed with the greatest care, or pockets of air will remain in containers and sterilization will be imperfect. This kind of apparatus requires skilled management if it is to be satisfactory.

At the end of a sterilizing run a load of dressings must be dried without contaminating it, and a vacuum must be drawn to achieve this. Finally, air must be admitted to break the vacuum before opening the autoclave, and this air must enter from a clean source through a bacteriological filter. Instruments do not need a vacuum to dry them, and autoclaves in wards or theatres used solely for them can operate more speedily.

Although the autoclave is capable of absolute sterilization, reliance on its efficiency will be misplaced unless certain conditions are fulfilled. Once an efficient autoclave has been installed in hygenic surroundings, there are four people who are responsible for successful sterilization.

(1) The bacteriologist should accept the responsibility for autoclave techniques and test their efficiency at regular intervals. Investigations in this and other countries indicate that where there is no single authority for sterilization methods, reliance on them may be quite misplaced.

(2) The engineer must maintain the machine in first-class working condition, and small faults should be reported at once.

(3) The person who packs the articles must do so in a way that allows effective steam penetration. There is no reason why a nurse should do the packing; once a satisfactory pack has been decided, lay people can do this quite well, and free the nurse for more personal tasks.

Boiling

Boiling cannot be relied upon to kill spores, and so is not a true form of sterilization, but it is effective against all ordinary bacteria, and is still widely used in wards and in domestic-style nursing. Boiling for five minutes is effective, if the water really boils throughout that period, if timing is accurate and articles completely submerged.

Pasteurization is the immersion of articles in hot water at 75° C. for 10 minutes. It has the same drawbacks as boiling, but is sometimes used for cystoscopes, which are usually heat-sensitive.

SIMPLE DRESSING

The pack illustrated in Fig. 60a consists of these articles, in the order found on opening.

1. An outer paper bag, sealed. This is subsequently to receive the used dressings.
2. A paper bag containing two pairs of dressing forceps which are used to lay the other sterile articles. The bag goes into the bowl on the lower shelf to receive used instruments.
3. An enclosing paper towel. It can be opened by means of its everted corners to form a sterile cover for the trolley.
4. A small paper towel which is used as an unsterile surface on which the handles of instruments can be laid if they are put down temporarily during the course of the dressing.
5. Two pairs of dissecting forceps and a pair of scissors.
6. A gallipot.
7. Swabs.
8. Dressing of gauze and wool.

The trolley is laid in the following way. The dresser puts on a mask, if this is indicated, washes her hands and swabs the top shelf of the trolley with a little sudol 1%, or a preferred disinfectant, using a mop kept for the purpose. It must be dry before use, and a disposable towel may be used. On the bottom shelf are the dressing pack, lotions, bandages and strapping, and a receiver which will hold the paper bag for the used instruments. A clip for a bag for soiled dressings is attached to one side of the trolley, and if there are bandages to be changed, a second bag is added.

If an assistant is available, she has in the meantime donned her mask (if required), drawn the bed curtains, and prepared the patient in the way indicated above.

The dresser washes her hands, opens her pack, lays the inner pack on the trolley, and places the outer bag well opened, in the clip on the side. She arranges her trolley as in the illustration, and pours out the lotion. The loosened dressing is removed and disposed of with the dressing forceps, which are discarded into the bag which originally contained them, on the lower shelf. Using fresh forceps and moistened swabs, she cleans the wound and then the surrounding area, observing any

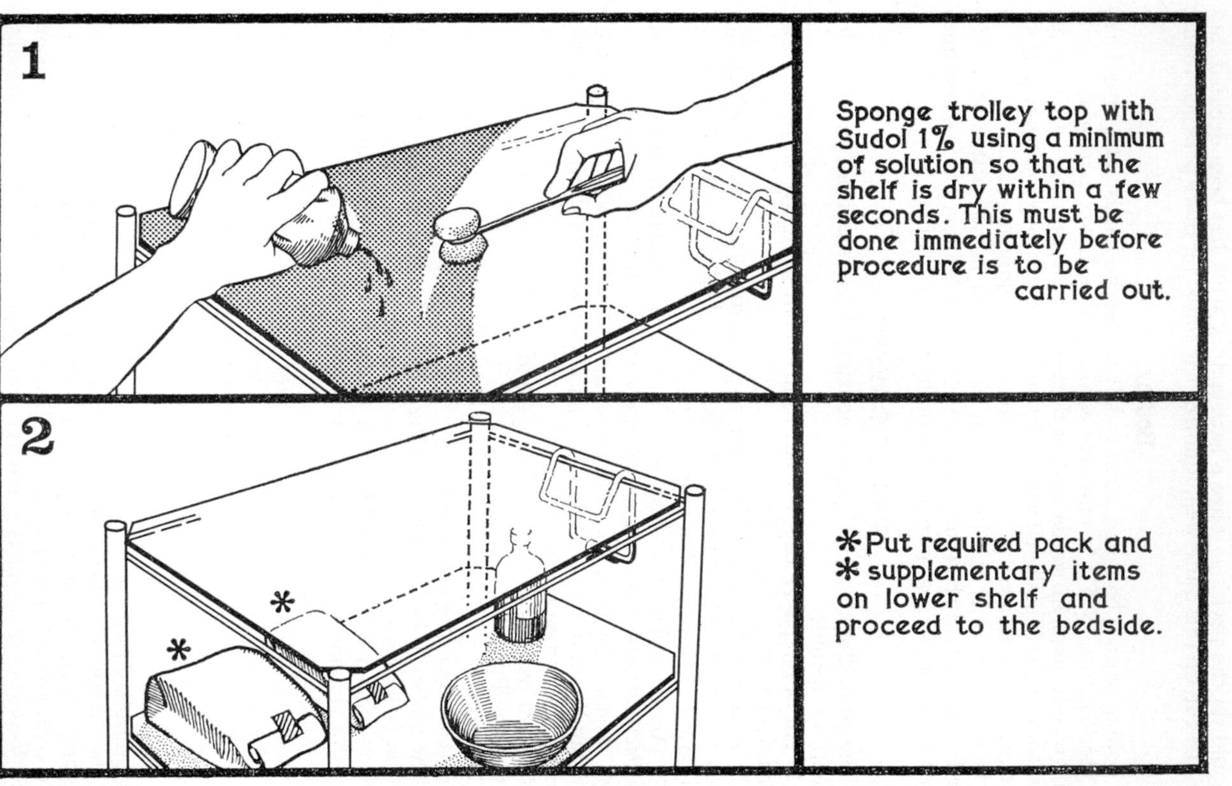
1
Sponge trolley top with Sudol 1% using a minimum of solution so that the shelf is dry within a few seconds. This must be done immediately before procedure is to be carried out.
2
*Put required pack and
*supplementary items on lower shelf and proceed to the bedside.
*
*

Fig. 60a.

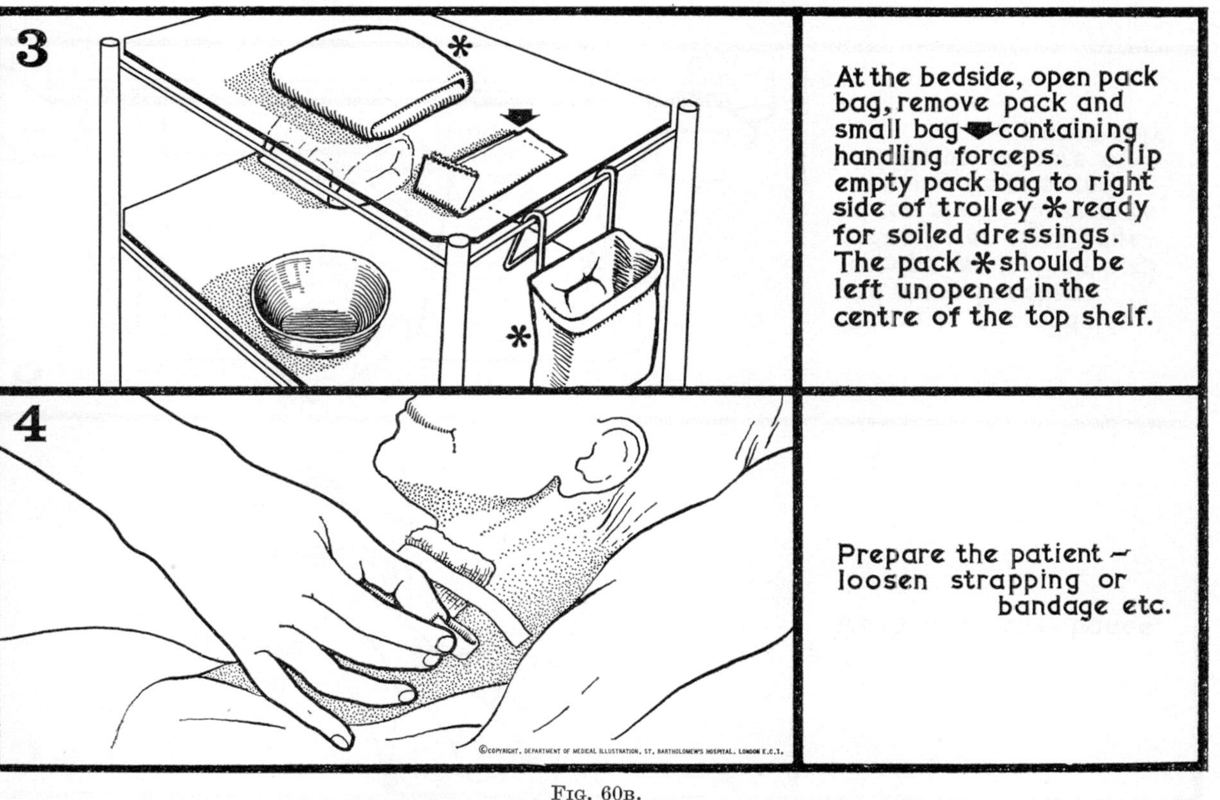
3
*
*
At the bedside, open pack bag, remove pack and small bag ➡ containing handling forceps. Clip empty pack bag to right side of trolley * ready for soiled dressings. The pack * should be left unopened in the centre of the top shelf.
4
Prepare the patient — loosen strapping or bandage etc.
©COPYRIGHT, DEPARTMENT OF MEDICAL ILLUSTRATION, ST. BARTHOLOMEW'S HOSPITAL, LONDON E.C.1.

Fig. 60b.

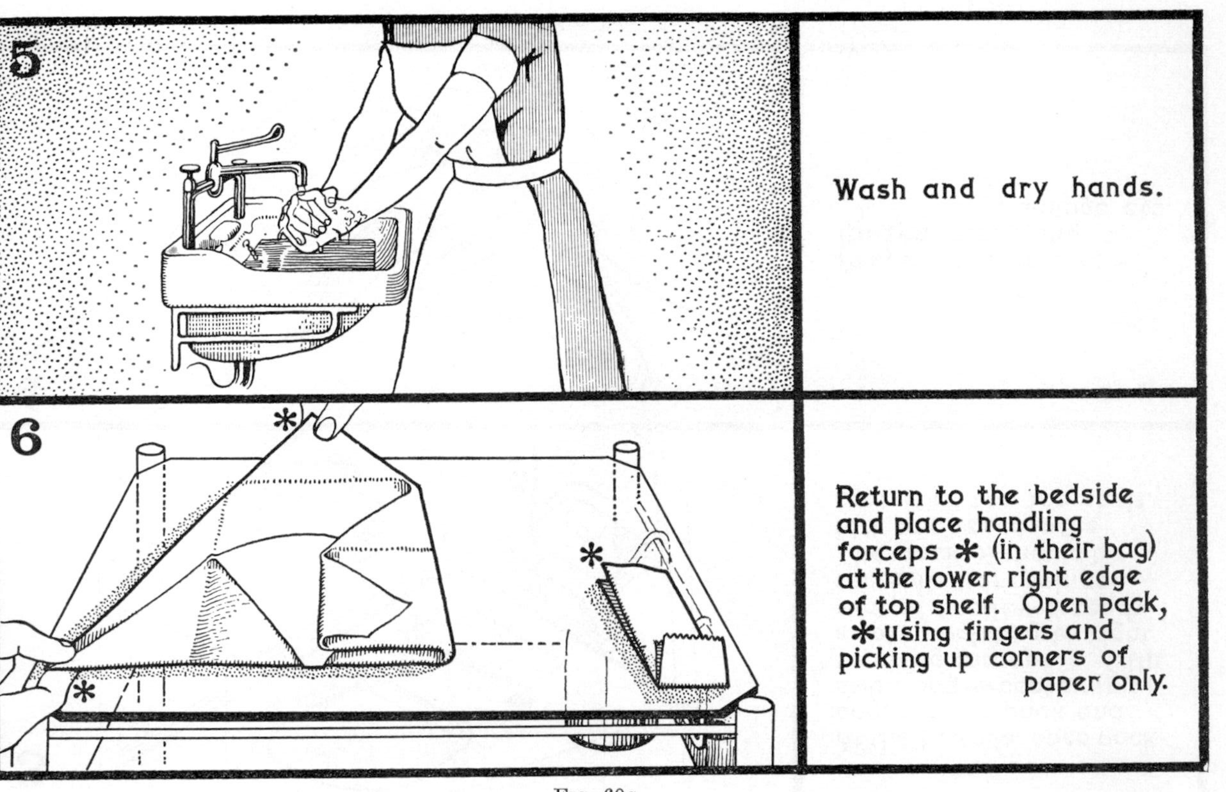
5
Wash and dry hands.
6
Return to the bedside
and place handling
forceps * (in their bag)
at the lower right edge
of top shelf. Open pack,
* using fingers and
picking up corners of
paper only.
*
*
*

Fig. 60c.

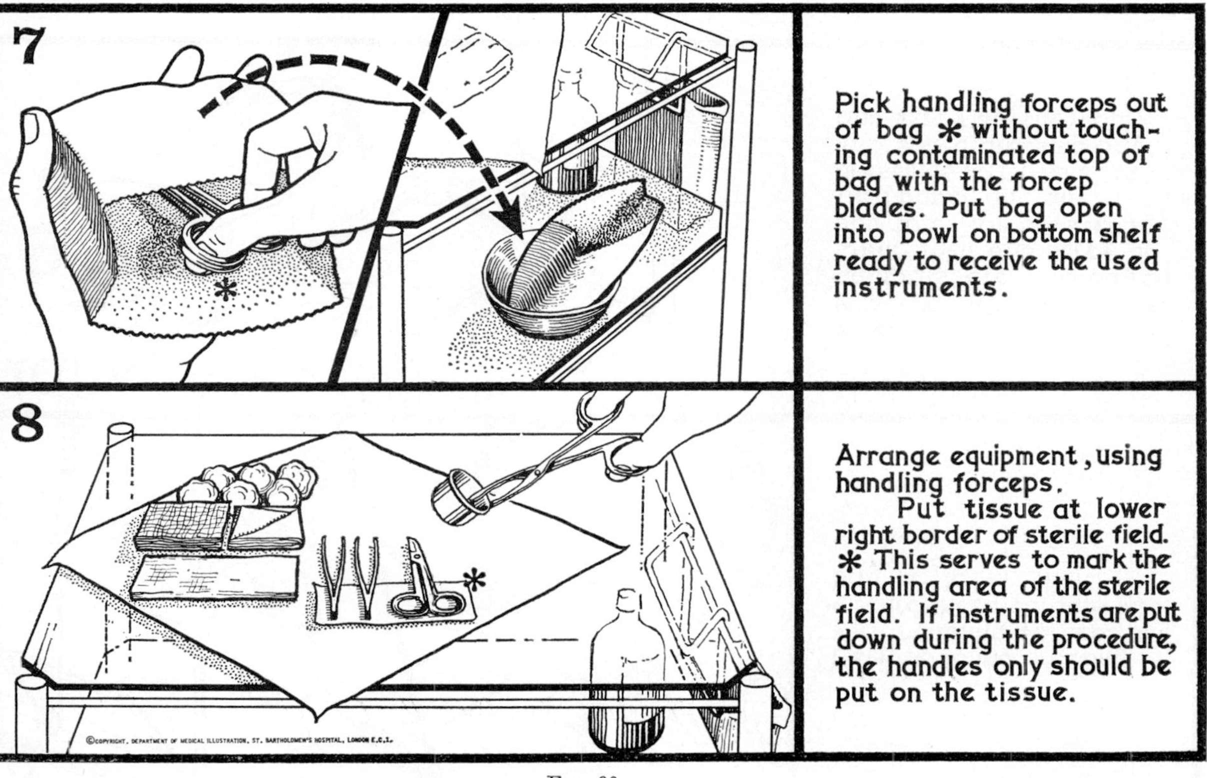
7
Pick handling forceps out of bag * without touching contaminated top of bag with the forcep blades. Put bag open into bowl on bottom shelf ready to receive the used instruments.
*
8
Arrange equipment, using handling forceps.
Put tissue at lower right border of sterile field.
* This serves to mark the handling area of the sterile field. If instruments are put down during the procedure, the handles only should be put on the tissue.
*
©COPYRIGHT. DEPARTMENT OF MEDICAL ILLUSTRATION, ST. BARTHOLOMEW'S HOSPITAL, LONDON E.C.1.

FIG. 60D.

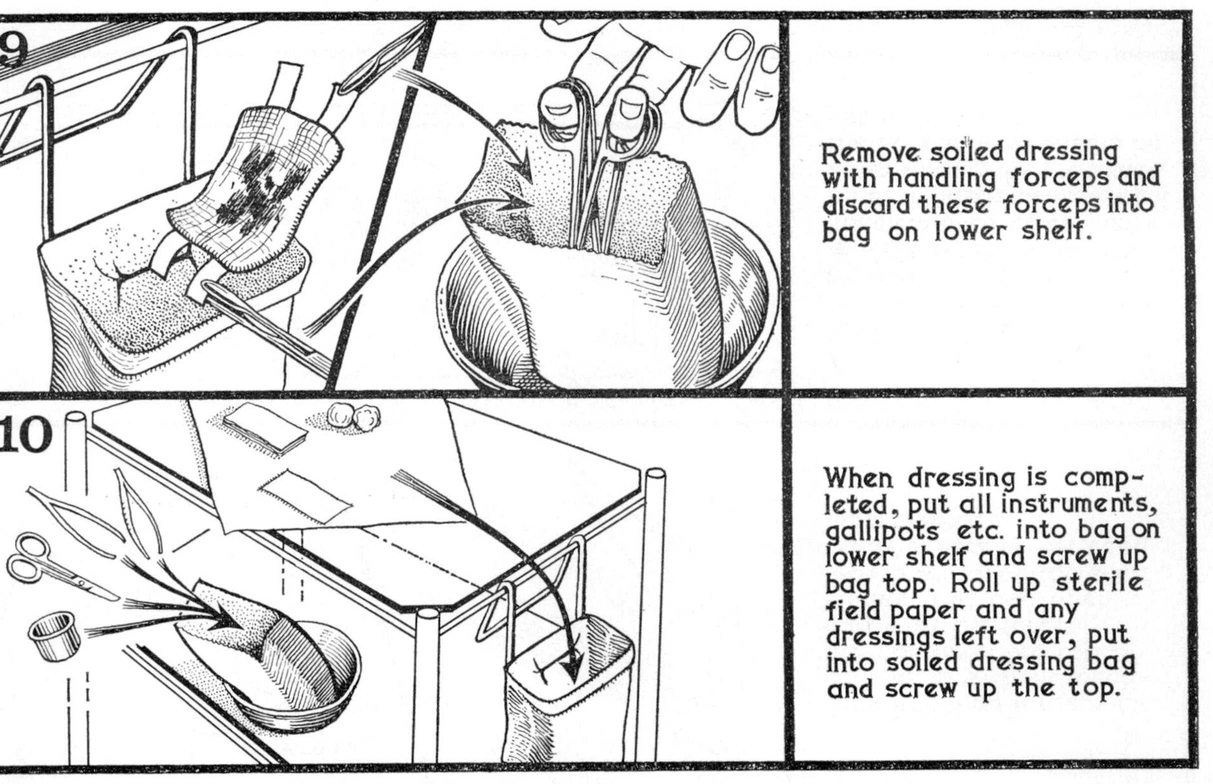
9
Remove soiled dressing
with handling forceps and
discard these forceps into
bag on lower shelf.
10
When dressing is comp-
leted, put all instruments,
gallipots etc. into bag on
lower shelf and screw up
bag top. Roll up sterile
field paper and any
dressings left over, put
into soiled dressing bag
and screw up the top.

FIG. 60E.

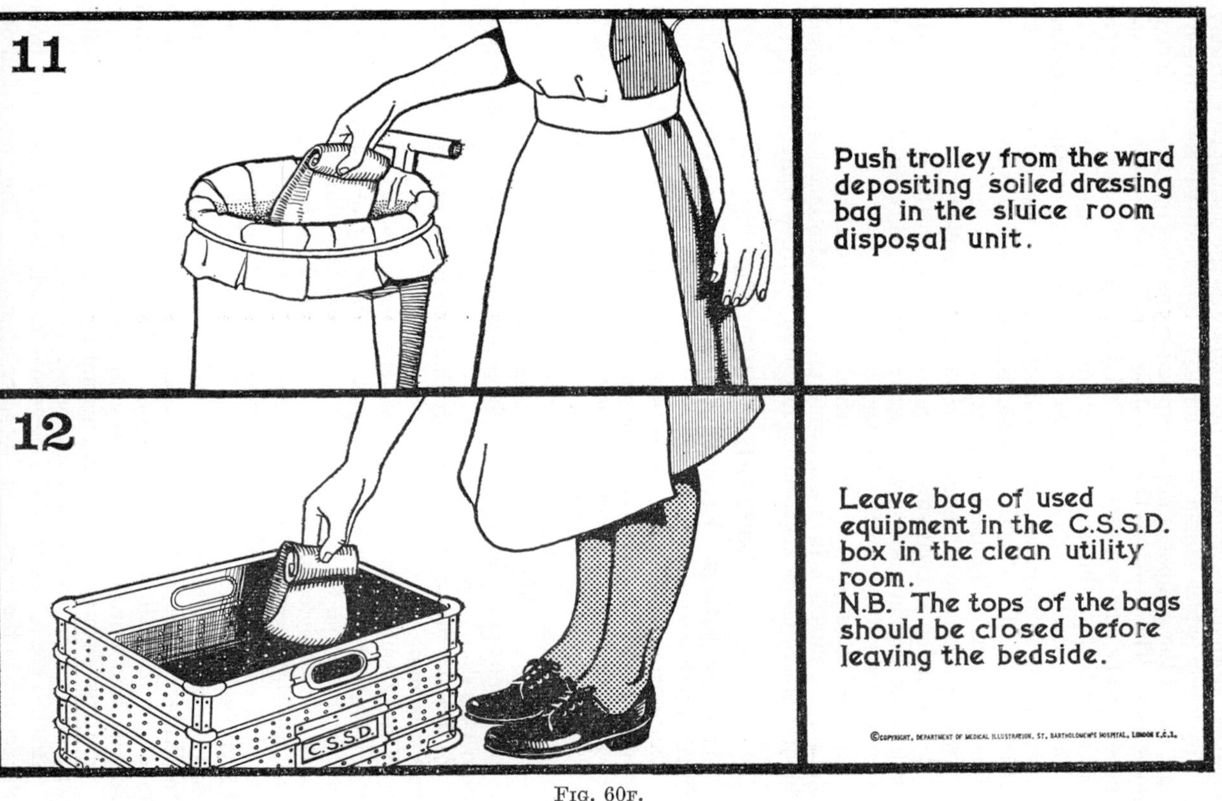
11
Push trolley from the ward depositing soiled dressing bag in the sluice room disposal unit.
12
Leave bag of used equipment in the C.S.S.D. box in the clean utility room.
N.B. The tops of the bags should be closed before leaving the bedside.
C.S.S.D.
©COPYRIGHT, DEPARTMENT OF MEDICAL ILLUSTRATION, ST. BARTHOLOMEW'S HOSPITAL, LONDON E.C.1.

Fig. 60f.

redness, tenderness or discharge. Gauze and wool are applied with forceps, then these are discarded into the lower bag and the dressing secured. Both nurses remake the bed and settle the patient comfortably.

Any lotion (which should be minimal) is tipped into the soiled dressing bag, and if the gallipot is not a disposable one it is put into the instrument bag. The towel on the top shelf is rolled up, together with any unused swabs, and put with the soiled dressings. This bag is unclipped and the mouth of this and the instrument bag screwed up.

Taking her trolley away, the dresser drops the bag of soiled dressings into a bin for incineration, and the instrument bag into a receptacle for return to C.S.S.D. Washing her hands, she again swabs the trolley top in preparation for the next dressing.

Two points are worth notice in clearing the trolley:

(1) Salvaging unused swabs is not economic, so the number in the pack must be the minimum; if extra are needed, a small packet of extra swabs is taken by the dresser.

(2) The instruments are not washed in the ward, in order to avoid a build-up of infection in the dressing area. It also enables the supply department to check that the set has been returned complete.

SPECIAL TECHNIQUES

Removing Sutures. Required (in addition to dressing trolley) Sterile stitch scissors.

The commonest skin sutures are interrupted, i.e. each is tied separately and the ends cut. The continuous and the mattress suture are also illustrated. Tension sutures, which are stitches designed to withstand strain, have a piece of narrow rubber tubing threaded on to them, to prevent the suture cutting into the skin.

There are two principles in stitch removal:

(*a*) Do not draw through the tissues any portion of the suture from above the skin.

(*b*) Do not cut any stitch in more than one place, or a part of it may be left behind.

When about to remove stitches, the nurse places with forceps a sterile swab to receive the pieces on the dressing towel, and takes a pair of dissecting forceps in the left hand and the stitch scissors in the right. Unless infection is present no pain will be caused and the nurse can truthfully assure the patient thus. The knot always lies against the skin on one side of the stitch, and it is taken by the forceps and lifted gently so that a millimetre or two of the stitch from below the skin is drawn above it. The points of the scissors are passed beneath the knot and the stitch is cut. Gentle traction with the forceps is made and the stitch slides easily out. The scar is inspected for sound healing, and a dressing may or may not be necessary.

Mattress sutures and continuous sutures are removed in a similar way, in accordance with the two principles above.

Stitches are removed on the surgeon's instructions, at any time from the second to the fourteenth day after operation. They are taken out early from the face and neck where cosmetic appearances are important, and later where stitches are subject to strain, or if the patient is elderly or suffering from malignant disease.

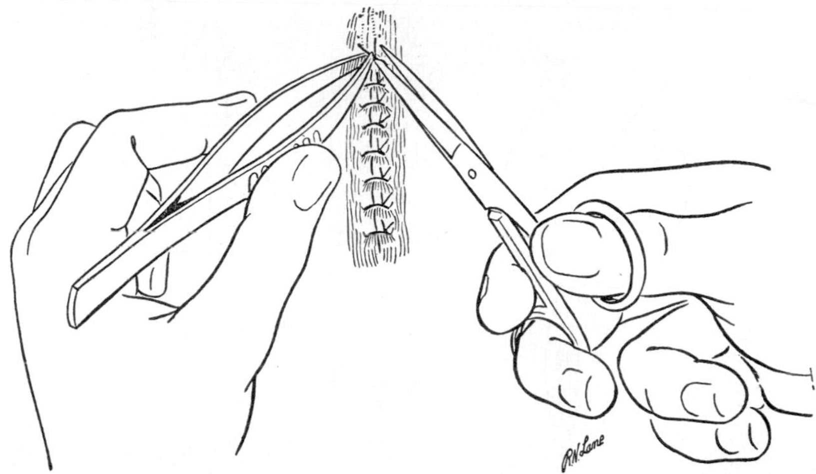

FIG. 61. Removal of stitches. The knot is lifted, and the stitch cut beneath it.

Removing Clips. Metal clips may be used for superficial incisions (e.g. after thyroidectomy). They are retained in place by sharp points which enter the skin, and two types are commonly seen, the Michel and the Kifa. Kifa clips are removed by pinching the centre tabs together with a pair of dissecting forceps held vertically, and disengaging first one point and then the other. Michel clips are taken out with a special remover. The lower blade is inserted below the clip, and the blades closed, when the points of the clip disengage themselves.

Shortening or Removing Drainage Tubes. Drainage tubes are usually a piece of corrugated tubing if superficial, or of round plastic tubing if intraperitoneal. They are usually secured with a stitch, and if intraperitoneal will have a safety pin fastened in the free end as well. To remove a tube, the stitch is taken out and the tube gently withdrawn. The sensation is unpleasant but not usually painful, and the patient's co-operation should be asked.

If a drainage tube is to be shortened, sterile stitch scissors and a sterile safety pin are needed on the dressing trolley. The stitch is removed, and the end of the tube drawn about half an inch out of the wound. The new pin is inserted through the tube with forceps just above skin level, and closed. The protruding portion of the tube is cut off. The tube must be held until the pin has been put in, or the tube may slip into the peritoneal cavity.

T-tubes are tubes whose short limb has been inserted into the common bile duct to drain it. These tubes remain in for some time—often several weeks—until the bile has resumed its normal channels. They cannot be shortened, and are removed by traction. The process is painful, and an injection of pethidine or morphine beforehand is indicated in many cases.

Redi-vac Suction Drainage Apparatus. Prevention of hæmatoma formation is important because collections of fluid delay healing,

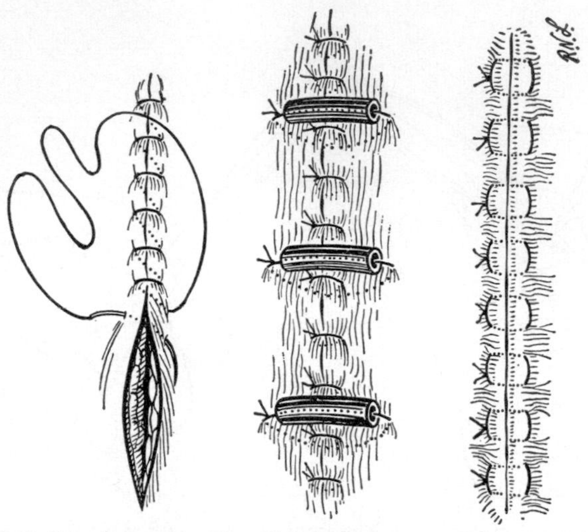

FIG. 62. Varieties of suture. The illustration shows (left to right) continuous suture; interrupted and tension sutures; mattress sutures.

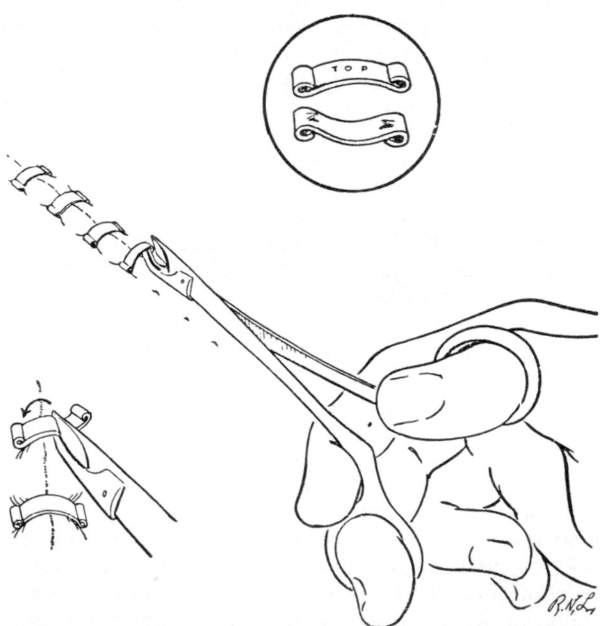

FIG. 63. Removing Michel clips. Notice the way in which the forceps are held. *Inset.* A Michel clip, showing the plain upper surface and the teeth which keep the skin edges together on the under surface.

predispose to infection, and spoil the appearance of the scar. Insertion of Redi-vac suction drainage at the time of operation lessens the likelihood of such collections.

The wound drainage tube is a fine plastic one with perforations at its distal end; this end is laid in place in the operation site. The preparation of the suction apparatus is as follows:

1. The stopper of the drainage bottle is squeezed a few times under running water to eliminate air locks, and is then pushed home into the bottle neck.
2. A syringe and needle are charged with a little coloured water, and used to fill the indicator tube in the stopper. Bubbles are eliminated, and the screw cap of the bottle tightened.
3. A vacuum pump or aspirator is attached to the tubing of the stopper, and air evacuated from the bottle to create a vacuum of 600 mm. of mercury. The coloured water will disappear from the tube when the pressure is about 400 mm. Hg.
4. The tube to the stopper is clamped, and the pump detached.
5. The drainage tube is connected to the bottle and the clamp released. Fluid should now begin to drip into the bottle.

The vacuum gradually disappears, as can be seen by the slow rise of the coloured water in the indicator tube. If it must be replaced, the rubber coupling between the drainage catheter and the stopper is clamped. A new vacuum bottle can then be attached. The amount of drainage is measured and recorded. The apparatus is sterilized in the autoclave. A portable plastic type is available; instructions are on the pack.

Wound Irrigation. Sinuses and granulating wounds are often irrigated. Lotions used should be sterile, at a temperature of 100° F. Hydrogen peroxide 1 in 6 is useful in infected wounds, but must be followed by normal saline. The apparatus used depends on the amount of lotion required. Small quantities may be given with a Dakin's syringe; for larger quantities a can, tubing connection and catheter (all sterile) is useful. Sterile dissecting forceps are used to direct the catheter into the wound, and the outflow is received into a kidney dish placed on a mackintosh.

Dressing Septic Wounds. Infected wounds must be dressed with the same aseptic technique as clean ones. Lotions containing spirit are painful and should not be used; Eusol is a useful substitute. Dressings unlikely to adhere to raw areas—tulle gras, or gauze soaked in flavine and liquid paraffin, or eusol and paraffin—are used if indicated. Red lotion is effective in promoting granulation when the wound infection is declining. As soon as a septic dressing has been completed and the patient's bed has been remade, the dresser and assistant should wash their hands before removing the trolley and drawing back the curtains. When the patient has been discharged all his bedding should be disinfected and the curtains changed.

Granulation tissue sometimes grows too exuberantly, and if it rises above skin level may be reduced by the use of the silver nitrate stick. It should be rubbed over the granulations, and a swab dipped in normal saline afterwards applied for a few seconds to the area.

CHAPTER 20

NURSING OF SOME SURGICAL CONDITIONS

THE problems that beset every surgeon in the performance of an operation and the after-care are the same, but the solutions depend on the circumstances under which it is performed, which of the post-operative complications seem most important to the surgeon, and perhaps on his past experience and temperament. Such decisions as to whether a wound is drained, how long the patient is to stay in bed, and when his stitches are to be removed, admit of many answers. The nurses' responsibilities and difficulties, however, are very similar whoever the surgeon is, and in this chapter these difficulties are briefly discussed, and an indication of the likely course of pre- and post. operative management given.

OPERATIONS ON THE STOMACH AND SMALL INTESTINE

A large number of patients are admitted from the waiting list for such operations as hernia repair, interval appendicectomy and partial gastrectomy. For these the routine preparation described in Chapter 19 is used, but an enema is not a routine unless constipation is present, or it is expected that rectal fluids will be given after operation. Others enter as emergencies, requiring operation at short notice, and among these will be cases of acute intestinal obstruction, and the pre- and post-operative care of these makes a great demand on the skill and powers of observation of the nurse.

Acute Intestinal Obstruction

On admission, the patient is received into a warm bed, where he will usually be most comfortable if sitting up adequately supported. Relatives are asked to give their consent to operation if the patient is a minor, and in any event may like to wait until a decision has been reached about the necessity for surgery, and the time at which it will be undertaken.

A vomit bowl, towel, mouth treatment tray and treatment board are kept at the bedside, and all nurses are told that nothing is to be given by mouth, and that all vomit is to be measured and separate specimens saved. This may give valuable information as to the stage the obstruction has reached. The pulse is recorded every fifteen minutes, the temperature, respiration rate and blood pressure hourly. A urine specimen is obtained as soon as possible, and in addition to the routine tests an estimation of the urinary chlorides (p. 47) may be requested. It is usual to pass a Ryle's tube transnasally into the stomach to avoid vomiting and gastric distension, and the necessary articles are collected.

Indwelling Ryle's Tube

Requirements. Ryle's tube in a receiver.
Gallipots with liquid paraffin and swabs.
Red and blue litmus paper.
50 ml. syringe.
Pint jug.
Strapping and spigot.

The tube is lubricated and passed transnasally as far as the second mark. Attempts to pass the tube often cause vomiting ; the patient is encouraged and told of the relief that will be experienced when it is in place. Once it is in position the syringe is attached and all the gastric contents aspirated, and the tube spigotted and strapped to the cheek. The amount and reaction of the fluid is recorded on the treatment board, and aspiration is repeated often enough to prevent the accumulation of fluid.

If there is any doubt about diagnosis, the two-enema test may be used. The nurse is asked to give an enema to clear the bowel of fæces and any flatus, and to repeat it half an hour later, staying with the patient while it is returned and noting if any flatus is passed, which would indicate that complete obstruction was not present.

In some cases (e.g. strangulated femoral hernia) operation is urgent because delay will lead to perforation and peritonitis. Pre-operative drugs are given, the operation area shaved, and the patient taken to the theatre as soon as possible. In others (e.g. obstruction by adhesions), delay in order to remedy thedehydration of an ill patient by intravenous fluids is possible and may be advisable.

Non-operative Treatment of Intestinal Obstruction

While mechanical obstruction is susceptible to operative cure, obstruction due to paralysis (*ileus*) of the intestinal muscles cannot be so treated, and conservative methods are adopted. The principles of these are :

1. To rest the gut until function is restored.
2. To supply intravenous fluids of the quantity and composition needed to make good the normal fluid loss, and that aspirated from the intestine.
3. To treat peritonitis, if present, by antibiotics.
4. To relieve discomforts by all nursing methods, and to collect the information that will lead to the correct performance of paragraph 2.

Routine records are made, and in addition the nurse notices the dryness of the tongue, if there is any sweating, and whether distension is increasing. Measurements of fluid loss by the urine, intestinal aspiration, and vomiting are meticulously kept, and the rate of intravenous flow is maintained at the rate ordered. Urinary chlorides are often estimated, though the blood chloride is a very much more reliable guide. The mouth is frequently treated, and regular blanket bathing and care of the pressure areas should be undertaken with as little disturbance as possible. Unfavourable signs that should be reported are a rising pulse rate, hiccough, very dry tongue, increasing distension or clouding of consciousness.

The doctor orders morphine six-hourly, and if an antibiotic is necessary, a broad-spectrum one like tetracycline is given. The amount and kind of intravenous fluid is decided from examining the blood chemistry and the nurses' records, and the principles used are described on p. 163.

The stomach is kept empty either by intermittent syringe suction on a Ryle's tube, or by continuous suction.

Continuous Gastric or Intestinal Aspiration

A simple apparatus is illustrated for maintaining continuous suction on an indwelling Ryle's tube. Water is allowed to flow from an upper bottle to a lower one, extracting the air necessary to permit this flow from a Woulfe's bottle, to which the Ryle's tube is connected by tubing. The rate of flow must be fast enough to keep the stomach

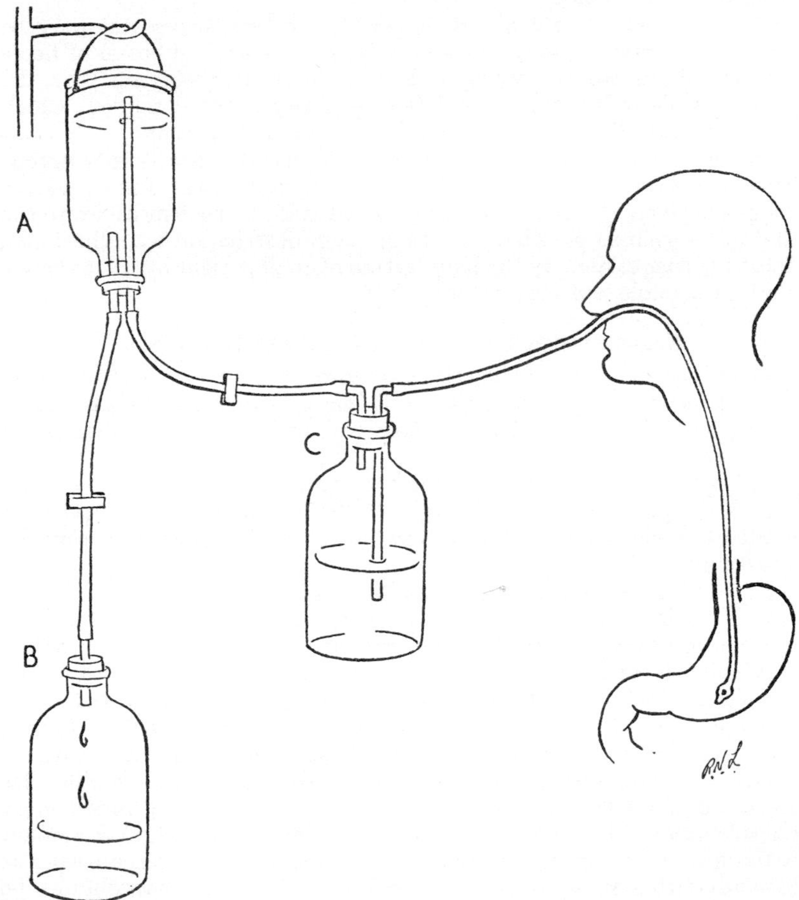

FIG. 64. Continuous gastric suction. Water flows from bottle A to B, creating a vacuum in bottle C, into which the stomach contents are aspirated.

empty, and when the upper bottle is empty, the corks of this and the full one are changed over, and the position of the bottles reversed. The Woulfe's bottle is emptied regularly, and the reaction and amount of its contents recorded.

Intestinal tubes have been devised which will travel through the stomach under favourable conditions and pass along the intestine to the site of obstruction. Perforations at the top allow continuous suction, and bags that can be inflated with air, water or mercury prevent fluid regurgitating backwards, and are also thought to stimulate peristalsis.

The Miller-Abbott tube is a double-lumen one, 6 ft. in length, with perforations and a rubber balloon at one end, and at the other a metal fitting with two outlets marked " suction " and " filling." Before setting it up, the amount required to inflate the balloon is tested with a syringe, and then the following articles are assembled at the bedside :

Miller-Abbott tube coiled in a receiver.
Lubricant and swabs.
50 ml. syringe.
Woulfe's bottle, tubing and glass connections.
Linen thread and scissors.
Electric sucker or water-suction apparatus.
Cocaine spray.

The nose should be sprayed with cocaine before beginning, as the end is rather bulky for nasal passage, the tip of the tube is lubricated, and passed nasally until the stomach is reached. The tube is anchored by passing round it a loop of thread which can be fastened to the patient's ear ; strapping must not be used, since the tube is meant to travel. The balloon is inflated with air (or water if the surgeon prefers) and the inlet closed with thread. The tube is connected to one side of the Woulfe's bottle, and to the other suction is applied by one of the means suggested. It is now hoped that the tube will pass through the pylorus and into the small intestine, and to this end the patient may, if he is fit enough, lie on the right side for an hour or two. If it does not pass through, it can, however, still perform the same function as a Ryle's tube in the stomach. If peristalsis returns before the tube has travelled far the balloon can be deflated and the tube withdrawn, but if it has penetrated to any distance, it must be allowed to pass on until the tip appears at the anus, when the upper end can be detached, and the whole tube allowed to travel through.

Care After Gastro-Intestinal Operations

After all operations affecting the continuity of the intestinal tract (e.g. resection of gut, partial gastrectomy, repair of peptic perforations) it is usual to withhold fluids by mouth, and to give them by the intravenous or rectal route until peristalsis returns. A Ryle's tube may be kept in the stomach, and frequently morphine is ordered to rest the intestine. Nurses should notice that if a doctor orders morphine (10 mgms.) six-hourly he intends it to be given at that interval; if he allows it to be given at the nurse's discretion he orders morphine (10 mgms.) six-hourly if necessary (p.r.n.). During this period attention to the mouth is required. When fluids by mouth are begun, water in small quantities is given, and the stomach aspirated before the next drink to ensure that fluid is not collecting. If progress is satisfactory the amount is increased, the Ryle's tube withdrawn and the intravenous or rectal fluids discontinued. This type of care will be referred to for convenience as " conservative."

Notes on Some Gastro-Intestinal Operations

Appendicectomy. Interval appendicectomy is performed in a quiescent period after an attack of appendicitis ; it is a minor procedure, after which the patient may get up on the following day, and go home as soon as the stitches are removed on the 5th or 6th day.

Acute appendicitis may, after operation, be similarly treated if the appendix was intact, but if it was gangrenous or perforated a drainage tube is usually inserted, and " conservative " treatment is maintained till peristalsis returns. An antibiotic is ordered if peritonitis is feared. Residual infection can lead to an abscess in the Pouch of Douglas, indicated by diarrhœa with mucus ; a subphrenic abscess (below the diaphragm) usually causes severe constitutional upset. Fever, tachycardia, pain, distension or diarrhœa should be reported at once.

If a patient when first seen has a well-localized abscess in the appendix area, it is drained, and appendicectomy undertaken at a later date when there is no risk of exciting general peritonitis.

Partial gastrectomy. Ascorbic acid is given pre-operatively, whether the operation is for relief of peptic ulcer or of cancer, and a Ryle's tube passed. " Conservative " treatment is used post-operatively, and while a well-prepared patient may be maintained on rectal fluids, intravenous infusion is often necessary. Vomiting or excessive fluid aspiration may indicate paralytic ileus or mechanical obstruction ; collapse and abdominal pain may be due to leakage from the suture line or duodenal stump. As soon as water is well taken, milk may be given and a suitable gastric diet built up. Feeds must be small and frequent at first until capacity increases, but in most cases a return to a normal diet can be anticipated. Patients on discharge should be given an appointment for re-examination ; feelings of faintness may occur after meals which are due to hypoglycæmia, and can be relieved by taking smaller, more frequent meals and resting after them. Years later, a proportion of patients develop anæmia, and instead of partial gastrectomy, division of the vagus nerve (vagotomy) combined with a drainage operation such as pyloroplasty, is often used. It is still too soon to know what the late results of vagotomy will be. Patients should be advised not to eat oranges after operation, as pith sometimes causes obstruction. The juice should be squeezed and drunk.

Perforated Peptic Ulcer. Operation is undertaken urgently, after the minimum preparation described for intestinal obstruction, and the perforation may be merely closed, or partial gastrectomy performed if the peritoneum is not grossly contaminated. Ascorbic acid is given by intramuscular injection ; " conservative " treatment is instituted, and the drainage tube left in position till discharge ceases, usually after three to five days.

Gall-bladder Operations. Removal of the gall bladder (cholecystectomy) is performed for gall stones or chronic inflammation. Patients are often middle-aged and obese, and deep breathing is begun early after operation to avert pneumonia. Nausea is common, and drinks should be of water or soda water, orange juice being badly tolerated for some unknown reason. A low fat diet is desirable because of the flatulence, but need not be long continued unless it is desired to reduce the weight. Fried food is best avoided. The drainage tube to the gall bladder bed is taken out at some time after forty-eight hours.

If the common bile duct has been opened, it is closed round a T-tube whose end projects from the wound. On return to the ward the spigot is at once removed from the tube which is drained into a sterile disposable plastic bag. The amount drained is measured and recorded,

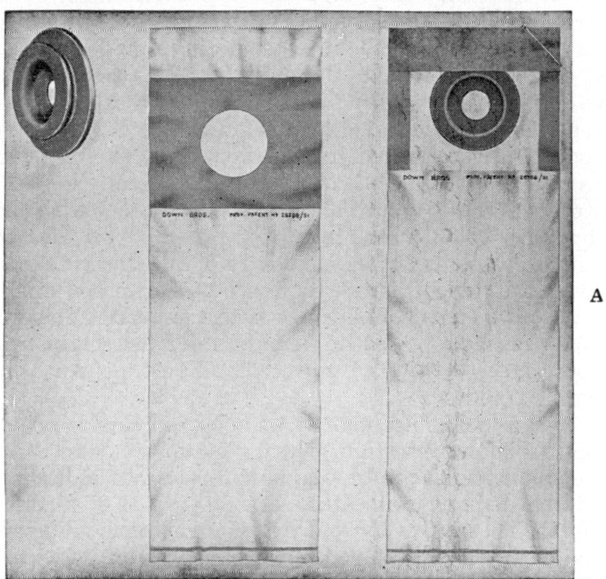

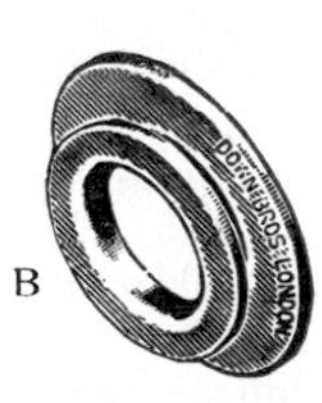

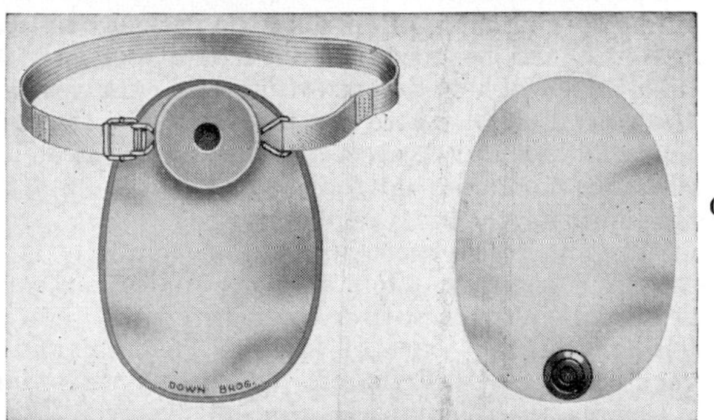

FIG. 65. Ileostomy appliances.

A. Chiron disposable bags, applied direct to the skin or to a flange.

B. and C. Kœnig-Rutzen bag with flange and belt.

(*Reproduced by courtesy of Down Brothers and Mayer and Phelps Ltd.*)

and the tube remains in place for two to three weeks until bile ceases to drain, and the colour of the stools indicates that bile is passing down the normal channels. Removal is not pleasant, and if reassurance is not felt to be sufficient preparation, morphine (10 mgms.) may be ordered before the stitch is cut and gentle traction made until the tube emerges. Leakage of bile may occur for a day or two from the fistula, but this usually heals rapidly.

It is preferred not to operate on patients with jaundice, but if this is necessary vitamin K is given before and after operation to raise the prothrombin level of the blood and prevent hæmorrhage. After all operations on the bilary tract any sign of jaundice must be noted, and the colour of the stools observed.

Ileostomy. The terminal ileum is sometimes made to discharge the intestinal contents on to the abdominal wall as treatment for acute ulcerative colitis. Since many surgeons believe that such an operation should be permanent (as it must be if colonic resection is also necessary), the instruction of the patient in the ways of managing it so that life may be as normal as possible is of great importance.

The introduction of bags which are kept in contact with the abdominal wall by adhesive has much improved prospects for the patient with an ileostomy. A hole is cut in the centre of an adhesive square, which is fitted over the flange of the appliance and trimmed flush with the rim after the protective backing has been removed. The skin around the ileostomy must be perfectly clean and dry before the apparatus is stuck in position, a dusting of powered Indian tragacanth is excellent for preventing soreness.

The greatest nursing problem is to keep the skin from excoriation by the fluid from the intestine, which contains enzymes. Sore skin is painful, depressing to the morale, and will prevent the fitting of a type of bag suitable for an active life. Such a bag is of plastic, with an opening for the ileostomy guarded by a flange, either joined to the bag or detachable. The flange is fixed to the skin with adhesive, and usually only needs changing twice a week, or less. There is a tap at the bottom for emptying the bag, which should be of such a size that it does not require emptying more often than the patient empties her bladder.

Patients must be encouraged to take as nearly normal a diet as possible; this will help them to think of themselves as normal members of the community. There are usually a few things that cause loose actions and these can be avoided. The efflux from an ileostomy contains much more fluid than do the normal stools, so patients must drink freely. Patients who have an ileostomy established are often young, and time taken to teach them how to live normally is well spent. The Ileostomy Association offers support, advice and companionship, and puts patients in touch with manufacturers with new appliances.

Hernia. Surgical cure of inguinal, femoral and umbilical hernia is very commonly undertaken. Early movement and exercises will help to strengthen the muscles that must prevent the hernia recurring. Inguinal hernia, which is the most common, is usually seen in men, and they may find a suspensory bandage of comfort after operation. This also appears to reduce the likelihood of hæmatoma formation in the wound, a not uncommon post-operative complication.

OPERATIONS ON THE RECTUM

Abdomino-Perineal Excision of Rectum. Patients with cancer of the rectum are often anæmic, undernourished, tired by pain and apprehension, and with fæcal accumulation in the colon above the growth, so that extensive mental and physical preparation is required. The surgeon explains in language that the patient can understand what the operation entails, and optimism with regard to the future is justified by the results. The nurse must be prepared to answer questions on the management of a colostomy and how far normal life may be maintained ; she should know that there are many men and women leading happy, busy lives, and that their acquaintances are quite unaware that they have a colostomy.

Investigations include the hæmoglobin and blood group ; chest X-ray, and an intravenous pyelogram to exclude involvement of the ureters in the disease. The diet should be high in calories and low in residue, and ample fluids must be given. Local preparation may mean daily enemata or rectal washouts until the bowel is cleared. A course of an insoluble sulpha drug (e.g. phthalysulphathiazole) and streptomycinis, given to sterilize the intestine and administration of vitamin C must accompany it. A complete abdominal and perineal shave is performed on the day before operation, and the immediate pre-operative care includes the passage of an indwelling Ryle's tube, and for men a self-retaining catheter in the bladder to minimize the risk of damage to the urethra during operation and to avoid post-operative retention of urine.

Blood transfusion is begun in the theatre, and the patient returns with the transfusion continuing. He is put to bed on an air ring, with the foot of the bed raised, and serial observations are begun on the pulse and blood pressure. The dressings are examined ; the abdominal binder covers a middle incision, sometimes with a drainage tube, and the colostomy, which is separated from the main wound by an oiled silk dressing. A T-bandage holds in place the dressing over the perineal wound, which is mostly stitched, but contains at one end a corrugated drainage tube or a pack. The urethral catheter is connected to a sterile irrigation apparatus (p. 361) or allowed to drain into a jar.

The problem for the first twenty-four hours is resuscitation. "Conservative" treatment is maintained until bowel sounds return, and during this time intravenous therapy continues. Vitamins are administered as long as antibiotics are given and a high fluid intake is pressed. As soon as possible the patient sits up in bed to obviate pneumonia, and can be turned from one buttock to another to prevent pressure on the perineum.

With regard to the wound management, no special problems arise about the laparotomy incision, which heals without trouble and from which the stitches are removed about the tenth day. The perineal wound takes longer, and drainage may continue from it for some time. Healing must take place from the apex, and a corrugated drain should be kept in place till this is well under way. Irrigation of the sinus with Eusol, Milton or hydrogen peroxide, followed by normal saline may be required to hasten the process.

The colostomy will not act until after about forty-eight hours when peristalsis recommences and then actions are scanty and frequent, as there has been no intake by mouth and regular rhythm is not established. The week or so during which the perineal wound is unhealed and the colostomy acting so irregularly is a time of great discouragement and depression which the patient must be helped to surmount. A plastic bag of the Chiron type is very useful as an application to the colostomy.

During the convalescent period and before discharge, the patient is taught the principles of colostomy management. If before his illness he had a regular morning bowel action, he may hope that the colostomy will act in the same way. The stimulus to peristalsis in the morning is activity and the taking of food, and he must allow time for the colostomy to act before getting dressed. Two cups of hot tea or coffee should be taken with the morning meal, and cellulose is the most convenient dressing to receive the discharge, as it can afterwards be flushed away in the water closet.

Care must be taken with the diet until the colostomy rhythm is stabilized, and usually afterwards as well. The escape of flatus cannot be controlled, and foods that cause flatulence—such as onions, brussels sprouts and large amounts of starch—may have to be permanently avoided. Large quantities of soft fruit cannot usually be taken without diarrhœa, and it is usually wise to begin with a plain diet, and to increase it by one article at a time to observe the effect. Kaolin powder is useful if there is any looseness of action.

Once the colostomy is acting regularly, only a small dressing need be worn during the day, such as a small square of gauze moistened with soft paraffin, a little wool and a piece of jaconet. It is retained with a belt or binder, and women often find that a roll-on corset is sufficient. The patient is asked to report regularly for examination, and, if necessary, for advice on his colostomy.

EMERGENCY COLOSTOMY

In acute-on-chronic obstruction, it is sometimes advisable to make an opening above the obstruction, and remove the growth later after measures to improve the general condition.

A temporary colostomy may be performed by bringing to the surface a loop of either transverse or sigmoid colon (these two being the mobile portions), opening the loop, turning back the mucous membrane and suturing it to the skin. Alternatively, a Paul's tube is sometimes used. This is a right-angled glass tube made in a range of sizes, with a single flange at one end over which is slipped wide, thin tubing, and a double flange at the other, which goes into the colon and is held by a purse-string suture of catgut. This dissolves in a few days and allows the Paul's tube to fall out. If opening the colostomy is not urgent it is delayed for a day or two, and then may be opened by cautery. No anæsthetic is required, as the colon is not sensitive to such stimuli.

Hæmorrhoids. Piles can cause a chronic anæmia if blood is lost from them, and are painful and distressing. They may be treated by injection at the base of 5% phenol in almond oil through a proctoscope,

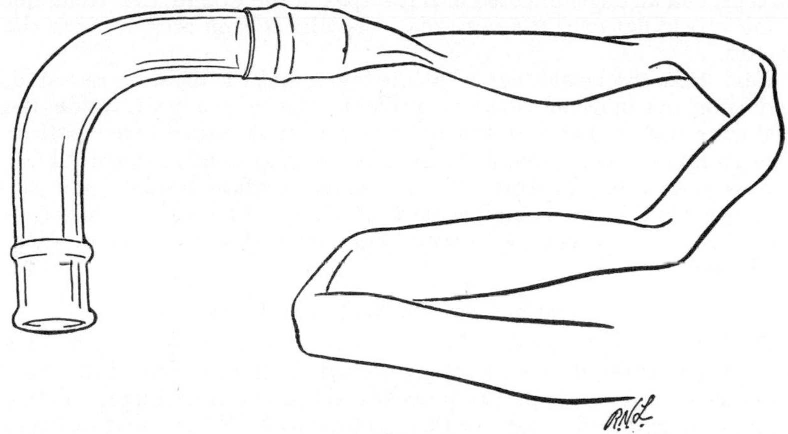

FIG. 66. Paul's tube.

or by surgical removal. The bowel must be empty before operation, and the perineum shaved.

After operation gauze dressings are arranged around the anus, with the apices tucked into the sphincter, and wool held over them with a T-bandage ; drainage tubes are painful and not usually considered necessary. Reactionary hæmorrhage must be watched for by inspection of the dressing and recording of the pulse rate, while morphine is the usual post-operative drug. Retention of urine may occur in men, and can usually be relieved by getting the patient out of bed.

The bowels are opened with aperients and an enema if necessary on the third day, and a bath is taken before the dressing is renewed. A daily bowel action is aimed at, always followed by a bath and a fresh dressing, which should not be inserted into the sphincter after the fifth day. After this time daily dilation of the sphincter with a well-lubricated gloved finger will prevent stricture formation, and the patient is taught how to perform this himself for a few weeks after his discharge. Regular bowel action should be established by training, and excessive taking of aperients avoided, especially liquid paraffin.

Fistula-in-ano. Such a fistula is a track, often complicated in extent, which opens into the anal canal at one end and on to the skin near the anus at the other. It must be completely opened up if it is to be cured, and this involves incising the anal sphincter. The bowels are kept confined for about three days, during which a low residue diet is given, and then opened with aperients and an enema. The dressing is passed at the same time, and watch should be kept for faintness. A bath is now taken, a sterile towel is applied under a T-bandage, and the patient returns to bed for the dressing. A large triangular raw area will be seen, of which the apex projects into the anal canal, and the aim is to secure healing from the apex outwards. Square gauze dressings are used (often called after St. Mark's Hospital where they are extensively used) and those in contact with the wound are moistened in Eusol or some bland antiseptic. They are held diagonally in dressing forceps, and an angle directed into the apex of the wound, the remainder being spread flat over the raw area ; the aim is even pressure over the wound.

Each time the bowels act a bath is taken and the dressing repeated, and soon granulation becomes evident. Once the part inside the sphincter has healed and the only raw part is outside, the patient may go home if it is possible to get the dressing done satisfactorily.

Fissure-in-ano. Excision of the fissure is often needed, and the wound resembles on a small scale that for a fistula and is dressed in the same way. Advice as to bowel regulation should be given before discharge.

Operations on the Neck and Breast

Partial Thyroidectomy. Most patients with thyrotoxicosis are women, and if the disease is of any severity a course of medical treatment as described on p. 194 precedes operation, and Lugol's iodine is given by mouth for fourteen days beforehand. Since the dressing is usually retained by a piece of elastoplast passing round the neck and crossing over the chest, the axillæ should be shaved before operation. The premedication should be adequate to allay anxiety, some surgeons prescribe heroin for toxic cases. If conscious, she should be accompanied to the theatre by someone she knows well.

The post-operative bed is unheated, a blanket is not put next to the patient, and in hot weather a body cradle and sheet are sufficient covering. Consciousness is quickly regained, and the patient is sat up as soon as possible, with the nape of the neck well supported by a jaconet-covered soft pillow. The usual records are kept, and special note made of the rate and rhythm of the pulse. Unless a Redivac drain is used, there is danger of bleeding under the skin flaps leading to increasing pressure on the treachea. Restlessness, dyspnœa, cyanosis and tachycardia indicate that the surgeon must be summoned, and a dressing trolley prepared with stitch scissors or clip removers and sinus forceps in order to evacuate the hæmatoma. It is possible, but not probable, that the nurse might have to do this herself if help was not promptly available.

The other major complications are : (1) Injury to the recurrent laryngeal nerve, which if bilateral can cause dyspnœa that may necessitate tracheotomy. Some surgeons like to assure themselves by laryngeal examination that all is well. (2) Tetany is due to parathyroid deficiency, and care in preserving these glands has made this complication rare. Tingling of hands and feet are premonitory signs that should be reported, and administration of calcium gluconate will then prevent the major muscular spasms, in which the feet are plantar-flexed, and the hands flex at the wrists, while the finger joints extend. (3) Thyroid crisis is heralded by hyperpyrexia, tachycardia of over 150, and extreme exhausting restlessness. The temperature must be lowered by sponging or fanning ; sedation and Lugol's iodine are prescribed, and nursing in an oxygen tent is often required. This is a rare complication if the patient is well prepared.

Lugol's iodine, phenobarbitone and if necessary digitalis are usually given post-operatively, and aspirin mucilage is useful before meals.

For a day or two the patient may be in some distress from a wave of toxicity—flushed, sweating, tremulous, and most apprehensive of moving her head. She is given full nursing care, with a daily blanket bath and frequent adjustment of the drawsheet. When she is moved, the nurse supports her neck from behind. With regard to the wound, the elastoplast is usually cut on the first evening, the upper part of the dressing changed and the strapping pinned. The Redivac drain is removed when drainage ceases, and the stitches or clips one or two days later, when a simple gauze bib may be worn as a dressing. When healing is sound, a little cold cream may be smoothed on to the scar daily, and the patient is assured that the final cosmetic result will be excellent, with only an imperceptible linear scar at the base of the neck. The time of getting up and discharge depends on the pulse rate and general condition.

Mastectomy. Though innocent tumours (fibro-adenomata) are not infrequently removed from the breast, the commonest operation is for cancer, which involves amputation of the breast, often accompanied by removal of the axillary glands and sometimes of the pectoralis major muscle if that is involved. The amount of tissue removed means that the superficial tissues on each side must be undermined in order to stretch them over the space, and if this cannot be accomplished without tension a skin graft is often used. Drainage is always necessary to prevent hæmatoma formation under the flaps, and a Redivac drain is the best method of securing this.

When consciousness is regained, the patient is sat up with a pillow on the affected side on which the forearm rests with the shoulder slightly abducted. Breathing exercises and movements of the hand and forearm are begun at once, but shoulder movements are not encouraged for a few days. The return of full use of the shoulder is important, but is not assured by over-early movement which may indeed contribute to hæmatoma formation.

The drainage tube is taken out when discharge ceases, and stitches are removed from the tenth to the fourteenth day. When the dressing is done the opportunity should be taken to wash and powder the breast and axilla on the unaffected side, and directions on bandaging will be found on p. 436. If there is any swelling of the hand or arm it should be elevated.

The patient may get up a few days after operation with the arm in a sling, and should be ready for discharge or the commencement of deep X-ray therapy in a fortnight. Before discharge she is measured for a brassière with an artificial breast, and is given an appointment for follow-up in a month, and thereafter at regular and decreasing intervals as no recurrence is found.

Operations on the Limbs

Varicose Veins. This common condition can be treated in suitable cases by the injection of sclerosing fluids, but there is some risk of the fluid entering the deep veins and causing thrombosis. After injection a pressure bandage is applied, and is worn for a fortnight. Operation is also common, and two main methods are in use: the veins can be exposed and tied at their communication with the deep ones, or they can be stripped out through conveniently placed incisions.

Many means have been tried of shortening the length of stay in hospital so that a larger number of people may be treated, and in some clinics operation is performed under local anæsthesia in out-patient departments and the patient is sent home by ambulance. Experience suggests, however, that the best results are achieved by a stay of some days in hospital. Bruising is extensive after a stripping operation, and may alarm the patient.

At operation the legs are firmly bound with crepe bandage and while these may need adjustment the dressing need not be done until the stitches are removed on the eighth day. The end of the bed is kept elevated, and walking (but not sitting) is encouraged from the second day onwards. On discharge the patient is provided with crepe bandages and taught how to apply them (p. 439). Bandages should be worn for six weeks, and an elastic stocking may be necessary afterwards to prevent œdema, which must not be allowed to become chronic. Advice on weight reduction is given if indicated.

Amputations. Amputation is occasionally required for new growth or injury, but the majority of cases seen by the nurse have disease of blood-vessels which interferes with the nutrition of a leg and necessitates amputation.

In such cases the nurse must realize that if the circulation is unable to sustain life in one leg, it is almost invariably affected in the other, and that her aims will be to produce a firm, well-shaped stump in a good position to take an artificial limb, and to preserve the other leg from any harm while the patient is in bed.

From the time of admission the sound heel must be protected from pressure by a small pillow beneath the ankle, or a sorbo pad under the heel. Smoking may well be forbidden, since nicotine is a vaso-constrictor, but to compensate, the patient may, if he likes, have a bottle of beer a day as a vaso-dilator. If possible, measurements should be taken before operation for the artificial leg, so that it can be fitted without delay.

At operation a Redivac drain is inserted if oozing is anticipated and the patient is returned to a post-anæsthetic bed. Œdema of the stump must be avoided if the new limb is to fit well, and flexion deformity of the hip prevented. Twitching of the severed muscles is sometimes troublesome after a mid-thigh amputation, and the stump can be steadied under a roller towel held in place by sandbags, but there is no need for this if the symptom does not occur. A body cradle keeps the clothes off the lower part of the bed, and the stump should be accessible for easy inspection. The nursing staff must know how to exert pressure on the femoral artery in the groin if major hæmorrhage occurs, and should not let this knowledge slip from mind because it is very rarely put into practice.

Patients normally " feel " the leg to be present still, and the time when they first see the stump is a disturbing one that needs tactful handling ; they should not be encouraged to look at the dressing being done until they are accustomed to the idea of their loss. Activity is encouraged from the first, and a pulley and chain is provided over the bed so that he may help to lift himself.

The drain is removed when drainage ceases, and the stitches on the tenth day. The patient can be taught how to walk with crutches as soon as his general condition permits, and must then be told to take care when getting up, as it is quite easy to attempt to step out with the leg that is no longer there, and sustain a fall.

Operations on the Sympathetic Nervous System

The action of the sympathetic nervous system on the blood-vessels is constrictor, and the removal of the sympathetic ganglia from alongside the vertebral column will allow the blood-vessels supplied from these ganglia to dilate, if they are capable of doing so. Cervical sympathectomy may be used in the treatment of Raynaud's disease, and in favourable circumstances will convert a cold, blue hand into a warm, red one. The commonest of these operations, however, is lumbar sympathectomy which is now most used to enhance the effect of arterial reconstruction.

Since the circulation is always impaired, careful attention should be paid to the heels from the time of admission onwards. The preoperative enema should not be omitted, because abdominal distension is always well marked after lumbar sympathectomy. Post-operative pain can usually be relieved by compound codeine mixture, and the stitches can be removed about the eighth day.

Operations on the Arteries

Such operations have only become feasible since the introduction of the anticoagulant drugs. Anastomoses between the pulmonary and systemic arteries, and resections of stenosed parts of arteries are practised by the chest surgeon (p. 305) and anastomosis between the portal vein and the inferior vena cava is performed by some surgeons in the treatment of cirrhosis of the liver.

The blood supply to the leg may be diminished by widespread arterial disease (Monckeberg's sclerosis), or by localized blocking of the great vessels such as the aorta, femoral or popliteal, and if it is possible to overcome this obstruction relief may be obtained. The material used to supply the graft may be a length of one of the patient's own superficial veins, reversed so that its valves do not obstruct the blood flow.

The alternative is a synthetic material (e.g. orlon or teflon) and it has the advantage that it can be made into any size required. It is not usual now to excise the obstructed portion, but to insert the graft above and below it to act as a bypass. After operation the administration of the anticoagulants ordered is punctually undertaken, the leg pulse and skin colour is checked, and the care of the heels necessary to such patients is given.

Sepsis

The infections which come within the province of the surgeon vary from small, well-localized ones like boils to the extensive and therefore dangerous infections like peritonitis or empyema. The principles which underlie the treatment and nursing care are similar in all cases, and may be considered under these headings :

General. 1. *Antibiotics.* Unless the infection is trivial, the organism is determined and the specific drug to which it is sensitive is given.

2. *Diet.* Plentiful fluids are given to dilute the circulating toxins and flush out the kidneys. In severe infections with fever the basal metabolic rate is raised and, therefore, the caloric intake should be adequate. Protein intake should be good, especially if there are extensive lesions like infected burns, vitamin C may be helpful, and any anæmia should be corrected.

3. *Hygiene.* Septic organisms are always found on the skin if an infection is present, so a daily bed bath is given. The bowels should be kept acting normally.

4. *Analgesics.* Pain should be relieved so that sound sleep can be attained.

Local. 1. *Rest.* Movement increases pain and the likelihood of spread. If acute peritonitis is present, morphine is given to reduce peristalsis ; if a limb is affected, it is rested in a sling or on a splint.

2. *Elevation.* If an arm or leg is involved, raising it will decrease the pain by allowing œdema fluid to flow away.

3. *Drainage.* If pus is present and localized, incision is required The wound is drained until all the pus has been discharged.

4. *Heat.* Warmth soothes pain, dilates the local blood-vessels that are bringing the phagocytes and hastens resolution. Short-wave diathermy (p. 507) is suitable for deep-seated infection ; hot soaks or fomentations will help the discharge from open wounds ; kaolin poultices are comforting and assist localization. Moist heat, such as by fomentations, should not be applied continuously or the surrounding skin will become sodden.

5. *Dressings.* An aseptic technique must be used, since super-infection can occur far more readily in an open wound than in one that has been made and sutured in the theatre. Squeezing boils and carbuncles will break up the leucocyte ring that has formed around the area and spread infected fluid further along the tissue planes.

Burns

The majority of burns are preventible, and this is an aspect that nurses as parents, health visitors or industrial nurses should always remember. These are some of the outstanding precautions against accidents.

1. Paraffin heaters should never be filled while alight, and are best if attached to a wall. Children should never be left alone in a room with such a heater, and paraffin should be locked up.

2. Children's night wear should be flame proof, and all fires must have a guard.

3. Work on electrical appliances should only be undertaken by those who understand them. Everyone should know the position of the main electrical switch in their house or flat.

4. Smoking in bed is highly dangerous; even the able bodied easily fall asleep with a lighted cigarette in the hand, and the old are very vunerable.

5. Corrosive fluids must be treated with respect, and those who use them at work must not allow familiarity to cause carelessness.

The first aid treatment of burns is described on p. 524. When the patient arrives in the casualty department, the clothes are removed if this is easy, but if material is stuck to the skin nothing should be done about it at this stage. The extent of the burn is ascertained, and figure 000 indicates the way in which this is calculated as a percentage of the body surface. Burns involving more than 15% of the total area are always serious, and the depth of the burn cannot be accurately assessed at this stage. Blood is taken for grouping, since transfusion will always be needed for a serious burn, and in the meantime an intravenous infusion is begun. Records of the temperature, pulse, respiration and blood pressure are started. The burnt areas are covered with sterile towels, and an analgesic is given. Morphine is commonly ordered but not all surgeons like it because of its tendency to cause vomiting; if it is used, it is given intramuscularly, because the skin circulation in a shocked patient is too poor to allow absorption of a subcutaneous injection.

If the patient is a child, the relatives will not only be alarmed and anxious, but full of remorse and self-reproach, and must be treated with understanding. The patient is transferred as soon as possible to the ward. The treatment time falls into three stages, each with its own problems, and these will be considered in turn.

The first two days. This is the time of resuscitation. The patient is nursed in a cubicle or single room to lessen the risk of infection. Fluid and salts will leak from the burnt area and red blood cells will have been destroyed, so the electrolyte level and the hæmoglobin are regularly ascertained, and the intravenous fluids adjusted accordingly. An indwelling catheter is often used, so that an up to date figure for the urinary output can be recorded. A Ryle's tube may be passed into the stomach, so that the fluid intake can be supplemented by this route. Analgesics and sedatives are given. Nursing toilet of the eyes and mouth is important.

Loss of skin means that a wide area is open to infection, as well as allowing fluid loss. The first burns toilet is often performed in the theatre under a general anæsthetic. The ideal dressing is one that will seal off the fluid loss quickly, and since serum will crust rapidly under good conditions, the best treatment if the nature of the burns allows is exposure to the air. The burnt parts are laid uncovered on sterile towels or plastic foam, or tulle gras, changed whenever necessary, usually two or three times a day. Strict barrier nursing techniques will help to limit the risk of infection.

Burns are not suitable for exposure treatment if they pass completely round the limbs or trunk, and these are treated by the closed method, with tulle gras dressings, wool and bandages. The dressings are lengthy and painful, and the risk of infection is increased.

During this phase, frequent records of the temperature, pulse and blood pressure are kept. The large quantities of fluid given intravenously in severe shock may cause strain on the right side of the heart, and such signs as engorgement of the superficial veins, dyspnœa or pulse changes should be reported early. Special nursing problems may be produced by burns of the buttocks or perineum, which must be kept uncontaminated by excreta.

The next 2 weeks. This is a very testimg time for patient and medical staff. Antibiotics will be required to prevent pneumonia and minimize wound infection. The hæmoglobin level continues to fall, and more transfusions will be required. Physiotherapy is given to the unburnt parts.

The patient may be febrile, toxic, perhaps irrational and incontinent, and as the sloughs separate the extent of full-thickness burns will become apparent. A high protein diet must be taken, and the morale maintained at a reasonable level. Fits of depression and anger are common, and constant encouragement will be required.

The next 2 months. This is the time of surgical treatment, when raw areas are covered with skin grafts, and repeated anæsthetics and operations will be a severe strain on the patient, who now has plenty of time to contemplate the social results of his accident. He may fear ostracism because of disfigurement or loss of earning power. Contractures begin to appear as scars tighten, and loss of weight and depression are common.

Convalescence away from hospital will improve the general health and the morale as well, but most patients have to return at intervals for minor procedures to improve the appearance, or to release contractures. Patients are assured that the red angry scars will become white over the course of two or three years.

SKIN GRAFTS

Skin grafts are used to repair losses due to burns and injuries, and to replace scar tissue, and since skin from one person does not survive when transferred to another, the graft must come from the patient himself. Skin which is completely severed from its attachment and moved elsewhere is called a free graft, and three kinds are used :

1. Split skin graft (Thiersch graft). The upper layers of the skin are removed, leaving the deeper portions around the papillæ intact so that regeneration takes place. Such grafts may be cut with a knife from flat areas, or removed with a dermatome. The skin can be transferred in sheets, or cut up into smaller pieces in order to economize in its use. Split skin grafts are used where cosmetic result is not of prime importance, or as a temporary measure.

2. Full thickness graft. The skin is entirely removed, and is stitched into place where required. A better appearance is produced in the final result. The donor area must in its turn be covered, and if the graft is a narrow one, it may be possible to draw the edges together and suture them ; if not, a split skin graft must be supplied from a second donor area.

3. Pinch grafts. Fragments of skin are raised on a needle, separated with a knife and transplanted. Their thickness varies considerably and the final result is not a level one. It is not a method much used by the plastic specialist, but the general surgeon finds it of value.

Skin grafts obtain their nutriment first from the fluid in the tissues to which they are applied, and afterwards from capillary loops which grow into them. The most important point in the aftercare is, therefore, to see that the dressing does not move, or the grafts will be rubbed off before they can become attached. Tulle gras, wool and a crepe pressure bandage are applied in the theatre, or a plaster splint may be used. The dressing is not done for ten days if no infection is present, at the end of which time it should have "taken." Masks should be worn, a scrupulous non-touch technique used, and no rubbing of the area with swabs is permitted. Some experience is required before the nurse can judge how successful the graft has been.

If subcutaneous tissue as well as skin is to be transferred, a pedicle graft is raised. The graft is left attached by one side to the donor area, while the remainder is laid over the wound that is to be grafted and sutured. When union is satisfactory the remaining side is freed and stitched into place. Pedicle grafts can be taken from distant parts of the body; for instance, a pedicle may be transferred from the abdominal end wall to the arm, and when it is attached there, the abdominal end is severed and moved to the face. This type of graft entails two or more operations, but gives great scope to the plastic surgeon in refashioning damaged structures.

The nurse who works with a plastic surgeon should regard herself as helping an artist. She must thoroughly understand the principles of his work, have a faultless dressing technique, be skilled in bandaging, and have the ability to inspire her patients to sustain their courage and optimism in face of repeated operations interspersed sometimes with long periods of waiting and frustration.

CHAPTER 21

GYNÆCOLOGICAL NURSING

A HIGH proportion of patients in a gynæcological ward are women in the child-bearing time of life, and their illnesses affect a system which is of the deepest psychological importance to every woman. Such symptoms as vaginal bleeding and discharge, which are so common in these wards, give rise not only to fears about their health, but about their married life or their prospects of marriage, and the possibility of having a family. No other branch of surgery requires more local treatment pre- and post-operatively than gynæcology, and this treatment is by its nature liable to cause embarrassment and discomfort unless performed with intuitive sympathy as well as technical efficiency. To be a first-class gynæcological nurse demands not only deft performance based on a sound knowledge of anatomy, but insight into the patient's emotional needs, and the ability to answer questions or the sense to refer them to those who can. Many women are not very articulate on the subject that is worrying them, or lack the vocabulary to express their questions. A sister is very often asked questions that the patient may be shy of addressing to the surgeon.

The conditions that bring patients to a gynæcologist may be summarized as follows :

1. **Congenital abnormalities** of the vagina and uterus.

2. **New Growths.** Those of the ovary are common and varied in type. Cancer of the uterus is regrettably frequent, and the uterine fibromyoma is a very common innocent growth.

3. **Infections.** Inflammation of the Fallopian tubes (salpingitis), uterine mucosa (endometritis), vagina (vaginitis) and vulva (vulvitis) are common. Venereal disease (p. 465) which is increasing in incidence, is of prime importance.

4. **Prolapse.** This means descent of the uterus and neighbouring structures from their normal position, and is usually met as a sequel to childbearing.

5. **Functional Disorders.** In these the primary complaints are disorders of function rather than of structure, and are often related to menstruation. In this group come a number of women more often met with in consulting rooms than in wards, whose symptoms of pain, backache or bleeding are a symptom of emotional tension and anxiety or frustration rather than their cause.

6. **Accidents of pregnancy,** e.g. pyelitis ; albuminuria of pregnancy ; threatened or inevitable abortion ; ruptured ectopic pregnancy.

GYNÆCOLOGICAL EXAMINATION

On admission to the ward, the patient will be fully examined. This is not only a pelvic examination ; the patient must be considered as a whole if a correct diagnosis is to be made. Patients often present with gynæcological symptoms when suffering primarily from diabetes or some other endocrine condition, or a carcinoma of breast with pelvic metastases.

Shave. It is common for patients admitted with a view to surgery to have a pelvic shave on admission. This encourages local cleanliness and facilitates pre-operative preparation, but is not essential to examination, and is never performed only for this reason.

The hair must be shaved from the abdomen and the vulva. The dry method may be used for the hair on the mons veneris, but soap and lather must be used for the vulva, and many would prefer it also for the abdomen.

Tray. Safety razor with new blade.
Powder shaker.
Bowl of wool swabs about 10 cm. square.
Bowl of warm water.
Soap.
Receiver.
Mackintosh and cover.

The patient lies on her back, with the bedclothes folded singly on to the thighs, while the upper parts are covered with a blanket or bed jacket. The pubic hair is thoroughly dusted with powder, or lathered well with soap, and then shaved downwards towards the vulva, the hair being collected with a swab. The patient is asked to flex and abduct her thighs and the hair on the labia majora is well soaped and rubbed to a lather. A swab is taken in the left hand and placed over all the vulva except the left labium majus, the skin of which is kept taut by this swab. The left side is shaved, and another swab is used to stretch the right labium as it is similarly treated. Finally the patient is turned on to the left side, and the shave is completed by removing any hair around the anus.

Preparation. It is desirable that the rectum be empty before a vaginal examination is made, but if the patient's habits are regular no special preparation is needed. The bladder should be emptied shortly before examination for the patient's comfort, unless a urethral discharge is present from which a swab is to be taken. It is imperative that the urine is tested, especially for albumin and sugar, and if there is a history of frequency or the urine is not clear, a clean specimen should be sent for bacteriological examination.

The instruments used must be boiled before use and sterile swabs and lotion used, but a full aseptic technique is not necessary except in the later months of pregnancy.

The patient's nightgown is removed, and she lies on her back with one or two pillows under her head. A blanket covers her, and the bedclothes are folded down to the level of the symphisis pubis. The doctor looks at the conjunctivæ and the inner surface of the lips for obvious signs of anæmia, and then feels the thyroid gland, since thyroid disorders commonly produce menstrual symptoms.

The chest is uncovered and the heart and lungs examined. The breasts are inspected and palpated with care, since breast activity is an early sign of pregnancy, and breast cancer may cause secondary growths in the ovaries. Abdominal examination follows; many tumours of the ovaries and uterus are palpable from the abdomen, and

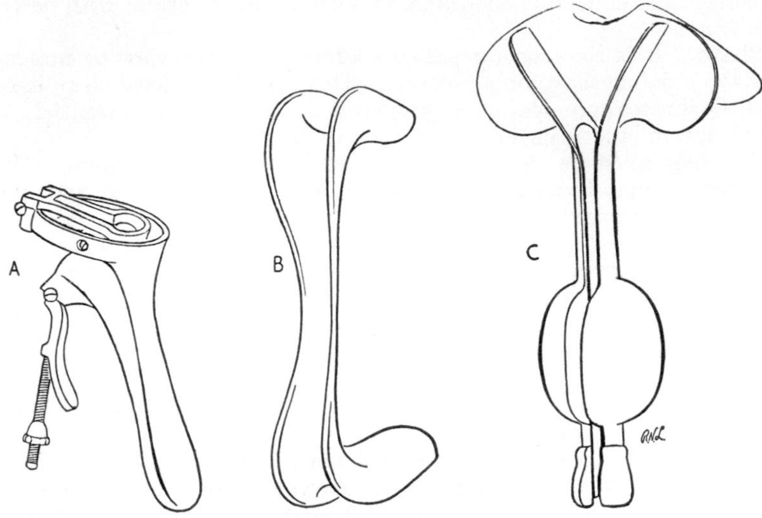

FIG. 67. Vaginal specula.
A. Cusco. B. Sims'. C. Auvard.

so is the pregnant uterus after the twelfth week. Internal examination follows, and the following should be available if a complete examination is being undertaken.

Trolley. Bowl of antiseptic, e.g. chlorhexidine (Hibitane).
Bowl of swabs.
Instrument tray with specula, e.g. Cusco's, Sims', Ferguson's.
Sponge-holding forceps.
Volsellum forceps.
Proctoscope.
Lamp.
Gloves, powder and lubricant.
Rectal tray.
Receivers for soiled dressings and used instruments.

For taking swabs : Rack with throat swabs.
Platinum loop.
Spirit lamp and matches.
Slides and coverslips.
Stuart's transport medium and charcoal swabs (for gonorrhœa).

The nurse prepares her trolley on the right-hand side of the bed, places the patient in the position liked by the doctor (see p. 287), and stands on the patient's left where she can help maintain the position. She assures her patient that no pain will be felt and uncovers the hips. After inspection of the vulva, and swabbing if necessary, the doctor makes first a digital and then a speculum examination. If he finds discharge he may take a swab. Rectal examination is often indicated, especially if carcinoma of cervix is present. When it is finished the nurse sees that her patient is dry and comfortable and gives her a clean pad if necessary. If a swab has been taken, she asks the doctor to sign the request form, and sends it to the laboratory without delay.

POSITIONS USED IN GYNÆCOLOGY

1. **Dorsal.** The patient lies on her back with one or two pillows under the head. Her trunk should be straight and her arms by her side. The chest and abdomen are examined in this way, and vaginal examination may also be done if the patient is asked to flex the knees and abduct the thighs.

2. **Left Lateral.** The patient lies on her left side, with the knees and thighs flexed and the buttocks at the edge of the bed. The trunk is slightly flexed to relax the abdominal muscles and one pillow placed under the head. This is the most commonly used position for rectal and vaginal examination, and for giving enemata.

3. **Sims' position** is a modification of the left lateral that gives a better exposure of the vulva, and of the vagina when a speculum is used. The left arm is drawn behind the patient so that her chest lies on the bed. The right knee is flexed until it lies on the bed above the left one. The nurse must see that both arms are comfortable.

4. **Lithotomy.** The patient lies on her back, with the thighs flexed and abducted and the knees flexed. Its commonest use is in the theatre for operations on the vagina, perineum and rectum, and for forceps deliveries. The end of the table is dropped and the buttocks brought to the edge. The legs are supported by webbing straps round the feet and ankles fastened to lithotomy poles, or by metal troughs. Both legs should be raised together when the anæsthetized patient is put into this position. A special lithotomy chair with metal troughs for leg support is much used in clinics for investigating and treating vaginal discharge. Lithotomy means " stone-cutting," and reminds one that stone in the bladder was in pre-Listerian times always approached from the perineum to avoid the risk of peritonitis.

5. **Trendelenburg.** The head of the patient is lower than the pelvis to permit upward displacement of the abdominal organs and a better view of the contents of the pelvis. The patient must, of course, be secured against a fall from the table. Methods include :

1. Pelvic crest supports.
2. Shoulder supports. These bring a risk of brachial palsy, and are best avoided.
3. The end of the table may be dropped, the knees flexed and the ankles secured. The weight of the patient presses the calves against the table, and is a cause of venous thrombosis.
4. Langton-Hewer corrugated mattress. This rubber mattress has transverse corrugations and the patient is supported by the adhesion of the skin of the back. The skin must be dry. Cushions of foam rubber are put beneath the neck, loins and ankles and the corrugations of these must fit those of the table. There are rubber straps on the lumbar cushion to secure the arms. Before tilting the table the nurse must ensure that the mattress is hooked to the end of the table.

6. **Knee-chest** or genupectoral. This position is occasionally used in obstetrics, e.g. following prolapse of the umbilical cord. The patient's weight is distributed between the knees and the folded arms. The head is turned to one side on a pillow, and the thighs must be vertical, so that the pelvis is as high as possible. It is used sometimes during the injection of hæmorrhoids. It is exhausting and cannot be sustained for long periods.

GYNÆCOLOGICAL OPERATIONS

The terms used of operations on the female genital tract are these :

Oophorectomy. Removal of an ovary.

Salpingectomy. Removal of a Fallopian tube.

Hysterectomy. Removal of the uterus.

(*a*) *Subtotal.* The body is excised and the cervix is left. This operation is not now very common, since removal of the cervix ensures that carcinoma cannot occur in it.

(*b*) *Total.* Body and cervix are included in the operation.

(*c*) *Pan-hysterectomy* was the term once used to describe removal of uterus, tubes and ovaries. It has fallen into disuse because it is ambiguous. One would now speak of hysterectomy with bilateral salpingo-oophorectomy.

(*d*) *Wertheim's Hysterectomy.* An extensive operation involving removal of the uterus and its appendages, the tissues around the uterus, the pelvic glands and the upper part of the vagina. It may be more rapidly performed, and the whole of the vagina removed, by a synchronous combined abdomino-perineal operation; two surgeons work in the same way as in performing a similar operation on the rectum.

Colporrhaphy. Repair of the vagina, anterior or posterior.

Perineorrhaphy. Repair of the perineum.

Dilation of Cervix and Curettage of Uterus. Curettage means scraping. It is a diagnostic procedure, primarily for patients suspected of uterine or cervical cancer, or with functional uterine bleeding. It can be used for the removal of retained products of conception.

PREPARATION FOR OPERATION

The *consent* of the patient is necessary as in all operations, but it is especially important that both she and her husband understand clearly what is involved, and if the operation involves sterilization the husband as well as the wife should sign the form. The *hæmoglobin* must be estimated, since anæmia is a common finding, and the *blood group*, including the *Rhesus* sign, must be ascertained before major surgery. the *menstrual history* is obtained, since it is not advisable to operate during menstruation. If anæmia is present it must be corrected ; if it is due to heavy menstrual loss, transfusion is performed and operation undertaken before the next period.

The *fluid intake* is measured, and should be 2–3,000 ml. to help avert urinary infection. The *urinary output* and *frequency* is recorded, and the usual ward tests made. If there is evidence of infection, a *clean specimen* is taken to identify the organism and the antibiotic to which it is sensitive. *Potassium citrate* with hyoscyamus may be ordered to keep the urine alkaline. An intravenous *pyelogram* is necessary if there is a cancer of the cervix, to exclude involvement of the ureters. The bladder must always be emptied by catheter immediately before any gynæcological operation to avoid the risk of injuring it.

Rest in bed is helpful to a tired woman, but enough exercise to keep the circulation moving in the legs is necessary for venous thrombosis and pulmonary embolism are not uncommon in gynæcology. *Breathing exercises* are always undertaken and smoking is discouraged.

The *rectum* and *sigmoid colon* must be empty, since the rectum lies so close to the vagina. An aperient forty-eight hours before, and an enema or suppository the night before operation is usual. If the operation is on the vagina the bowels will be kept confined for four days afterwards, and a *low residue* diet is given for twenty-four hours beforehand.

Preparation of the skin is usually limited in the ward to a *shave* and a *bath*. If the vagina is to be opened, some vaginal preparation is needed, e.g. *vaginal douche* ; *painting* of the vagina ; use of soluble *pessaries* ; inserting a *sterile pack*.

The emotional attitude of these patients has been referred to. They ask many questions and need much encouragement, but they respond well to it.

Vaginal Douches

Douches are less commonly used than formerly. They are not recommended for regular use simply as a hygienic measure, since they change the bacteriological flora of the vagina. Douches are used:

1. As a pre-operative cleansing measure. Lactic acid 1%, flavine 1 in 1,000 or normal saline are suitable, and the temperature should be 105° F. (or 40° C.).

2. To check bleeding. Sterile water or normal saline is used when the surgeon orders such a douche. The temperature should begin at 110° F. (44° C.) and be slowly raised to 120° F. (50° C.). This will feel uncomfortably hot to the patient, and a layer of vaseline should be applied to the perineum and anus over which the solution will run.

3. To remove discharge, e.g. in a patient wearing a vaginal pessary. Any of the solutions mentioned in (1) are satisfactory. If the discharge is caused by ulceration from a retained foreign body, sodium bicarbonate 1 drachm to a pint is effective. If used for sepsis in the vagina following operation, a douche is not usually ordered till after the eighth day, and is really an irrigation, given with a rubber catheter at very low pressure.

Equipment for a pre-operative douche.

Douche can, 1 metre of tubing, clip and douche nozzle in a bowl, sterile.
Lotion thermometer.
2-pint jug of selected lotion.
Bowl of lotion for swabbing.
Bowl of large-size swabs, sterile.
Mackintosh and towel (which may be disposable).
Warm douche pan and cover.
Blanket or shawl.

The curtains are drawn and the patient is assured that there will be no discomfort. The bedclothes are folded on to the thighs, the blanket put over the patient, and the mackintosh and towel and douche pan slipped underneath her. The pillows are left under the head and shoulders so that she is lying flat.

The nurse washes and dries her hands, pours the lotion into the can, and allows a little to run through before tightening the clip. The temperature is checked. The can is arranged at a height of not more than a foot above the vagina ; if the trolley is a low one, the bowl can be inverted and the can stood on it. If too much force is used, infected material may be carried into the uterus or even the Fallopian tubes. It is also possible to force air into the uterus and thence into the circulation, causing air embolus.

The patient is asked to lift the blanket and to flex and abduct her thighs. The nurse parts the labia minora with the first two fingers of the left hand and swabs the introitus with warm lotion. She takes the douche nozzle in her right hand, inspects it to see that it is not cracked, and passes it into the posterior fornix of the vagina along the posterior wall, which runs upwards and backwards in the direction of the sacral promontory. The clip is undone and the lotion allowed to run in.

When it is finished, the nozzle is removed and returned to the can. The patient is sat up, and asked to cough to drain any remaining fluid out of the vagina. The douche pan is taken out, and the vulva and groins dried. The patient is then asked to turn on her side and the perianal region dried. The mackintosh and towel are taken out and the bed made.

Vaginal Pack

Equipment. Sterile dish with gauze roll 2 metres long, and large gallipot.
Sterile Sims' speculum and lubricant. Sterile sponge-holding or dressing forceps.
Penicillin 60 ml., 1,000 units per ml., or desired antiseptic.
Warm lotion and swabs.
Receiver for dirty dressings.
Blanket, mackintosh and towel.

If the pack is a pre-operative one following a douche, the patient will already be lying on a mackintosh and towel covered with a blanket and there will be no need for swabbing. The left lateral position is the most useful and the buttocks should be brought to the edge of the bed. An assistant pours the penicillin over the gauze roll. The speculum is lubricated and introduced along the posterior vaginal wall, and the blade is used to draw back the wall in order to open the upper part of the vagina. Several loops of gauze roll are gathered into the forceps, and are introduced along the speculum into the posterior fornix. The vault of the vagina is packed closely but not tightly, and then the rest is filled. A sterile pad may finally be applied.

A vaginal pack may be used to check bleeding, reactionary or secondary, after operation. This can only be done effectively under an anæsthetic and in aseptic theatre conditions, but it is possible that there are circumstances in which a nurse may have to do this pending the arrival of a doctor. The bladder should be emptied beforehand, since an efficient pack will prevent micturition. Dry gauze must be used, and the vault packed as firmly as possible.

Painting the Vagina

This procedure may be performed pre-operatively, and is also used occasionally in the treatment of vaginal infections.

Equipment. Receiver with sponge-holding forceps and gauze-covered swabs.
Sims' speculum and lubricant.
Gallipot of required antiseptic (e.g. Bonney's blue paint pre-operatively).
Pad.
Mackintosh and towel.
Gloves.
Light.

The patient lies on the left lateral or Sims' position, with the mackintosh and towel beneath her. The solutions used are all apt to stain, and they must be used neatly. The light is adjusted to give a good view, and the speculum lubricated and inserted. Sims' or Cusco's are suitable, as they give a wide exposure of the vault of the vagina. Ferguson's cannot retract the posterior vaginal wall and is not a good one for this purpose. A swab is dipped in the antiseptic, and the whole vagina thoroughly painted. The posterior wall is painted as the speculum is withdrawn. A pad is supplied to prevent soiling of the clothes.

Soluble Pessaries

Pessaries are extensively used in vaginal treatment, and as pre-operative measures. Sulphathiazole and penicillin are frequently used, and stilbœstrol pessaries are often ordered before operation on patients of post-menopausal age. The reason is that this hormone promotes the production in the vagina of lactic acid, which is a powerful barrier to infection. This protective acid reaction is lost after the menopause and can be stimulated by stilbœstrol pessaries.

Equipment. Right-hand glove, or caped finger stall.
Swabs.
Pessary.
Pad.

The pessary must have been checked with the prescription. The left lateral is the most usual position, and the pessary is introduced by the gloved right hand over the perineum, and pushed up into the posterior fornix. Its position is important.

If a patient has pessaries prescribed as an out-patient treatment, she must be taught how to introduce them. She should put it as high as possible when she is in bed at the end of the day, so that the upper part of the vagina will have prolonged contact with the drug.

POST-OPERATIVE CARE

Shock is only likely to be met after extensive operations for malignant disease. It is dealt with by the methods described on p. 242.

Pain will necessitate morphine 10 mgms.(gr. $\frac{1}{6}$) or pethidine 100 mg. Pethidine appears especially suitable for gynæcological patients. Neither need be used for more than twenty-four hours generally, and tabs. Codeine Co. B.P.C. are useful afterwards. Pain in perineal stitch lines is often caused by œdema a few days after operation, and the removal of a stitch may give much relief.

Vomiting may be treated on the usual lines. *Distension* is more marked than might be expected, since the intestines are little handled. Vomiting and distension occurring together suggest *intestinal obstruction,* either mechanical or paralytic. Vomiting in excess of intake and a rising pulse rate must be reported urgently.

Sepsis occurs readily in vaginal and perineal stitch lines. The nurse hopes to avert it by careful pre-operative preparation, an aseptic dressing technique, and giving a diet adequate in protein and vitamin C. Slight pyrexia and offensive vaginal discharge are indications for gentle vaginal irrigations and an appropriate antibiotic. If not controlled, it may lead to secondary hæmorrhage.

Bleeding is one of the commoner major complications, and is usually vaginal and evident. Intraperitoneal bleeding is diagnosed by the signs of internal hæmorrhage (p. 242). *Reactionary* bleeding usually necessitates a return to the theatre to secure the bleeding point, or to insert a pack. *Secondary* bleeding is due to sepsis, and if severe is also best treated in the theatre. If a hæmorrhage occurs the house surgeon is informed, and the patient kept at rest in bed with one pillow and the foot of the bed on blocks. Morphine is usually ordered at once. A mackintosh and pad are placed beneath the buttocks, and the pulse rate is taken at five-minute intervals. The nurse may be asked to prepare, and give, a hot douche.

Thrombosis in the deep veins of the leg must be watched for. It is signalled by slight fever and tenderness in the calf. Prevention is better than cure, and the means are given on p. 247. Anti-coagulant drugs can be given if there is no risk of provoking hæmorrhage, e.g. heparin 10,000 units six-hourly for twenty-four hours, and phenindione 100 mg. b.d., decreasing as the prothrombin time falls.

Pulmonary embolus is sometimes a much-feared complication of venous thrombosis (p. 247). Though not now very common as a fatal sequel to surgery, such cases as are seen are often in the gynæcological wards.

Chest complications are a comparatively minor problem. The incisions are low in the abdomen and do not hinder diaphragmatic movement ; morphine, a powerful respiratory depressant, is little used in large doses, and women are seldom heavy smokers.

Urinary complications are undoubtedly the commonest of all. An accurate chart of frequency and output will give timely warning of many. *Infection* has already been mentioned. *Retention* is very common, and if it is to be treated by catheterization, a meticulous technique must be used, since retention and instrumentation both predispose to infection. *Retention with overflow* must not be allowed to develop, and correct interpretation of the output chart will prevent it. Re-establishment of micturition after an indwelling catheter has been removed is not always easy, and after twenty-four hours the *residual* urine is discovered by passing a catheter after the patient has endeavoured to empty her bladder. If the amount is more than an ounce or two the test should be regularly repeated until the bladder is emptying normally.

Suppression of urine may indicate injury to the ureters, and if no urine has been passed within sixteen hours of operation the patient is catheterized. If no urine is found in the bladder the diagnosis of this dangerous condition is confirmed. Incontinence may be the result of a fistula between bladder and vagina. Fistulæ have to be dealt with surgically later, and in the meantime the skin must be kept from excoriation by a barrier cream or ointment.

SOME GYNÆCOLOGICAL CONDITIONS

1. **Congenital Abnormalities.** These usually involve absence of or duplication of genital organs, and some are amenable to plastic surgery. *Imperforate hymen* is not uncommon ; the hymen completely closes the vaginal orifice, resulting in retention of the menstrual flow in the vagina, or cryptomenorrhœa.

2. **New Growths.** (*a*) *Ovary.* Ovarian cysts are frequent and of many kinds, and often bilateral. They are nearly always removed because of a marked tendency to malignancy and other complications. Cancer of ovary results in ascites and inoperable cases need frequent paracentesis.

(*b*) *Uterus.* Cancer of the cervix is one of the commonest cancers in women. Treatment may be by radium, or by Wertheim's hysterectomy or a similar operation. Cancer of the body of the uterus is always treated surgically and has quite a good prognosis.

Early Detection of Cancer

Cancer of the cervix is the cause of death of many women. In its early stages, when it is confined to the cervix, a high cure rate can be expected, but once the disease has spread into the bladder or rectum, there is little hope of effective treatment. The earlier the condition is diagnosed, therefore, the more lives will be saved, and the more pain and misery averted. Nurses may often help by advising women who consult them about slight bleeding at unusual times to consult a doctor at once.

For some time (perhaps years) before symptoms appear or a lesion can be seen, there are changes in the epithelium of the cervix. If at this stage the surface of the cervix is scraped with a wooden spatula, the cells detached can be examined microscopically, and this pre-malignant phase detected. Simple hysterectomy will at this stage effect a cure.

In order to detect this non-invasive stage, women without symptoms must be induced to attend clinics where this cytological service is available. At many such clinics examination is made to exclude carcinoma of breast, another major cause of death. Nurses can help this important health work by telling women that the examination is painless, and mostly results in assurance that all is well. In the very small minority who have an early lesion, cure can be confidently expected.

Fibromyomata are innocent growths, practically confined to the uterus and often numerous. Their importance is in their association with sterility, and the fact that they give rise to anæmia from bleeding.

3. **Infections.** (*a*) *Salpingitis.* Acute salpingitis is treated conservatively, since there is no danger to this vascular organ of gangrene, as in the appendix. It should be treated urgently or sterility may follow from adhesions in the tubes. Penicillin (until the results of a vagina swab are known), rest in bed, high fluid intake, alkaline mixtures and warmth to the abdomen are indicated. If a discharge is present, the patient must have her own bedpan. Cure is rapid, but if neglected chronic sepsis follows with much ill health and usually an operation.

(*b*) *Vaginitis* is commonly caused, either by thrush or by trichomonas vaginalis, and is usually seen in out-patient departments.

Tampons are occasionally used to absorb vaginal discharge, or to apply medication to the cervix. They are made by folding in half an 8-in. strip of wool 1 in. wide. Linen thread is passed through the loop and knotted, the ends being left free for withdrawing it. To insert one a nurse needs :

Sims' speculum.
Sponge-holding forceps.
Tampons, all in a dish.
Lubricant.
Lotion and swabs.

With the patient in the left lateral position the vulva is freed from discharge. The tampon is clipped into the forceps with the thread hanging down. The posterior vaginal wall is retracted and the tampon passed into the posterior fornix. It cannot be felt if correctly placed, but if it rests on the perineum it is painful. The patient must be instructed in its removal. Proprietary makes of tampon are preferable if available.

Vulvitis or inflammation of the vulva is commonly due to irritation from a vaginal discharge, or a urinary condition. Testing the urine for sugar is vital.

4. **Prolapse.** Prolapse of the uterus is often accompanied by descent of the anterior vaginal wall and bladder (*cystocele*) or of the posterior wall (*rectocele*). Surgery is incomparably the best treatment. Fothergill's or the Manchester operation involves amputation of cervix, tightening the transverse ligaments, and repair of the vagina and perineum. Mayo's operation is vaginal hysterectomy with vaginal repair. Even elderly patients are now successfully operated on.

The alternative is support of the organs by a ring pessary, and it is usually only tolerated by the patient until operation is possible. The ring is made of plastic, which does not irritate the tissues, and it is inserted into the vault of the vagina which it stretches and sustains.

Equipment. Warm lotion and swabs.
Pessary, boiled.
Gloves.
Lubricant.
Mackintosh and towel, blanket.

The pessary is inserted with the patient in the left lateral position. The labia are cleansed, and the pessary touched with lubricant at one side. It is taken in the right hand and compressed until it can be introduced through the introitus. If difficulty is found in compressing it a piece of tape secured with artery forceps is helpful. Once it is released it disappears into the vagina, and the first two or three fingers of the right hand are used to push it into position in the vault, with the cervix lying in the middle.

The patient must be told to return to have it changed in a month or six weeks, and if the patient is elderly and inattentive a relative should be told. Douching at regular intervals is necessary to irrigate away the discharge that will be provoked. Most patients find it most convenient to sit in the bath for this. The help of the district nurse must be sought if the patient is unable through age or infirmity to do it for herself.

A variety of other pessaries are very occasionally used for this purpose, but they are largely of historic interest. Looking at diagrams of such apparatus as a cup and stem pessary, the nurse will wonder at the fortitude of women who had to wear such an appliance which rendered hygiene almost impossible, before modern anæsthetic and operative techniques made surgery feasible for most patients.

A Hodge pessary is a rigid one designed to maintain a retroverted uterus in place. It is put in by the doctor after manually replacing the uterus in its normal position.

5. **Functional Disorders.** The terms used of menstrual disorders include :

Menorrhagia—excessive menstruation.
Amenorrhœa—failure to menstruate.
Dysmenorrhœa—painful menstruation.

6. **Accidents of Pregnancy.** The commonest in gynæcological wards is abortion.

ABORTION

Abortion is the termination of pregnancy before the twenty-eighth week, the date at which it is capable of independent existence. The patient, who is usually in the first three months of pregnancy, begins to lose a little blood per vaginam and to experience colicky pain. This stage is known as *threatened abortion* and the loss of the pregnancy is by no means certain. The patient is put to bed with only one or two pillows, and morphine 10 mg. is often ordered to allay her pain and anxiety and allow her to rest. Pads must be saved and any increase in bleeding or rhythmic pains reported. The diet should be low residue ; aperients and enemata must be avoided, since they stimulate uterine contractions. The patient should stay in bed till all bleeding has ceased, and should lead a quiet life till the pregnancy is firmly established.

Once the cervix is dilated, or any part of the fœtal membranes is passed, the abortion is *inevitable*, and the doctor will hasten its conclusion by ordering ergometrine 0·5 mg. The products of conception that are passed must be saved for inspection, to ensure that nothing is retained in the uterus. When the abortion is over, the thighs should be well washed with soap and water, and the vulva swabbed with antiseptic and dried. Sterile pads should be used. Vulval swabbing is repeated twice a day until bright bleeding has ceased, and the patient may then go home if the temperature is normal.

Uterine infection may follow any abortion, especially those that are not complete, or have been induced by criminal methods. The patient has high fever, with bloodstained offensive discharge. A cervical swab should be obtained to find the infecting organism, but penicillin may be begun at once since it is often a streptococcus. The patient is nursed sitting well up, and with precautions to prevent the spread of infection to others. The fluid intake must be high, and aseptic toilet of the vulva regularly undertaken.

In 1967 the Abortion Act was passed, making the termination of pregnancy legal if two registered medical practitioners agree that

(*a*) the continuation of the pregnancy would involve risk to the life of the pregnant woman, or of injury to her physical or mental health, or of any existing children, greater than if the pregnancy were terminated or

(*b*) there is a substantial risk that if the child were born it would suffer from such physical or mental abnormalities as to be seriously handicapped.

The operation must take place in a Health Service hospital or approved nursing home, and must be notified. Subject to the proviso that there is a duty to participate in treatment necessary to save the life, or prevent injury to the physical or mental health of the pregnant woman, no one is required to take part in any treatment authorized by the Act to which he has a conscientious objection. This applies to nurses as well as doctors.

MATERNITY NURSING

Although the conduct of labour and the delivery of the baby is the province of the doctor or trained midwife, the student or trained nurse may assist in the care of the pregnant woman and nursing her during the *puerperium* or lying-in period.

Good antenatal supervision has a major role to play in making pregnancy happy and free from many discomforts and complications, in educating the mother-to-be, and in making labour safe for mother and baby. The patient should visit her doctor or hospital department regularly once a month for these purposes.

1. **Reassurance.** The knowledge that all is going well is important, and the pregnant woman may have doubts and fears that can be allayed. She may have more material anxieties, which the welfare worker may advise about.

2. **Examination.** At each attendance the urine is tested, the blood pressure estimated and the patient weighed. The hæmoglobin, Rhesus group and Wassermann reaction are ascertained, and perhaps the chest X-rayed. Her previous medical history may have an influence on her present condition.

3. **Education.** She may need advice on :

(*a*) *Diet.* Plenty of fluids (including milk), adequate protein, and the inclusion of salads in the diet is recommended. Excessive weight gain is discouraged.

(b) *Clothes.* The type of brassière should be one that does not compress the nipples. There should be no constriction of the legs that would encourage varicose vein formation.

(c) *Exercise.* Moderate exercise is desirable, and the physiotherapist will conduct classes to strengthen muscles and teach relaxation.

(d) *Baby Care.* Mothercraft classes are extensively held, especially at welfare centres. Some encourage fathers to attend as well.

(e) *Teeth.* Dental decay may occur if the growing fœtus is making excessive demands on the mother's calcium, and the dentist should be consulted.

(f) *Financial* benefits available.

4. **Assessment of Presentation.** The most favourable presentation is by the vertex, i.e. the baby's head is the lowest part. It is usual to endeavour to correct any other presentation (e.g. persistent breech presentation) before delivery.

LABOUR

The course of labour can be divided into three parts :

1. The first stage. This begins with the onset of labour (with rhythmic pain in the back and abdomen and the discharge of a little mucus and blood). It ends when the cervix is fully dilated. This stage may last up to eighteen hours with a first baby.

The patient is usually admitted to the maternity unit in this stage. The lie and presentation of the baby are checked, and whether the head is engaged in the pelvis. The temperature, pulse and blood pressure are recorded, and a specimen of urine obtained and examined for protein, sugar and acetone. The strength and regularity of the pains, and the interval between them is checked. An enema is given (since a loaded rectum prolongs labour), a vulval shave and a shower. During the early stages, the mother may walk around or lie down as she wishes, and the company of the husband will be a comfort. Solid food should not be given once labour is well established, since the stomach empties very slowly at this time, and if need for an anæsthetic arises unexpectedly, this will cause trouble. Fluids should be given freely.

If the contractions are painful, an analgesic is given and sometimes towards the end of the first stage gas and oxygen may be given. The fœtal heart rate and maternal pulse are checked with increasing frequency as labour progresses. The first stage is usually rather a tiresome one for the patient, since nothing can be done to hasten it. The mother needs encouragement, the company of her nurse, and watchful care to detect any signs of impending danger to mother and child.

2. The second stage. Once the cervix is fully dilated, the descent of the baby through the vagina and its expulsion to the exterior begins. It may occupy one to three hours in a primipara, or only a few minutes if the patient has had babies before. This stage ends with the birth of the baby.

The onset of this stage is normally greeted with relief by the patient, who can now take a more active part. Once the cervix is fully dilated the baby begins to leave the uterus, and if the membranes have not ruptured before, they do so now. The patient begins to hold her breath and bear down with each contraction, and nitrous oxide and oxygen given by the " Entonox " apparatus will relieve the pain and enable the patient to cooperate with her attendants.

Delivery can be effected with the mother lying on her back or on the left side, and is conducted with aseptic technique. Only an outline of the technique of delivery is given here. The aim of the accoucheur when the baby is presenting by the vertex in the usual way is to keep the head well flexed, by pressing with a sterile pad over the perineum, so that the smallest diameter of the head distends the vulva. Once the occiput has passed under the symphysis pubis, the forehead and face are drawn out from under the perineum, and the head is free. With the next pain the shoulders are delivered, first the anterior and then the posterior, and the rest of the trunk follows easily.

The baby usually begins to breathe and cry at once, but it may be necessary to aspirate mucus from the pharynx before breathing is established. The mother is told the baby's sex, the cord is clamped and divided, and the baby laid in a cot with the head low, and attention returns to the mother.

3. The third stage. The contractions of the uterus separate the placenta and it is expelled along with the fœtal membranes.

Conduct of the third stage is directed to ensuring that the placenta is delivered intact, and with the membranes complete, and that bleeding is minimal. The mother should if possible be allowed to hold her baby, and after a short rest is washed, changed into clean clothes and taken to the ward along with her baby.

Nursing in the Puerperium

The number of deliveries taking place in the home is decreasing since even in apparently normal cases a sudden emergency may arise which requires hospital facilities for its treatment. Women who are booked for hospital delivery normally remain for about eight days. It is also quite common for women to come into hospital when labour begins with their general practitioner or midwife, and to return home a few hours later for domiciliary care.

The basic considerations for nurses working in maternity wards is the vulnerability of both mother and baby to infection, and all nursing techniques should be devised with this in mind. The baby has lived hitherto in a sterile environment, and now is exposed to infection of the intestinal tract, umbilical cord and skin. The mother has a raw area in the uterus to which the placenta was attached, and although puerperal fever through infection of the site is not now the common and fatal disease it once was, it is still a danger to be remembered.

The temperature, pulse and respiration rates should be charted four-hourly for the first three days, and subsequently twice a day. The fluid intake should be recorded, and a high one encouraged. The height of the fundus of the uterus above the symphisis pubis should be measured daily, and if progress is regular it should no longer be palpable from the abdomen by the tenth day. The uterine discharge, or lochia, which is mostly bright blood immediately after delivery, should become first brownish and then almost colourless by the time the patient leaves hospital. At no time should the lochia be offensive.

Toilet of the perineum has been simplified by early rising. Mothers may take a bath or shower the morning after delivery, and if bidets are available local hygiene is easy. Graded exercises are begun the day after delivery to improve the tone of the abdominal muscles and pelvic floor, and to ward off venous thrombosis.

The breasts become tender and enlarged soon after delivery, but milk secretion is not really established until the third day after a first baby is born. The mother is taught how to hold her baby while feeding him, and to wash her hands and nipples before feeding. Breast feeding should be supervised until it is free of difficulty both for mother and baby.

The mother must obtain as much sleep as possible. Early and late feeds curtail her night's rest, and a quiet time should be observed in maternity wards after lunch so that extra sleep can be obtained Only her husband and mother should visit her for the first day or two, and large numbers of visitors should never be encouraged.

Babies are not now bathed in hospital as frequently as formerly; baths are difficult to disinfect, and regular immersion in early days seems unnecessary. Cleaning with swabs moistened with hexachlorophane emulsion is substituted. The cord is swabbed daily with spirit until it separates. Record should be made when the bladder and bowels act. He is weighed daily, and when lactation is well established test feeding may be used to establish that the amount taken at a feed is satisfactory. The mother need not be told the weight on each occasion. Babies always lose weight during the first few days, and do not usually regain the birth weight for a fortnight, but young mothers need much reassurance before accepting this as normal. The nurse should put on a mask, and should wash her hands before attending to each baby.

Before going home the mother is shown how to bath her baby, and is given an opportunity to do it herself under supervision, and to ask questions. On her return home the health visitor will call on her to offer advice or help. Many problems arise at home which cannot be visualized in hospital, and these can be solved for her. The husband has not played a prominent part during the stay in hospital, but now he becomes very important. The hospital nurse's concern has been to send home a confident mother and a healthy baby. The health visitor helps to ensure that they settle without difficulty into the home environment and begin a happy life as a family.

CHAPTER 22

THORACIC SURGICAL NURSING

THE lungs are kept in contact with the chest wall and diaphragm by the fact that there is a negative pressure in the pleural cavity that surrounds each lung. As the rib cage expands and the diaphragm descends during inspiration, the lungs are stretched, pressure within them falls, and air is drawn in along the trachea. In order to operate on the lungs or heart, the thoracic surgeon must open one or sometimes both pleural cavities, and as he does so the lung would collapse against its root if the anæsthetist did not inflate it through an endotracheal tube. Were he to close the chest wall as his colleague does the abdomen, the lung would remain collapsed and infection would inevitably follow. Provision for re-expansion must be made, and this is done by inserting into the chest a drainage tube of which the distal end passes under water, to prevent air entering the pleural cavity along it. This is called closed or waterseal drainage, and the nurse in the thoracic ward must understand its purpose, management and dangers.

At the close of the operation, the surgeon puts one end of the tube into the base of the pleural cavity, secures it with a stitch, and passes round it a suture which can be tied when the tube is removed in order to close the hole. The tube is attached by means of a wide-bore plastic connection and rubber tubing to a jar (illustrated) which is sterilized and contains sterile water or saline. The long tube in the bung (to which the closed drainage is attached) has its end 1 in. below the water level. The short tube acts as an air outlet (Fig. 68).

As the patient breathes in, the pressure in his chest and his drainage tube falls, and the water level rises ; as he breathes out it falls. As he is returned to the ward, the jar is carried by a nurse who keeps it below the chest level in order to prevent the water being drawn into the chest, and when he is in bed the jar is placed on the floor beside him. Blood-stained serum will escape into the jar as it drains away from the operation site.

Each time the patient coughs or breathes deeply a little air is expelled along the tube, and as air cannot enter, the lung expands a little to fill the vacant space. If the pleural cavity is uninfected and movement and coughing is encouraged after operation, the lung will be fully expanded in twenty-four to seventy-two hours, as will be shown by an X-ray and the fact that the water level in the glass tube is stationary. When expansion has occurred and the air leak is stopped, the tube is removed, and the stitch at once tied by an assistant to close the wound, and an occlusive dressing applied.

While closed drainage is in operation, these points are vital :

1. The jar must never be raised above the chest level ; ward cleaners must be told never to pick it up.

2. The bung must not be taken out of the bottle without first clipping the tube, or air will enter the chest. The jar is emptied twice daily, and

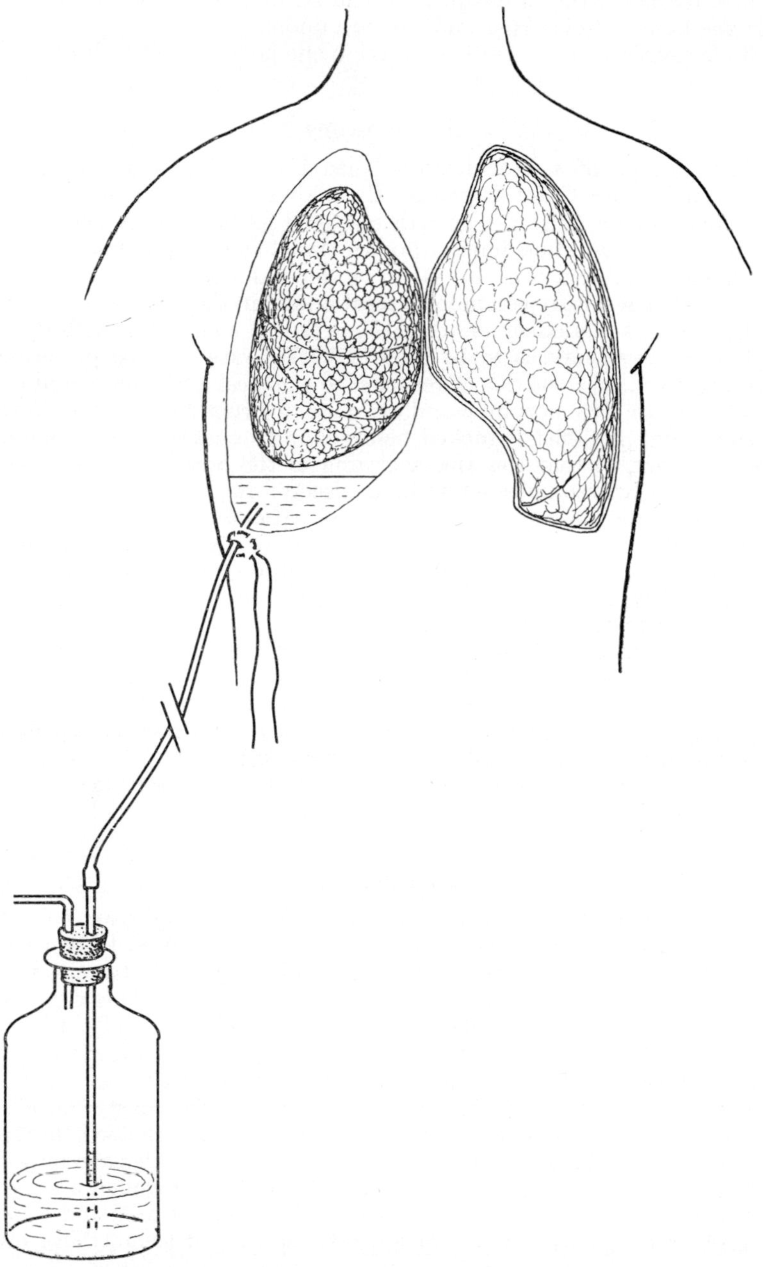

FIG. 68. Closed drainage of the pleural cavity.

when this is done a clip is applied; the bung is removed and placed in a sterile receiver; the drainage is measured and fresh sterile fluid put in; the bung is re-inserted and the clip undone.

3. Disinfectant must never be used in the jar in case it is drawn into the chest.

Bronchoscopy

The passage of a bronchoscope into the trachea and bronchi is performed mainly to aid diagnosis ; the main air passages can be inspected, and specimens from a growth removed for section, or pus can be aspirated. In addition foreign bodies that have been inhaled can be removed. Children will be given a general anæsthetic, and it is becoming increasingly common to treat adults in the same way because of the alarm and anxiety many patients feel in connection with it.

If local anæsthesia is to be used, a barbiturate may be prescribed overnight to lessen the risk of reaction to the local anæsthetic, and it is customary to give morphine and atropine or drugs similar in action as preparation. A tablet is sucked beforehand to anæsthetize the mouth and pharynx, so that the anæsthetizing of the larynx in the theatre can be rapidly accomplished without discomfort.

As the bronchoscope is passed, the patient's head is extended, and must be supported on a special rest, or by an assistant, over the end of the table. On return to the ward, the pulse and respiration are regularly observed, and any difficulty in breathing or stridor is reported to the surgeon at once. Fluids must not be given until feeling returns to the mouth and throat, but mouth washes are appreciated as the mucous membrane is very dry. When sips of water are swallowed without difficulty, larger amounts can be given, and aspirin mucilage to relieve the sore throat. Those who have had a general anæsthetic receive the usual post-operative care.

Bronchoscopy is sometimes required as a therapeutic measure to remove retained secretions after operation.

Thoracoscopy

Inspection of the pleural cavity by a thoracoscope can only be accomplished if a pneumothorax (p. 469) exists. It used to be necessary when adhesions between the lung and chest wall prevented the successful collapse of the lung by artificial pneumothorax in the treatment of pulmonary tuberculosis. The obsolescence of this form of therapy has made thoracoscopy for this purpose correspondingly less common, but it may be performed to help diagnosis.

A trocar and cannula are introduced through the chest wall after infiltration with local anæsthetic, and the thoracoscope passed through the cannula. Adhesions are inspected and if not too extensive may be divided by the cautery, which is usually introduced through a second cannula. After thoracoscopy the patient is nursed at rest, and watch is kept on the pulse and respiration rates in case of hæmorrhage into the pleural cavity, which is the main complication to be feared. Escape of air into the subcutaneous tissues (surgical emphysema) may also occur.

Empyema

This term means pus in the pleural cavity, and is most commonly seen as a complication of pneumonia. During or after an attack of pneumonia the temperature rises, there is respiratory embarrassment, and an X-ray shows fluid in the chest. A few millilitres are withdrawn for examination and identification of the organism.

Successful treatment of pneumonia has considerably reduced the incidence of empyema, which is not now common. The appropriate antibiotic is given as soon as the condition is diagnosed, and each day the chest is aspirated and usually antibiotic is injected into the pleural cavity. With such treatment a proportion of patients can be cured without operation, but sometimes an abscess cavity remains that must be drained.

A portion of rib is resected at the bottom of the empyema (though this is not always needed in children), and a drainage tube inserted and closed with a water seal established as described above. All measures appropriate to the care of a patient with a septic focus are used, and energetic breathing, coughing and arm exercises are taught to expand the lung and close the abscess cavity as quickly as possible. Fairly soon the lung becomes adherent to the chest wall around the drainage tube, which may then be cut short near to the chest wall without fear of allowing the lung to collapse. This tube must not be removed without the surgeon's instructions, and the final stages of closing the track may be rather tedious, but if the general condition is well maintained and exercises conscientiously performed, healing should take place with a minimum of deformity.

Thoracoplasty

Thoracoplasty is an operation designed to allow the structures of the chest wall to collapse on to the lung after removal of sections of the ribs, and is a measure that will collapse a lung more selectively than artificial pneumothorax. The collapse is permanent, and is used for cavitation of the lung. It has shared in the eclipse of all methods of collapse therapy, but is still sometimes needed for extensive disease not suitable for resection.

Thoracoplasty is usually now performed under general anæsthesia, and portions of the upper ribs are removed first. Following it, the complication of paradoxical chest movement may occur, and must be watched for and prevented. As the patient breathes in, the chest expands on the sound side, but the part deprived of the support of the ribs is sucked inwards. As he breathes out, the operated part is blown outwards instead of sinking down and inwards like the rest of the chest. The consequence of this is that during inspiration air is drawn into the sound side not only from the trachea, but also from the opposite lung, and that when he breathes out, expired air passes across into the diseased side as well as out by the trachea. This to-and-fro movement of air from one lung to the other results in increasing oxygen lack, with dyspnœa, cyanosis, agitation and restlessness. The surgeon endeavours to prevent it by applying firm pressure with a pad and strapping to the operation site, and the nurse can help to stop it by pressure over the site when the patient coughs.

A second operation to remove further ribs may be required, and the large incision and alteration of the chest contour can cause considerable deformity unless physiotherapy is adequate.

Lobectomy

Removal of a lobe of lung is practised in the treatment of localized bronchiectasis, of certain new growths, and of tuberculosis. For this last condition, smaller amounts of tissue may be removed by segmental resection.

The preparation is related to the condition for which lobectomy is performed ; if bronchiectasis is the cause, as much sputum as possible should be removed by postural drainage, and reduced in quantity by antibiotics. If tuberculosis is present, isoniazid, P.A.S. and streptomycin are given, and in all cases the general condition is made as good as possible by a high protein diet.

After lobectomy, the anæsthetist expands the remaining parts of the lung as much as possible before the chest is closed, but it is usually necessary to institute closed drainage for a day or two. The basal drain is linked to the water seal, and since it is possible for the lung to expand sideways to meet the chest wall and leave some air trapped at the top of the pleural cavity, an apical drain is usually inserted and attached to a Robert's electric sucker. Oxygen is not usually needed after operation on young adults, but it is sometimes required for a few hours, when it is given by a plastic mask. Postural drainage to promote expectoration of sputum is necessary, and coughing and deep breathing is encouraged from the outset.

An X-ray of the chest is taken in the ward on the following day, and should show good expansion of the remaining lobes. The drains are taken out as soon as full expansion is reached and the air leak stopped, and the stitches tied to seal the openings. Patients may get up in a few days' time, unless bed rest has been prescribed for the tuberculous.

The main complication is broncho-pleural fistula which occasionally occurs. Bubbling occurs in the underwater tube, and the basal drain must be left in until the fistula closes.

A full recovery of function can be expected, and the result is due to the combined efforts of surgeon, nurses, physiotherapists and the patient.

Pneumonectomy

Excision of a lung is usually undertaken for carcinoma of bronchus, and since this disease has increased twenty-fold since the 1920's it is a common operation in thoracic units. Surgery offers at present the only hope of a cure, and in those cases which are not too advanced for operation when seen, the prognosis is fair. Since it seems right to presume that some new factor has been operating in the last thirty years or so to cause the calamitous rise in incidence, research has been undertaken to identify the cause, and it is now clear statistically that those who smoke cigarettes heavily for some years are much more likely to get a cancer of the lung than non-smokers. It is the duty of all health workers to make this known to young people. The figures cannot be denied, though not all pathologists place the same interpretation on them, and some think that smoking does not actually cause cancer, but determines the site at which it will appear.

Operation should be undertaken as soon as possible after diagnosis, and on admission the hæmoglobin and blood group are ascertained and the sputum investigated. Bronchial infection is cleared as far as possible by antibiotics, and breathing exercises are taught to increase the vital capacity and encourage chest movement after operation.

The patient returns from the theatre in his bed with oxygen and a blood transfusion running. The space from which the lung has been removed must fill gradually, and not be completely drained so that the heart and great vessels are drawn over into the empty space, or heart failure will result. Closed drainage may be set up in the theatre and a clip kept on the tube which is released for ten seconds hourly so that blood-stained serum may be drained into the bottle. Some surgeons close the chest completely, and rely on chest aspiration and air replacement if indicated. Fluid is not allowed to accumulate up to the level of the severed bronchus within the first few operative days.

Deep breathing and coughing is encouraged as soon as consciousness returns, and analgesics (such as pethidine) are given in sufficient quantity to allow this to be done without too much pain, but not to such an extent that breathing is depressed. Postural drainage may help expectoration, but if it is not effective, suction through a bronchoscope is performed. If the pericardium has been opened, the patient must not be allowed to lie on the operated side, or the heart may dislocate from the pericardial sac, and circulatory collapse will occur.

Venous thrombosis and pulmonary embolism are much-feared complications ; massage to the calves is given regularly from the time of the return from the theatre. It is customary to get the patient up on the second day to avert such troubles. The transfusion is stopped as soon as fluid loss has been made good and the patient can drink, for fear of overloading the heart. Chest X-rays are taken regularly and antibiotics are continued as long as is necessary.

Rehabilitation by exercises and occupational therapy is an important part of the treatment and after convalescence a gradual return to normal life begins. Heavy manual labour will not again be possible for older patients, but ordinary activity is.

OPERATIONS ON THE HEART AND GREAT VESSELS

One of the less rare forms of congenital heart conditions is the persistence after birth of the ductus arteriosus which in fœtal life passes the blood which the unexpanded lungs do not need from the pulmonary artery to the aorta. A persistent ductus arteriosus leads eventually to heart failure and bacterial endocarditis, and it is desirable to close it during childhood before these complications can occur. This was one of the earliest operations designed to affect the heart, and it is usually a simple and safe one. A basal closed drain is inserted and managed as described previously, and in young patients complications are rare.

Following this, the operations of Blalock and Potts came into use for " blue babies " with Fallot's tetralogy, in whom the ventricular septum is deficient, the aorta arises from both ventricles and the pulmonary artery is stenosed. The mixing of the arterial and venous blood in the heart could not at that time be corrected, but the blood supply to the lungs was improved by joining one of the great systemic vessels (aorta or subclavian artery) to the pulmonary artery.

It was then found practicable to introduce a finger into the heart, and an instrument alongside it, and so acquired heart lesions came within the scope of surgery and stenosed mitral valves could be dilated. Finally, the introduction of hypothermia (described below) and the heart-lung machine have enabled the heart's action to be interrupted without damaging the brain, so that open cardiac operations can be performed, and lesions such as septal defects can be repaired, or valves replaced. The artificial valve most commonly used is the Starr-Edwards valve, a ball and cage pattern (Fig. 69).

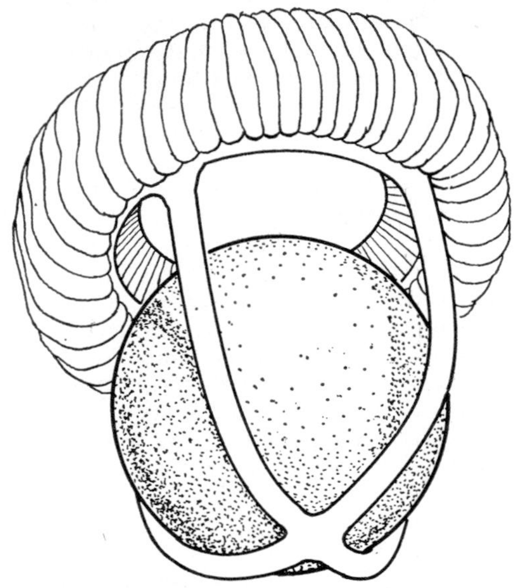

FIG. 69. The Starr-Edwards mitral valve prosthesis.

Thorough investigation of the lesion, the heart capacity and the general condition is made beforehand. X-rays, electrocardiogram, erythrocyte sedimentation rate, hæmoglobin, blood grouping, cardiac catheterization and sputum investigation give the required information. If there is any heart failure, a low salt low fluid diet and diuretics are given, and even if the pulse is regular a full course of digitalis is given so that when atrial fibrillation occurs the ventricular rate will be controlled. When the surgeon has decided that operation is possible he discusses it fully with the patient, and presents the alternatives to him, since the operation is too serious to be undertaken without the confident co-operation of the patient.

Breathing exercises are thoroughly taught and practised beforehand, but no unusual pre-operative measures are required except the medical treatment described above. The patient returns from the theatre in his bed receiving oxygen and with a slow intravenous infusion of dextrose saline or blood. Closed drainage of at least one pleural cavity will be necessary and if both have been opened there will be two basal drains. The blood pressure is taken every half-hour and the pulse every fifteen minutes until satisfactory, and examination is made of the limb movements and of the pupils in case cerebral embolism has occurred from blood clot in the heart. Papaverine is given by intramuscular injection, if there is any paralysis, to dilate the cerebral arteries.

Morphine or pethidine is given to allay anxiety and to enable coughing to take place without too much pain. Fluids by mouth can be given when consciousness returns, and the intravenous fluids are stopped. A low salt diet is resumed as soon as the patient can take it.

Leg massage, deep breathing and arm movements are practised to avoid thrombosis, and fever, pain in the chest or bloodstained sputum should be watched for and reported at once. Anticoagulants can be administered without too much risk of bleeding, but the prothrombin level should not fall below 20%. The stitches are removed on the eighth day, and continued vigilance should be exerted against thrombosis and embolism throughout the next week.

The amount of activity and the time of getting up will be decided by the heart capacity. It may be necessary to return the patient to a medical ward for further rest before discharge, or the surgeon and nurses may have the pleasure of seeing a patient who had led a severely restricted life beginning to return to activity.

HYPOTHERMIA

At normal body temperature the cerebral cells are unable to survive for more than three minutes if the circulation is interrupted, since they are very sensitive to oxygen lack ; but the oxygen needs of the brain decrease as its temperature falls until at 30° C. (86° F.), the circulation may be stopped for ten minutes without causing irreversible damage. The application of this principle to heart surgery has been of immense importance, since ten minutes allows time to open the heart and repair defects in the atrial septum. An account of the use of hypothermia in the ward in connection with head injuries is given on p. 393.

The stages in the employment of hypothermia in the theatre are as follows :

1. **Premedication.** A conscious patient will endeavour to neutralize the effects of cooling by shivering, and sedation is given (usually by chlorpromazine, pethidine and phenergan) that will enable anæsthesia to be conducted at a desirably light level without the risk of shivering.

2. **Anæsthesia.** Induction is begun with thiopentone and curare, a cuffed endotracheal tube is passed and a light anæsthetic given through it.

3. **Records.** Preparations are now made for the continuous observations of the temperature, heart action and blood pressure that are so important. Indwelling electrically-recording thermometers are placed in the rectum ; the œsophagus (via the mouth) to indicate the temperature in the chest ; the pharynx (via the nose) to register the tempera-

ture as near the brain as possible. Leads for an electrocardiogram are attached, likewise a cuff for the sphygmomanometer and the diathermy leads. An intravenous infusion is begun, which can be changed to blood when the necessity arises.

It will be seen that good team work is essential if confusion is to be avoided when so many workers are engaged.

4. **Cooling.** The body temperature may be lowered by cooling either the skin or the blood.

(*a*) *Surface Cooling.* The patient is stripped except for a loin cloth, and such methods adopted for cooling the skin as immersing him in a cool bath ; laying him on a water-cooled mattress covered with a second one ; applying ice bags to the trunk and limbs ; or using a fan. The skin must be carefully observed, especially if ice bags are used, to forestall frostbite. Pallor or cyanosis is a dangerous sign.

Surface cooling is time consuming (it may take two hours in an adult) but comparatively safe. It is a wise precaution, however, to have an operation set ready and a surgeon in gloves in case of cardiac arrest so that the heart may be massaged or the defibrillator applied.

(*b*) *Blood-stream Cooling.* Blood is led from a vessel, e.g. the superior vena cava, pumped through a cooling unit, and returned to another vessel, usually the inferior vena cava. It is a quicker method, but entails an increased incidence of ventricular fibrillation.

Cooling is therefore usually stopped at 32° C., and re-warming at 34° C.

Deep Hypothermia

Blood is taken from the left atrium, cooled through a heat exchanger, and pumped back to a systemic artery. By the time the heart has cooled to 30° C., and the beat is failing, blood is taken from the right atrium, and pumped back to the pulmonary artery via the right ventricle. This is in effect extracorporeal circulation, using the patient's own lungs as an oxygenator. When the temperature has reached 15° C. or lower, the pumps are stopped, and operation carried out on the cold, still, empty heart. At the end of the operation the heart is closed and the process reversed. Blood is pumped through a warming heat exchanger until the heart beats again, when the tubes in the right heart are removed. The warming is continued to about 35° C., when the left side tubes are removed.

When the septa are intact, or have been repaired, and the heart is paralysed, blood from the bronchial circulation returning to the left side cannot escape, and unless it is removed by a vent-tube, the heart will distend and be permanently damaged.

Extracorporeal Circulation

If an operation on the heart cannot with certainty be concluded in ten minutes, it cannot safely be performed under orthodox hypothermia, and a means other than the heart must be found of circulating the blood. This involves passing it outside the body through a pump-oxygenator which will take over the functions of the heart and lungs while the heart is opened and repaired. By means of such a "heart lung" machine defects of the ventricular septum, stenosis of the aortic valve and Fallot's tetralogy are susceptible to surgery.

The principle of all those in use at the moment is similar. Blood is drained by gravity into the machine, oxygenated, and pumped back into a systemic artery. The machine must be primed with about 6 pints of blood before it can be brought into use, and the amount needed for perfusing an adult may be 16 pints. There are several means by which blood can be oxygenated, and disposable plastic bubble oxygenators are being increasingly used. These can be primed with 5% glucose or Hartmann's solution.

When the by-pass machine is to be brought into action the right atrium or venæ cavæ are intubated, and the blood led into the machine. From the oxygenator it is returned to an artery, usually the femoral. Suction is used to return the blood from the coronary and bronchial circulations to the machine. There is a reservoir from which additional blood can be fed into the circulation when any is lost during operation. The blood must be heparinized to avoid clotting, and the heparin inactivated with protamine at the close of operation.

The physiological problems involved are of great complexity. The rate of blood flow must approach that of the output of the resting heart; the blood must be returned to the body at the same rate as it is withdrawn; blood pressure must be maintained; oxygen saturation must be adequate; the blood pH must be within normal limits; the heart action must be watched on a continuously recorded electrocardiogram; infection, thrombosis and air embolism must be averted. In addition to all these the anæsthetic and surgical difficulties that may be present at any operation may arise. Not infrequently it is necessary to perform a tracheostomy, using a positive-pressure ventilator, as described on p. 323.

Cardiac pacemakers. In heart-block, the impulse from the sinuatrial node fails to reach the ventricles which contract at an independent and very slow rate. This rate can be raised by means of a pacemaker. If the block is thought to be temporary, the electrodes are placed over the right ventricle, and the pacemaker is kept on the locker. Where the block seems likely to persist, and the circulation is inadequate, a pacemaker is implanted in the axilla, or in the abdominal wall, with electrodes either passed via a vein into the right ventricle, or attached to the surface of the heart.

Recovery Room

Patients who have undergone cardiac surgery require observation and treatment in a special recovery room. The temperature (skin and rectal), pulse, arterial and central venous blood pressure, respiration rate and colour are recorded every 15 minutes. A complete progressive fluid balance chart is kept. A continuously recording electrocardiograph checks the heart rhythm, and if heart block causes a slow ventricular rate an artificial pacemaker must be used.

Cardiac arrest. If it is suspected that the heart has stopped, as shown by cessation of the pulses and change in the electrocardiograph, resuscitation must be carried out within two minutes. The surgeon must be informed at once and the sterile pack of instruments for thoracotomy opened. The circulation is restored by cardiac massage, and it may be necessary to defibrillate the heart before a normal beat can be established. Such drugs as 5 ml. of 10% calcium chloride or 5–10 ml. of 1 in. 10,000 adrenalin may be injected into the ventricle to improve or restore the beat

CHAPTER 23

EAR, NOSE AND THROAT NURSING

THESE three structures are related to each other not only anatomically but also in their pathology. Infections of the middle ear, for instance, usually come from the naso-pharynx via the Eustachian tube, and nasal infections spread readily into the accessory nasal sinuses or down into the larynx and trachea. The nose and throat lie at the entrance to the respiratory and digestive tracts, which are protected by the abundant lymphoid tissue there, and the oro-pharynx is common to both tracts, so that the reflexes of swallowing and breathing are closely related to each other.

In order to understand some of the operations performed on the ear, it is necessary to recall a few facts of elementary anatomy. The external auditory meatus is the canal leading into the ear. It is a curved tube, closed at its inner end by the tympanic membrane, which separates the meatus from the middle ear. This chamber is a narrow cleft only 2–4 mms. from the tympanic membrane to its medial wall, and 15 mms.

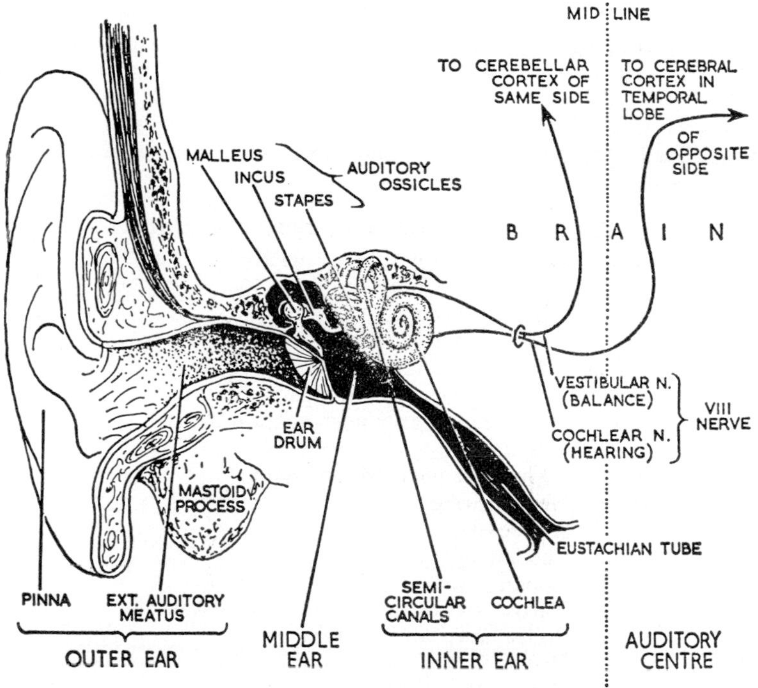

FIG. 70.

in its other dimensions. Three small bones (ossicles) are strung across it; the lateral one (malleus) is attached to the tympanic membrane; the middle one is the incus; the medial one (stapes) has a foot piece resting in an opening, the oval window, in the lateral wall. The movements of stapes are transmitted through the oval window to the fluid in the internal ear in which are the endings of the auditory nerve (Fig. 70).

Below the oval window is the round window; the membrane closing it vibrates in unison with the movements of stapes. The middle ear is air-filled, being connected with the naso-pharynx by the Eustachian (pharyngo-tympanic) tube. Behind the middle ear and opening into it are the air cells that fill the mastoid process of the temporal bone. The facial nerve supplying the muscles of the face can be seen running above the oval window.

The middle ear is so small that operations on it are performed with the help of the operating microscope.

The internal ear consists of two parts, both of which are supplied by the eighth (auditory) nerve. The semi-circular canals are concerned with balance, the cochlea with hearing. Conditions that affect the internal ear may therefore cause giddinesss (vertigo) or loss of hearing.

Loss of Hearing

Hearing is diminished or lost in these circumstances.

1. The external meatus is blocked with wax.

2. The tympanic membrane cannot vibrate because air cannot enter the middle ear due to obstruction in the Eustachian tube. Large perforations of the tympanic membrane will also stop its vibration.

3. The ossicles may fail to vibrate e.g. because of infection in the middle ear. Another important cause of deafness is overgrowth of bone around the foot plate of the stapes (otosclerosis), a disease which often affects quite young people, and for which several operations have been devised.

Examination of the Ear, Nose and Throat

Requirements. Large instrument tray with :

- Aural specula.
- Aural forceps.
- Wool carrier or applicators.
- Nasal speculum.
- Nasal dressing forceps.
- Laryngeal and post-nasal mirrors.
- Spatula.
- Gallipot with Staché wool.

Head mirror.
Auriscope.
Cocaine spray.
Tongue cloths.
Throat swabs, labels and request cards.
Spirit lamp and matches.
Receivers for swabs and used instruments.
Bowl for dentures.
Paper towels and gauze swabs.

A head mirror reflects the light from behind the patient into the nose and mouth, and is a necessity for all but the most superficial treatment. The patient should be asked to remove any dentures before examination, and sits facing the surgeon, who usually begins by looking at the throat. He asks the patient to open the mouth and breathe steadily, while a spatula is placed on the tongue, and the tonsils and oro-pharynx examined and perhaps a swab taken. The nasal cavity is next inspected with the aid of a speculum, and were all nurses able to see the interior and its intricate architecture they would treat it with more respect and understanding when passing catheters and tubes through it. The ear is examined through the auriscope, which gives a magnified and illuminated view of the ear drum. It is not always necessary to inspect the larynx or the post-nasal spaces, but if it is, the mucous membrane is sprayed with cocaine and the mirrors warmed over the spirit lamp before use.

Cocaine is a Dangerous Drug and must be handled with the appropriate precautions. It is more used in this department than in any other, and the victims of addiction not infrequently come here in the hope of obtaining supplies. Only the smallest quantities should be put into sprays, and patients must not be left alone with a trolley with cocaine on it.

Syringing the Ear

Requirements. Instrument tray with :

- Aural syringe.
- Aural specula.
- Aural forceps.
- Wooden wool carriers, dressed.
- Wax hook.

Head mirror.
Lotion thermometer.
Jug of lotion at 100° F. (38° C.).
Kidney dish.
Staché wool.
Mackintosh or cape and towel.

The lotion used can be normal saline, sodium bicarbonate 1 drachm to a pint, or plain warm water. The temperature of the lotion is important, because the introduction of fluid into the ear at a temperature much different from that of the body will set up convection currents in the semi-circular canals and cause intense giddiness and vomiting. The temperature that matters is that of the lotion given, so the syringe must be well warmed by drawing lotion in and expelling it again several times until it no longer feels cold to the hand. The size of the syringe should be convenient to the operator, since the use of a syringe too large for the hand causes lack of control. Syringing should not be undertaken by a nurse without a doctor's instruction, since syringing can be very dangerous if an acute perforation of the eardrum is present.

The patient should sit up for this procedure in a chair which supports the back ; his clothes are protected and he may hold the kidney dish himself to catch the lotion, making sure that there is firm contact

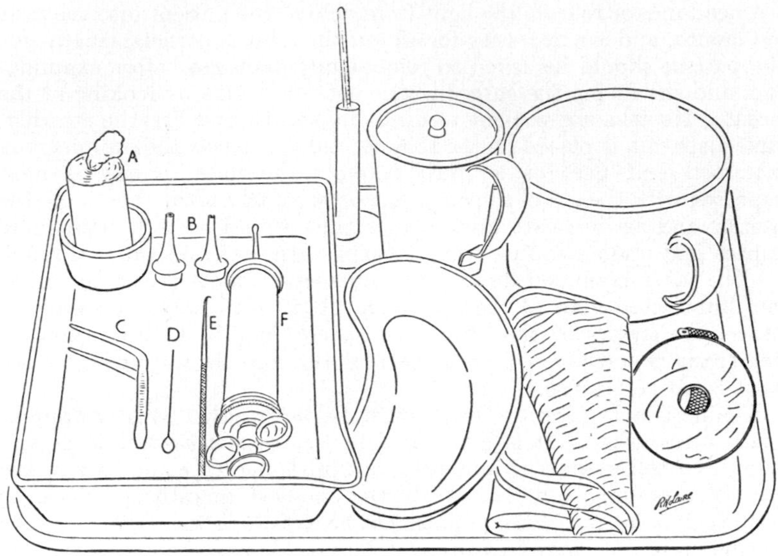

FIG. 71. Tray for syringing the ear.

A. Staché wool.
B. Aural specula.
C. Aural forceps.
D. Wire wool carrier.
E. Wax hook.
F. Aural syringe.

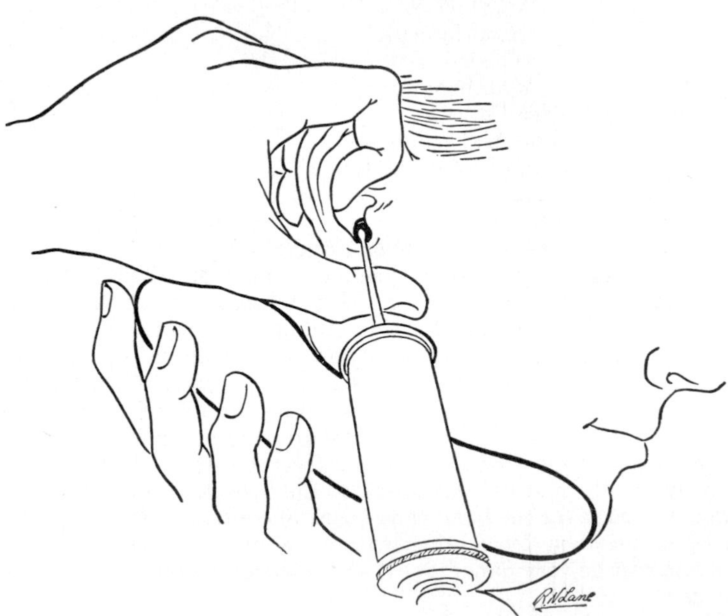

FIG. 72. Syringing the ear. Showing the method of retracting the pinna and steadying the syringe. The lotion is being directed along the upper wall of the meatus.

between the margin of the dish and the skin. The head is tilted slightly away from the operator. The nurse fills her syringe from the jug, puts on the nozzle, and holds the syringe upright while expelling the air ; the upright position ensures that all air is got rid of, and that no water remains in the barrel beyond the piston. If the right ear is the affected one, she takes the upper margin of the pinna firmly but gently between the first and second fingers of the left hand, draws it slightly upwards and backwards to straighten the meatus, and steadies the syringe against her thumb. She thus has complete control of the syringe, and no unguarded movement of the patient can allow damage to the ear drum. She directs a steady stream of lotion against the upper border of the meatus, and the fluid flows out along the floor of the passage into the receiver, carrying with it any accumulations of wax. Two more syringefuls of fluid may be used if the first is ineffective. Finally the ear is well dried internally with wool and externally with a towel.

Nurses are normally only asked to syringe ears to remove wax, though the doctor may use this method to extract foreign bodies. If the syringing is ineffective, ear drops of sodium bicarbonate may be used at home to soften the wax before the procedure is repeated.

Ear Drops

Drops must be warm when they are inserted, or they are highly uncomfortable ; if they are being used in small quantities it suffices to rinse the dropper in boiling water and draw the drops up while it is hot. The patient lies on the unaffected side, with the chin higher than the vertex. Sodium bicarbonate 6% is recommended for loosening wax, or cerumol can be used twice daily for three days. Oil is not much liked today because it melts the wax and allows it to run further into the meatus.

NURSING OF SOME EAR CONDITIONS

Boils in the External Meatus

Boils in this situation are very painful because the skin is closely adherent to the underlying cartilage, and there is no room for swelling, and boils may occur here in series. The skin of the meatus should be wiped with Vaseline Brand Petroleum Jelly, and then a gauze wick dipped in magnesium sulphate paste inserted. When the boil has healed the meatus may be painted with gentian violet 2½% in water to prevent recurrence.

Otitis Media

Acute inflammation of the middle ear usually follows naso-pharyngeal infection which has ascended the Eustachian tube. If the drum has not perforated, glycerine and phenol ear drops may be ordered ; if it has, a swab should be taken of the discharge, and the appropriate antibiotic ordered. If the drum is bulging, incision (*myringotomy*) may be undertaken under a general anæsthetic, and the patient nursed after operation on the affected side to promote drainage. Dry mopping of the meatus is practised until the incision heals. The commonest acute complication is extension of the infection into the mastoid process, and

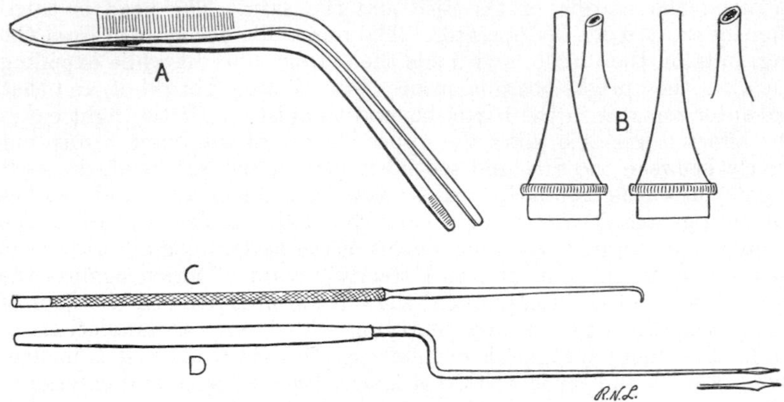

FIG. 73. Some aural instruments.
A. Aural forceps. C. Wax hook.
B. Aural specula of two different sizes. D. Myringotome.

continued fever, mastoid tenderness and swelling behind the pinna are indications for operation.

Simple incision is now less commonly performed than the insertion of a plastic ventilating tube into the tympanic membrane. This admits air into the middle ear if the Eustachian tube is inadequate, and allows secretion to drain slowly away down the tube. The presence of the tube does not affect hearing, and it can be left in place for long periods. Chronic otitis media is common, and perseverance is needed in its treatment. Regular aural toilet to remove débris and discharge and the use of antiseptic powders such as boric and iodoform are generally used. Cessation of discharge, if accompanied by giddiness, headache or nystagmus, is an unfavourable sign and should be reported to the surgeon.

Mastoiditis

Infection of the mastoid process from the middle ear requires surgical treatment, since, if unchecked, it may lead to extradura abscess, meningitis, cerebellar abscess, or thrombosis of the lateral sinus which lies close to the mastoid. Pre-operative preparation of the area (taking care that the correct side has been chosen) is to comb the hair well back from the ear, and shave an area 2 in. wide behind it.

The Schwartze operation is most used for mastoiditis following acute middle ear disease in children, and the incision is a post-auricular one. The face is carefully examined after operation in case damage to the facial nerve has occurred, and the patient is nursed sitting up, turned towards the affected side. Giddiness is common on the first day, and the child will usually have to be fed, while codeine mixture or nepenthe is given for pain. The clips are removed after forty-eight hours, and the dressing is performed daily. The drain is removed between the second and fifth days, when discharge has ceased. Gentle syringing, with an aseptic technique, may be ordered to remove blood and pus. Once the temperature is normal the child may get up, and goes home when the ear is clean and dry. Headache, giddiness, vomiting or rigor should be promptly reported.

Radical mastoidectomy involves opening the middle ear and mastoid cavity into each other, and unlike the previous operation will entail impairment of hearing. It is only needed if long-continued infection of the middle ear has existed. Lining the cavity with Thiersch grafts is often practised to hasten healing, and if this is the surgeon's custom, the skin of the thigh should be shaved and cleaned to act as the donor area. An antiseptic pack (e.g. BIP paste) is put in, and is removed under an anæsthetic a week later, when the clips are also taken out. The cavity is repacked weekly under anæsthesia. The most usual approach to this operation now is endaural, i.e. through the meatus, but the nursing involved is similar wherever the incision is placed.

Ear bandages must be firm enough to retain the dressings in place without slipping, but not tight enough to cause headache or damage the skin of the forehead. Crêpe bandages are the most comfortable, and a piece of tape beneath the forehead turns will help to keep the eye unobstructed.

Treatment of Otosclerosis

Otosclerosis has been mentioned as a cause of deafness in young adults. The footplate of the stapes is imprisoned by overgrowth of bone and can no longer by its movements stimulate the internal ear. Several operations have been practised, but the one currently in use is to remove the stapes (stapedectomy) and insert a prosthesis to replace it. The results are very good, 90% of patients regain normal hearing.

The nursing of patients after this operation presents no special difficulties. The vertigo that used to be so troublesome after earlier types of operation is uncommon, but patients should be assisted when they first get up. The physiotherapist may give re-education in balance if giddiness persists, and dramamine 50 mg. is helpful.

NURSING SOME CONDITIONS OF THE NOSE

The common cold is a virus infection of which the symptoms are too well known to merit description, prevalent in cool, wet climates, especially in winter. In spite of much research, no cure has yet been found, and treatment is confined to alleviating the symptoms and preventing extension of the infection to the bronchi or the paranasal sinuses. It is wise in the acute stages to remain in a warm room at an even temperature, which makes the condition more tolerable and prevents the infection of colleagues, but this is a course of perfection that cannot always be followed. A copious fluid intake, aspirin, throat lozenges and the use of paper handkerchiefs can be recommended, and if bronchitis shows signs of developing, the treatment described on p. 211 is instituted.

Sinusitis

Infection may spread into any of the sinuses, but the one most usually involved is the maxillary antrum which is the largest. Fever,

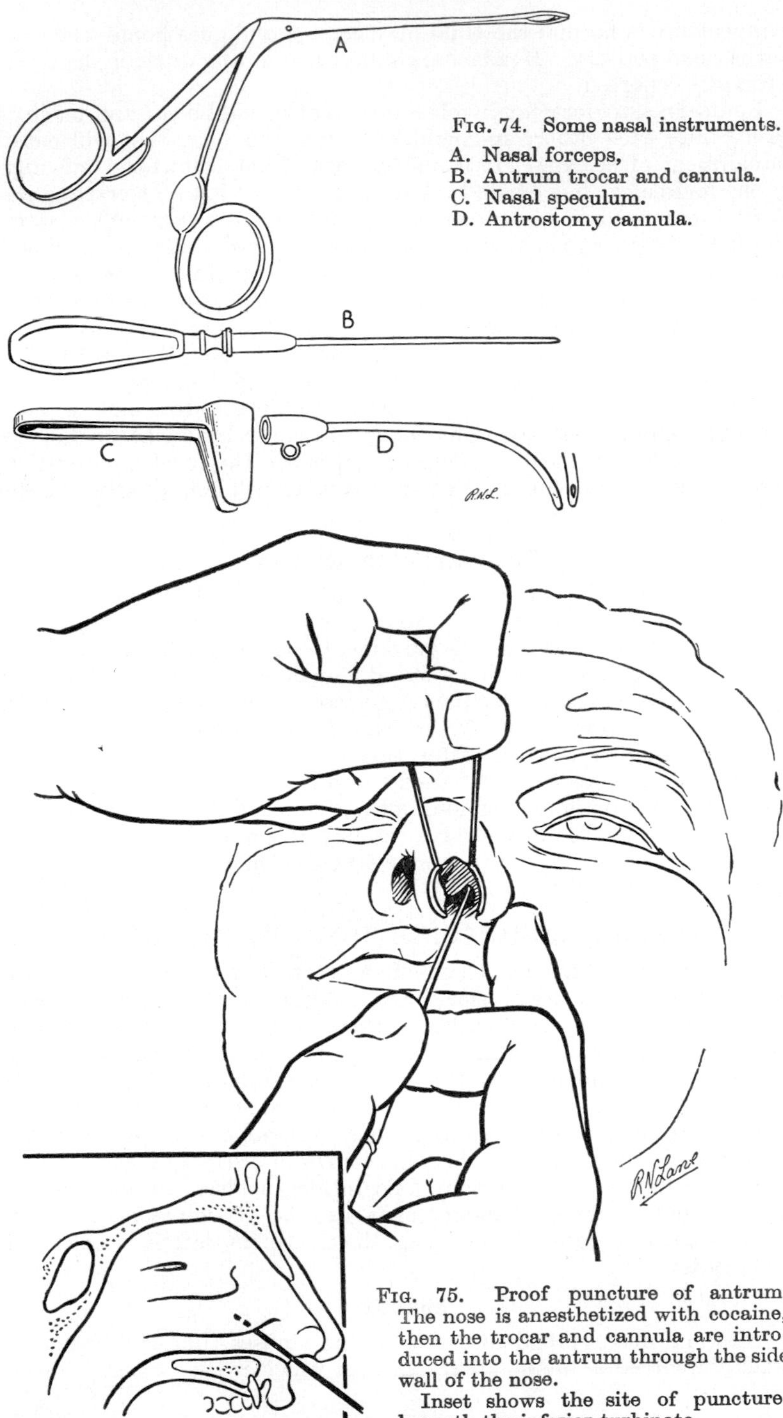

FIG. 74. Some nasal instruments.

A. Nasal forceps,
B. Antrum trocar and cannula.
C. Nasal speculum.
D. Antrostomy cannula.

FIG. 75. Proof puncture of antrum. The nose is anæsthetized with cocaine, then the trocar and cannula are introduced into the antrum through the side wall of the nose.

Inset shows the site of puncture, beneath the inferior turbinate.

pain in the face and purulent nasal discharge indicate its onset, and treatment must be vigorous if chronic infection is to be averted. The patient is kept in bed in a warm room and a nasal swab is taken to identify the organism and the appropriate antibiotic. Steam inhalations are important, analgesics will be necessary for pain, and ephedrine nasal drops may shrink the mucosa and open up the normal drainage channel. The patient should be nursed in a sitting position to avoid the spread of infection to the middle ear. If this treatment does not prove effective, puncture and washout of the antrum will be necessary.

Proof Puncture of Antrum

Requirements. Cocaine spray.
Dressed flexible wire wool carriers.
Cocaine 10%.
Sterile { Lichwitz trocar and cannula.
Nasal speculum.
Nasal forceps.
Sponge-holding forceps. }
Jug of normal saline, sterile.
Lotion thermometer.
Black kidney dish and Higginson's syringe with adaptor.
Staché wool.
Test tubes for specimens.
Receivers for used instruments and for swabs.
Gauze swabs or paper handkerchiefs.
Mackintosh apron.

The procedure is often performed in out-patient departments, and a local anæsthetic is used for adults. The patient sits facing the surgeon, wearing a mackintosh apron to protect the clothes, and after preliminary inspection of the nose, the surgeon inserts a wool-carrier soaked in cocaine into the nose, and leaves if there for ten minutes until the nose is anæsthetized. Watch must be kept for pallor or faintness at this stage.

When the nose is insensitive, the patient is asked to hold the kidney dish, and is told that there will be no pain, though pressure will be felt. The nurse fills the syringe with saline at 100° F. (38° C.), and the surgeon inserts the trocar and cannula, via the nose, into the antrum by puncturing its anterior bony wall, withdraws the trocar and attaches the Higginson's syringe to the cannula. The patient holds the kidney dish at chest level and inclines the head forward so that, as the surgeon fills the antrum, the lotion may run out of the opening of the antrum, through the nose, into the dish, carrying with it the pus and mucus from the antrum. The cannula is withdrawn, the nose dried, and the patient given a swab or tissue in case a little bleeding follows. A portion of mucopus is put in a test tube with sponge holding forceps and sent for examination. Antrum puncture is a trying and unpleasant, if not a painful, experience, and a rest is indicated until the patient feels well enough to leave the department.

Puncture frequently has to be repeated, and if after six weeks the antrum is not clear, antrostomy via the nose will usually be performed. Daily toilet of the nose with nasal forceps and normal saline is done, and a week later the antrum is washed out.

If this treatment is unsuccessful, a Caldwell-Luc antrostomy is usual. The antrum is entered above the teeth under the upper lip, the antrum curetted and an opening made into the nose to allow free drainage. Through this opening washouts can be performed, using an antrostomy cannula and a Higginson's syringe.

Nasal Drops

Drops for the nose, as for the ear, should be warm. The patient should lie with the chin higher than the vertex, and should breathe in and out through the mouth while they are being given, to prevent draining them into the air passages. Ephedrine is often used to shrink inflamed mucous membrane, and liquid paraffin is useful for crusting.

If it is desired to irrigate the nose, the easiest and safest way is to teach the patient how to sniff an alkaline solution into the nose and spit it out.

Ephedrine Replacement

The object of this procedure is to withdraw air from the sinuses and replace it with lotion (usually ½% ephedrine in normal saline) to shrink the mucous membrane and wash out infected material. A glass syringe with a tip to fit the nostril and a rubber bulb for filling is used. Some patients can be taught to perform this for themselves, but it must be carefully demonstrated to them, as it is most alarming if any of the lotion is inhaled.

Requirements. 1 oz. of warm lotion.
Syringe.
Mackintosh and cover.
Receiver.
Paper handkerchiefs.

Method. The patient lies on her back on a couch, with the head over the end so that the chin is vertically over the ear, and a mackintosh and towel over the chest. She is asked to breathe steadily through the mouth all the time, and on no account to bring the head forward; the eyes should be closed. The nurse then draws the lotion into the syringe, up to the 10-ml. mark, and holding it vertically by the glass part, drops the fluid slowly into the nose, distributing it equally between the two sides. With the bulb compressed, the nozzle is introduced into one nostril so that it fits closely, the opposite nostril is occluded, and the patient is asked to swallow, or to repeat " kik-kik-kik " while the bulb is allowed gently to expand and exert suction on the nostril. This is repeated three times for each nostril, and the patient then rolls over (without sitting up) and allows excess fluid to drain from the nose.

Epistaxis

Bleeding from the nose is very common, and minor degrees are treated by sitting the patient at a sink with a few swabs in cold water.

She must keep her head forward to allow the blood to run out and may keep a cold swab pressed to the nose. The classical rustic cure of applying a door key to the back of the neck indicates that no very active therapy is needed in most cases, but patients frequently arrive in the casualty department with more severe bleeding for which treatment is needed. The patient should be seated, a cork is put between the teeth at the side of the mouth to encourage mouth breathing and prevent swallowing of blood, and she leans over a bowl. A strand of wool is teased out and inserted into each nostril with the ends protruding. If this does not stop the bleeding, cauterization of the area with silver nitrate, chromic acid or an electric cautery is usually resorted to next. Alternatively the nose may be packed with BIPP gauze, of which about a yard of 1-in. ribbon gauze will be required. Some surgeons like to use a finger stall, tied firmly over the eye end of a catheter and inflated. If these measures fail a post-nasal pack must be inserted. A catheter is passed along the nose into the naso-pharynx, the patient is asked to open the mouth, and the catheter is caught with sponge-holding forceps and drawn forward into the mouth. The pack is tied to the end of it, and traction on the part still protruding through the nostril will draw the pack up into the post-nasal space.

Nasal packs, if properly placed and secured, may slip down the pharynx and even block the air-way, and every precaution must be taken to see that this cannot occur. Unpleasant drying of the mouth occurs due to breathing through it, and mouth washes are appreciated.

Bleeding from the nose in patients who have sustained head injuries may indicate a fracture of the anterior part of the base of the skull, and toilet of the nose should be conducted with sterile forceps, wool and instruments.

Adenoidectomy

The lymphatic tissue in the nasopharynx may hypertrophy, and is removed by curetting. The operation is sometimes confined to this region, but frequently the tonsils are removed at the same time. The post-operative nursing is similar to that for tonsillectomy, and the patient, who is always a child, may go home on the third day.

Submucous Resection of the Septum

A grossly deviated nasal septum interferes with breathing, and is corrected surgically under local anæsthesia by raising a flap of mucous membrane and excising the crooked part. Healing without hæmatoma formation is the aim.

Most such patients are men, since they take part in sports that produce blows on the nose. Nasal toilet is performed, and it is best to shave off a moustache, though if this seems a hardship to the patient it may be vaselined flat. The operation is usually performed under a general anæsthetic given by endotracheal tube.

The patient will return to the ward with a splint or pack in each nostril to compress the membranous septum and prevent the formation of a hæmatoma. Lake's rubber splints are often used, or the finger of a glove packed with ribbon gauze. Whichever is used, the two are fastened together (over a swab, to prevent painful pressure) under the columella. This will prevent accidental inhalation of a pack or splint. The packs are removed after twenty-four hours, and daily nasal toilet begun, and if there is no fever or hæmatoma formation the patient may go home on the eighth day.

NURSING OF SOME THROAT CONDITIONS

Tonsillitis

Infection of the tonsils, usually by a streptococcus, is the commonest throat ailment, especially in the young who have yet to acquire immunity, and it should be promptly treated, since acute nephritis and rheumatic fever occasionally follow tonsillitis. The patient has a sore throat, fever, difficulty in swallowing, and usually the backache and headache often associated with any infection. On inspection, the fauces and tonsils are seen to be reddened and swollen.

A swab is usually taken to determine the organism. The doctor needs a spatula and a sterile swab, and the patient sits facing him in a good light. If the patient is too young to co-operate, a nurse should hold the child on her lap, or standing between her knees, with one arm round its chest and arms, and the other hand on its forehead, steadying its head against her chest. The patient is asked to breathe steadily and open the mouth widely, the tongue is depressed with a spatula, and the swab rubbed against each tonsil in turn.

The patient should stay in bed in a warm room. Aspirin mucilage will be ordered to enable him to drink freely, and hot gargles or mouth washes are comforting. If the tonsillar glands enlarge, kaolin poultice or a warm woollen wrapping round the neck will be useful. One of the sulpha drugs may be ordered, but unless the organism is a virulent one, antibiotics are not usually given except when the fever does not subside in three days.

A *quinsy* is a peritonsillar abscess and is an infrequent complication of tonsillitis. The temperature remains elevated, difficulty in swallowing and breathing is pronounced, and a swelling can be seen in the region of one tonsil. Penicillin is given, and is usually effective in relieving the pain and reducing the inflammation. Incision is only required in exceptional cases; it is an unpleasant procedure, and often fails to produce pus. The instrument used is a pair of quinsy forceps, which have sharpened points to enable them to penetrate easily, while the blades can be parted to widen the incision. A cocaine spray is used to produce local anæsthesia, and the operation is performed with the patient sitting upright.

Chronically inflamed or enlarged tonsils, or repeated attacks of acute tonsillitis are indications for tonsillectomy.

Tonsillectomy

Removal of the tonsils is most satisfactorily performed by dissecting them out, and securing any bleeding points with ligatures, if necessary. The tonsil guillotine, once widely used, is not now looked on with favour by most surgeons. The distal end of the guillotine is a metal ring, which is used to surround the tonsil, and a sharpened blade is then pressed home to amputate the tonsil. This leaves part of the tonsil behind, and causes free bleeding, and is an unsatisfactory operation. Some surgeons use it with a blunt blade, which when shut grips the tonsil and enables it to be twisted off. This is a better procedure, but not as satisfactory as dissection.

Preparation is confined to omitting a meal, and administering an atropine-type and a sedative drug. The anæsthetist inspects the mouth of a child to make sure that there are no loose milk teeth which might be knocked out during the course of the operation. The patient should be laid on the trolley on his side for transport back to the ward, and put into bed with a mackintosh and towel under the head and a vomit bowl against the cheek. The semi-prone position is maintained by putting a pillow against the back and flexing the upper leg further than the lower one. If the lower arm is drawn through behind the patient it will prevent him rolling on to his back while semiconscious, which might allow obstruction of the airway by the tongue or by blood.

Reactionary hæmorrhage must be guarded against, and the pulse should be taken every half hour, and watch kept for pallor and frequent swallowing. Vomiting a little altered blood is usual, but if the blood is bright or the pulse rate rising, the surgeon is informed. If he finds a large blood clot in the tonsillar fossa he may remove it with sponge-holding forceps, and this sometimes stops the bleeding, but if it does not, the patient is taken to the theatre and the pillars of fauces are stitched together over a pack.

Mouth washes can be given, but gargling must not be attempted after tonsillectomy. Aspirin will reduce the pain of swallowing, and on the day after operation taking solids must be encouraged. If it is found to be very painful, the patient may press his fingers into his ears while swallowing ; meals are apt to be rather lengthy, but pain in the throat will diminish much more rapidly if solids are taken than if the diet is fluid.

Children are discharged from many hospitals after forty-eight hours, with instructions to the mother to return if there is earache or bleeding. It is more satisfactory, if the bed situation allows, to retain them for six days until the sloughs have separated. A child having tonsillectomy is often paying his first visit to hospital, and if he only stays forty-eight hours he has no memories of hospital except of alarm, discomfort, and separation from his mother.

Tracheostomy

A tracheostomy is an opening into the trachea, through which air enters and leaves. It is a procedure being increasingly used in medical and surgical wards, and though sometimes it has to be permanent, in many cases the tracheostomy is temporary, and is closed before the patient leaves hospital. The chief indications for this operation are as follows:

1. Obstruction of the larynx by œdema ; by inflammation ; (diphtheria, once a common cause of obstruction, is now rare); by paralysis of the vocal cords; by carcinoma.

2. Pulmonary management of the unconscious patient (e.g. one with head injuries) or the paralysed (e.g. in poliomyelitis). Tracheostomy is often used in connection with a respirator to maintain intermittent positive pressure breathing.

3. Reduction of " dead space " in acute or chronic chest disease. In breathing, air must not only be moved in and out of the lungs, but in and out of the air passages, where no gaseous exchange takes place. Tracheostomy reduces the volume of air that must be shifted by shortening the distance to the lungs. It also makes the aspiration of copious or viscid secretion easy.

4. Preparation for thoracic, throat and neurosurgical operations.

Occasionally this operation has to be undertaken urgently, and local anæsthesia may have to be used, but more often it is planned in advance and it is possible to pass an endotracheal catheter and give a general anæsthetic. If the patient is well enough, the operation should be

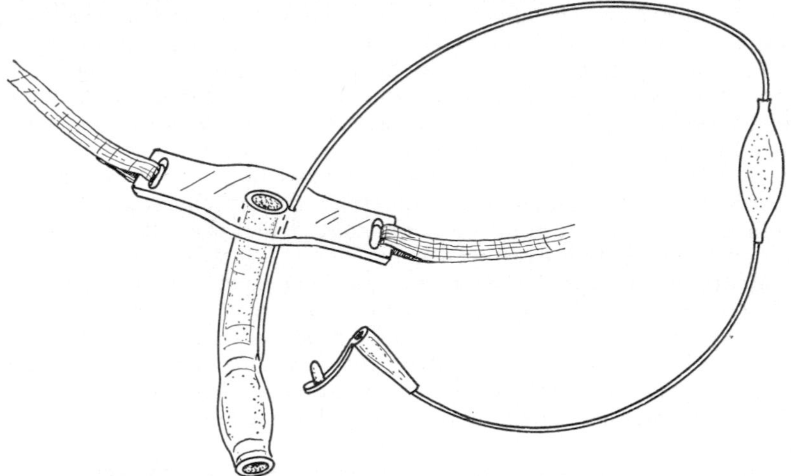

FIG. 76. Plastic tracheostomy tube, with inflatable cuff, for use with an intermittent positive pressure respirator.

explained, since speech will be lost, and coughing produces a loud, wheezing which is alarming at first. If the operation is only temporary, this must be stressed.

The opening in the trachea is kept patent with a tracheostomy tube. There are many patterns of tube, but only two important divisions.

(*a*) If the tracheostomy is temporary, a wide bore plastic tube is used. Such a tube is used too if radiotherapy is being given. An inflatable cuff, by occluding the space around the tube, allows the use of a respirator with the tracheostomy (Fig. 76).

(*b*) Metal tubes are used with permanent tracheostomies. They consist of three parts.

1. The outer tube, which has slots at the side for carrying tapes by means of which it is tied in position around the neck. The tapes should be put through double and fastened by a clove hitch.

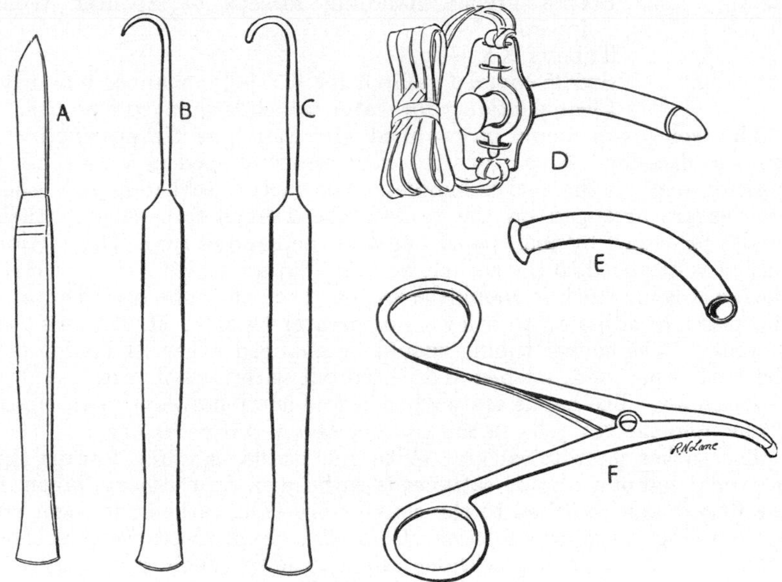

FIG. 77. Tracheostomy set.

A. Scalpel.
B. Sharp hook.
C. Blunt hook.
D. Tracheostomy tube, with pilot and tapes.
E. Inner tube.
F. Tracheal dilators.

2. The pilot, which fits the tube and has a solid end. It is only used while introducing the tube.

3. The inner tube, which is worn within the outer tube, and can be removed for cleaning. Some are attached by catches or screws to the outer tube, but it is usually safest to use one which only fits in, so that it can be removed or coughed out easily if it is blocked.

The operation of tracheostomy is usually performed by cutting a flap in the trachea, and turning this down. The patient who has had a tracheostomy cannot clear his airway by coughing, and has lost the protection against infection afforded by the nose and pharynx in ordinary people. The most important point in post-operative care is therefore the clearing of the airway from mucus to prevent asphyxia, and the use of a sterile technique that will prevent chest infection. The method of suction described depends on a supply of prepacked sterile articles, and uses a fresh sterile catheter each time the trachea is cleared.

Apparatus. Table or trolley for equipment.
Electric sucker or Smith-Clarke foot sucker.
15 in. no. 10 suction catheters sterilized, in paper bags.
Sterile suction tubing and straight connection.

Sterile French handling forceps or Spencer Wells forceps.
Tube of KY jelly.
Sterile covered gallipot for KY jelly, changed 6 hourly.
Clean container for water, which is changed 6 hourly.

The trolley top should be swabbed with Sudol, as if preparing for a surgical dressing. A bag for used catheters is clipped in a convenient position (e.g. on the sucker handle). The suction catheters and other articles are arranged on the trolley, the French forceps with their blades protected by their paper bag and the handles free. The suction tubing is attached to the sucker, and an adaptor added. If an electric sucker is being used, it should be switched on, the tube occluded, and the pressure adjusted to a level not greater than 10 M. (25 cms.) of mercury. The sucker tubing should be changed every 24 hours, and the bottles emptied, washed and rinsed out with hypochlorite.

Procedure. The hands are washed before suction except in an emergency, and the KY jelly in the gallipot renewed if necessary.

The sucker is switched on. With the sterile handling forceps the proximal end of a suction catheter is withdrawn from its bag, taken in the fingers and attached to the connection. The catheter is occluded by doubling it against the connection. The tip of the catheter is then withdrawn from its bag without allowing it to touch anything, and seized with forceps. It is dipped in KY jelly, and (still occluded) inserted into the tracheostomy as far as it will go. Pressure on the catheter is then released, and suction is exerted as the catheter is slowly withdrawn. When the airway is clear, the catheter is sucked through with water, detached, and put into the bag ready for re-sterilization. Oral suction may also be required in certain patients (e.g. the unconscious). After performing suction the hands are washed, and this point must never be omitted.

While suction must be performed thoroughly and completely, the nurse must remember that while the catheter is in the trachea the patient cannot breathe properly. A useful rule is not to continue suction for longer than the nurse can comfortably hold her breath.

Should the tube come out, the tracheal dilators must be at once inserted and the blades parted to keep the tracheostomy open. The patient is told that he is quite safe, and asked to lie quietly, since restlessness will also cause breathlessness and increase his alarm. An experienced sister can insert the spare tube herself, but in her absence the house surgeon should be summoned.

As soon as the patient is fit enough, he should be given a pad and pencil and encouraged to communicate with his nurses, who must always allow him to write everything he wants to say. Once the tracheotomy is stabilized, the nurse may give him a bell to summon assistance, and not remain entirely at his bedside, though she must of course be within hearing. Tracheitis may be troublesome, and a steam kettle often gives relief.

Patients often have to visit other departments and if they have a metal tube they should always take with them the pilot so that the outer tube can be reinserted should it inadvertently come out.

Many patients go home with a tracheostomy, and they and their relatives must have its management fully described and demonstrated, so that they have no fear of it. The relatives should be shown how the inner tube is taken out and cleaned, and should also be shown the reinsertion of the tube with pilot, in case the whole tube should inadvertently come out at home if the tapes part. The patient is provided with the following:

1. 2 brushes, medium and small.
2. Bicarbonate of soda.
3. Liquid paraffin.
4. Gauze roll.
5. 5-oz. enamel bowl.
6. 2 tracheostomy dressings consisting of :
   (*a*) 2 pieces of tape, 1 × 19 in. and 1 × 17 in. for the tube.
   (*b*) 1 piece of jaconet $5\frac{1}{2}$ in. × $4\frac{1}{2}$ in., covered with gauze both sides. This should have a small hole for the inner tube 1 in. from the top centre.
   (*c*) One bib 8 in. long when doubled.
   (*d*) 2 small pieces of gauze.
7. Pilot. Tubes are of silver, and if kept wrapped in chamois leather will be preserved from scratches.

Plastic tubes are worn if deep X-ray is being given.

It may be helpful to give them printed instructions in simple terms about how to clean the tube, and such a sheet might run as follows :

Instructions to clean your inner tube when at home.

1. Take out your inner tube and rinse well under the tap.
2. In the bowl provided mix $\frac{1}{2}$ teaspoonful of Bicarbonate of Soda with 4 oz. of warm water.
3. Dip the brush in this fluid, and run it up and down through the tube dipping frequently in the solution until all mucus is removed.
4. Rinse under the cold tap thoroughly.
5. Dry the tube on a small piece of gauze.
6. Lubricate the outer surface of the tube with a small amount of Liquid Paraffin on a piece of gauze, shaking it well before re-inserting it in the outer tube. (Drops left on the tube cause coughing.)
7. Replace the veil of gauze.
8. Once a day boil, in a pan kept for this use only, the two brushes and small bowl for five minutes. Then fold them in a clean cloth and keep all the things together ready for the next time.

Rubber tubes are all in one piece and there is no inner tube to change.

Patients are instructed to take their meals quietly, without talking or laughing. They usually wear a thin scarf or muffler round the neck, but a collar and tie can be worn when confidence is established. In suitable cases, an inner tube with a valve which permits speaking can be worn during the day. Further discussion of speaking will be found in the next section.

Laryngectomy

Radiotherapy is often effective in curing carcinoma of larynx, and in selected cases laryngectomy is undertaken. It is quite a severe operation, entailing the loss of laryngeal speech, and the patient must have its implications fully explained to him beforehand. Speech need not be permanently lost, since it is possible to learn to swallow air into the upper part of the œsophagus, and to speak with this, modified by movements of the tongue and lips. Mastering œsophageal speech requires some effort, and the old or discouraged rarely succeed at it, but men of employable age and reasonable intelligence usually master it, and may be able to use the telephone. It is a great incentive if his firm are ready to re-employ him when he can speak, and an old patient who will return to the ward to demonstrate his abilities is a great asset.

Before operation the chest should be X-rayed to confirm that no secondary growths are present, and the hæmoglobin and the Wassermann reaction should be ascertained. Any dental sepsis should be treated, and a high protein diet given. Since swallowing is often difficult, milk, eggs and semi-solids with added Casilan should be given. The area of the pre-operative shave extends down to the nipple line.

At the beginning of the operation a tracheostomy is performed, and the anæsthetic subsequently administered through it. The larynx and trachea above the tracheotomy are removed and the anterior wall of the œsophagus joined to the back of the tongue. A small drain or two is inserted in the wound, and finally a plastic catheter of adequate bore is passed through the nose into the œsophagus, where it must remain until the anastomosis is soundly healed.

After operation, the nursing is that described for tracheotomy. Nasal feeds are given four-hourly, and the superficial wound drains are removed after the second day. About the eighth day, if healing appears satisfactory, small drinks of distilled water may be given with the nasal catheter still in place, and if there is no leakage into the airway the feeds may be gradually increased and the catheter withdrawn.

The diet may become a full one, but should be smooth in texture, since leakage at the anastomosis is dangerous and troublesome. The progress of those patients for whom laryngectomy is feasible is good, and they should be constantly encouraged to believe that they can overcome the disability with regard to speech and breathing, and make a social recovery as good as their physical one.

Deafness

The public sympathy accorded to the blind is not generally given to the deaf, who are under a severe social handicap, perhaps because their sensory loss cannot be seen. In addition to the isolation due to their hearing defect, deaf people may have other troubles like nausea, vertigo, and head noises due to disturbances of the labyrinth.

Some deafness is preventible, and early diagnosis and effective treatment of ear disease, especially in young children, is important. Streptococcal tonsillitis, measles, scarlet fever, rubella and meningitis may cause ear complications, and should be prevented or energetically treated.

Children who are deaf from birth will also be dumb unless specially taught from an early age. People with some hearing may benefit from the use of a hearing-aid. This should be selected for them by a trained person, and instruction given in its use. Deaf people are often disappointed to find that the aid magnifies all sounds, including background noise, and they may find the clamour confusing, and give up. They need encouragement, and regular attention to servicing and batteries.

CHAPTER 24

OPHTHALMIC NURSING

THE eye is the smallest part of the body to be the subject of specialist skill, and yet is of vital importance to everyone. It is the centre of the most important sense, and the means by which we communicate with each other. A large part of its structure is visible from outside, and the observant nurse may see as readily as anyone else abnormalities of these parts.

The globe of the eye is seen between the two lids, which are made of skin, fringed by the lashes, and with many sebaceous glands along the margins. The lids and the whole of the visible globe is covered by a transparent membrane, the conjunctiva. The white part or sclera is a dense fibrous layer into which are inserted the muscles that move the eye. Over the anterior section of the eye lies the cornea, which must be perfectly clear if it is not to impede the passage of light into the interior of the eye. Behind the cornea is the coloured iris, a muscular sheet with a central hole, the pupil. The movements of the iris enlarge or constrict the pupil, and so control the amount of light admitted into the eye. Behind the pupil, the lens, and again this structure must be clear to transmit light fully, and correctly shaped to focus its rays. The retina, in which lie the light-sensitive cells, cannot be seen except with the aid of an ophthalmoscope, which directs a light into the eye through the pupil.

If the lower lid is gently drawn down to expose the lower fold, or fornix, a small dot will be seen near the inner angle. This is the

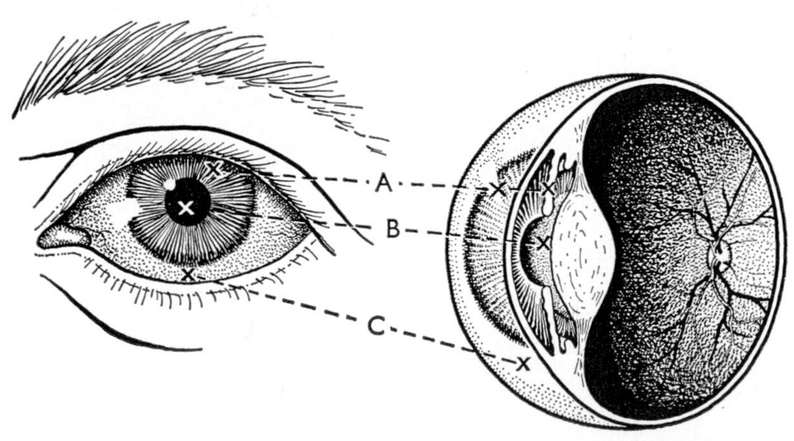

FIG. 78.

A. Iris
B. Pupil
C. Sclera

The section shows how the iris is covered by the cornea.

punctum, and is the orifice of the channel by which the tears drain from the conjunctival sac into the nose.

Both eyes normally open and close together ; it is difficult to open one if the other is held tightly shut, so that if the nurse is carrying out a procedure on one eye, the patient is asked to keep both eyes open.

THE NATURE OF EYE DISEASE

The kinds of damage and disease to which the eye is subject are the same as those of the rest of the body and may be classified in the same way.

1. *Congenital.* The fœtal eye develops most rapidly in the 8th to 12th week of pregnancy, and it is then most vulnerable. Should the mother-to-be develop Rubella (German Measles) at this stage, her baby may have as a result of the infection various congenital defects, of which cataract, or opacity of the lens, is one.

2. *Infective.* Any part of the eye may become infected, but since the conjunctiva is the outer layer, it is the part most commonly invaded. Trachoma is a form of conjunctivitis that is an important cause of blindness in countries where it is endemic. Sometimes the organisms ascend the lacrimal duct from the nose. Infections may be carried

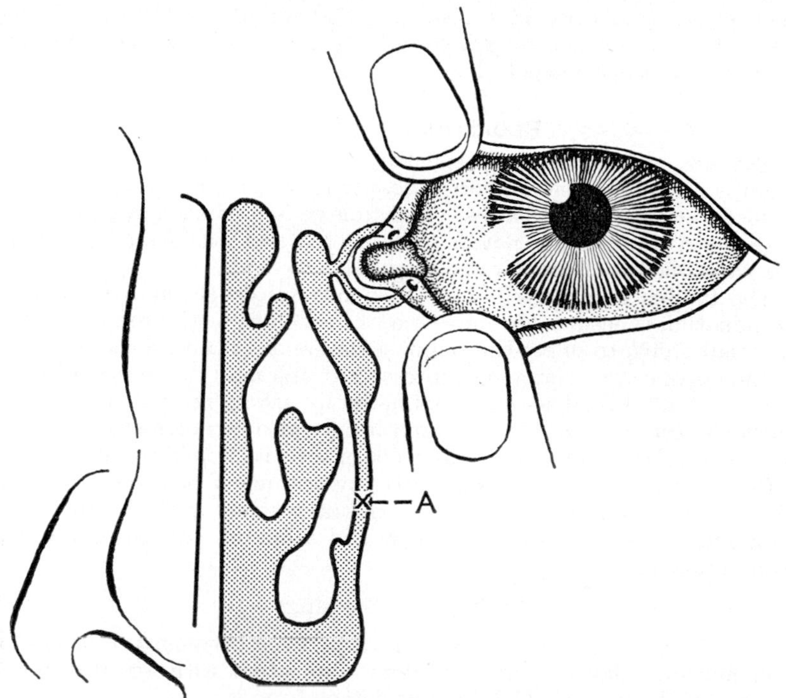

Fig. 79. The tears are drained from the conjunctival sac by the naso-lacrimal duct (A) into the nose. It is possible for infection to reach the eye from the nose by this route.

into the eye by foreign bodies, or may gain entry to operation wounds.

3. *Traumatic.* Injuries are not uncommon, especially in industrial communities.

4. *Neoplastic.* The new growths of the eye are not numerous, but since they usually entail loss of sight, if not the eye itself, they are grave. A melanoma is a coloured growth which sometimes arises in the pigmented choroid that supports the retina, and it is highly malignant.

5. *Nutritional.* A diet grossly deficient in vitamins (especially A and B) may result in loss of sight. There are still many emergent countries in which deficiency states of this kind occur.

6. *Degenerative.* With advancing age many structures become less efficient. Frequently the lens becomes increasingly cloudy (senile cataract), and may become such a barrier to sight that it has to be removed surgically. Diabetes, arteriosclerosis and hypertension are general diseases that often cause degenerative eye lesions.

Ophthalmic Patients

Patients in an eye ward are of all ages from the very young to the very old, and both these groups make special demands on the nurse. The tempo and style of ophthalmic nursing is quite different from that in a general surgical ward. The dressing technique is a meticulous and delicate one in a very small field, and the nursing problem is how to make the patients so comfortable in body and mind that they can rest quietly until the eye has healed.

Examination of the Eye

The lids and lashes are inspected, and then the conjunctiva. If there is reddening, the doctor notices if it is uniform, greatest in the fornices, or around the cornea. If discharge is present, a swab may be taken, and its nature is noted. The cornea and lens should be clear, the pupil black and circular and responsive to light.

The fundus is inspected with an ophthalmoscope, and if detailed examination is needed, the nurse may be asked to instil drops of cyclopentolate 0·5% to dilate the pupil beforehand. If abrasions or ulcers of the cornea are suspected, fluorescein drops may be needed as described below. Visual acuity is estimated by asking the patient to read Snellen's test chart at 6 metres, and it may also be necessary to find if the intraocular pressure and the extent of the visual field are normal.

Complaints about the eyes are often symptoms of such conditions as diabetes, hypertension, nephritis or cerebral tumour, and the nurse may be asked to test the urine for sugar and albumin, and to record the blood pressure.

Ophthalmic Dressings

Eye Pads. These are oval and made of wool between two layers of skin muslin. Gauze is little used in connection with eye dressings, because of the way in which threads detach from it.

Swabs. Wool may be used for bathing, but for cleaning the lids, commercial medical wipes are in general use. Orange sticks dressed with wool and sterilized are also useful for cleaning the lashes.

Dark glasses. Cheap dark glasses are used when the eye needs covering, but a pad and bandage are not indicated; a discharging eye, for instance, must not be bandaged as infection will increase rapidly in the warm moist conjunctival sac from which secretions cannot escape. Such glasses afford some protection to the eye, but do not allow retention of infected material.

Protective Shades. A guard to prevent pressure on an eye may be included in a dressing. *Cartella* shields are made of perforated card-board, and are attached with cellotape. They are marked " L " or " R " for the appropriate eye, and the letter should be uppermost.

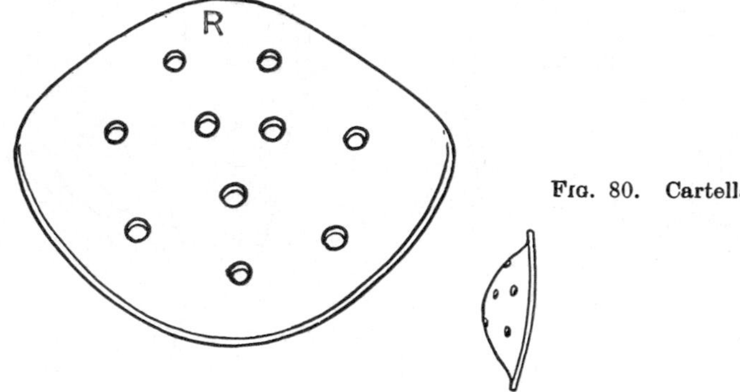

Fig. 80. Cartella shield.

Similar shields are made in aluminium which can be boiled. Wire cages are also used, especially after eye operations, to prevent the patient inadvertently knocking or pressing on the eye.

Buller's eye shield is a watch glass enclosed in a square of jaconet by strapping. They are occasionally used to protect an uncontaminated eye from being infected from the other. An air outlet is left on the temporal side to prevent condensation on the inside of the glass.

If a pad is to be used on the eye, it must be bandaged in position firmly enough to prevent the eye being opened behind it. Various types will be needed for different conditions and patients, and some of them are described below.

Roller Bandages. 1. *Single eye* (A). A 2-in. roller bandage, an eye pad and a safety pin are needed. If the bandage is for the left eye, the nurse begins the bandage over the affected eye and takes a fixing turn round the head. The bandage then passes down the back of the head, and under the left ear, over the eye pad on the nasal side and straight up over the head, under the left ear and up over the eye pad, covering the remainder of it, across the head overlapping the previous turn, behind the occiput and up above the left ear, round the head in a fixing turn, ending in the centre of the forehead.

The turns across the eye should cross each other and the head turn at the same point if neatness is to be obtained. The good eye must not be obscured at all, and the left ear not incommoded. The safety pin should go through all the turns in the centre of the forehead, and is more effective in keeping the bandage firm than is a piece of strapping.

2. *Single eye* (B). The nurse stands behind the patient, leaves 6 in. of bandage free under the occiput and passes the bandage round the forehead from the right side to the left to the back of the head again. Holding the tail of the bandage in the left hand, she passes the head of the bandage round it, thus reversing its direction. She passes the

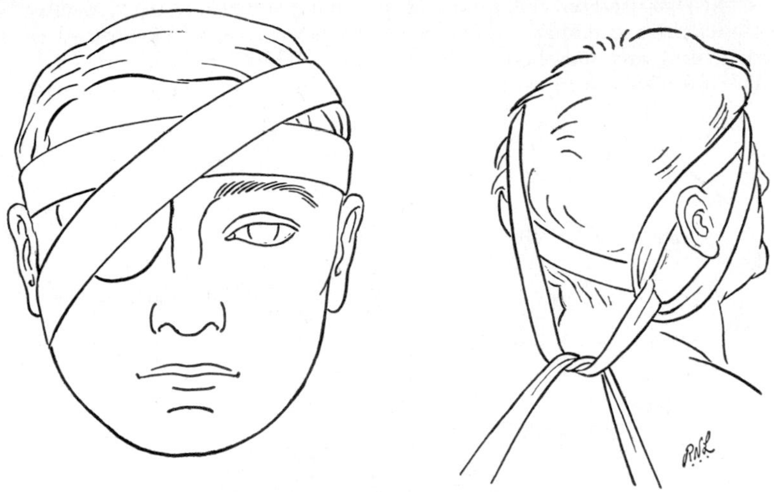

FIG. 81. The knotted eye bandage.

bandage back below the left ear, up over the eye pad and across the vertex to the occiput again. The bandage is cut off, and the two short ends firmly knotted.

This is a bandage that is economical of material but is not suitable for bed patients because of the knot at the back.

3. *Double eye*. The fixing turn passes round the head, and then below the left ear, up over the left eye pad and across the head to the back, round the head and over the right eye in a downward direction. For those people in hospital who have both eyes bandaged and must keep their heads at rest against their pillows, application of a roller bandage would involve too much movement. A *many-tail* bandage would be suitable for these. It is made of four strips of 1½-in. fast-edge

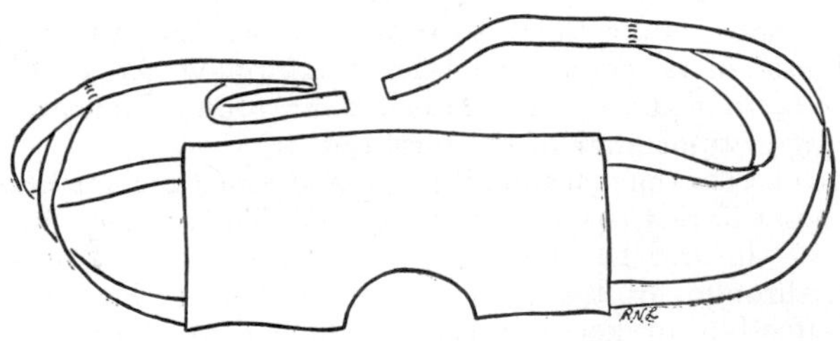

FIG. 82. Moorfield's eye bandage.

bandage joined at their centres diagonally. It is put under the back of the head, and the lower slips are drawn up alternately over the eyes, while the upper ones pass round the forehead.

A *Moorfields* bandage is a double strip of material with tapes at the corners, made as in the illustration. The tapes cross at the back of the head and are tied on the forehead over a swab. A " bandage " can also be made by knitting a 3 in. × 2 in. white strip, decreasing at both ends. Tapes are attached for retaining the dressing in place. They are most used for out-patients.

Eye Drops

Drops (guttæ) are extensively used in eye work, and some of the more useful are described here. The usual strength is ½ or 1% and they may be made up in water or oil. The containers are of glass, the pipettes usually of glass and rubber, and they must be sterilized at regular intervals.

Mydriatics dilate the pupil. They are used in examination, for corneal ulcers, and extensively after intra-ocular operations. Atropine is the commonest ; sometimes sensitivity to it is shown by swelling and reddening of the lids, and then hyoscine can be used. Cyclopentolate is useful in examination because its effects can be neutralized by eserine.

Miotics constrict the pupil. Eserine and pilocarpine are examples.

Anti-infective drops are usually of chloramphenicol or neomycin, or of a soluble sulphonamide, sulphacetamide 10%.

Plain *lubricants* are sometimes needed, and paroleine or castor oil is commonly used to prevent drying of the cornea, or sticking of the lids by discharge.

Local anæsthesia is of especial value in ophthalmic conditions, because minor procedures, like removal of embedded foreign bodies from the cornea, can be conveniently done with a local anæsthetic. Cocaine, which was formerly widely used, has been replaced by amethocaine 1%, since the latter neither damages the corneal epithelium nor dilates the pupil.

Cortisone is a hormone of the suprarenal cortex which among other effects controls the inflammatory process, limiting swelling and exudation. Some of its most important uses are in iritis (inflammation of the iris) and keratitis (inflammation of the cornea). It may be given as drops (½%), as an ointment, or by subconjunctival injection. Many of these drugs can also be used as ointments. Fluorescein is a useful *diagnostic* substance; it is put up in individual sterile packs, or as impregnated filter paper strips, since in bulk it easily becomes contaminated. If an ulcer or abrasion is present on the cornea, it will retain the yellow-green dye and become visible.

SOME NURSING TECHNIQUES

Most ophthalmic techniques are most conveniently performed from behind the patient, who lies on a couch or in his bed. The couch should be of a height suitable for the operator to work comfortably, while for minor treatment, such as the insertion of drops, a chair with a rest for the head can be used.

The nails should be short, filed to a round shape and well manicured. The hands are washed and the nails scrubbed before each treatment. Deft hands with a smooth skin are a great asset to the surgeon and the nurse.

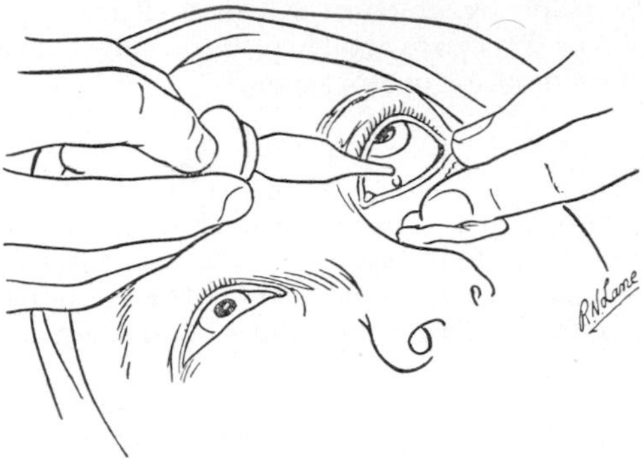

Fig. 83. Putting diagnostic drops in the eye.

Giving Eye Drops

Requirements. Drop bottle.
Medical wipe.
Prescription.

The prescription is read as carefully as if a medicine were to be given, noticing the drug, the strength, and whether oily or watery drops are to be given. If the pipette is one with which the nurse is not familiar she should fill it, raise the end just above the level of the fluid, and see how much pressure is needed to release a single drop promptly. It is equally undesirable to flood the eye, and to keep the patient waiting an inordinate time for the drop to fall.

If the drops are for diagnostic purposes, the patient is asked to look

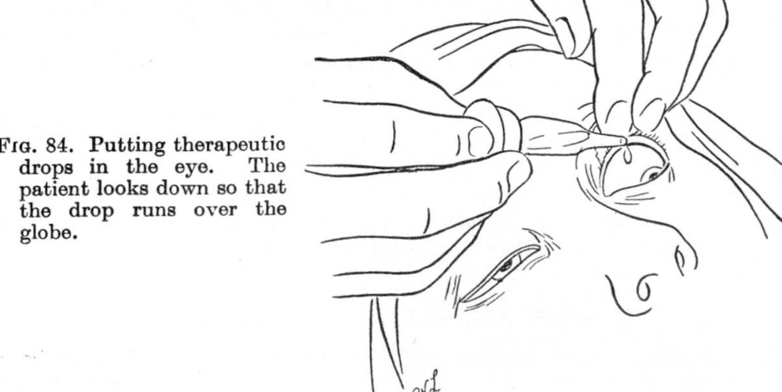

Fig. 84. Putting therapeutic drops in the eye. The patient looks down so that the drop runs over the globe.

up, the lower lid is depressed, and the drop allowed to fall into the lower fornix. The eye closes reflexly, and the lids are dried with the lint square. If the drops are therapeutic, the patient is asked to look down, the upper lid is drawn up and the drop placed on the sclera above the iris.

Application of Ointment

Requirements. Ointment prescribed.
Small sterile glass rod.
Medical wipe.

The nurse collects a small portion of ointment on the top of the glass rod, and standing behind the patient asks him to look up. She uses the rod in her right hand for the right eye and vice versa. She draws down the lower lid, lays the end of the rod gently along the lower fornix and asks that the eyes be closed, then puts the swab over the lid and withdraws the rod sideways, rotating it slightly as she does so, so that the ointment is left in the conjunctival sac. Individual tubes of ointment allow the ointment to be squeezed out straight into the lower fornix.

If ointment is to be applied to the lid margins, it should be carefully and thoroughly applied after a warm bathing to remove crusts and scales. An orange stick dressed with wool is a convenient applicator. The lashes should not be left loaded with ointment.

Everting the Lids

The lower fornix is shallow, and easily exposed by asking the patient to look up, drawing down the lower lid and rolling it slightly outwards. The upper lid is the larger of the two, and a little dexterity and practice is needed to turn it outwards and expose the upper part of the eye and

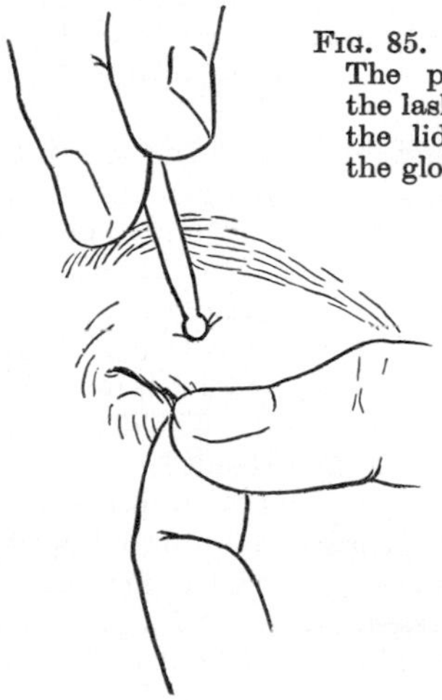

FIG. 85. Everting the lid 1. The patient looks down the lashes are grasped, and the lid lifted away from the globe.

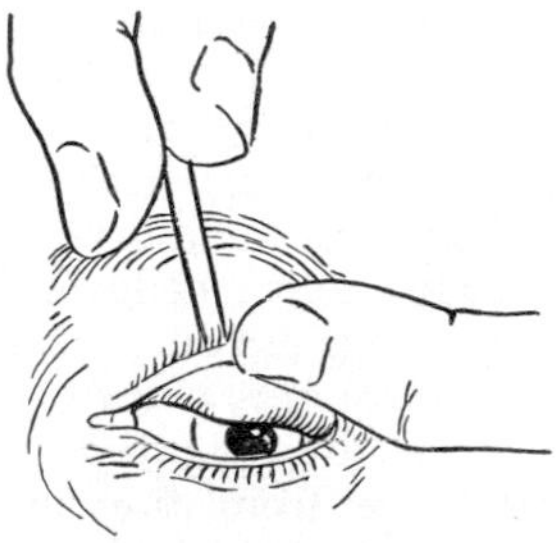

Everting the lid 2. The lid is turned over the glass rod, which is then withdrawn.

the interior surface of the lid. Two methods can be used, of which the first is the easier, and the second the quicker and more expert.

(*a*) With the patient looking down, the upper lashes are taken between the left thumb and forefinger and a small glass rod laid along the lid above the lashes. The lid is drawn up across the rod and held with the left forefinger while the rod is withdrawn.

(*b*) Standing behind the patient, the nurse asks him to look down, then puts the tip of the left forefinger below the lashes and the thumb just above the lash margin. The thumb is used as a fulcrum, and the lid margin rotated back over it and secured with the finger tip. Whichever manœuvre is used, it should be executed with the left hand, leaving the right hand free for treatment.

Irrigating the Eye

Eye irrigation with an undine is less practised than formerly because infected eyes can be more efficiently treated with drops of chloramphenicol or sulphacetamide. Splashes of chemicals in the eye must be promptly washed out, but much larger volumes are required than can be accommodated in an undine, and in works where such accidents may occur, a douche can and tubing should be kept ready for use.

Requirements. Undine, sterile, and a kidney dish.
Jug of lotion (e.g. normal saline) at 100°F. (38° C.).
Lotion thermometer.
Lint swabs in bowl.
Bowl of lotion.
Receiver for used swabs.
Mackintosh and towel.

Method. The patient should lie on a couch or in his bed, with the mackintosh and towel against his neck. The kidney dish is held against the cheek to collect the lotion, and if the patient cannot do this efficiently himself an assistant will be needed. Triangular dishes with unequal sides are used in ophthalmic units and are useful for hollow-cheeked patients for whom the most suitable side can be selected.

The undine is filled from the jug by pouring lotion into the opening. Standing behind the patient, the nurse asks him to look up and keep *both* eyes open, then she tilts the undine and allows the lotion to fall on the inner margin of the orbit, then directs it upwards into the eye. If the lotion is allowed to fall at once on to the eye, spasmodic closure of the lids will make irrigation difficult. The lower fornix is irrigated by drawing down the lower lid, then the patient is asked to look down, the upper lid is drawn back and the upper fornix washed out. The direction of flow should be always from the nasal to the temporal side.

After the irrigation, wet lint swabs should be used to remove any discharge from the lid margins, and these should be meticulously cleaned. Every lash should be clean and separate when the procedure is complete. Finally the eye and cheek are dried.

The hole in the undine is for filling, and to allow air to enter so that the lotion can run out. Flow is controlled by the angle of the undine, and not by keeping a finger over the airhole ; this only results in an awkward grip on the undine. If the patient through age or infirmity seems unlikely to co-operate, the ulnar border of the hand holding the undine should be in contact with the patient's forehead, so that a sudden movement will not allow the glass nozzle to injure the eye.

If a baby has to have an eye irrigation, it should lie on the nurse's lap wrapped in a towel. It is not now common to use anything but drops for an infected eye in an infant. Chloramphenicol is very effective, especially against gonococcal infections, which were once a cause of blindness, and which have fortunately now become rare.

Cutting the Lashes

Before intra-ocular operations it is usual to trim off the lashes. A pair of blunt-ended, well-sharpened scissors should be used, and a layer of soft paraffin ointment should be applied to both blades. The patient should be asked to keep the eyes closed but not screwed up. Applying a little traction to the upper lid will separate the two rows of lashes without opening the eye, and they should be trimmed separately to the level of the skin. It is an easy manœuvre, only taking a few seconds, and if the scissors are well greased and the eye kept closed there is no danger of a lash entering the conjunctival sac and causing damage.

Applying Heat

Hot steaming is commonly prescribed for styes. A pad of gamgee tissue is tied to the bowl of a wooden spoon with thread, and the patient sits up with a bowl of boiling water in front of him. He dips the spoon in the bowl, and lifts it to within a few inches of the eye to allow the steam to reach it. As the water cools it may be replenished, or the hot gamgee may be held against the eye. If a patient is having such treatment four-hourly his own spoon and bowl may be kept for him, and sterilized when the treatment is discontinued.

Short-wave therapy is the most efficient way of applying heat to the eye and surrounding tissues. It will be given by the physiotherapist and is the treatment of choice for the more serious eye conditions (e.g. glaucoma) for which heat is prescribed.

The Maddox heater is a small electric pad operated at the bedside, which is enclosed in an eye pad and bandaged in place. It may be used for one hour in four, and has been to a great extent superseded by the use of short-wave diathermy.

Removing Conjunctival Stitches

Stitches in the conjunctiva are removed in exactly the same way as stitches elsewhere, but an anæsthetized eye, a confident patient and manual dexterity are needed. A drop of amethocaine is put into the eye once every five minutes on three occasions, and a pair of conjunctival forceps and fine scissors are used. An assistant should hold back the upper lid, and the patient directs the eye so that the stitches come into view. It will be found convenient to rest the ulnar border of the right hand lightly against the cheek or nose, so that if the patient moves the hand does too and there is no danger of the scissors hurting the eye. The minimum of traction that will enable the scissor point to pass under the stitch should be made with the forceps. After removing the stitches, a pad should be kept over the eye until the effects of the cocaine are past.

Ophthalmic Instruments

The instruments used in ophthalmic work are small and delicately made, and scrupulous attention must be paid to their maintenance and sterilization. Joints of scissors must be lubricated at intervals, and small forceps must not be roughly handled, or the blades may not meet truly.

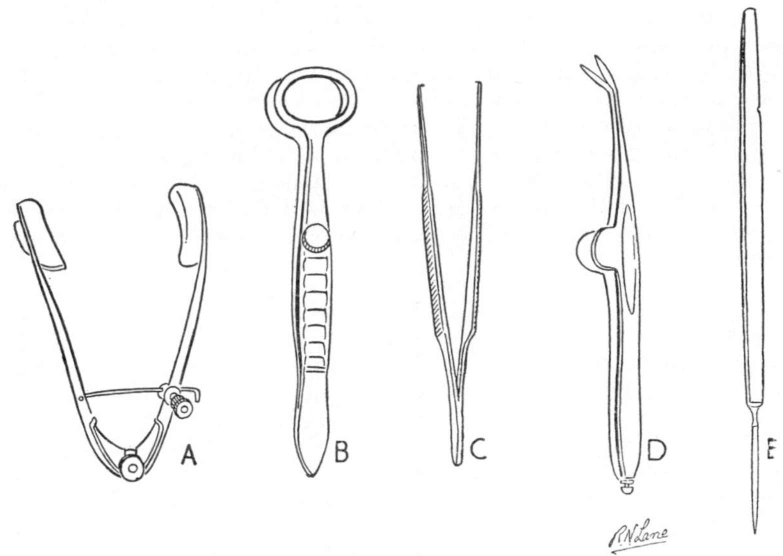

FIG. 86. Some ophthalmic instruments.

A. Speculum.
B. Chalazion clamp.
C. Toothed conjunctival forceps.
D. De Wecker's iridectomy scissors.
E. Graefe knife.

The most important instruments are the knives (e.g. Graefe) used in intra-ocular operations. A theatre nurse who watches a cataract operation will realize her responsibilities. The knife must pass in at exactly the right spot, and cannot be withdrawn if it is faulty. In three or four movements it must emerge at the top of the eye, having completed an incision which is very small, but one of the most crucial in surgery.

Every blade must be minutely inspected before being sterilized. The knives should be locked in a holder, so that the blades cannot be touched and autoclaving is the method of choice. If boiling is the method, distilled water should be used, or furring from hard-water deposits may occur.

SOME COMMON EYE CONDITIONS

The Lids

Styes. Like hair follicles everywhere, the root of a lash may become infected by staphylococci, and a small abscess, called a stye or hordeolum, is formed. It is painful out of proportion to its size, and causes swelling of the lid which restricts vision. Hot bathing will hasten the process, and chloramphenicol ointment is applied to the lids. Penicillin should not be used for eye infections, since many organisms are resistant to its action, and manv patients are sensitive and may show allergic reactions.

Styes sometimes recur, because staphylococci have become resident in the lash follicles, and the persistent disfiguring infection is not only painful but unsightly, and lowers the morale. Chloramphenicol ointment should be applied twice a day for six weeks, whether styes are present or not. General measures include a good fluid intake and avoiding undue amounts of sugar in the diet. The urine must be tested to exclude diabetes mellitus, which is often accompanied by sepsis.

Meibomian Cysts. A chalazion is a retention cyst in one of the sebaceous Meibomian glands. It forms a rounded swelling, occasionally inflamed, within the lid. It is evacuated through the inner surface of the lid by anæsthetizing the eye and applying a chalazion clamp to the lid encircling the cyst, which is opened and curetted free from its contents. A pad and bandage should be worn until the next day.

The Conjunctiva

Foreign Bodies. Specks of dust may commonly enter the conjunctival sac, and usually fall into the lower fornix whence they are easily removed. Should they lodge in the cornea, they may be irrigated away, but if they are adherent it will be necessary to anæsthetize the eye and extract the foreign body with a spud. After this a pad and bandage are applied until the abrasion is healed. If no foreign body can be seen, but the patient feels it to be there, it is almost certainly adhering to the upper lid, and if the lid is everted it can be seen and removed.

Foreign bodies that enter the eye with force penetrate into its interior, and must be removed. The outlook for the eye depends on the structures traversed and what the foreign body consists of.

Conjunctivitis. Inflammation of the conjunctiva is common and causes muco-purulent discharge and brick-red congestion which is most marked at the periphery. The eye feels " gritty " rather than painful, and there is no interference with sight. This will spread to the other eye, and be transmitted to other people unless the patient receives some instruction on how to avoid this. A swab is taken, and hot bathing begun. Some women get an allergic conjunctivitis from the use of mascara, and must subsequently avoid this cosmetic. Dark glasses may be worn, but a pad and bandage must never be used, or infected material is retained in the conjunctival sac.

The worst form of conjunctivitis is ophthalmia neonatorum, a gonococcal infection of the eye of the newly born. In countries where gonorrhoea is common, a drop of chloramphenicol should be instilled into each eye at birth as a prophylactic. If swelling and purulent discharge from the eyes should develop in a baby, a swab should be taken, and treatment is begun at once. Chloramphenicol drops are instilled every minute for half an hour ; once every 5 minutes for an hour ; once every 15 minutes for 2 hours ; once every half hour for 3 hours ; every hour for 6 hours, and every 2 hours for 12 hours. This intensive therapy will save the sight if begun promptly, and rigorously followed. The nurse should wear gloves as well as gown, and must take the greatest care not to transfer infected material from her hands.

The Cornea

Corneal Ulcers. A simple corneal abrasion which fails to heal and becomes infected may give rise to a corneal ulcer. More severe and intractable forms are seen in which infection and poor general health play a part. These irregular and sometimes extensive ulcers are called dendritic. Sometimes complaints by ill patients of a sore or red eye may seem of minor importance, but these signs must be reported and investigated. Treatment must be promptly undertaken, since ulceration over the central part of the cornea may produce scarring that will limit vision. Mild cases of simple ulcer may be treated with atropine and sulphacetamide drops and a pad and bandage to stop movement of the lid over the raw area. More severe types may respond to subconjunctival soframycin, or to carbolization of the ulcer, which is dried with blotting paper, and touched with a glass rod dipped in pure carbolic.

Corneal Grafts. If the cornea is opaque, vision will be lost just as a frosted window obscures the view. In some cases the sight can be restored by inserting a transparent corneal graft. There are three difficulties in connection with this simple statement.

1. The donor graft must be human, taken from a healthy cornea within four hours of death under aseptic conditions, and of the same blood group as the patient. The Corneal Graft Act, 1952, made the legal position easier, but the technical difficulties of obtaining the grafts, except in hospital, are great.

2. The operation is not an easy one. A non-penetrating graft is the easiest to apply, but is not very clear, and can only be used if the corneal opacity is superficial. If a full-thickness graft is used, there is danger of injuring the iris, or adhesion formation between the cornea and iris later.

3. Unless blindness is of fairly recent onset, merely letting light into the eye will not restore the ability to see, and in a proportion of cases that are at first successful, the corneal graft slowly becomes opaque.

The patient who has had a penetrating graft is nursed flat with both eyes covered for two weeks ; the stitches normally remain in place for at least 3 weeks, and steroid drugs are given to reduce the risk of inflammatory reaction.

The Iris

Iridocyclitis. Inflammation of the iris (iritis) and of the ciliary body (cyclitis) frequently but not necessarily occur together. The eye is painful, with redness around the margin of the cornea, photophobia and watering. The pupil is small and often irregular, the fibres of the iris are swollen, and the cornea hazy. The congestion interferes with the drainage of the aqueous humor from the anterior chamber, and if it is not effectively treated, glaucoma (see below) may ensue.

The cause is usually an infection elsewhere, and tuberculosis, syphilis, gonorrhœa, dental or upper respiratory sepsis may produce it. On admission to hospital, treatment on these lines will be ordered :

1. Atropine drops to dilate the pupil and improve drainage from the anterior chamber.
2. Cortisone to decrease the inflammatory reaction.
3. Heat, by short-wave diathermy or bathing.
4. A lint flap, to keep light from the eye.
5. Antibiotic drops if indicated.
6. Examination to determine the cause if possible.

The investigations and history taking give rise to anxiety in many patients, who will need much encouragement and reassurance.

Glaucoma. This term means a rise of intra-ocular pressure, and is due to failure of the aqueous humor in the anterior chamber of the eye to drain away by the canal of Schlemm. If this rise of pressure is not relieved, blindness will eventually be caused by optic atrophy. Some cases are secondary to iritis, but others are primary.

Acute glaucoma is sudden in its onset, though mild symptoms are often present before. Sometimes the precipitating cause seems to be anxiety or grief which might increase ocular congestion, and sometimes a visit to the cinema with its effects on the pupil's reactions to light precedes an acute attack. The patient notices coloured rings round lights, and the eye becomes very painful, with headache and often vomiting, and the eye is found to be red and hard, with an oval dilated pupil that does not respond to light.

The patient must be admitted at once to hospital, and morphine can be given immediately to allay the natural anxiety, relieve the pain and perhaps help to constrict the pupil, since pressure on the canal of Schlemm is greatest when the pupil is dilated. Eserine drops are used for the same reason. Heat by short-wave diathermy, or bathing is helpful for pain. An oral diuretic is directly helpful in lowering the intraocular pressure. Medical treatment is usually successful in relieving the pressure, but peripheral iridectomy is usually necessary.

Chronic glaucoma is insidious in its onset, and the patient's usual field is sometimes much restricted by the raised pressure before he comes for treatment. He complains of headache and failing vision, and on palpation through the closed lid the eyeball is felt to be hard. The pressure can be measured by a tonometer. Pilocarpine drops ½ to 2% three times a day will be helpful. An operation is avoided wherever possible. The patient is seen every 3 months, and the intraocular pressure and visual fields tested. Only if deterioration cannot be halted by medical means is operation considered.

The Lens

Cataract. Opacity of the lens is called cataract, and if the opacity is central or extensive, gross interference with sight is caused, though the patient does not lose all perception of light. Three kinds are met in ophthalmic wards.

1. *Congenital Cataract.* The patient is a child, and one of the commonest causes in countries with adequate dietetic standards is infection of the mother by German measles about the third month of pregnancy. The condition is bilateral, and is treated by discission, i.e. piercing the front of the lens with a needle. The results obtained are variable.

2. *Traumatic Cataract.* If the lens is pierced by a foreign body, it will become opaque, and must be removed. The treatment is the same as described for the next group.

3. *Senile Cataract.* Developing opacity in the lens appears to be part of the aging process in some people, as changes in the arteries are in others. Diabetics are more prone to this condition than the average. Although one eye is usually affected before the other, eventually the cataract will be bilateral. The only method of treatment available is operation.

Pre-operative Treatment. These patients are usually over 60 years old, and should be admitted two days before operation. Elderly people who are alert and self-supporting in their own environment are easily confused in strange surroundings, and need a little time to learn them. A conjunctival swab must be taken, the lashes are cut, and some surgeons like the lacrimal duct to be syringed through. The chest is examined, and the urine tested. General cleanliness is ensured, and women should be given a shampoo. Men should be introduced to the use of a urinal, or difficulty with post-operative micturition may be encountered. Disorientation at night, or a tendency to get out of bed should be noticed, as this will be more marked when the eye is bandaged after operation.

Straining, as in post-operative vomiting or restlessness, may cause hæmorrhage into the eye and lead to loss of sight. If a general anæsthetic is used, it is because good anæsthetic resources and post-operative care is available and quiet recovery can be confidently expected. Probably most patients still have their operation under local anæsthesia, and if this is so, careful explanation must be given. She is told that she will not be asleep during the operation, but that it will be quite painless ; her eye will be bandaged, and she must not touch it, but rest quietly with her head and shoulders resting against the pillows.

A sedative may be given on the night before operation if necessary, but otherwise should be avoided, as elderly people are easily confused by drugs. Morphine is avoided pre-operatively, since it often causes vomiting. Women patients should have their hair well brushed and divided into two plaits if it is long ; the hair will not be brushed again for a day or two.

Operation. If a general anæsthetic is used, sutures are placed at the upper margin of the cornea to close the wound afterwards, and a stitch is passed through the margin of the lid, to keep it firmly closed after operation.

Several operations are in use. The most popular now is to turn down a conjunctival flap, cut along the upper margin of the cornea with knife or scissors, and insert a cryoprobe. The iceball which forms makes firm adhesion between the probe and lens, which can then be drawn out of the incision. If cryosurgery is not possible, the lens is seized with capsular forceps and aided by pressure from below, is drawn out of the wound. Sometimes a small portion of iris is excised to prevent prolapse. The flap is then sutured into place. The stitches are tied, and a pad and bandage and Cartella shield is applied. Some surgeons think it is wiser to bandage both eyes, but most only cover the operated eye.

Post-operative Nursing. Most cataract patients are nursed in a sitting or semi-recumbent position, and while the operation is in progress the bed is made up with enough well-arranged pillows. There is no need to warm the bed in ordinary circumstances; patients are commonly warm after the theatre session in gown and socks. She is lifted gently into bed with the head supported, and the pillows carefully arranged until the back and head are in a completely comfortable position. She will probably be tense at first, and her nurse should stay with her until she is relaxed. Pain in the eye is abnormal, and the patient is usually amazed and relieved to find that it is all over.

If a general anæsthetic has been given, the nurse must stay with her patient until she is assured that she is not only conscious, but fully aware. The patient is encouraged to rest quietly; stooping and bending (as in searching in the locker) is dangerous.

Bowel action is not encouraged for three days, and then a suppository may be given, or liquid paraffin started twice a day. On approaching the patient the nurse should speak to her before touching her to avoid startling her.

The food should be of soft consistency that needs no chewing—minced meat, pounded fish, scrambled or poached eggs, vegetable purées, crustless bread and butter, soft puddings. The patient must be fed, and this must be done thoughtfully if it is to be the pleasure it should. The nurse may sit if the patient is lying down, but if the patient is nursed sitting up, it will be more convenient to stand. A teaspoon is the best utensil, and the nurse tells her patient what she is going to give her and arranges a napkin on her chest. The speed of feeding should be such that the patient is neither kept waiting nor hurried. She is unable to see when a spoonful is ready, and the nurse will find that it is convenient to touch the patient's chin with her little finger as a signal to open the mouth. Water is offered with lunch, and bread if it is liked. Fluids can be given in a cup or glass, not over-filled, if the patient is sitting up, or a feeder if she is lying down.

Watch should be kept on the temperature, pulse and respiration. A chest infection, with the coughing it involves, could be disastrous for the still-unhealed eye. The first dressing is often postponed for forty-eight hours, but if the eye is painful or there is any discharge from the nostril on the operated side, it should be done earlier.

Requirements. Medical wipes and eye pads.
Stitch scissors and forceps.
Atropine 1%, warm.
Chloramphenicol.
Light.
Cellotape.

At the first dressing, the lid will be found closed by a suture whose ends are strapped to the cheek. The strapping is gently removed, and the stitch taken out in the usual way. The normal eye is swabbed first, then the lid of the operated eye lightly cleaned. The patient is asked not to squeeze the lids at all, is warned that a light is to be shone on the eye, and then the lid is gently lifted and the eye inspected. The pupil should be black, and the cornea clear and the iris in position, and if all is well the patient is warned that a drop is coming, and the atropine is instilled, and chloramphenicol. A pad is applied and the bandage replaced.

If all is well with the eye, the patient may feed herself with soft meals with a spoon. On the next day she may sit beside her bed, and a week later may dress, but no real activity is undertaken, and she should still be washed by the nurse. Stooping (to get slippers from the locker, for instance) is especially harmful to the healing eye.

After the first week, steroid drops are often given, and at the end of the second week the corneo-sclerotic stitch is taken out. The patient may go home, with the eye protected by dark glasses, and must not undertake any strain until she returns to be seen in a month's time.

The results are in most cases excellent, but in many remote parts of the world old people suffer from blindness only because there is no surgical assistance available.

The description of post-operative care after a cataract removal applies to all patients who have had operations on the interior of the eye. The complications that are feared and the precautions by which they are averted are :

1. Infection. (Pre-operative conjunctival swab ; skin cleanliness ; care in cocainization ; sterile dressing technique.)

2. Prolapse of Iris. (Iridectomy before the close of the operation ; pad, bandage and absolute rest for a week; careful inspection at each dressing, since if prolapse occurs a return to the theatre is needed.)

3. Hæmorrhage. (Prevention of straining ; protection of the eye from inadvertent knocks by cartella shields or similar devices.)

The Retina

Retinal Detachment. The retina is normally in contact with the choroid but in this condition there is a hole or tear in the retina, which is lifted off the choroid by fluid formation. Many such detachments are traumatic ; for instance they are not uncommon in boxers ; and some are associated with high degrees of myopia. The patient complains of restriction of sight in one eye, as if a curtain were being drawn over it.

The method of treatment is to apply a cryoprobe or diathermy to the sclera immediately above the detachment, in the hope of making it adhere again. The patient must rest quietly in bed with the eye bandaged, usually for a week. Since many of these patients are vigorous adults, the lack of activity is very irksome, and the fortitude exhibited by most is the measure of the importance of sight. In hospital practice, the most popular form of diversional therapy is talking, and a perceptive patient will be able to give his nurse many practical hints. He will say that he can tell by her movements if she is in a hurry, and if he feels this is so will hesitate to ask for her services. He can tell by her voice if she is smiling or no, and is glad when she is.

Extra Ocular Muscles

Squint. When the eyes are at rest, and looking straight ahead, the visual axes should be parallel. Deviation of one or both eyes is strabismus or squint. The most important squints from the point of view of treatment are those occurring in children, in whom the affected eye usually deviates inwards ; a divergent squint indicates short sight.

Nurses are often asked by parents for their advice on squints in small children, and the answer should be that treatment should be undertaken at once. The lay belief that the child " will grow out of it " has little foundation in fact. In order to avoid seeing double, the child must ignore the image from the squinting eye, which becomes amblyopic, or lazy. Someone with a squint has a very unsightly defect of which he is constantly reminded because people find difficulty in deciding which eye to look at when speaking to him, and usually select the amblylopic one.

Parents must be told that treatment may have to last for years. The refractive error is most carefully corrected, and the child must wear glasses constantly. If there is no sign of improvement the good eye is kept covered, and vision may then be regained in the squinting eye. Orthoptic treatment may then enable the patient to regain binocular vision by eye exercises. In many cases, however, a simple operation will be needed. For the usual convergent squint, the internal rectus tendon may be divided and set further back on the eyeball ("tendon recession") or advancement of the external rectus tendon can be performed.

Other varieties of strabismus are :

1. Sensory squint. If an eye becomes blind it often deviates, usually outwards in an adult, and an operation may be performed for purely cosmetic reasons.

2. Paralytic squint. Damage to one or other of the nerves that supply the extrinsic muscles of the eye will produce a squint. Head injury and meningitis are examples of causes.

The operation is done under a general anæsthetic, and dressings are not usually applied after the operation. Glasses must be worn again at once. Free visiting by the mother makes the post-operative period happy for small children.

Loss of Sight

Fear of loss of sight is felt by many patients in an ophthalmic ward, and they often appeal, directly or indirectly, for reassurance. While this can often be given, one contribution to success that the nurse can always give is careful technique and alert observation, so that infection is avoided and early symptoms noticed and reported.

Possession of two eyes is an advantage in judging distances, relations and speeds. The patient who has lost the sight of an eye not only suffers a shrinking of the visual field, but finds it difficult to go downstairs, and hazardous to cross the street, and a great handicap in playing tennis or cricket.

Prevention of Blindness

This is of course a situation in which prevention is better than cure, and might be considered again under the headings used in classifying the nature of eye disease.

1. **Congenital Blindness.** Unless it proves feasible to prepare a vaccine against German Measles, girls should not be protected against infection, so that they may gain immunity before pregnancy. If not, they should be guarded from infection during the first half of pregnancy. Gonorrhœa must be diagnosed and if necessary treated during pregnancy, to avert infection of the baby's eyes during birth.

2. **Blindness Due to Infection.** The last patients might be included also under this heading. Trachoma is a variety of conjunctivitis still common in the Middle East, which can now be effectively treated with sulphacetamide. Scrupulous ward and theatre technique will avert postoperative infections, which must always be considered completely avoidable.

3. **Traumatic Blindness.** Industrial injuries from sparks or foreign bodies can cause blindness, and many of these are preventible if the visors and eyeshields which are provided are worn. Industrial nurses constantly seek to encourage workmen to use the protection provided for their sight.

4. **Neoplastic Blindness.** Of this one can only say that the search for a cure for malignant disease seems likely at some time to be successful.

5. **Functional Blindness.** Blindness is a not uncommon hysterical complaint, and its management is the province of the psychiatrist. Under this heading might be included the early detection and treatment of glaucoma, before it can cause loss of sight. This means that ophthalmic advice must be widely available and easily sought.

6. **Nutritional Blindness.** It is the duty of all people of developed countries to help those of emergent countries to raise their standard of diet.

7. **Degenerative Blindness.** Cataract is the main condition in which the surgeon can restore sight. In such conditions as diabetic and hypertensive retinitis the physician may by effective treatment prevent blindness.

Removal of Eye

The entire eye may be removed (*enucleation*), or the contents of the globe evacuated (*evisceration*). If the muscles of the eye can be retained and sutured, they will impart a suggestion of natural movement to the artificial eye which will later be fitted. It has already been said that the loss of an eye is a great blow to anyone, and since in many cases the operation is performed with little warning following injury or a diagnosis of malignant growth, the patient has had no time to prepare his thoughts. Relatives too will be much upset, and the brighter side of the picture must be presented to them when their first shock has subsided.

Artificial eyes are now made that match the good one very well. They must be taken out and washed daily, and the socket should be bathed clean. The utmost care must naturally be taken of artificial eyes when not being worn, e.g. if the patient has to go to the theatre.

WELFARE OF THE BLIND

Blind people are entered on the Blind Persons' Register after certification, and become eligible for the special welfare facilities provided for this group.

Babies need their mothers, and nurses can help the mother of a blind baby to understand his special difficulties. He finds it hard to learn to feed himself, and to recognize people and things. The baby who can see reaches out for things he sees and explores them. The blind baby must have objects presented to him to feel, and is encouraged to keep in touch with his surroundings by all the other senses he possesses. In cases of especial difficulty there are resident homes.

There are special schools for blind children in which they are educated by methods not involving the power of sight. They are prepared to earn a livelihood, and many are capable of this, either in a protected environment or in the ordinary labour market.

Local Authorities must make provision for providing workshops for the blind, and selling their products ; for providing residential homes where required, and hostels ; for arranging recreational facilities, and information. Blind people in this country are eligible for the Retirement Pension at the age of 40.

CHAPTER 25

UROLOGICAL NURSING

Affections of the urinary tract are much commoner in men than in women. Enlargement of the prostate gland in elderly men usually necessitates surgical treatment, and in addition new growths of the bladder, both innocent and malignant, affect men more frequently than women. Deposition of salts from the urine to form stones in the kidney, ureter or bladder is commoner in men than in women, probably because of the short wide female urethra which allows easier passage of minute fragments.

The work involved in a urological ward calls for keen observation and clinical insight, and efficient care and knowledge of the apparatus involved. It is sometimes thought that this apparatus is complicated and that a knowledge of physics is necessary to understand it, but this is not so. The main facts that a nurse needs to recognize are how a syphon works, and (more important still) that water normally tends to run down hill.

Investigations

All patients are investigated with a view to establishing their diagnosis, but in many urological patients it is necessary to know whether kidney function has become impaired to any extent that affects their general health. Kidney efficiency is of the greatest importance in deciding what treatment should be given.

Clinical Observations. The *temperature* indicates if infection is present, and how the patient responds to it ; the *pulse* is always important ; irregularities of *breathing* (e.g. Cheyne-Stokes respiration) should be reported at once. The *blood pressure* is often raised in association with chronic kidney disease. The record of fluid *intake* and *output* is probably the most important single observation that can be made. It must be complete if it is to be of any use, and now that so many patients are allowed up for toilet purposes, it is essential to have a system of marking urinals for subsequent measurement that patients can conveniently use. Metal numbers for attaching to handles are suitable. Frequency of micturition is another record that can be valuable ; stone in the bladder, for instance, may cause greatly increased frequency by day, but disturbs the patient little by night, because the stone moves away from the sensitive base of the bladder. Routine urine *tests* must be regularly carried out ; those for reaction, specific gravity, albumen, pus and blood, being the most informative. Inspection of the tongue is thought a little old-fashioned by some today, but a dry, brown tongue will suggest that a patient is dehydrated or uræmic faster than the pathologist can supply the information.

The *blood urea* should be estimated on admission, and whenever required afterwards. The normal range is 20 to 40 mg. per cent in an adult, and this amount comes from the breakdown of protein from the food, and from the normal wear and tear of body tissues. After physical injury or stress (e.g. operation) the blood urea may rise because of the increased breakdown of tissues, but this effect is transient, and in the absence of such a cause a rise in the blood urea indicates that the kidney is failing to remove this substance from the blood into the urine. It is dangerous to do an extensive operation, or to give by mouth or injection substances that have to be excreted by the kidney, if the blood urea is raised.

X-rays of the urinary tract may be plain, or a contrast medium can be used. Retrograde and intravenous pyelograms are described on p. 128, and from the last paragraph it will be seen that it is not wise to perform an intravenous pyelogram unless the blood urea is normal, since the failing kidney will not be able to excrete the dye. A cystogram alone may enable a diagnosis of bladder conditions, such as a diverticulum, or new growth, to be made. The dye is injected into the bladder after catheterization.

The tests of function, such as urea clearance (p. 115), are less used now than formerly. The results depend too much on such factors as the patient's ability to empty his bladder completely, and the accurate timing of specimens. Blood urea estimation is to most surgeons an adequate overall test of renal function.

Where there is any cause for belief that the bladder is not completely emptied by each act of micturition, the *residual* urine remaining in the bladder must be measured. A catheter is passed into the bladder immediately after the patient has endeavoured to empty it, and any urine is withdrawn and measured. This investigation may also be made during examination of the bladder by cystoscopy.

Cystoscopy

The cystoscope is a lighted instrument by means of which the bladder may be inspected after it has been distended with lotion. The maintenance and sterilization of these delicate and costly instruments is discussed on p. 416.

Cystoscopy may be performed under general anæsthesia, but a simple examination can be readily made after instillation of a local anæsthetic into the male urethra, while not even this is necessary for a female patient. If cystoscopy is done in the theatre, a sedative injection is often ordered beforehand to allay uneasiness, but in the less alarming atmosphere of an out-patient clinic this is omitted.

If cystoscopy alone is contemplated, a local shave is not necessary, but if it may be the prelude to operation, an abdominal and perineal shave should be given. Just before the examination (e.g. when the theatre trolley comes for the patient) the bladder must be emptied, so that any which is removed from the bladder when the cystoscope is inserted is residual urine.

The condition of the bladder walls, prostate gland and ureteric orifices can be observed, and the presence and nature of growths or stones noticed.

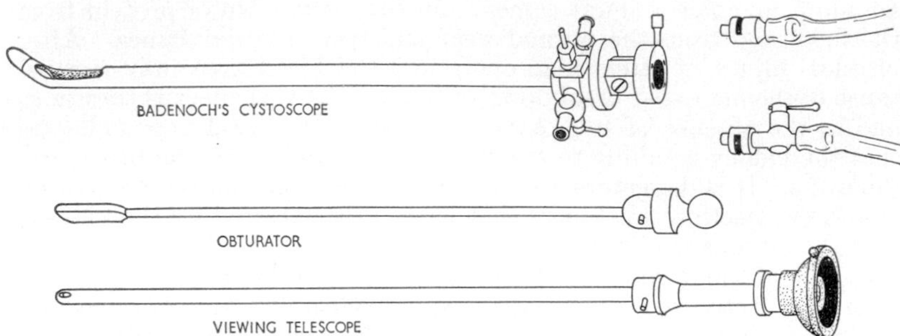

FIG. 87. Badenock's cystoscope (*from Urology for Nurses, James Robinson, Heinemann*).

UROLOGICAL SIGNS AND SYMPTOMS

Suppression and Retention of Urine

A patient who is not passing any urine is suffering from one of two conditions.

(*a*) *Suppression* of urine, or *anuria*, when no urine is being formed by the kidneys and the bladder is empty. It can be seen in acute nephritis, crushing injuries, following involvement of the ureters in new growth or injury, in toxæmia of pregnancy and in blockage by sulphonamides and some other drugs of the ureters. It is always a grave condition, since if unrelieved it will be fatal, and the cause must be found and appropriate treatment given (e.g. irrigation of the ureters through a catheterizing cystoscope in sulphonamide obstruction). The electrolyte balance is assessed daily, and if a favourable result can be hoped for, peritoneal dialysis or hæmodialysis is used in the hope of maintaining life until urine secretion returns.

(*b*) *Retention* of urine means inability to void it from the bladder where it accumulates. Relief is usually a fairly simple mechanical problem, and the importance of this condition depends on its cause, and whether it has been present long enough to cause dilatation of the ureters, and of the kidney pelvis (hydronephrosis) and perhaps renal failure.

Retention of urine, apart from the reflex retention seen in gynæcological wards, is uncommon in women because of the short urethra. In men, retention may occur acutely, with severe low abdominal pain, because of prostatic enlargement, urethral stricture, spinal injuries or following rectal operations. In urological wards the most important acute form is *clot retention* caused by bleeding into the bladder. The patient is unable to pass water, is in great pain, and in addition shows pallor, sweating and a rising pulse rate to indicate that hæmorrhage is taking place. Morphine 15 mg. is usually prescribed for the pain and to slow the bleeding, and the blood clot must be removed via a suitable catheter in the way described on p. 360.

Chronic retention is almost confined to men with slowly increasing enlargement of the prostatic gland. It is painless or nearly so, but the risk of kidney failure and uræmia supervening is great. It was at one time customary to pass a catheter into the bladder of such a patient, and decompress it by some apparatus that allowed the urine to drain away slowly. Quick emptying was thought to lead to uræmia, but now most surgeons prefer to perform the surgery that will be needed before the bladder is infected, which will be the inevitable result of catheterizing that atonic organ.

Hœmaturia is a common urological complaint ; it may be due to renal tuberculosis ; new growths of kidney or bladder ; stones in kidney, ureter or bladder ; injuries ; and to many medical conditions, such as acute nephritis, hæmorrhagic diseases or renal infarct. When it arises as a new symptom, a specimen of all urine passed should be saved to see whether bleeding is increasing or decreasing, and the possibility of clot retention, or the need of transfusion, must be borne in mind if the loss is more than slight.

Frequency of micturition is most often seen in cystitis ; the inflamed bladder walls give rise to pain as urine accumulates, and initiate the desire to micturate. Very acid urine may cause a similar state ; stones in the bladder ; new growth arising in its wall or infiltrating it from the cervix ; or chronic retention with overflow. *Precipitancy* means that the patient must empty the bladder as soon as he feels the desire ; it is a symptom of some nervous conditions, like disseminated sclerosis. *Strangury* is a continual painful desire to empty the bladder without the ability to do so, and is characteristic of severe cystitis.

CATHETERS

Catheters are extensively used in urology, and are made in a very great variety of materials, shapes and sizes. There are three main groups :

(*a*) Urethral catheters, used in the way their name implies.

(*b*) Suprapubic catheters, which are passed into the bladder through a suprapubic incision. They are larger than urethral catheters, since their purpose is to ensure adequate and free drainage. The indications for their use have markedly declined since the number of operations involving opening the bladder is much smaller than formerly. The only catheter now commonly used is a Foley-type one.

(*c*) Ureteric catheters are fine plastic graduated catheters used for passing into the ureters with a catheterizing cystoscope. They are also used for cardiac catheterization (p. 129).

Materials. Red rubber was for many years the commonest material for catheters, but it should not be used for urological purposes, since it sets up a reaction in tissues with which it is left in contact. Latex or plastic are the usual materials, they are inert when in contact with the urethra, and can be boiled as well as autoclaved.

Silver catheters are still occasionally used for female catheterization. They are easy to handle, and if the normal relations of the urethra are disturbed (for instance by an operation for stress incontinence) it may be easier to follow the lumen. It is in precisely these cases, however, that damage can be caused by a rigid catheter, and silver ones should be considered outdated.

Shapes. Catheters are made in five shapes :

(*a*) *Straight.* This kind has an eye near the tip, which is solid to prevent material from collecting in it, and to facilitate introduction. This is the commonest catheter shape; all the ones used for enemata, etc., are made like this.

(*b*) *Coudé.* Rigid catheters may be made with an obtuse angle behind the eye, said to assist passage through the prostate gland.

(*c*) *Olive-headed.* The solid tip is moulded to an oval shape that may enable narrow passages or strictures to be negotiated. *Bougies,* which are solid implements of catheter shape and size used to dilate the urethra, are usually olive-headed.

(*d*) *Whistle-ended.* The tip is open at an angle generally with one or two openings below it. Such catheters are used where drainage must be free, as in hæmaturia.

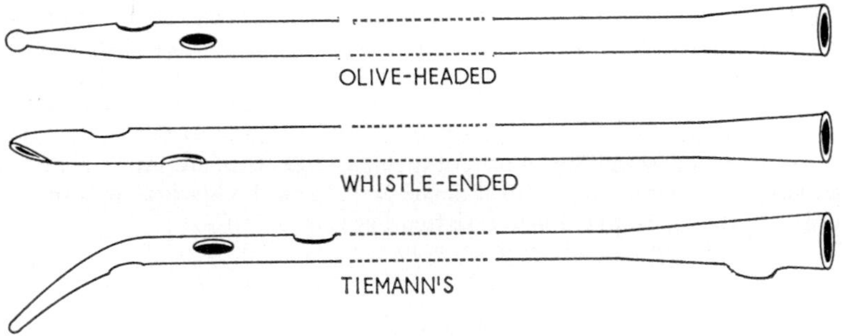

FIG. 88. Some types of urethral catheter.

The *Jacques* catheter is the familiar straight soft one with a single eye ; the *Harris* has two larger eyes, and is suitable for a bladder with blood clot in it. The Tiemann is a male catheter with a coudé end and an olive head ; at its distal end is a small ridge which indicates the direction in which the coudé end is pointing. It is useful for surmounting difficulties in passage, but not usually comfortable if left in the bladder. Many other varieties are made for special purposes; a flexible whistle-ended plastic catheter is useful as an indwelling catheter after prostatectomy.

Catheters are made in patterns which will enable them to remain in the bladder without external fixation, i.e. they are *self-retaining.* The Foley is popular for both sexes, and is a plastic catheter with a balloon beneath the eye that can be distended with water via a side-tube which must afterwards be secured. These balloons take 5, 10, etc., ml. of water, and the amount required is printed on the catheter; it is uncommon to use more than 30 ml., and most surgeons find the 5 ml. size adequate.

Non-disposable catheters must be most carefully cleaned; traces of protein congealed in them may lead to severe reactions if they are used

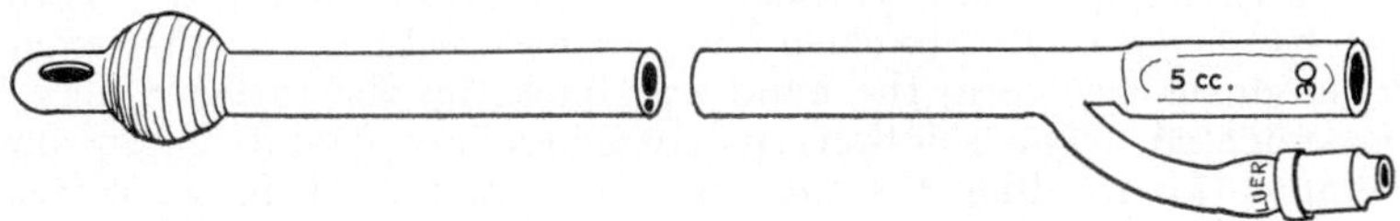

FIG. 89. Foley Catheter. The balloon can be inflated by inserting the nozzle of the charged syringe into the side arm. The amount required is printed on the catheter.

again in that state. They should at once be rinsed through under running water from the narrow (eye) end down, and the great advantage of semi-transparent ones is that any soiling of the interior can be seen. If blood was present, catheters may be syringed through with cetrimide, or soaked in hydrogen peroxide. Finally soap and water is used for the exterior, and hard brushes likely to scratch the surface must be avoided.

Sterilization. Disposable catheters are being used in increasing quantities, and these are supplied by manufacturers in sterile packs. The penalty of inefficient sterilization is bladder infection, and such methods as boiling or chemical disinfection should not be relied upon.

CATHETERIZATION

A catheter is passed into the bladder for these reasons :

1. To obtain a specimen for bacteriological examination. This used to be the commonest indication, but catheterization is rarely used for this purpose now. A clean specimen involves no risk of bladder infection and usually provides adequate information.
2. To relieve retention of urine.
3. To measure the residual urine.
4. As a precaution against urinary complications before resection of the rectum.
5. To ensure that the bladder is empty before pelvic operations.
6. To enable bloodclot to be evacuated, or a bladder washout to be performed.

The fact that it is such a common occurrence should never blind nurses to the fact that it carries with it a very serious risk of bladder infection. Cystitis means pain and discomfort to the patient, and if the bladder is atonic or paralysed an ascending infection may lead to pyelitis, which may become chronic, and eventually cause renal failure and death from uræmia. The infection can arise in three ways:

1. The part of the catheter entering the bladder may be contaminated by the operator's hand.
2. Ineffective cleansing of the meatus may lead to the introduction of organisms from the patient's skin.
3. The technique may be aseptic, but minor trauma to the mucous membrane or urethra or bladder may allow the bacteria that occasionally pass through the normal urinary tract without infecting it to settle in the inflamed mucosa and establish themselves.

All training schools devote much thought to the most effective way of dealing with these problems. The real point of difficulty is that both hands are needed to clean the meatus effectively, so that even if sterile gloves are worn, the hand that picks up the catheter may be contaminated. The solution lies in using forceps and a non-touch technique for handling the catheter, or picking it up in some sterile material (e.g. gauze). With regard to the third point, a lubricant such as sterile liquid paraffin or catheter jelly should be used for both sexes to facilitate introduction. A full-sized catheter should always be used ; it is not less traumatic than a fine one, and makes it easy to ensure that the bladder is empty.

The chief difficulty in catheterizing the female bladder is adequately to expose the meatus, and to prevent the labia minora touching it once it has been cleansed. In men the meatus is obvious, and the problem is to introduce the catheter along the long narrow urethra without trauma, a problem often intensified by the fact that an enlarged prostate gland or a stricture may have to be negotiated during passage. The account of catheterization given here represents only one solution ; there are others that are effective. The use of a non-touch technique, which does not rely on the " sterility " of the bare hand, is, however, one with which student nurses are familiar in doing dressings, and is readily understood.

Catheterizing the Female Patient

Trolley.

Top Shelf. Two sterile towels and about 8 swabs, in a dish or sterilized in a packet.
2 Jacques' or Harris' catheters (size 14 F for an adult) and a gallipot for lubricant, 2 kidney dishes, all sterile.
Kidney dish with 2 pairs dissecting forceps and 1 pair dressing forceps or Spencer Wells' forceps, sterile.
Covered jug of warm lotion.

Lower shelf. Sterile liquid paraffin or catheter jelly.
Sterile jar if a specimen is to be taken.
Jug or container for used instruments.
Jug of warm chloroxylenol lotion.
Waterproof and cover.
Treatment blanket.
Receiver for swabs, or pedal bin on floor.
Light, adequate and capable of being directed on the vulva.

Method. Catheterization can be done by a nurse singlehanded, if she arranges her equipment carefully, works methodically and has a co-operative patient. An assistant is however highly desirable.

The trolley is taken to the right side of the screened bed and must be within easy reach, so that the nurse has access to all the equipment on the top shelf with her right hand, while the left is holding the labia apart. The patient lies on her back with not more than two pillows, and if there is an air ring it is taken out. She may be feeling apprehension and embarrassment and while preparing her the nurse indicates that this small procedure is painless and soon over, and that the patient will be exposed as little as is necessary for effective work and for the minimum time. A relaxed patient is necessary for successful catheterization, and if necessary a few extra minutes spent in reassurance are well repaid.

The bedclothes are folded singly to knee level, the blanket put over the patient and the nightdress rolled neatly and securely up to the waist. The warm mackintosh and cover are slipped under the buttocks ; the patient is asked to flex the knees and abduct the thighs and the light is carefully adjusted. The blanket is replaced until the operator is ready ; protracted exposure is unpleasant and unnecessary.

The nurse passing the catheter should always help her assistant prepare the patient, so that she is satisfied that everything is correct. Some doctors will prefer that she now puts on a mask. She then goes and scrubs her nails and hands in warm running water for three minutes, while her assistant prepares the trolley. She removes one of the covering kidney dishes, handling it only on the outside, and fills it with warm lotion from the jug (Chloroxylenol 1 oz. to a pint; cetrimide 1%; and many similar lotions of antiseptic or other qualities have their advocates). A little liquid paraffin is put into the gallipot, and the sterile towels and swabs exposed.

When the operator returns she takes a sterile towel, dries her hands on it and discards it. This aseptic preparation is not strictly necessary in view of the fact that a non-touch technique is used, but if a self-retaining catheter is to be used (vide infra) some handling of the catheter is necessary, and it is confusing to have two different hand-preparations for such similar procedures. The assistant lifts the blanket on to the abdomen and places a sterile dish between the thighs, again being careful only to touch the exterior.

The operator transfers with forceps five of the sterile swabs to the lotion, picks up a sterile towel with forceps and lays it over the right thigh across which she is to work. Two dry swabs are taken in the left hand and used under the first two fingers of the left hand (or the index finger and thumb if that appears more natural) and these are inserted deeply between the labia minora, which are parted widely and drawn slightly upwards so that the fingers are supported against the pubis. The urethral meatus should now be visible with the clitoris above it and the vaginal orifice below. Full and adequate exposure is necessary for successful catheterization and unless the meatus is well exposed and confidently identified the position of the fingers is adjusted. After this the left hand must not be moved until the procedure has been completed.

A wet swab is taken with forceps, excess lotion is drained off against the inside of the dish, and the inner surface of the right labium majus cleaned with a downward movement of the swab, which is then thrown away. The left labium majus, the inner surfaces of both labia minora and lastly the urethral orifice are similarly treated, and if any excess moisture remains a dry, sterile swab is used on the meatus.

A catheter is lifted from the dish, with dressing or Spencer Wells forceps, about 1½ in. (4 cm.) from the eye end, which is dipped in liquid paraffin. The catheter is held at right angles to the blades of the forceps and must be secure. The open end of the catheter is dropped into the dish on the bed, and the eye end is passed gently and directly unto the orifice without touching the labia and passed inwards until the urine begins to flow. If by mischance the catheter should touch anything before insertion it is discarded and the second one used. When urine ceases to flow, the catheter is taken out and the labia dried with sterile swabs. The mackintosh is removed, the bed remade and the patient thanked.

The urine is measured and a specimen saved. All equipment is washed and boiled, special care being taken that all liquid paraffin remaining is thoroughly washed off with soap and hot water before the gallipot goes in the sterilizer.

Indwelling Catheters. If a catheter is to be left in the bladder, it must be a self-retaining one of a special pattern. The Foley catheter is popular for both sexes, and its management is described under male catheterization.

Infection is almost inevitable if an indwelling catheter is used. It may be minimized by scrupulous working technique ; the avoidance of rubber catheters ; cleaning the catheter once or twice a day with cetavlon or liquid paraffin where it leaves the urethra ; careful toilet of the vulva ; maintaining a high fluid intake ; and perhaps the administration of a sulphonamide or antibiotic.

CATHETERIZING THE MALE PATIENT

The chief problems in connection with passing a catheter into the male bladder are that at least 8 in. of catheter must be passed along the urethra which is narrow in calibre, and that in a great many cases the patient is suffering either from an obstruction which necessitates skilful passage, or a paralytic lesion that demands the most scrupulous technique if infection is to be avoided. Doctors and male nurses in particular have devoted much thought to the problems involved, and the solutions reached have included the following :

1. The hands are scrubbed, dried on a sterile towel, and the catheter passed with the bare hand. This is the oldest way, but sterility of the skin cannot be relied on.
2. A sterile cotton mitten is drawn on to the right hand before using the catheter, after cleansing the meatus.
3. A non-touch technique using forceps is adopted, which ensures sterility of the catheter. If the catheter is flexible, as are the majority today, care must be taken not to allow the distal end of the catheter to become unsterilized, and a well-known spinal injuries unit advocates that an assistant supports this end with sterile forceps while the dresser inserts the catheter.
4. Sterile gloves are used. This method is especially useful where obstruction is severe, since the fingers alone are more sensitive than through the mediation of forceps.

The method chosen will depend on the circumstances of the unit and the type of staff performing the catheterization. Whichever is used, a lubricant is necessary ; liquid paraffin or catheter jelly is reliable

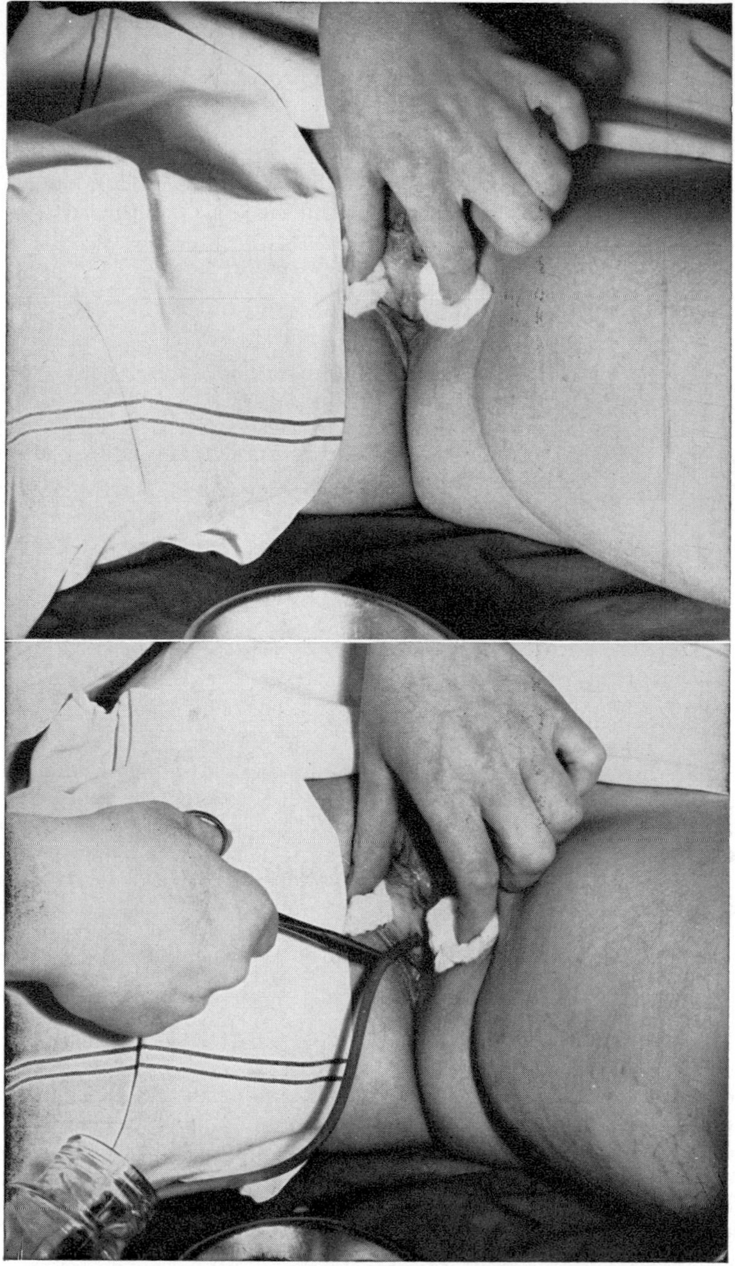

FIG. 90. Passing a catheter by a non-touch technique.

and cheap, but if difficulty is likely to be met, an anæsthetic lubricant like xylocaine ointment may be preferred. The equipment listed below is for catheterization by the forceps technique. Local cleanliness is ensured with soap and water before the procedure begins.

Trolley.

Top.

Sterile.
- Catheter pack with necessary catheters.
- 2 kidney dishes.
- Instrument tray with 3 pairs forceps, 2 gallipots and 2 gauze swabs for holding the penis and the catheter.
- Packet of towels and swabs.

Sterile jar if a specimen is required.

Bottom.

Waterproof and cover.
Blanket.
Container for used forceps.
Cetrimide, sterile liquid paraffin, catheter jelly.
Receiver for swabs, or pedal bin.

If a Foley catheter is being used, add these articles for inflating the balloon. Sterile water is used in case rupture of the balloon occurs.

Sterile.
- Syringe, 5 ml. or required size.
- Tubb's adaptor.
- Distilled water.
- Gallipot.
- Introducer.
- Spencer Wells' forceps.

Bladder Irrigation

Bladder washouts are far less frequent than formerly ; infection can be more effectively dealt with by chemotherapy, and the trauma associated with repeated catheterization or an indwelling catheter is in itself conducive to infection. Should such a washout be required, the following will be needed once a urethral or suprapubic catheter is in position :

Sterile.
- Sterile Barrington bladder syringe, or sterile disposable syringe.
- Jug of sterile lotion, e.g. Hibitane 1 in 5,000.

Lotion thermometer.
Mackintosh and towel.
Treatment blanket.

The temperature of the lotion should be 100° F. (38° C.), and a thermometer should always be used. Great care must be taken to exclude air from the syringe, with the point uppermost. Not more than one syringeful must be injected at a time, and if a bladder operation has been performed, or the patient's capacity is limited, 2 oz. (60 mls.) is enough.

If a catheter is blocked by blood clot, injection of fluid into the bladder is dangerous (see p. 368, prostatectomy), and must never be undertaken without the surgeon's direct instructions.

Irrigation. The apparatus illustrated shows a closed system for bladder irrigation, which may be set up in the theatre, Sterile lotion drips from the upper bottle into the bladder at a rate controlled by the

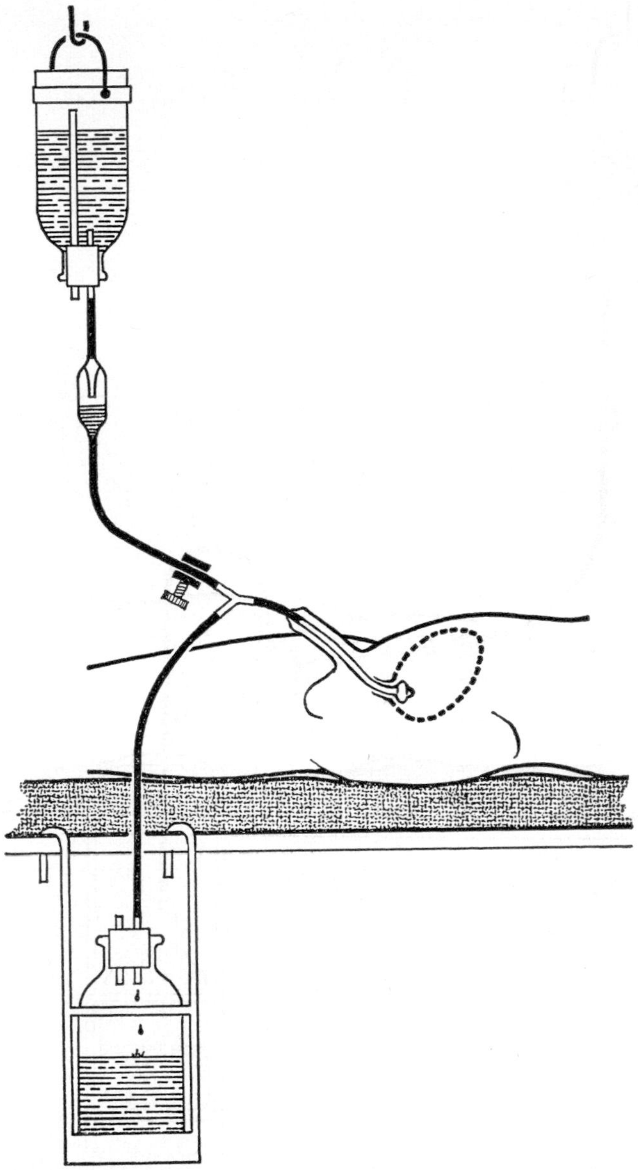

FIG. 91. A closed sterile apparatus for post-operative irr igation of the bladder.

clip. From the bladder it flows out into the lower bottle, displacing the air through the short tube. When this is full, the bung and its glass tubes should be transferred without contaminating it to a fresh sterile bottle. The amount of irrigating lotion should be substracted from the total to find the amount of urine secreted.

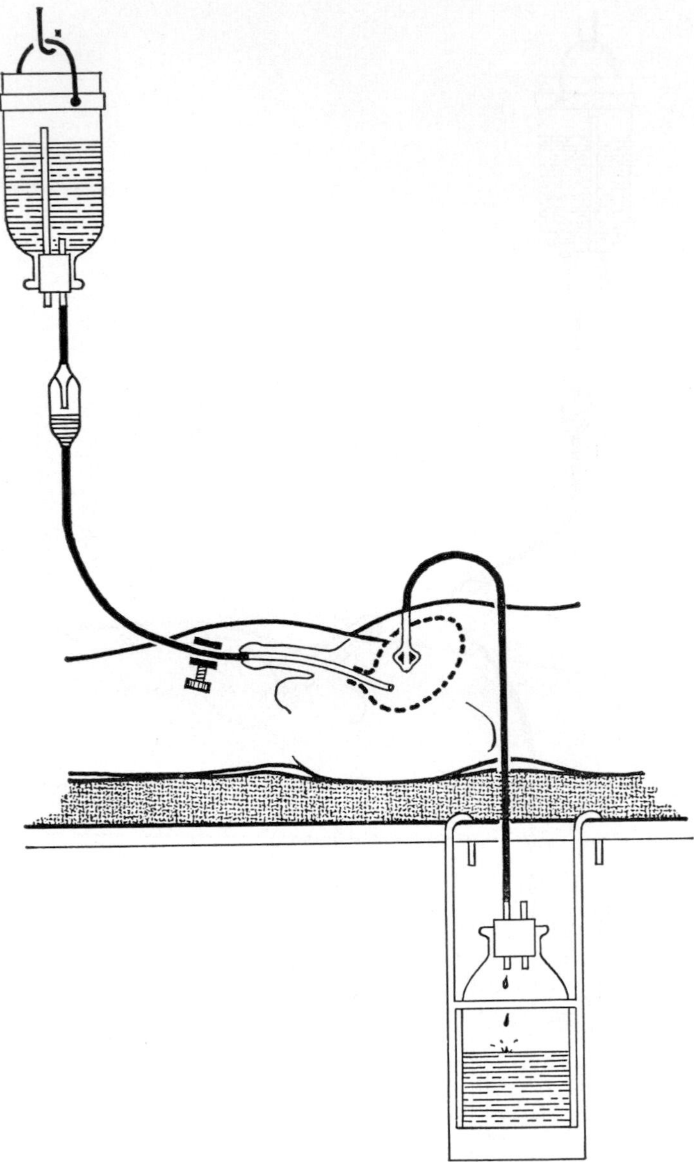

Fig. 92. A method of irrigation to prevent clot-retention of urine after bladder operations.

Decompression of the Bladder

It was once the custom, when patients presented with chronic retention of urine, to insert a urethral catheter and decompress the bladder slowly. Such cases are usually men with prostatic obstruction, and in this country men now present earlier than at one time for surgical treatment, and it is not common to see patients with gross distension of the bladder and impaired renal function. Those who wish to decrease gradually the amount of urine in a distended bladder either spigot the catheter and release 10 ozs. (300 ml.) of urine 2 hourly, or control the rate of outflow with a clip on the tubing. Whatever method is used, the nurse must see that a confused patient does not pull the connection or spigot out of the catheter, and so allow the bladder to empty at once.

Indwelling Male Catheters

The management of an indwelling catheter is of great importance for the patient's comfort and freedom from infection. Its presence causes irritation of the urethra with increased secretion, and if this secretion is allowed to dry on the catheter it will damage the mucous membrane, and possibly lead to stricture formation later. An antiseptic and lubricant dressing, such as flavine and liquid paraffin gauze, is wound around the catheter where it enters the penis and kept lightly in place. Toilet of the catheter must be performed daily. Crusts are removed with cetrimide or liquid paraffin, and the dressing changed.

A self-retaining catheter needs no extra means of securing it, but others will have to be tied in place. Two pieces of tape, each 9 in. long, are knotted at their centres below the catheter dressing, and the four ends brought up alongside the shaft of the penis, to which they are secured by a ½-in. strip of elastoplast. This must be applied with no stretching at all, or œdema of the gland and intense discomfort will be caused.

The catheter dressing must be changed daily, and any signs of inflammation reported. Sedation at night is usually necessary or confused or elderly patients will pull out their catheters.

The glass connection to the drainage tubing must be straight-sided, not tapering, to allow free flow, and the tubing long enough to permit movement, but secured to the drawsheet. The drainage receiver may be a sterile jar, or a graduated disposable plastic bag. Most ward sisters prefer to use a jar in the immediate post-operative period, when it is important to see clearly the amount of hæmaturia, and whether drainage is continuous. The best position is about a metre from the foot of the bed. If the tubing passes straight over the side of the bed into a jar, it is easy to tuck it in with the drawsheet, and so cause acute retention of urine, and if the jar is at this level, it will be knocked by anyone attending to the patient. Supports are available for attaching jars to the bedside where they are visible, but not exposed to the hazards met on the floor. Tubing and jars should be sterilized daily.

If urine is not draining, the nurse should first assure herself that the tube is not obstructed in some way, as by a clip left closed on it. If an intermittent irrigating apparatus is being used, solution is run into the bladder, in the hope that this will free the catheter. If it does not, the drainage tube should be " milked ", which will exert suction on it, and if this is ineffective a sterile Higginson's syringe with the valve reversed may be used.

SOME UROSURGICAL CONDITIONS

Certain principles apply to all patients with surgical conditions of the urinary tract.

1. The intake and output of all patients must be accurately and regularly recorded.
2. The fluid intake must be kept high (5 or 6 pints or about 3,000 ml. per diem for adults). This is of especial importance if drugs of the sulpha group are being given, in order to keep them in solution in the urine.
3. The urine should be tested daily.
4. Hæmorrhage, both reactionary and secondary, is excessively common after bladder operations, and nurses must be vigilant to detect its early beginnings. Urinary infection is the other troublesome complication.

Operations on the Kidney

Nephrectomy. Removal of a kidney may be performed for cancer ; for tuberculosis, somewhat less frequently than formerly and after adequate medical preparation ; for suppuration (*pyonephrosis*) and for injuries. Investigation beforehand is directed towards ensuring that the kidney remaining is a healthy one. The pre-operative shave should cover the area from shoulder to pelvis, from the midline in front to the spine and including the axilla.

The patient will return with a round or corrugated drain in the wound, which is a large one following the lower border of the ribs. He should be given a post-operative injection early, as this incision is a very painful one, and it is desirable to keep him lying towards the operated side to promote drainage and prevent hæmatoma formation. Intravenous fluid is rarely needed, and fluid intake should not be unduly pressed for the first day or two, so that the sound kidney may be able to adjust gradually to the increased work. The ube may be removed after the second day.

Heminephrectomy is removal of part of a kidney. There is an increased liability to hæmorrhage after operation from the kidney and careful watch on the dressing and pulse must be kept. As the operated kidney secretes, small blood clots will be washed down the ureter causing renal colic. If severe, it can be treated by the methods mentioned below, but usually if the patient understands the cause of the pain, he does not find it too uncomfortable. An indwelling catheter in the bladder is often used to avert the possibility.

Pyeloplasty is performed to reduce the size of a dilated renal pelvis, and to widen the pelvi-ureteric junction. If the kidney substance is normal, good results will be obtained, but where it has atrophied from pressure by the hydronephorsis, nephrectomy will be the operation selected.

Surgical Conditions of the Ureter

Small stones formed in the kidney pass into the water, and the peristalsis they provoke initiates severe pain called *renal colic*, felt along the course of the ureter, and often accompanied by restlessness, sweating, pallor and vomiting. Morphine will relieve the pain, and probanthine or atropine will relax the ureter and probably allow the stone to pass into the bladder and thence to the exterior. Fluids must be freely taken, and the urine collected to observe when the stone is passed.

Should the stone fail to pass out of the ureter, it will have to be removed. The first method tried will be by means of an operating cystoscope, by which the surgeon endeavours to pass a catheter past the stone in an attempt to dislodge it, or a minute basket to catch it. Failing this, ureterolithotomy will have to be performed from the abdomen. In either case, an X-ray is taken on the morning of the operation to ensure that the stone has not moved.

Cancer of the Bladder

Cancer of the bladder is a disease with a bad prognosis, and for many cases surgical relief is impossible. If retention of urine occurs, a urethral catheter may be necessary, and the chief nursing problem will be adequate relief of the pain which is intense with bladder growths. Deep X-ray or radium treatment is sometimes tried, but these growths are not normally very sensitive to radiotherapy. The cobalt bomb appears to give slightly better results than older methods.

In a suitable case, partial cystectomy may give relief, and if a ureter is involved, it may be transplanted into another part of the bladder. In a few cases it is possible to transplant the ureters elsewhere, and remove the bladder completely (total cystectomy). The ureters may be implanted :

(*a*) Into the sigmoid colon. Pre-operative sterilization of the bowel with antibiotics will be ordered, with vitamin supplements, and the prothrombin level of the blood is checked since a fall may indicate the possibility of hæmorrhage. The great dangers are ascending pyelitis and œdema of the ureteric openings leading to suppression of urine. After operation a rectal tube is kept in place, draining the urine into a jar until secretion is well established, when the patient is gradually encouraged to gain control over the rectal passage of urine.

(*b*) Into an ileal conduit. Such an artificial bladder is also constructed in connection with pelvic exenteration, and for children with incontinence due to spina bifida. A loop of ileum and its mesentery is isolated and continuity of the bowel re-established. One end of the ileal conduit is closed, the ureters are transplanted into it, and the other end is brought out on to the abdominal wall to discharge the urine into a polythene bag.

(*c*) The sigmoid colon can be detached from the rectum, and brought out onto the abdominal wall to discharge the fæces through a colostomy. The rectum is thus isolated, and can serve as a " bladder " if the ureters are transplanted into it.

Following operation, treatment centres on the re-establishment of bowel function, following what is virtually a resection of gut and the draining of the ileal bladder. An indwelling intragastric Ryle's tube, and intravenous fluids are used and the blood chemistry is constantly checked. Such symptoms of electrolyte unbalance as drowsiness, muscle weakness and dry tongue must be watched for, and the urinary output meticulously measured. After the first week the patient may be fitted with a bag of a more permanent kind ; Koenig, Salt, and Rutzen are examples. These adhere to the abdominal wall which must be perfectly dry when they are applied and the urine drains into a bag with a tap at the bottom.

Papilloma

The commonest new growth is the papilloma, a growth which is potentially malignant. It causes hæmaturia and must be treated early and thoroughly by diathermy with an operating cystoscope, for though this growth is innocent at first, it shows a pronounced tendency to recur, and the ones that do this frequently become cancerous later. The patient must return every three months for a year for cystoscopy, first under general anæsthesia and then later in an out-patient clinic if results are negative. The intervals between reporting are gradually lengthened as a permanent cure appears to have been achieved.

Stones may be crushed and small foreign bodies removed via the urethra, but removal of big stones, or treatment of large papillomata, or relief of chronic retention of urine with impaired kidney function entails opening the bladder from above the symphysis pubis.

Suprapubic Cystotomy

Suprapubic cystotomy, as this operation is named, is less common than once, now that few prostatectomies are performed by this route. In order to heal the bladder wound without fear of urine leaking into the peritoneal cavity, the bladder must usually be drained for ten days until healing is complete.

If a transverse incision into the bladder below the peritoneum has been used, a urethral catheter will suffice, while a small corrugated drain is inserted between the bladder and the symphysis pubis. The patient returns with a spigot in the catheter, which must be released at once.

If the bladder has been widely opened, a suprapubic catheter may be stitched into place for forty-eight hours and then removed. The small retropubic drainage tube will be taken out in three to five days, and the urethral catheter will remain up to ten days.

Suprapubic cystotomy for enlargement of the prostate with the purpose of improving impaired kidney function by free drainage entails keeping the suprapubic catheter in place for some months. Before discharge the patient is fitted with a narrow rubber belt, which maintains the catheter in position, and a bag into which the urine constantly drains. The catheter must only be changed by a doctor, but the patient may be shown how to insert it in case it accidentally comes out. In most cases it is hoped that the prostate gland that is causing the obstruction can be removed later, but sometimes the apparatus must be retained permanently.

Suprapubic Fistula

When a suprapubic catheter is removed, a fistula remains between the bladder and the abdominal wall. Although urine will leak from this, provided that flow via the urethra is unimpeded the hole will rapidly close, and usually in twenty-four hours there is no further leakage. An adequate intake of vitamin C is helpful to healing. When such a catheter is taken out, therefore, a piece of tulle gras is put over the opening, and a firm wool dressing strapped on, and a good result may be expected. If there is any obstruction to urethral drainage, or the fistula is large and the patient very elderly, urine may discharge via the abdominal wall, and recourse to another method must be had. This will usually be a Chiron bag, of the kind used for patients with an ileostomy. The skin must be dry before the bag is applied.

If the fistula fails to heal, it must be repaired by the surgeon.

ENLARGEMENT OF THE PROSTATE GLAND

Any but minor degrees of prostatic enlargement are treated by surgery. These patients may present as emergencies, with acute or chronic retention of urine, or may be admitted for a planned operation. In all of them careful assessment by the nursing and medical observations at the beginning of this chapter should be made, and three types of operation exist.

(*a*) Retropubic or Millin operation. The incision passes between the symphysis pubis and the bladder, which is not opened. This is the commonest type of prostatectomy today because it does not entail the use of a suprapubic catheter.

(*b*) Transurethral resection. The operation is performed via the urethra with a diathermy loop or a cold punch. The gland is not dissected out, but the middle lobe is pared away to allow uninterrupted passage of the urine. It is especially suitable for the old and frail.

(*c*) Classical suprapubic operation. The bladder is opened and the prostate enucleated from within it, and the prostatic bed closed and left dry. A suprapubic catheter is used.

After retropubic prostatectomy, the patient returns to the ward with an indwelling urethral catheter in situ and a small drain in the retropubic space. Sometimes the surgeon leaves an antiseptic (e.g. hibitane 1 in 5,000) in the bladder, and likes the spigot to be kept in the catheter for an hour. Whichever method is used, the catheter is joined with a sterile straight-sided connection to rubber tubing draining into a jar. The circulatory and respiratory functions are carefully assessed, and as consciousness returns and the condition warrants, pillows are gradually inserted. A blood transfusion is quite often needed.

Meanwhile continuous observation of the fluid draining is maintained, and a little experience is needed to decide whether anything but pure blood is flowing. If the drainage is interrupted, steps must be taken at once to re-establish it, and a five-minute record of the pulse is instituted to ensure that the bleeding in quantity into the bladder does not take place unnoticed. The surgeon should be informed, and the bedclothes divided so that easy access to the catheter is secured without uncovering and disturbing the patient. The surgeon may adopt the method illustrated here to ensure that clot retention does not occur. Sterile lotion drips into the bladder through the urethral catheter and out through a suprapubic one. When the urine is free of blood, the suprapubic catheter is first spigotted and then removed at about 48 hours. On the fourth or fifth day the wound drain is removed, and if all is well the urethral catheter is taken out the next day.

Bladder washouts (p. 148) are falling into disuse in connection with clot retention and bleeding from the bladder. It is easy to force fluid through a catheter containing loose clot, but the fluid does not return, and the bladder is still further distended. Suction on the catheter by means of a Barrington bladder syringe or a disposable syringe with a well-fitting bulb is more effective and less dangerous. If blood clot is allowed to distend the bladder, pain will render still worse the shock associated with the blood loss.

Although reactionary hæmorrhage is common, many patients pass through this period with only moderate loss. By the next day the patient should be sitting up on an air ring, drinking well and eating light meals if he feels able. The flavine and paraffin dressing round the catheter is changed and the connection and tubing washed and boiled on this and every subsequent day in which they remain in use. The blood in the urine should be less bright than on the preceding day.

The retropubic drain is removed between the 4th and 5th post-operative day, and if the urine is free from blood and the condition satisfactory, the patient may get up on the following day. On the sixth day the catheter is taken out, and on the eighth day the stitches will be removed. After a fortnight the patient should be discharged to convalescence, emptying the bladder easily and not too frequently.

From the fifth day to the fifteenth, however, there is a risk of secondary hæmorrhage due to infection of the prostatic bed. Such bleeding may be slight or alarming in proportions, and it is necessary in all but the minor cases to pass a catheter and evacuate the blood clot from the bladder.

Apart from hæmorrhage and bladder infection, complications are not numerous. Pulmonary embolism is rare now that patients can be got up early, and pneumonia is uncommon. A high fluid intake, meticulous catheter cleanliness and watchfulness for the first signs of bleeding should keep the incidence of trouble to a minimum.

SURGICAL CONDITIONS OF THE URETHRA

Few surgical conditions affect the female urethra, but rupture of the male urethra is a well-known complication of fracture of the pelvis. If it is suspected that injury to the urethra has occurred, the patient should be taken to the theatre, and a urethrogram performed. The treatment for rupture of the urethra is to establish a suprapubic cystotomy and to repair the urethra later. Subsequently bougies will be passed regularly to ensure that a fibrous stricture does not develop at the site of rupture.

Urethral stricture from gonococcal urethritis is becoming uncommon, but a patient with a stricture, whatever the cause, is encouraged to attend regularly for dilatation of the stricture.

Circumcision is needed when the foreskin is too tight to be retracted behind the glans. It is performed as a ritual on all Jewish boy babies, without an anæsthetic, and with little subsequent inconvenience apparently to the baby. Older boys have an anæsthetic, while local anæsthesia can be used for adults. The operation involves removing part of the foreskin on its dorsal aspect, and uniting skin and mucous membrane with a stitch or two. Friar's balsam and a little ribbon gauze is a satisfactory and convenient dressing.

CHAPTER 26

ORTHOPÆDIC NURSING

THE word "orthopædic" would seem to imply that this branch of surgery is concerned only with straightening children, but patients of all ages and many sorts of complaints are seen in the orthopædic wards, with lesions of bones, joints and their associated structures, and muscles. The diversity of causes can be seen from the following examples :

1. **Congenital.** Bones may be missing or imperfectly developed, extra fingers or toes may be present.

2. **Traumatic.** This is a very large group, comprising fractures, dislocations, injuries to tendons, ligaments and cartilages.

3. **Infective.** There are acute conditions like osteomyelitis and chronic ones of which tuberculosis is the most important. Tuberculosis of bones and joints is a bovine infection, and children are the usual victims. Pasteurisation of milk has greatly reduced the number of such infections, which often entailed years of treatment in orthopædic hospitals.

4. **Neoplastic.** Tumours, both innocent and malignant, occur in bone.

5. **Degenerative.** Such acquired deformities as bunions can be considered as part of this group, and osteoarthritis, especially of the hip, provides many long-stay patients.

The methods of treatment and of auxiliary therapy that are available are :

(*a*) Immobilization.
(*b*) Operation.
(*c*) Manipulation.
(*d*) Physiotherapy.
(*e*) Occupational therapy.

Reference to the last two items is made in Chapter 34, and the ways in which the first three are used and the nursing problems involved are discussed below.

IMMOBILIZATION

Rest allows inflamed or injured tissue to heal, and since in orthopædic conditions the parts involved are often bones or joints, movement must be completely prevented if healing is to take place following a fracture, or after a joint operation. The means used to achieve this are splints, plasters, or internal fixation.

Splints

Splints have been less commonly used since the introduction of plaster of Paris, and many types which were bulky, unphysiological or unable to produce perfect immobilization have now become obsolete. Among the ones which the nurse may meet are these :

1. *Thomas's* splint is a metal one used for fractures of the femur and

some hip conditions. At one end is a padded ring which fits into the groin, at the other is a kink in the metal frame round which cord or bandage can be secured. When it is required for use, one must be selected which is correct for length and ring size and prepared by fastening strips of material about 4 in. in width across the splint, and pinning or clipping them to form a cradle on which the leg can rest. Flannel is the traditional material, but stitched calico bands can be laundered and re-used, and do not stretch like flannel does. The heel must project over the edge of the lowest strip, and a pad is placed under the knee to relax it a little.

If immobilization of the leg with the knee straight is undesirable a flexion iron is screwed on to the sides of the splint (as shown in Fig. 99, p. 377) at the level of the joint, and splint dressing is continued along the flexion piece. A footpiece is also available which is fixed to the flexion piece and dressed in the same way, but is not as much used as the other parts of this valuable splint.

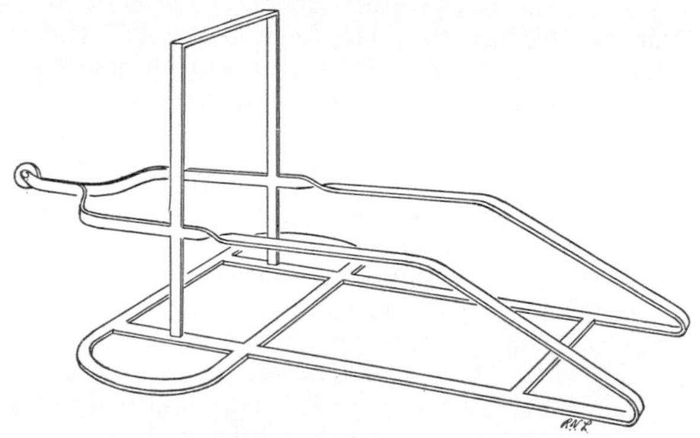

FIG. 93. Braun's splint.

2. *Braun's* splint is a metal frame, dressed like a Thomas's splint, which rests on the bed and supports the leg with the knee partly flexed. The upper part of the splint serves to keep the bedclothes from the dorsiflexed foot, and there is a pulley at the end for traction purposes. It is used for fractures of the lower leg and of the femur just above the knee.

3. The *gallows* splint is a wooden frame which is often used to immobilize the legs of infants under the age of two. It is placed over the trunk at hip level, and the legs are fastened by skin traction (p. 372) to the overhead beam. The traction must be enough to raise the buttocks clear of the bed, since this splint is used to reduce the nursing problems of keeping apparatus clean and dry in a child who has not yet achieved continence.

4. *Denis Browne* splints are used to correct the deformity of club foot in infants. Two metal supports for the foot and ankle are attached to a cross bar, and are adjustable.

5. The *straight* splint is a rectangular wooden one which is padded. It is widely used to support the hand and forearm during a blood transfusion, but the orthopædic surgeon no longer requires it.

6. The *back* splint is similar, but has a foot piece and is used for the ankle and knee if temporary immobilization is necessary. For instance, if a loose body is to be removed from the knee joint, the knee should be X-rayed with the leg firmly bandaged to a back splint which is not taken off until the patient is anæsthetized, when the loose body should be found in the situation indicated in the X-ray.

7. A *cock-up* splint is a metal one, mitten-shaped, and useful for resting a hand in the dorsi-flexed position. Injured or septic hands can be supported on it, and there are right- and left-handed varieties.

8. *Plastic* splints. Light-weight splints can be moulded from plastic sheets. They are very useful for supporting paralysed parts which could not bear the weight of a heavy splint or plaster.

9. *Inflatable* splints are useful and comfortable first aid equipment. If over-inflated there is a risk that they may interfere with the blood supply to the limbs, but if the splint is blown up by mouth rather than with a pump this risk is avoided.

An efficiently applied splint suitable for its purpose should be capable of immobilizing a fracture that has been reduced. There are some fractures, and some other conditions, in which traction must be exerted during the period of immobilization.

TRACTION

Traction means " pulling," and is a process used by the orthopædic surgeon for such purposes as to keep inflamed joint surfaces apart (as in infective arthritis) ; to maintain unstable injuries (as in fracture-dislocation of the thumb) ; and especially in the treatment of fractures of the shaft of the femur, where spasm of the strong thigh muscles causes over-riding of the broken ends unless it is overcome.

The means by which this pull is to be made and maintained involve an understanding of the mechanical principles involved, which are apt to be discouraging to female students, though men find no difficulty in it. This is perhaps because the fractured femur fully equipped with splint, cords going in different directions, weights and pin and pulleys, looks confusing, but if the essentials are considered, the difficulties should disappear. Since traction is most used for the leg, this is the kind which will be described.

If a pull is to be exerted on the leg, the apparatus making it must be attached to the leg in some ways, and there are two structures which may be used—the skin and the bone—and on this basis traction may be thought of as *skin* or *skeletal.*

Skin Traction

This pull is usually made by means of elastoplast applied to the side of the leg, and before it is used a patch test to eliminate the possibility of skin sensitivity is a wise precaution.

Requirements. Shaving tray.
Friar's balsam, gallipot, brush or swab.
Traction elastoplast.
Tape measure.

Requirements (contd.)

Scissors.
Orthopædic felt.
Spreader.
Blind cord.
4-in. Domette or crepe bandages.
Gamgee or brown wool pads to cover leg.
Receiver.

Traction elastoplast is inelastic in its length so that it will not stretch when pulled out, but can be stretched crosswise so that it can be moulded to fit flat on to the limb. The spreader is a square of wood, with a hole in its centre and a piece of webbing with buckles at each end fastened to it, as shown in the illustration. Its function, as the name implies, is to spread apart the strapping which forms the skin traction, and to provide somewhere to which to attach the cord by which the pull is made.

Method. The strapping is usually applied to both sides of the leg from the level of the head of the tibia to above the malleoli, and this length is measured. The leg is shaved, and then painted with Friars' Balsam to obviate skin irritation from the elastoplast. Two strips of plaster are cut, each 20 in. longer than the length of the leg, laid sticky side uppermost on a flat surface, and the excess 20 in. is folded in half so that the sticky surfaces adhere evenly to each other. Each

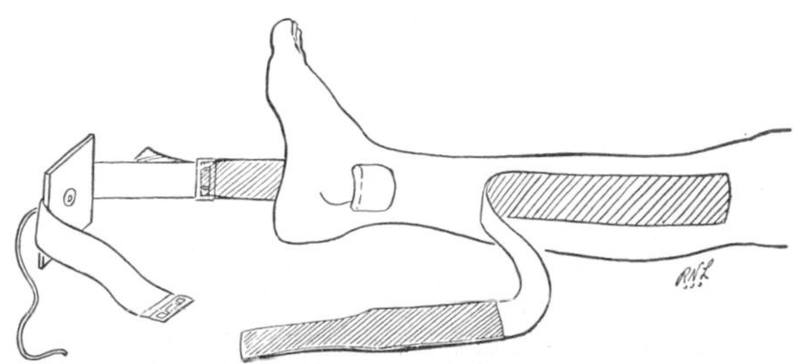

FIG. 94. Applying the extension plaster for skin traction. The plaster must not adhere to the malleoli, which receive additional protection from a pad proximal to them.

is then applied to the leg, starting at the ankle just above the malleolus where the margin adjoining the folding portion is attached. It must be without wrinkles, and must on no account adhere to the malleoli or the skin will be pulled off them. If they are very prominent a strip of orthopædic felt or wool can be laid above them, and care must be taken to use a spreader large enough to keep the strapping clear of them.

Bandages are applied evenly and firmly over the strapping to help keep it in place ; encircling turns of plaster must not be used. The loose ends of the elastoplast are trimmed to the size of the buckles on the spreader and fastened into them ; a length of cord is knotted into the hole in the centre of the spreader, and this cord can be used to exert traction in one of two ways.

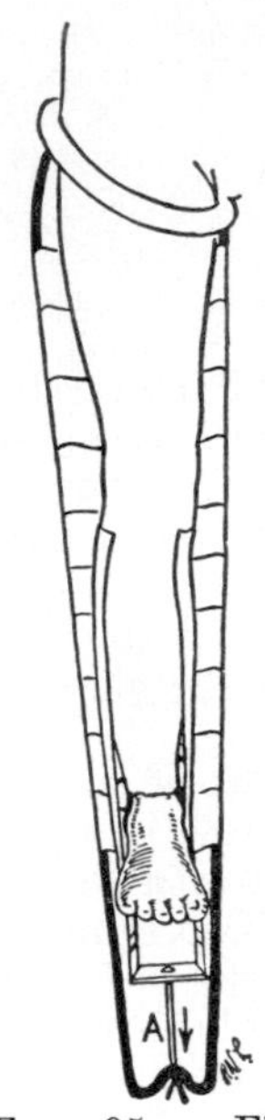

FIG. 95. Fixed skin traction. Tightening the cord A increases the traction.

Fixed Traction. A Thomas's splint is prepared with flannel bandages and put on the leg. If the traction cord is passed over the splint and tightened, the ring of the splint is pressed into the groin and the foot is drawn down towards the end of the splint and traction is exerted on the leg. The pressure in the groin would be very uncomfortable, but can be obviated by tying the end of the splint to the foot of the bed, which is then raised on blocks. The tension on the leg remains the same, but the patient's weight now tends to move away from the ring of the splint, and the pressure is relieved.

The amount of traction cannot be accurately estimated by this means, so it would not be suitable for a fractured femur, but might be used to straighten an arthritic knee, or is useful as a means of immobilizing a leg before a patient is transported to another hospital.

The next method is more useful.

Sliding Traction. A splint is not necessarily used for this. A bed-end pulley of the pattern illustrated is fixed to the foot of the bed, the traction cord is passed over the wheel, and a weight attached to it. As before, the end of the b ed must be raised on blocks, as in all forms of traction, so that the patient is not pulled down the bed. It will be

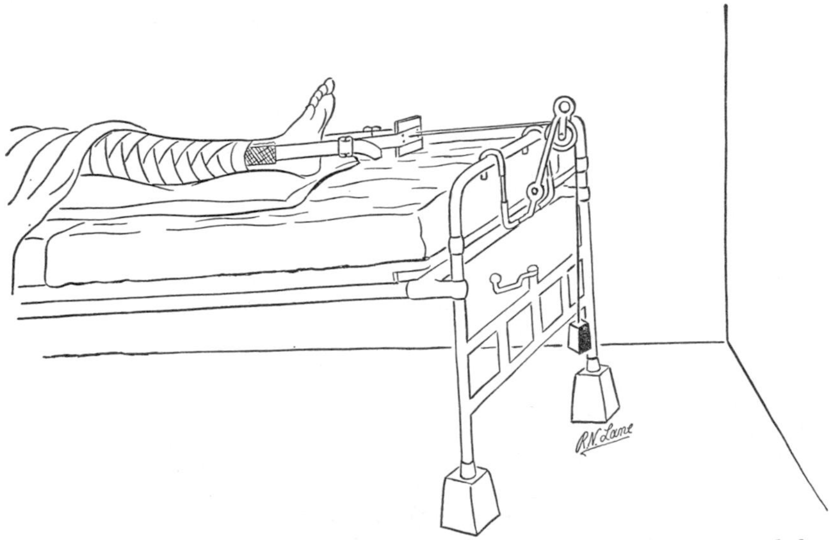

FIG. 96. Sliding traction. Skin traction has been applied to the leg, and the weight hangs over a pulley on a bed-end extension. Notice that the foot of the bed is raised.

seen at once that this allows a change of position without altering the amount of traction ; if the patient sits up in bed, the weight is drawn up the bed because the cord can move over the pulley, and if he lies down the weight sinks again.

In both of these cases the foot is unsupported, and must be constantly exercised to avoid foot drop, while a cradle is used to prevent hindrance of movement by the bedclothes. If a weight is used it must hang freely without touching the bed. It should be noticed that in both cases the knee is kept straight and if it is desirable to have the knee flexed, as it is during long periods of immobilization, skeletal instead of skin traction will have to be used.

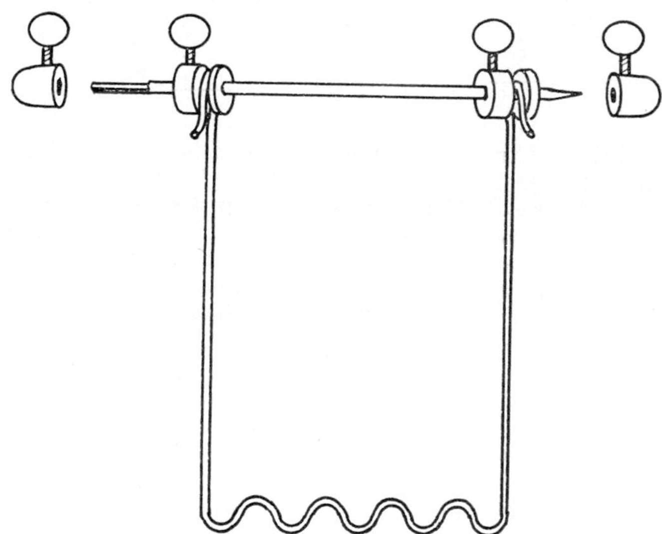

FIG. 97. Steinmann's pin and stirrup.

Skeletal Traction

This form of traction is attached to bone, and the points which may be used are the lower end of the femur, the head of the tibia, and the os calcis, and of these the tibia is the most usual. The bone is pierced from the outside by a pin or wire which supports on its protruding ends a stirrup to which the traction cord is attached. Kirschner wire is liable to fracture, and generally the stouter Steinmann pin is preferred. It is a stainless steel pin about the thickness of a metal skewer, with a sharp point at one side, and a square end at the other to fit into the introducer.

The site chosen is shaved, and the pin is generally introduced under thiopentone anæsthesia in the theatre, but it is a short and simple operation to perform in the ward. The skin is cleaned, and the pin is pushed through by means of an introducer, and a dressing of collodion may or may not be applied to the puncture holes. The stirrup is fastened to the pin, and older types of stirrup leave exposed the sharp end of the pin, which should be shielded with a cork. The patient returns to the ward

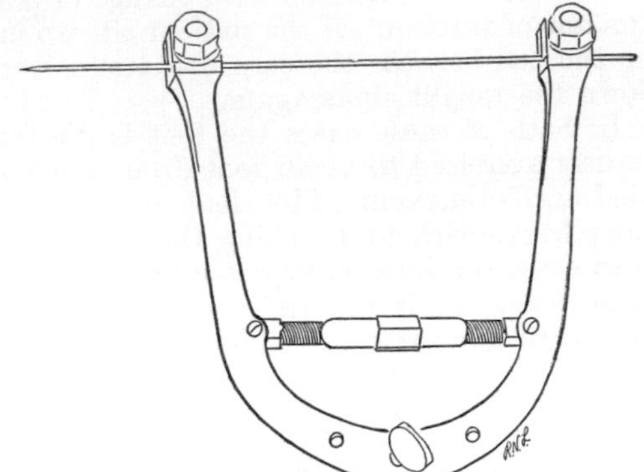

FIG. 98. Kirschner wire and stirrup.

for application of traction to the pin, and this will almost certainly be balanced traction.

Balanced Traction. This is the kind of apparatus that nurses may find difficult to understand at first sight, because it involves two or three sets of pulleys and weights. One of these is concerned with the pulling ; one is for keeping the Thomas's splint balanced clear of the bed, and there may be another helping dorsiflexion of the foot.

Requirements. Bed with overhead beams and rising foot or blocks.
Thomas's splint, with flexion iron.
Footpiece if required.
Flannel or calico strips.
Clips.
Traction cord.
Weights.
Gamgee or brown wool pads.
Scissors.
Pulleys.

The Thomas's splint is dressed with flannel or calico strips and clips as far as the knee, and the strips are then continued down the flexion iron and the foot piece. Not every surgeon likes the foot piece, and there are many ways of keeping the foot dorsiflexed if it is felt that any support is necessary. The splint is manœuvred into position.

Cord is attached to the centre of the ring of the splint, passed upwards over a pulley fixed in the overhead beam, over a second one level with the end of the splint and downwards to the end of the splint, where its length is adjusted, before tying it to one that will suspend or balance the splint at a suitable level. It is then continued down to the end of the flexion piece, where again its length is adjusted so that the whole splint is clear of the bed and the desired amount of knee flexion is maintained. These cords and pulleys are solely for the purpose of balancing the splint, and the position of the limb is now inspected to ensure that there is no internal or external rotation of the leg, and that the limb is nowhere pressing on the iron part of the splint.

There are many other ways of balancing the splint, one of which is illustrated.

Traction is now applied by tying a cord to the stirrup, running it over a pulley at the end of the bed (passing round the end of the splint on the way if preferred), and then attaching the main weight to the end of the cord. The pull is now being exerted in the axis of the femur, and the end of the bed must be sufficiently raised to prevent the patient being drawn downwards.

Dorsiflexion of the foot by some means is necessary in most cases except the very young. A foot piece is an effective support, but limits movement and so is losing popularity. A common and satisfactory method is to apply extension elastoplast to the sole of the foot, fastening cord to it and passing this across an overhead pulley and

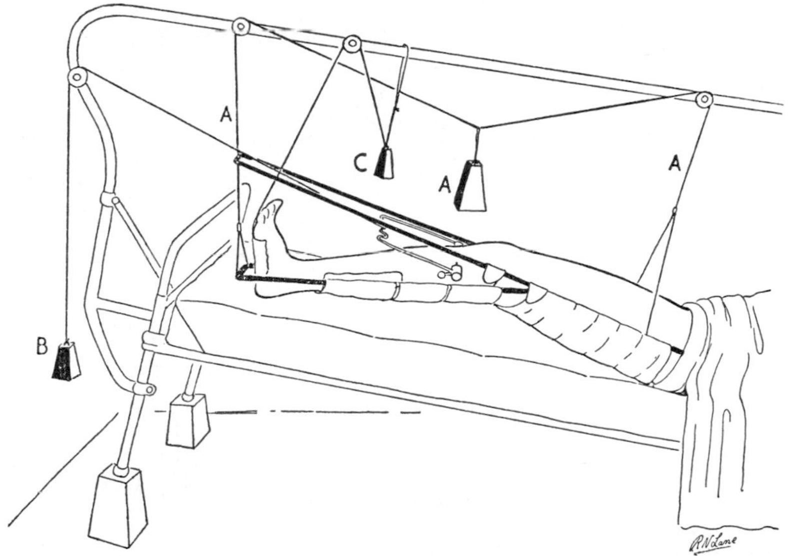

Fig. 99. Balanced skeletal tractions with a Thomas's splint and flexion piece.
A. The cords and weight which balance the splint off the bed.
B. The main weight exerting the traction on a Steinmann pin through the head of the tibia.
C. A small weight, with safety loop, for dorsiflexing the foot.
The end of the bed is raised to prevent the patient being pulled down the bed.

attaching a weight, large enough to keep the foot dorsiflexed, but not so heavy as to prevent plantarflexor movements. Finally, the limb is covered with pads to keep it warm, and later a quilt can be made which fastens to the splint with tapes.

The bed is made up by putting a blanket over the trunk and sound limb, then making the bed in two halves. A second blanket and a counterpane are passed under the splint to cover the good leg and complete the lower half of the bed. The upper is made by folding a small blanket in a sheet to form a packet which covers the chest and abdomen. A pulley and chain is necessary so that the patient can help lift himself for toilet purposes, and an air ring is usually supplied. Enough pillows are given to maintain a semi-recumbent position, but the patient must lie down at night, or a flexion deformity of the hip may ensue.

The splint must be inspected regularly to ensure that the correct position is maintained and that the leg is not pressed against the metal part of the splint. In a day or two, when the apparatus has been finally adjusted, long ends of cord or webbing are trimmed off to give a neat appearance. The principal nursing problems are the care of the pressure areas, including the heel of the sound leg and the skin under the ring of the splint, and the maintenance of bowel function. The position is one which encourages constipation, and in elderly patients impaction of fæces occurs readily.

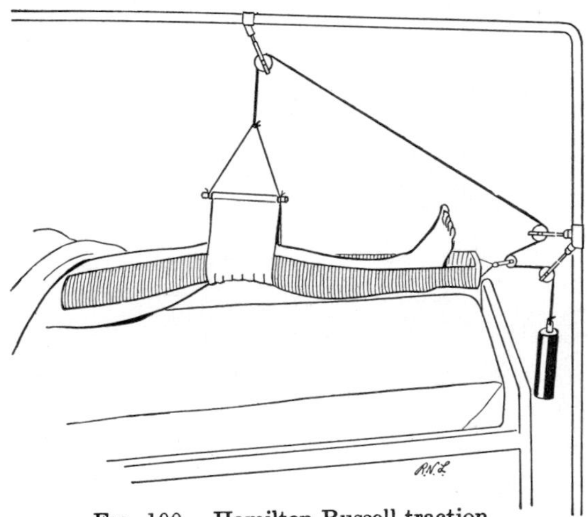

FIG. 100. Hamilton Russell traction.

Russell Traction

This type of balanced traction can be used for transtrochanteric fractures of the femur, and as a post-operative treatment for hip arthroplasty. No splint is used ; skin extension plaster is attached to the leg and a sling passes below the knee. A cord is attached to the sling and passes up vertically to a pulley on the overhead beam ; then over two pulleys as illustrated to join the traction cord. A pillow supports the thigh, and the end of the bed is raised. Traction is exerted along the line of the femur, and the knee is flexed at a comfortable angle.

Skull Traction

Fractures or subluxation of the cervical spine and some post-operative spinal conditions are treated by applying skeletal traction to the skull. Calipers are applied whose points pierce the outer table of the skull, and from these a cord crosses a pulley on the bed-extension piece and supports a weight. The head of the bed is raised to keep the patient in position.

The view which a patient has in this position is restricted to the ceiling and what he can see by moving the eyes. If the bed position is reversed he will be able to see more, and the traction apparatus is more readily available for inspection.

PLASTER OF PARIS

Plaster of Paris is a white powder made from dehydrated calcium sulphate or gypsum. When water is added to it it undergoes a chemical change, becoming hard and solid with evolution of heat. Splints can be made for almost all parts of the body by applying wet plaster bandages and allowing them to harden. Such casts are made to fit the patient, and therefore provide much more efficient immobilization than a splint can. Plaster is very extensively used, and its application, maintenance and nursing difficulties have to be appreciated not only by nurses in orthopædic wards.

Plaster bandages can be made by tearing into strips 3 in., 6 in., or 9 in. wide a packet of book muslin, which is twelve yards long. The marginal threads must be frayed off along the whole length, or the bandage will have a hard edge. Each is loosely rolled and then is passed from one end to another through a tray of plaster of Paris, which is thoroughly pressed into its meshes. The loaded bandage is rolled evenly up as it is impregnated. It takes practice to make high-class bandages of consistent quality, and is time-consuming. Most hospitals now use proprietary ones.

Plaster may be applied without padding, and this is sometimes used for fractures. It should be applied by an experienced surgeon. A layer of stockinette is normally drawn over the limb, before it is applied, and this prevents the plaster from sticking to the hair on a limb. Failure to take this precaution may occasion much pain to the patient who has to have his plaster removed for any reason shortly after application. If there is anxiety about bony prominences becoming sore, a layer of orthopædic felt can be applied near them and under large plasters that include the trunk a thin layer of wadding is used. Padded plasters sometimes have to be used temporarily over fractures involving much swelling, and when this has subsided a close-fitting plaster is applied.

Nurses in their student days are concerned only in assisting in applying plasters, but graduates working in fracture clinics make them themselves, and do it with the skill and neatness that might be expected. Applying plaster bandages is quite different from putting on other bandages. When the plaster is finished it must set into a smooth homogeneous mass with no ridges inside or out, so that reverses or constrictions that make uneven pressure must be avoided.

The basis of a plaster is a slab which is laid on one aspect of a limb and held in place with simple spirals of wet bandage. This bandage is rolled smoothly round the limb with one hand, while the other smooths into the cast the redundant folds under the limb, which must result from applying a straight bandage in spirals to a shaped part.

Application of a Plaster

Requirements Plaster bandages.
Deep bowl or bucket of tepid water.
Stockinette.
Orthopædic felt.
Strong scissors.
Tape measure.
Rolls of wadding.
Metal strips, if plaster is to be bivalved.
Plaster shears.
Skin pencil.
Mackintoshes.
Plaster apron.
Soap, water and towel for patient.
Floor rug.

The floor and the clothes of the patient and operators must be protected from plaster splashes, which are very difficult to remove. Articles must be arranged in a business-like way ; for instance the bowl or bucket in which the bandages are immersed should be at a convenient working level close beside the person applying the bandages. With a very little experience the number of bandages required for any cast is known, and excess should not be put out, since if they are splashed with water they are spoiled.

The limb should be washed before applying or renewing a plaster, dried, and measured to find the length of slab required. A piece of stockinette 3 in. longer than this is cut off and drawn on to the limb. A dry 6-in. bandage is unwrapped, and a slab made by folding over six layers of dry bandage of the required length. This is drawn through water, excess is removed by running it through the hand, and it is applied to the back of the hand and forearm for the arm, along the calf and sole if it is a leg. While this is being smoothed into place the nurse immerses another bandage in water, waits a few seconds until the bubbles cease to rise, then takes it out, squeezes it gently by the ends to get rid of excess water without losing plaster, loosens the end of the bandage and hands it to the operator, who runs it smoothly on in the way described above.

After the first layer has been put on, the edge of the stockinette is doubled back at the top and bottom to form a neat finish, and subsequent turns should be put carefully on so that this folded edge just appears on the finished plaster. As the plaster sets it begins to give off heat, and the hands are rinsed free of dried plaster and used to smooth and polish the surface of the cast. This must not be compressed at all during drying or uneven pressure will result.

The plaster is dated with a skin pencil, and must be protected until it is dry. If it has been put on for an out-patient, a card of instructions should be given and the important points emphasized. The plaster must not be allowed to get wet, or to receive hard knocks but all joints not immobilized must be fully exercised. This is especially important in the case of the fingers. Those with leg plasters should not spend long periods close to the fire, since if the plaster gets overheated it will not be appreciated until the heat has penetrated to the flesh beneath and burns can occur. If pain is felt the patient must report at once.

Nursing Care

In-patients are returned to bed in a position which puts no pressure on prominences ; the heel of a leg plaster, for instance, must be kept clear of the bed. Heat is not needed to dry it, and may indeed be dangerous, but a current of warm air is useful, and a leg plaster should be covered with a cradle and the bedclothes left open. The extremities must be regularly inspected for colour, temperature and mobility. Such symptoms as pain, cyanosis, coldness, anæsthesia or inability to moves toes or fingers must be promptly reported to the surgeon.

Pain over such prominences as the malleoli may indicate the onset of a pressure sore, and in general the plaster will be split to relieve the pressure. If the edge of the plaster is tight, elevation of the part should be tried first, and then the edge of the plaster should, if necessary, be split. It should be self-evident that if the plaster is tight pushing pieces of wool inside will only make it tighter.

Those who have the trunk enclosed in plaster feel uncomfortable—sometimes severely so—because of abdominal distension after meals. It is due to a combination of oppression and anxiety caused by the plaster, having to lie flat, and perhaps the morphine which may have been used pre- or post-operatively. The meals should be small, dry, and frequent for a day or two until adjustment has been made. The shoulders must not be propped up with pillows until the plaster presses into the epigastrium.

Immobilization of large parts of the trunk and limbs in plaster results in calcium being withdrawn from the bones and lost in the urine. This may result in renal calculi if precautions are not taken. Fluid intake should be high, and twice daily the patient should be turned over on to his face for half an hour. This prevents pooling of high-calcium urine in the pelvis of the kidney, and improves the circulation in the lungs and through the pressure areas over the buttocks. These can be adequately washed and treated while the patient is prone.

Bowel action is difficult in this unnatural position, and it is wise to bind the edge of the plaster in the nursing area with waterproof strapping. The patient's worst problem, however, is boredom, in a ward of patients who are all making a long stay. Results are slow as compared with other surgical and medical wards, but faithful supplying of the patient's basis needs while he is a prisoner in the plaster may make the difference between a bedridden state and a normal life to her patient.

Removing a Plaster

Taking off a plaster is more formidable to the patient than putting it on, and is a task requiring some strength and a good deal of skill and of insight into the anatomy of the part concerned and into the patient's natural fears.

A good pair of plaster shears is required, with a shallow lower blade $\frac{1}{8}$ in. longer than the upper. Electric shears save the time and energy of the operator.

The line along which the plaster is to be cut should be one which does not traverse any bony prominences on which the shears might exert painful pressure. The patient is told that he must complain at once if pain is felt. The lower blade is kept parallel to the skin, and the upper blade closed on to it to cut a small bite in the plaster. After each bite the blades are opened by moving the upper one, not the lower, which is advanced a little after each cut. Thought must be constantly given to the position of the lower blade, which is the one that may damage the skin.

Some plasters are bi-valved as soon as they are dry, and if this is the intention a metal strip should be included inside the plaster as it is applied, and along this the plaster can be quickly and painlessly split.

INTERNAL METHODS OF FIXATION

A fractured bone may be fixed internally by means of screws, plates or intra-medullary nails inserted at operation. These internal fixatives

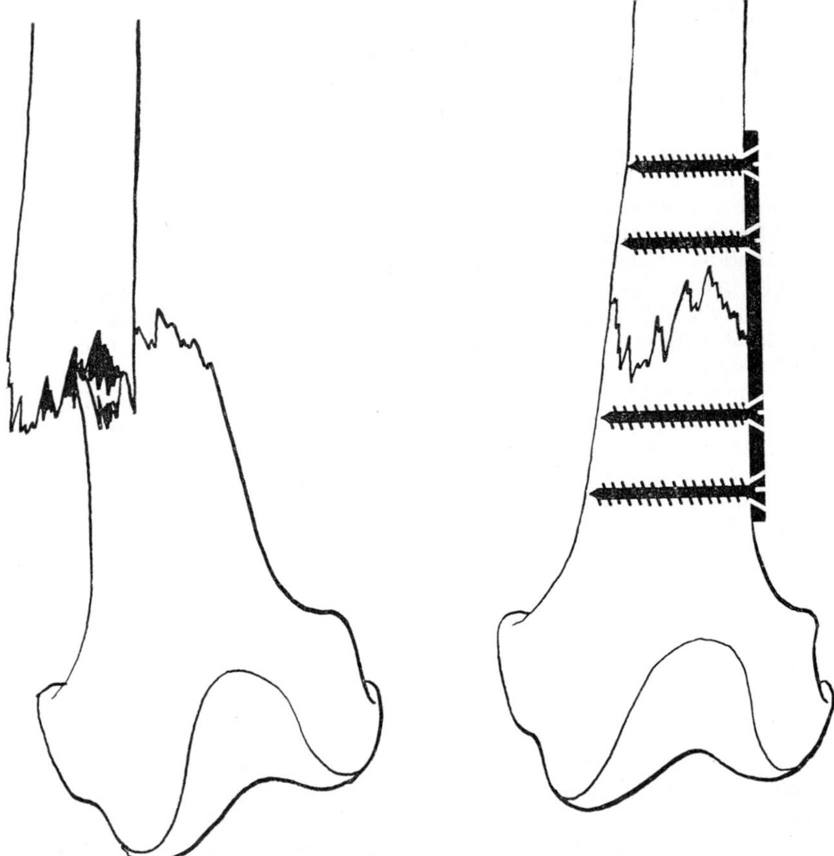

FIG. 101. Fracture of the shaft of tibia and fibula, showing reduction and immobilization by plating.

merely serve to keep the fracture reduced, and it must not be thought that no external support is necessary, or that weight can be borne on the limb.

The best-known means of internal fixation is the Smith-Petersen nail, which is used to maintain position in fractures of the neck of the femur. This is a fracture peculiar to the elderly and the old, and is often a terminal event from shock, pneumonia or uræmia. A method of treatment that involved a long period of immobility lying flat would

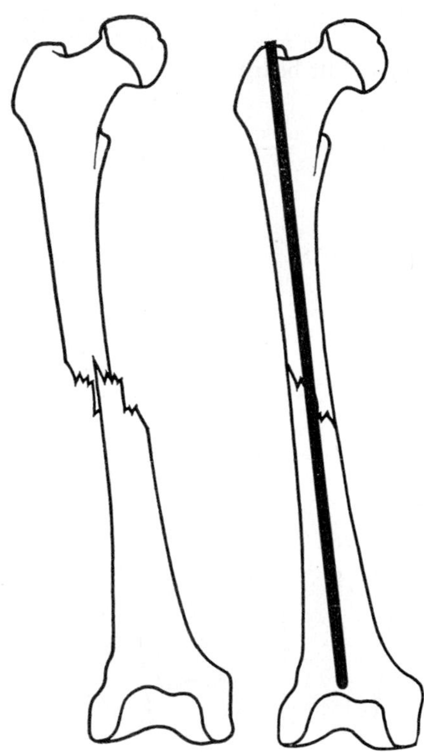

FIG. 102. Fracture of the shaft of the femur showing reduction and immobilization by an intramedullary nail.

claim many victims, but the introduction of a Smith-Petersen nail allows the patient to be sat up in bed immediately after operation.

The nail is trifid to prevent it turning in the bone. The great trochanter is exposed through a small incision, a guide wire is driven through it along the neck into the head of the femur, uniting the broken parts. If an X-ray shows its position to be satisfactory, the nail is hammered home along it.

Subsequently the patient can be sat up and allowed to move about the bed. In two or three weeks (or in much shorter times in the agile) she may be got out of bed, and walking with crutches but without weight-bearing is begun. No weight is taken by the injured leg until healing is sound, but by that time the patient is active and mobile.

Other Appliances

A walking *caliper* resembles a Thomas's splint with the end removed. The sides end by fitting into holes in the heel of the patient's boot, and the caliper is of such a length that when he stands his weight rests on the ring of the caliper, and from there is distributed to the boot by means of the side irons, and without allowing any weight to fall on the leg. A leather knee-guard prevents flexion of the joint.

Short steels begin below the knee, from which the weight is carried by the steels to the sole of the boot in the same way as in the caliper. They can be used when the knee joint is normal to save the lower leg from weight-bearing.

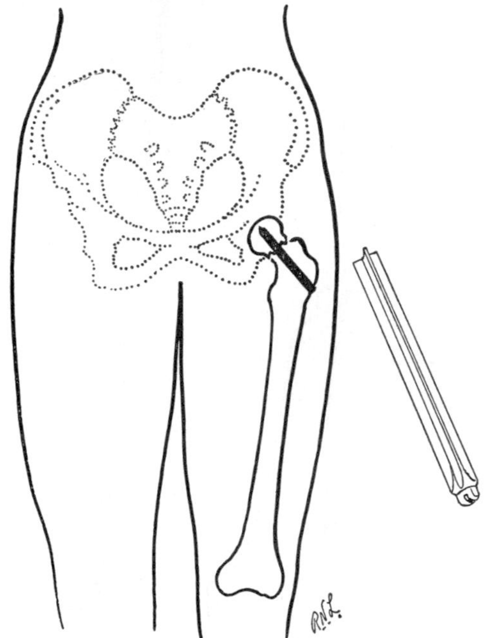

Fig. 103. Smith-Petersen nail showing the way in which it is used to immobilize a fracture of the neck of the femur.

Toe-raising springs are used for correcting the deformity of foot drop. Such a spring passes from a band round the calf to the ball of the foot and maintains it in a dorsiflexed position. It is inconspicuous in use when trousers are worn.

ORTHOPAEDIC OPERATIONS

The types of operation performed on orthopædic patients include the open reduction of fractures; lengthening, shortening and transplanting tendons; removing joint cartilages; re-fashioning joints (arthroplasty) or rendering joints immovable (arthrodesis). While the general principles of surgical care apply to these operations, there are some points of particular importance.

Pre-operative Treatment. While a careful aseptic technique is employed by the abdominal surgeon, he is aware that the peritoneal cavity is able to deal with minor contamination and has methods of localizing infections which can be successful even against major septic events like perforation of the appendix. The consequences of infection in a joint, even with antibiotics available, may be permanent stiffness. Fear of such infection produced the classic preparation that is described next.

At least two days of preparation are required before a joint operation. On admission, a bath should be taken, and then the limb is inspected by the nurse for any septic lesions which would be a bar to operation at that time. It is often necessary now to carry the toilet a stage further than the patient has done, with nailbrush, scissors, nail file and a detergent. Cetrimide is a good one, and if combined with Hibitane is very successful at cleaning the skin and reducing its bacterial flora.

A wide area of skin is prepared, and, therefore, the pre-operative shave should extend to the joints above and below the operation site, e.g. if the knee is to be opened, the whole leg should be shaved. It must be done meticulously for scratches or grazes may lead to infection. Apart from the skin cleansing, at least one antiseptic skin preparation is performed in the ward for the majority of orthopædic surgeons. The part is cleaned first with ether soap and then with spirit or some skin disinfectant, and wrapped in sterile towels which are secured with open-wove bandages. Sterile gloves may be worn, but more strict asepsis can be maintained with a non-touch technique, and the use of forceps. The preparation is repeated on the theatre table.

An increasing number of orthopædic surgeons feel that this stay in hospital before operation is unnecessary, and that the treatment described may increase rather than abolish risk of infection. They undertake the entire preparation in the theatre, including the shave. Small skin abrasions are not important, as there is no time for them to become infected.

Most operations on limbs are performed in a bloodless field obtained by means of an Esmarch's bandage. The leg is elevated, and the bandage applied firmly from the toes up to the mid-thigh where it is fastened and the lower part undone. Failure to take this off at the end of the operation will result in gangrene and the theatre routine should provide for a check to the removal of the tourniquet.

Post-operative Care. Following orthopædic operations on the limbs, an inspection of the circulation in the extremities should be made on return to the ward and at regular intervals afterwards, especially if plaster or pressure bandages have been used. Pallor, coldness, pain, cyanosis, anæsthesia or inability to move fingers or toes must be reported at once, and all measures will be taken to relieve them. Pressure areas must receive regular attention.

Pain is often quite severe, especially if a joint has been opened, and an adequate analgesic must be given in amounts sufficient to control it. After forty-eight hours this symptom should diminish markedly. Raising the foot of the bed helps to prevent pain after operations on the leg.

Turning Orthopædic Patients. When turning a patient painlessly for bedmaking or treatment of pressure areas after hip surgery, the patient should while lying on the back be asked to flex the good knee, and slip this foot under the knee of the operated limb. The foot is slid down under the ankle, and can then be used to support the operated limb while rolling on to the good hip.

After operations on the knee, quadriceps exercises should be encouraged immediately, so that when the patient is moved he can be contracting the thigh muscles and keep the knee extended.

Following operations on the back (such as laminectomy) patients should be rolled carefully from side to side so that the back is kept straight. Sitting with flexed hips, or reclining on a bedpan is painful; an easier method is to roll the patient onto her face, ask her to flex the knees and rise onto the hands and knees, so that the nurse can slip the bedpan between the thighs, when the patient can sit back onto it.

Crutches. Crutches are commonly used after operations on the hip, following amputation, or after injuries to the leg when mobility is desirable, but weight-bearing on the affected limb is not allowed, or is only partial.

It is important that crutches of the correct length are fitted. Full length crutches should reach to within an inch (2·5 cm.) of the axilla when the patient is standing upright; if they are too long they will press on the nerves in the axilla, and if too short they will cause stooping. The hand grips should be adjusted so that when they are grasped the elbows are slightly flexed. Patients are instructed that when standing, they should not allow the weight to fall in the axillary rests, or pressure on the radial nerve will cause crutch palsy. Elbow crutches are more suitable for elderly and feeble patients than axillary ones. Nurses should inspect the rubbers on patients' crutches and renew them when necessary, since worn rubbers may cause accidents through slipping.

The diet can be a full one for most patients after the first day or two, and since the period of immobilization and waiting after an operation may be long and rather tedious, interesting and varied meals are important in maintaining morale. Fluid intake should be high, to prevent concentration of the urine and stone formation in those at rest for long periods.

Apparatus must be kept in good order and regularly inspected in case adjustment is needed. Overhead beams, traction cords and splints that are in position for some weeks must be dusted regularly with a damp cloth. Weights must not be allowed to hang against the bed.

Patients may find time hanging heavily on their hands, with only mealtimes, the doctor's visit and physiotherapy to occupy them. Frequent visiting, a good library, occupational therapy and a cheerful nursing staff will help to shorten the time.

Two examples of orthopædic operations are given, to illustrate the type of treatment employed.

Internal Derangement of Knee

One or other of the semilunar cartilages in the knee-joint may become torn, and thenceforward is apt to be caught between the articular surfaces during movement and to lock the joint. It is an especially common sports injury, and will, if untreated, lead to arthritis and joint effusion, as well as the painful and inconvenient locking of the joint.

After preparation of the kind described above, the joint cavity is opened, and the torn cartilage extracted. A pressure bandage is applied over the knee to restrict movement and limit post-operative pain. The end of the bed is raised on blocks and a cradle is used over the leg. Pain is always severe unless properly controlled with analgesics, and is due not only to the joint disturbance, but to spasm of the large muscles around it. Morphine or pethidine may be ordered regularly for the first day, after which compound codeine mixture may suffice.

The patient is taught before operation to contract the quadriceps without moving the joint, and regular exercise must be given to this muscle post-operatively or the knee will tend to give way when later weight is borne on it. The dressing is done and the bandage reapplied about the third day, and progress should be normal until the stitches are removed about the tenth day, when the patient may get up if there is no effusion in the joint. Physiotherapy will be continued as an out-patient when he leaves after about three weeks in hospital.

Osteo-arthritis of Hip

The hip joints are often affected in the elderly by arthritis, which causes stiffness, pain on walking and at night a flexion-adduction deformity that may eventually prevent the patient from walking.

Medical treatment with diathermy and analgesics may slow down the degenerative process ; attention to diet may remove the strain of overweight from the affected joints ; but surgery is at the moment the only hope of restoring function. It is not offered to very large numbers of patients because it is only successful if the patient has the energy and determination to pursue the long and often painful rehabilitation course, and even in such people the results are sometimes disappointing.

Three types of operation are used :

1. *Osteotomy.* The femur is divided through the trochanters, and immobilized in its new position with internal fixation. An active patient may be allowed up on crutches in two or three weeks. For the more disabled, a preliminary period of traction is necessary until healing has commenced. It is one of the older operations and has no consistent effect on the disease process, but often succeeds very well because it relieves the pain.

2. *Arthrodesis.* The hip joint is obliterated and bony union encouraged between the femoral head and the acetabulum. It is quite a good operation for a patient fairly young in years or physique with one hip affected. Pain disappears, walking is possible, and in spite of the stiff hip the results are good in properly selected cases. The patient is nursed in plaster.

3. *Arthroplasty.* Several operations have been devised to make a new head of femur, or acetabulum, or both, either from plastic or metal. One currently practised is the McKnee Farrar. The head of the femur is excised, and a new metal acetabulum fixed in place with bone cement. The new femoral head has a blade portion which is pushed down the centre of the shaft of the femur, and fixed with cement. Until the patient is fully conscious, the legs are bandaged together to

prevent dislocation of the hip. Physiotherapy is begun at once, and fit patients may be up and sitting in a chair within a week. Walking with partial weightbearing soon begins, and the patient may in favourable cases leave the wards in three weeks.

Much perseverance and hard work is required of the patient if a successful result is to be obtained, and often he may feel that little advance is being made in spite of efforts that are sometimes painful. He should be reminded that improvement may not be visible from day to day, but that if he thinks of his condition a week ago he will see some. The hope of a return to normal life and activity should be kept before him.

Talipes

This congenital abnormality is commonly called clubfoot and there are several varieties of the deformity. The kind most frequently seen is talipes equino-varus, in which the foot is inverted and the heel drawn up so that only the toes reach the ground. It is often bilateral, and may be accompanied by other congenital deformities.

Treatment to be effective should be started soon after birth, and consists of gentle pressure to correct the deformity and splinting to maintain the improved position. The Denis Browne talipes splint which is commonly used, consists of two foot pieces each with an extension which goes up the outside of the leg, and a cross bar which joins them together. The angle at which the foot pieces are attached can be adjusted.

The foot piece is lined with orthopædic felt, the foot is fastened to it with elastoplast over felt, and the foot pieces are both attached. The splint must be removed twice a week for manipulation of the foot, and cannot be dispensed with for some months or even a year, and a night splint will be needed for some time afterwards. In persistent or neglected cases, operations on the bones are not usually performed under the age of 12.

MANIPULATION

Joints are manipulated (often under general anæsthesia) for two reasons. It may be done to break down adhesions, relieve pain and increase the range of movement. Feet, knees and backs are often so treated and the physiotherapist begins active treatment afterwards to maintain the benefits conferred.

The other purpose of manipulation is to improve the position of a limb or joint and to maintain that improvement by immobilizing it in its new position.

CHAPTER 27

NEUROSURGICAL NURSING

THE brain is enclosed by the meninges and cerebro-spinal fluid, and lies in a bony cavity which it completely fills. If hæmorrhage takes place within this cavity, or œdema occurs, or a new growth or abscess forms, space is taken up inside the skull which compresses the brain and causes a rise of pressure within the cranium. Whatever the cause, raised intracranial pressure gives rise to a well-marked group of clinical signs and symptoms, and from a battery of diagnostic tests at his disposal the neurosurgeon determines the cause and decides on his treatment, which may have to be undertaken urgently if life is to be saved.

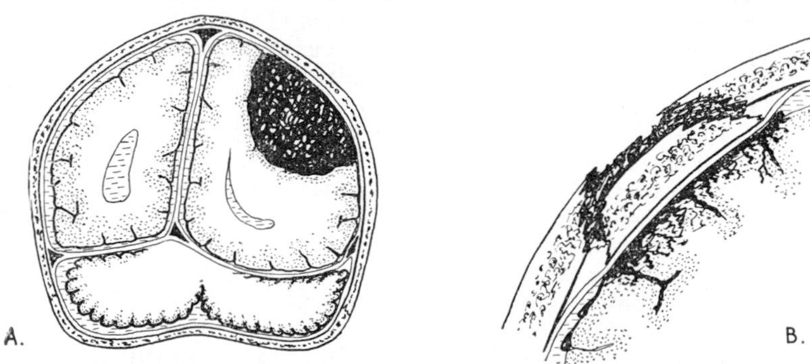

FIG. 104. The brain is in a rigid box. Any lesion (such as a depressed fracture, or haematoma) which takes up space will compress the brain and raise the intracranial pressure.

RAISED INTRACRANIAL PRESSURE

The speed at which the signs occur varies with the cause ; a hæmorrhage outside the dura will run its course in a few hours, while a slowly-growing tumour may cause months of slowly rising pressure.

The *temperature* is not usually raised except in traumatic or infective cases. Pressure on the medulla causes a *pulse* slow in rate and full in volume (until a very late stage), and deepening and slowing of the *respiration* ; irregular or Cheyne-Stokes breathing is a serious sign. The *blood pressure* rises in order to force the blood through the compressed brain. *Headache* is common and often very severe. *Consciousness* is progressively affected, with drowsiness, confusion and sometimes restlessness, leading to stupor. Dilatation of one *pupil*, with gradual failure of its reaction, is very important. *Papillœdema* is œdema of the optic disc due to obstruction of the venous drainage of the optic nerves, and can be seen with an ophthalmoscope ; failing sight or even *blindness* is due to the same cause. *Vomiting* occurs early and is often projectile in type. A localized lesion can cause weakness or paralysis of one side, most easily observed in slight cases as a weakness of the hand grip of one side. Progressive loss of consciousness produces retention or incontinence of urine and of fæces.

In acute cases serial observations at frequent intervals are of the utmost importance ; progressive slowing of the pulse and deepening unconsciousness may indicate the need for surgery.

Intracranial New Growth

New growths within the skull may be innocent (e.g. meningiomata) but many are malignant, and until the tumour is exposed its nature cannot always be known, though a long history raises the hope that it is innocent and a short acute one is typical of the malignant growth. In addition, there are tumours which though innocent, by their position or relation to important structures are not amenable to treatment.

Localization of the tumour must be as accurate as possible, since the neurosurgeon is not in the fortunate position of the abdominal surgeon who by a midline incision may reach any organ ; he must open the skull directly over the tumour. He makes his diagnosis from :

(*a*) Clinical examination.

(*b*) X-rays, plain or contrast. The ventriculogram (p. 130) is one of the most useful, and a carotid angiogram may give vital information.

(*c*) Electroencephalogram. The electric impulses generated by brain activity can be recorded in the same way as those of the heart, and multiple leads enable the whole surface of the brain to be covered. Disturbances of the waves in certain leads can indicate the site and sometimes the probable extent of the growth.

(*d*) Brain scan (p. 506).

If these investigations decide the surgeon that treatment is feasible, craniotomy is undertaken.

Pre-operative Preparation

The head must be shaved and in many cases the shave is total. For women this is a great trial, and if the tumour is in the posterior fossa, it may be possible to leave an inch or so of hair in front. The bowels are opened with magnesium sulphate by mouth. Magnesium sulphate is effective in lowering intracranial pressure by withdrawing fluid from the tissues into the intestinal canal, but has been replaced in general by intravenous mannitol. The blood group is ascertained, an electrocardiogram is performed if hypothermia is likely to be used during or after operation. The patient and the relatives should be informed as fully as possible of what the surgeon hopes to accomplish.

Anæsthesia in this country is usually a general one, but this is not true of all parts of the world, and minor operations such as the drilling of burr-holes can be done with a local anæsthetic. The usual fasting period is observed, and premedication is simple (e.g. scopolamine 0·45 mg.). Morphine is contraindicated because of its depressing action on respiration.

Head operations often last some hours. The patient must be placed most carefully in position on the table so that he may safely lie without moving for a long period, and that both surgeon and anæsthetist have easy working conditions. Opening the skull, too, is time-consuming and laborious. A scalp flap is turned back from the selected area, and the meninges are exposed either by removing the bone piecemeal or by cutting out an osteoplastic flap which can be replaced. If the tumour is an innocent one, it can sometimes be removed with some ease; if it is a malignant one the surgeon must decide if it can be removed without causing severe after-effects such as hemiplegia. Unlike other surgeons, the brain surgeon cannot sacrifice quantities of tissue, or the last state of the patient may be worse than his first.

Post-operative Care

The bed should be taken to the theatre to receive the patient after his operation; usually he is laid flat with one pillow, but after operations on the posterior fossa he may be sat up with his head secured to the pillow by a turn of bandage. Commonly an intravenous infusion is running at a slow rate.

On return to the ward, the temperature (per rectum), pulse, respiration rate and blood pressure are ascertained. Observations are made of the colour; the reaction of the pupils; the state of consciousness; the rate of intravenous infusion, which is usually given at a speed of two pints in twenty-four hours to avoid raising the intracranial pressure; whether there is any evidence of hemiplegia. If fits occur, the nurse should record their frequency, duration, where the movements begin and how they spread.

As consciousness returns pillows are gradually added and the head of the bed raised on blocks, and sips of water can be given when the swallowing reflex is well established. By the next morning the intravenous infusion can usually be discontinued, and an oral intake of 1,500 ml. instituted. Retention of urine is not uncommon after extensive operations, and the bladder should be catheterized with every aseptic precaution, a procedure that should be repeated as often as necessary. The rectal temperature is regularly noted, and if it rises more than a degree or two, steps should be taken to reduce it by removing blankets, raising the top sheet on cradles, the use of a fan and the administration of aspirin. If such measures are begun early they will be successful, but if the temperature is allowed to rise too far, hyperpyrexia can be dangerous and difficult to control. Breathing and limb exercises are begun.

On the second day the dressing is done, the drainage tube removed and the wound inspected for swelling that might indicate raised intracranial pressure and the need for lumbar puncture. The bandage used may be a triangular one, a capelline, or a tubegauz one.

The bowels may be opened by an enema, and in a favourable case progress will be uneventful. The patient may get up about the fifth day, and occupational therapy will improve muscular co-ordination. The stitches can be removed now, unless the operation was on the posterior fossa when they may remain until the 10th day. The time of discharge varies greatly, depending on the time needed for rehabilitation and the home circumstances.

Inoperable Tumour

Not all cases make such a recovery as this ; craniotomy may disclose that the growth cannot be entirely removed, or that its situation makes excision impossible, while sometimes such a diagnosis may be made without opening the skull. Deep X-ray therapy may be used, and is sometimes successful.

Plain aspirin is given for headache, and phenobarbitone or paraldehyde are other useful drugs for restlessness. The patient's head must be kept raised, since lying flat increases the intracranial pressure, as does a high fluid intake. Magnesium sulphate or a caffeine and sodium benzoate mixture or intravenous mannitol will help lower it.

The sight is sometimes lost from pressure on the optic nerves while the patient is still able to appreciate the magnitude of his loss, and if so he will need much help and encouragement. If vomiting is troublesome, the prescription of chlorpromazine may do something to mitigate it. When finally the patient is bedridden regular care of the pressure areas, turning, treatment of incontinence and feeding will be necessary. Even when the prognosis is hopeless, a great deal can be done in these ways to relieve symptoms and give comfort, and nurses working in neurological wards find the giving of such service most rewarding.

HEAD INJURIES

A person who has sustained a heavy blow to the head loses consciousness as a result of the shaking up, or *concussion* of the brain. The period of unconsciousness may be brief, as in boxers who have been knocked out, and the care of such persons presents no problems. Blows of some violence, however, cause œdema and swelling of the brain, and a rise in the intracranial pressure takes place, which can lead to prolonged unconsciousness, and to all the signs described on p. 389.

Cerebral Concussion

When a patient with such an injury is to be admitted, a bed is prepared ; bedsides will be needed and the pillow should be protected by a plastic cover. The position of the patient depends on the relative importance of the different aspects of his condition. Often the protection of the airway from obstruction by blood or the patient's tongue is vital, and he is therefore nursed flat in the semi-prone position. A sucker may be required to keep the airway clear, and the patient is turned regularly from one side to the other and the chest " clapped " to avert pneumonia. The temperature, pulse ($\frac{1}{4}$ hourly), respiration rate and blood pressure are recorded. The reaction of the pupils, and their equality or otherwise is of great diagnostic importance.

Blood or cerebro-spinal fluid coming from the nose or ear may indicate fracture of the base of the skull. Such fractures are always compound ; toilet of the nose or ear in such circumstances should be with sterile swabs, and antibiotic treatment is begun early to avert meningitis.

The depth of unconsciousness must be continually observed. In a minor case it may be of quite short duration. Return of consciousness is frequently accompanied by restlessness, dis-orientation, vomiting, photophobia and resentment of examination or treatment. Such a patient can be expected to make a fairly quick recovery and bed rest is not nowadays advised for long periods. He should be given plain aspirin for headache, and phenobarbitone for sedation ; the fluid intake must be only moderate, and magnesium sulphate is given daily by mouth or as an enema till signs of raised intracranial pressure have gone. If an X-ray was not taken on admission, the skull and cervical spine are X-rayed at a convenient time.

In more severe cases with no early sign of returning consciousness a nasal catheter is passed into the stomach, and nasal feeds to the amount of 1,000–1,500 ml. given in twenty-four hours. Either retention or incontinence of urine may occur and must receive appropriate treatment. Intravenous mannitol is given.

HYPOTHERMIA

In some cases of severe head injury, or after operations on the intracranial blood vessels, hypothermia may be used as a method of treatment. As the body temperature falls, the needs of the cells for oxygen and nutriment decrease, so that the cerebral cells may survive the difficult conditions associated with raised intracranial pressure or restricted blood supply, if the body temperature is artificially lowered. Hypothermia in connection with anæsthesia is discussed in the chapter on heart surgery (p. 805), for which it is widely used.

The patient should be nursed in a sideroom, so that the air temperature can be kept low, and where the nursing and medical attention required do not disturb other patients. Any artificial heating is turned off. A sorbo or ripple mattress is used, and the bottom bedclothes are the usual ones. Either the head or the foot may be raised, if the blood pressure necessitates it.

Equipment for lowering the temperature

3 washing bowls of ice.
4 sheets.
Small bath of cold water.
2 bed cradles; 2 electric fans.
Indwelling low-reading rectal thermometer.
Mackintoshes and floor rug.

Equipment for records and care

Suction apparatus ; sterile catheters ; bowl of water.
Oxygen and mask.
Rubber airway and lubricant jelly.
Tray for mouth toilet.
Sphygmomanometer ; stethoscope, torch.
Syringes (2, 5, 10 ml.) assorted needles.
Swabs and skin disinfectant.
Graph paper.

Induction. Cooling the skin normally leads to shivering, which prevents the temperature falling. Shivering must therefore be inhibited, and this is done by a lytic mixture, such as:

Phenergan 50 mg.
Pethidine 50 mg.
Chlorpromazine 50 mg.
} in 10 m.l of normal saline.

This is given by intravenous injection, and repeated subsequently in the amounts ordered when indicated.

An intravenous infusion is set up, the night clothes are removed except for a loin cloth, and the rectal thermometer inserted. The patient lies on one side and if he is unconscious an artificial airway is used.

Records should be kept of the rectal temperature (5 minutes), pulse, respiration, blood pressure and state of the pupils (15 minutes). Any movement or change in colour is noted. Three sheets are wrung out of iced water and packed over the patient, covering trunk and limbs completely. The fourth sheet is to enable the cold sheets to be changed in rotation. The fans are turned on. The most desirable temperature is 31.7–32° C. (89–90° F.), and since the temperature continues to fall after cooling measures have been stopped, the iced sheets should be removed when the rectal temperature is 33–32.7° C. (92–91° F.), and a sheet supported on bed cradles used instead. At 32° C. (90° F.) the fans are turned off.

Maintaining hypothermia. Once the temperature has become stable, it is kept there by means of the lytic mixture, and by adjusting fans or sheets to match slight variations. It is important not to allow the temperature to fall below the prescribed level—should it fall below 30° C. (85° F.) it will be difficult to reverse this process. The pulse and blood pressure will fall with the temperature, and sometimes drugs are given to raise the blood pressure, though this encourages a rise of temperature.

Nursing Care

Position. This is flat unless the surgeon instructs otherwise. Turning the patient half hourly or hourly is beneficial from all aspects.

Attention to chest. Pneumonia is a much-feared complication, and regular turning and gentle clapping will help avert it. Prophylactic antibiotics may be ordered, and the airway should be kept clear by suction. If there is any difficulty in coping with secretion, tracheostomy is usually performed. Oxygen may be required.

Intake. Nasal feeds are given by polythene œsophageal tube. Calorie needs are reduced when the temperature is low, and 200 ml. of water with 10 G. of glucose 5 times a day is enough. The temperature of the feed should be 35° C. (95° F.).

Bladder and Bowels. Retention of urine must be treated by catheterization. A small enema or a suppository every fourth day is often needed.

General Nursing. The mouth must be regularly treated, as must the pressure areas. Vigorous friction to these points will raise the temperature, and deep massage rather than superficial rubbing is indicated.

The relatives of this patient need special consideration ; to see a relative undergoing such treatment is difficult to bear, and they must be told about its aims and benefits.

When the surgeon judges that the cold treatment can be discontinued, the temperature is allowed to rise slowly without any artificial warming.

Fractures of the Skull

The skull is of two parts. The vault is made of flat bones which are slightly resilient when struck. If the vault is broken, the fracture may be *linear*, with no displacement, and no treatment beyond that of the concussion is required. If the blow is received on a fairly small area, a fragment of skull may be broken off and driven inwards, forming a *depressed* fracture. Such a fracture is usually compound, and the patient must be taken to the theatre for wound toilet, excision of the bone fragment and suture of the dura.

The base of the skull is of thick irregular bone and may be fractured by violence to the vault being transmitted to it, or occasionally by falls on the feet, which can cause fractures of the os calcis, lumbar vertebræ and the skull base. Since the cranial nerves leave the skull by the base, these are often damaged by such injuries, the olfactory and the facial being especially vulnerable.

If the fracture is an open one, some precaution against meningitis must be taken. Penicillin by intramuscular injection penetrates poorly into the cerebro-spinal fluid, so although it is useful for preventing pneumonia, one of the sulpha drugs is more effective against meningitis.

Extradural Hæmorrhage

A blow on the head sometimes ruptures an artery outside the dura (the middle meningeal artery being often involved) and bleeding follows. Sometimes the patient has recovered consciousness after the injury, and then as bleeding progresses and raises the intracranial pressure, drowsiness and a falling pulse rate indicate compression of the brain. If untreated, the patient will sink into unconsciousness and die. It is important to notice the first signs, since the neurosurgeon can open the skull, evacuate the blood clot and secure the bleeding vessel.

After operation, the patient is nursed with the foot of the bed on blocks and allowed a free fluid intake to help the brain to re-expand. The blood pressure and the pulse rate will indicate when the patient may be allowed to sit up.

Subarachnoid Hæmorrhage

Bleeding into the subarachnoid space may be due to injury or small congenital aneurysms, and until recently patients were admitted to medical wards where it was hoped that natural recuperative powers and careful nursing might promote recovery, but second and more serious hæmorrhages frequently happened. Now it may be possible to prevent repeated bleeding in favourable cases.

On admission, lumbar puncture is performed, and the presence of blood in the cerebro-spinal fluid confirms the diagnosis. The blood irritates the meninges, and causes such signs as head retraction and stiffness of the back. The patient is nursed flat at complete rest, and heavy sedation will be needed if he is conscious as headache is severe. The mouth and the pressure points need regular treatment, and a fluid intake of 1,500 to 2,000 ml. is given orally or by nasal feeds. If he recovers, carotid angiography is undertaken to ascertain if surgery is likely to be of use. Carotid ligation is a small and simple operation that may give good results. Following it the patient is nursed with the foot of the bed raised to increase the circulation to the brain following the cutting of the carotid contribution, and the blood pressure is taken every quarter of an hour until it has reached a satisfactory level. The bed blocks are kept in position for about five days, and pillows are gradually added until the patient is sitting up by the tenth day. It may also be possible to deal with the aneurysm itself by intracranial procedures.

Subdural Hæmorrhage

This condition follows injury, which is sometimes so slight as to be disregarded. Onset of neurological signs may be slow, but may eventually progress to hemiplegia. Evacuation of the blood clot will give a complete cure.

OPERATIONS ON THE SPINAL CORD

The spinal cord is enclosed in meninges like the brain, and by the neural arches of the vertebræ, and when lesions arise in connection with it, usually it is necessary to remove the posterior part of one or more neural arch, i.e. perform *laminectomy*. This operation may be undertaken to remove a spinal tumour or portions of a protruded intervertebral disc, or to divide the sensory nerve columns for the relief of intractable pain due to malignant disease (*chordotomy*).

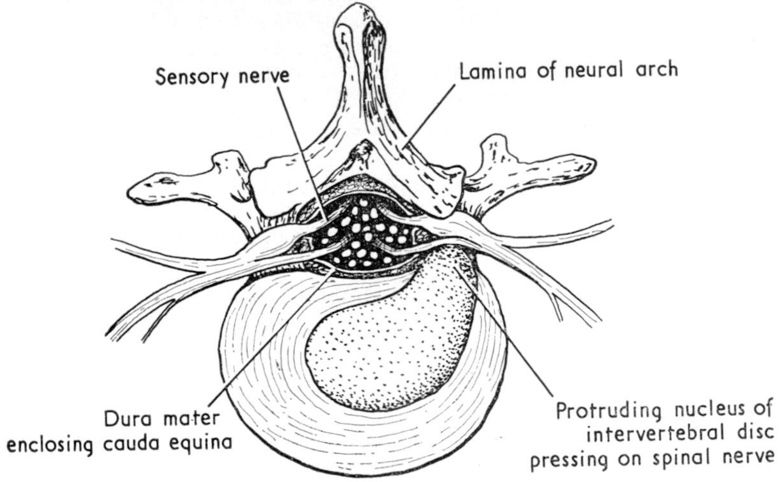

Fig. 105. Prolapse of an intervertebral disc causes symptoms by pressing on a spinal nerve

Before laminectomy, the level of the lesion is determined by a myelogram (p. 130). The bowels are opened by an enema and pre-operative sedation given. When the patient returns from the theatre he will have a head dressing if the operation was a cervical one, and if it was dorsal the upper arm will be included in the bandage to avoid pulling on the spinal muscles by movements of the arms. He is put flat in bed with pillows under the elbows and knees, and fluids are given freely as soon as consciousness returns. Retention of urine often occurs and catheterization of the bladder is performed eight-hourly until normal micturition returns. The pressure areas must be treated regularly, and if the operation was for chordotomy treatment should be two-hourly to avoid trophic ulceration. Abdominal distention is rather marked, for the same reason as retention of urine occurs, and an enema can be given after the third day. Drug treatment will include a sulphonamide, to prevent meningitis and urinary infection, and regular sedation with a barbiturate with a medium-long action, such as amylobarbitone. The time at which the patient gets up is decided by the nature and site of the lesion.

Injuries to the Spinal Cord

The spinal cord may be injured by fracture-dislocations of the spine, and if the cord has been severed permanent paralysis and sensory loss below the level of the lesion must occur since regeneration of nerve cells does not occur. An X-ray may indicate that the outlook for return of movement is grave, but in some cases the paralysis may be due to spinal concussion, hæmorrhage or œdema and improvement may be looked for.

There are three dangers that threaten the patient with a traumatic paraplegia :

1. Sepsis from trophic ulcers on the sacrum and heels. These occur very readily even with devoted nursing, unless this is done with insight and skill. The important point is the avoidance of pressure rather than frequent rubbing which may in itself devitalize the skin. The heels, for instance, must be prevented from resting on the bed by pads beneath the Achilles tendons, and pillows to keep the feet dorsiflexed. The bed may be made in sections which can be removed separately. Turning must be regular by night as well as day, especially in the early stages, if the first break in the skin (which can spread so alarmingly) is to be prevented.

2. Urinary infection, which may lead to pyelitis and death. At the time of injury retention of urine occurs due to spinal shock, but eventually reflex micturition will return, and although the patient will not have voluntary control over the act, he may be able to initiate the reflex by suprapubic pressure. It is in the early days, while the bladder is atonic, that the risk of infection is greatest, and administration of a urinary antiseptic with a copious fluid intake is begun at once. If catheterization is required, the technique must be faultless, but it should be avoided altogether if suprapubic pressure is effective in emptying the bladder.

3. At a later stage contractures may develop at the hips and knees, and this must be prevented by efficient management.

On admission, then, the main problems are to preserve the patient from pressure sores and urinary infection, but there will be a grave psychological problem as well. The patient will be stunned by the misfortune that has befallen him, and must be prevented from sinking into apathy. Above all, he must be encouraged to take a high protein diet and drink plenty of fluids. In those cases (the majority) in which the use of the arms is retained, he must be encouraged to use them, since it is by the development of these muscles that he will eventually regain some independence.

The bowels will give trouble, since voluntary control is lost and the abdominal muscles cannot contract to help expulsion. Aperients will produce incontinence of fluid stools that will make care of the sacral pressure areas more difficult. Regular manual evacuation of the rectum is the most satisfactory long-term method of management.

It is of inestimable benefit if the patient can be transferred to a unit for spinal injuries at a fairly early stage, where his difficulties can receive specialist help, and where there is an atmosphere of hope. He sees around him people who have met with a similar misfortune, and are overcoming them, and is spurred to emulate them. The social prognosis for someone who is well cared for in the early days, and is determined to lead as active a life as possible, is good. Many paraplegics hold jobs or do their own housework, have families, drive cars and pursue hobbies. The Chronically Sick and Disabled Persons Act, 1970, underlines the needs of the disabled to live at home, to be able to move about and gain access to public buildings, rather than to be kept in institutions.

If the lesion is high enough to cause paralysis of all four limbs (quadriplegia) all these difficulties will be present, and, in addition, the patient must be fed. If breathing is only conducted by the diaphragm, pneumonia is a real risk and treatment in a respirator may be needed, when the prognosis will be a poor one.

CHAPTER 28

OPERATING THEATRE TECHNIQUE

ALL students think a great deal about the operating theatre before they go there to work, and when on their first visit from the surgical ward they watch the smooth routine and swift but controlled activity, they wonder how they will fare when they are members of the theatre team, carrying some of the responsibility for the successful outcome of an operation. When they do so, they find that many hours of preparation have been made for the moment when the surgeon stands ready for the first incision, and may come to realize that the thought and work of thousands of people over many years has gone to the devising of the routines that make aseptic surgery possible. In this chapter some of these preparations and routines will be suggested.

The nurse who is successful in theatre work must be conscientious in adherence to these routines, and must have insight into the reasons for them. She must be able to think quickly, and have the confidence to act quickly as well, often in circumstances of great emotional tension and technical complexity. In ward work speed is desirable, but in the theatre it may be vital. Finally, since every operation is the result of very closely co-ordinated team work, she must be able to work happily and loyally in a group. Contact with patients is apt to be brief—most of those who come in are drowsy in the anæsthetic room ; and not all nurses find the satisfaction here that they do in patient-care in the wards, but some recognize at once a field of work offering great opportunities of service to those who are gifted in it.

Theatre Premises

Ideas on theatre layout are developing continually, and changes in sterilization technique and methods of working theatres have their influence on design. A theatre should not open off a corridor in which there is through-traffic, or bacterial contamination of the air will occur unless air-conditioning is installed. Theatres are ideally situated in a block, so that they can be conveniently supplied from a central packing and sterilizing department. Here trays of instruments, towels, swabs and dressings are assembled, autoclaved and despatched. Theatres in such a block are some distance from the wards they serve, and a recovery room is necessary, to avoid the hazards of a long journey by trolley for an anæsthetized patient. The block should contain an intensive care unit, where those seriously ill, or patients requiring close care for several hours or days can receive it.

The operating room itself is light, but should face north or east so that it is not exposed to long hours of sun, and must be capable of being darkened for endoscopic examinations. Many are built now without windows, with air conditioning, supplied under positive pressure to the clean rooms. The floor is smooth for easy cleaning, quiet to walk on and not slippery; the walls are washable, and meet the floor in a rounded curve, not an angle. There is an alternative lighting supply in case the main source fails, and all fittings are designed for easy cleaning.

The sterilizing room is equipped with boilers for providing sterile water for lotions, and with instrument autoclaves and there should be enough room for laying trolleys in comfort. There are dressing rooms for surgical and nursing staff, and scrub sinks where the hands and arms are prepared. These are equipped with elbow taps and a mixer for hot and cold water. A clock with a second hand should be in view and the surgeon should be able to see into the operating room while he is scrubbing. There should be sufficient room to put on sterile gowns without risk of brushing against fitments or other people. The sink room in which instruments and bowls are washed should provide comfortable working conditions.

An anæsthetic room in which induction is performed is a psychological advantage to the patient, who never sees the operating room itself. It should be quiet, and not contain any other equipment but that of the anæsthetist, so that there is no necessity for any coming and going that may disturb the patient waiting there. After operation the patient leaves the theatre by a separate exit. This room should have oxygen and suction equipment available, and space for storing blankets for the patient.

PREPARATIONS FOR OPERATION

On the day previous to the operating session, the theatre sister receives the case list from the house surgeon and prepares the stock she requires. Sterile gowns, masks and gloves will be needed for the surgeon and his assistants ; towels for the patient and the trolleys ; swabs, packs, and dressings ; instruments, sutures and needles ; and electrical equipment. If there is no autoclave in the theatre, apparatus like manometers is sent to be autoclaved the day before.

The advent of presterilized stock, prepared either commercially or by a central sterile supply department, has greatly lightened the work of the theatre staff. Disposable articles have replaced many traditional types ; masks are now always disposable, and gloves usually so, which saves much time formerly spent in washing, testing and packing them. Waterproof paper has replaced batiste as a protective, and paper has superseded textiles in many other ways. Sets of operation instruments can be preset and sterilized, and ordered by the theatre sister when she knows her list.

The instruments required will vary not only with the case but with the surgeon, each of whom has his own preferences. Every theatre keeps a list of the basic requirements for each type of case, known as a foundation set, and in addition, a book should be kept for each surgeon listing the instruments he likes for any type of operation he performs. This must be kept up to date. Since all theatre nurses work from such books it is not helpful to give detailed descriptions of the lists used in any particular hospital, but reference is made to the more important groups of common instruments.

OPERATING SESSIONS

The cleaning of the theatre should be done the night before the trolleys are laid. The walls should be washed as far as one can reach; all fixtures are damp-dusted and the floors scrubbed with detergent weekly. After this has been done, no one should enter the theatre except in foot-gear reserved for that purpose. The windows are closed and the air inlet turned on, so that incoming air is filtered and finds its way out under the doors, preventing the possibility of bacteria-laden air from the corridors finding its way in. Firms of contract cleaners are widely used. Sterile packs are put in position, and the anæsthetist's trolley is checked. He will require the following:

Face masks, assorted sizes, and harnesses.
Corrugated tubing and adaptors.
Airways.
Magill's tubes and introducer.
Endotracheal catheters.
Laryngoscope.
Bronchoscope for emergency tracheal aspiration.
Syringes and disposable needles for intravenous anæsthesia.
Throat packs.
Sucker with assorted nozzles and catheters.
Mouth gag, spatula, sponge holders, tongue forceps, mouth swabs.
Lubricant.
Throat sprays, and tongue cloths.
Spencer Wells' forceps and scissors.
Vomit bowl.
Parolene eye drops.
Stimulant tray.
Anæsthetic machine, fully stocked with cylinders, ether, trilene and the anæsthetics in use.

All nursing staff change their shoes and wear a theatre frock instead of their uniform clothes. The hair is completely covered by a cap, and a mask is worn which must be kept in position over the nose and mouth and not raised and lowered. Masks are changed between cases.

Trolleys can be laid by a nurse in sterile gloves. They are wiped over with Sudol 2% before the packs are laid on them. Packs are opened on the trolley, the gloved nurse unfolding the towels towards herself first. Should it be necessary for an unscrubbed nurse to open the pack with Cheatle's forceps, she unfolds it away from herself first.

The instruments can be put on the trolleys in the trays on which they were sterilized, or the instruments are laid directly on the towels. This can be done with Cheatle forceps, or the instrument nurse can scrub and put on a sterile gown and gloves to handle her equipment.

"Scrubbing" and Gowning

Having put on her theatre frock, shoes, cap and mask, the nurse cleanses her hands and forearms preparatory to putting on her sterile

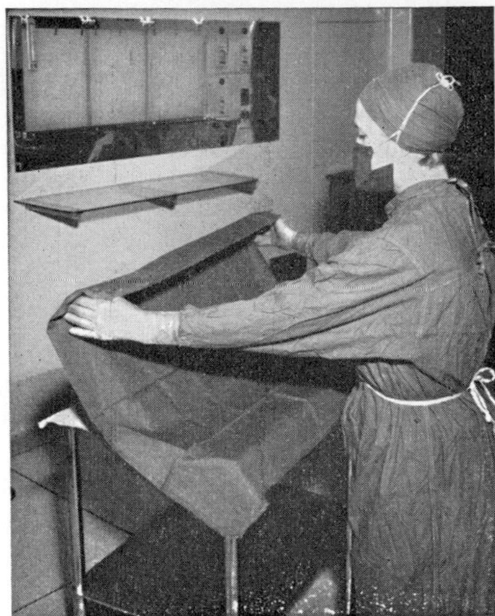

Fig. 106. When covering a trolley with a sterile towel the edge is cuffed over the gloves to protect them from contact with the trolley.

gown. The brush used is preferably a freshly autoclaved one for each case. The water is set running, adjusted to a comfortable temperature, and the nurse notices the time and begins washing with soap. She will continue for not less than five minutes, using the brush for the nails, and soaping and rinsing every part of the hands and arms.

After five minutes she rinses off the soap, allowing the water to run first over her hands, then over the arms. She keeps her hands up so that moisture cannot run on to them from the forearms, takes a sterile towel, dries her hands and then the forearms. The water is mopped up, since rubbing the towel up and down might carry bacteria from the upper parts of the forearms to the hands.

She takes her sterile gown by the collar, the inside of which was left showing when it was packed, and shakes it out in front of her. The arms are put into the sleeves, and an assistant takes the edges of the gown, draws them together in the midline and fastens the neck tapes. The scrubbed nurse holds up the waist tapes, and the assistant takes them by their ends (and not between the gown and the scrubbed hands) and fastens them behind.

The sterile gloves must be put on without touching the exterior with the bare hands, which are first powdered with the lint in the glove packet. The pictures illustrate the way in which it is done. The left glove is taken by the fold and drawn on to the left hand still leaving the cuff turned up. The right glove is picked up by putting the gloved left fingers into the turn-up, and is drawn on to the hand. The right sleeve is folded at the wrist and the fold held with the thumb while the fingers draw the cuff down over it. Finally, the left cuff is turned down.

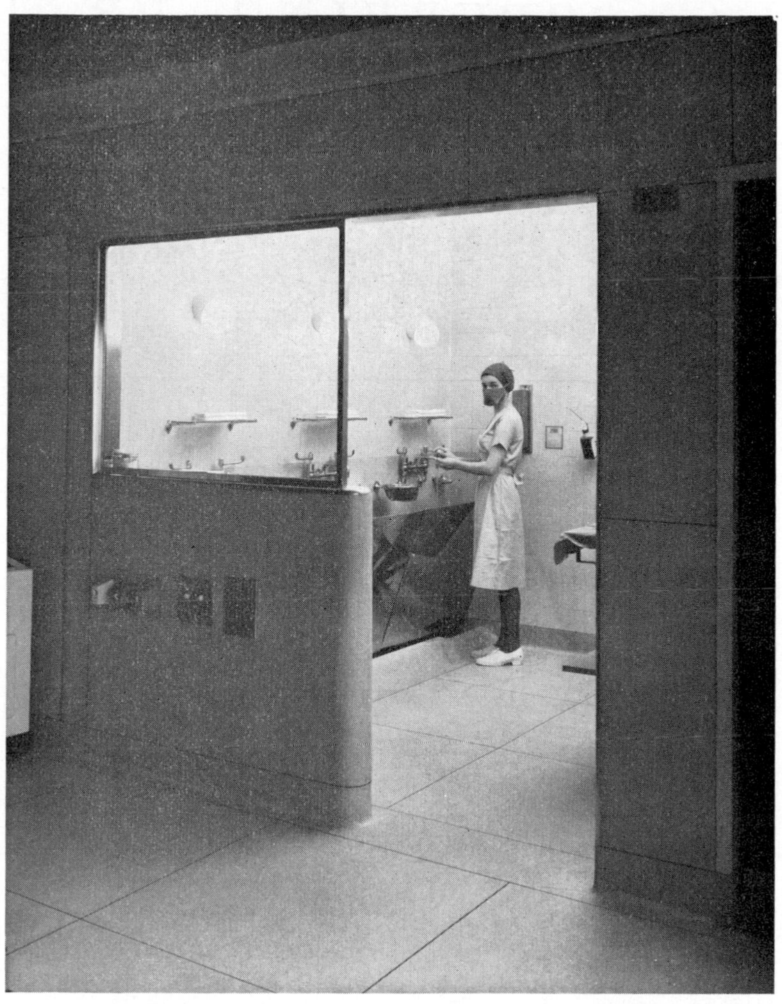

FIG. 107. Sister can see the clock and watch the theatre while washing her hands and arms.

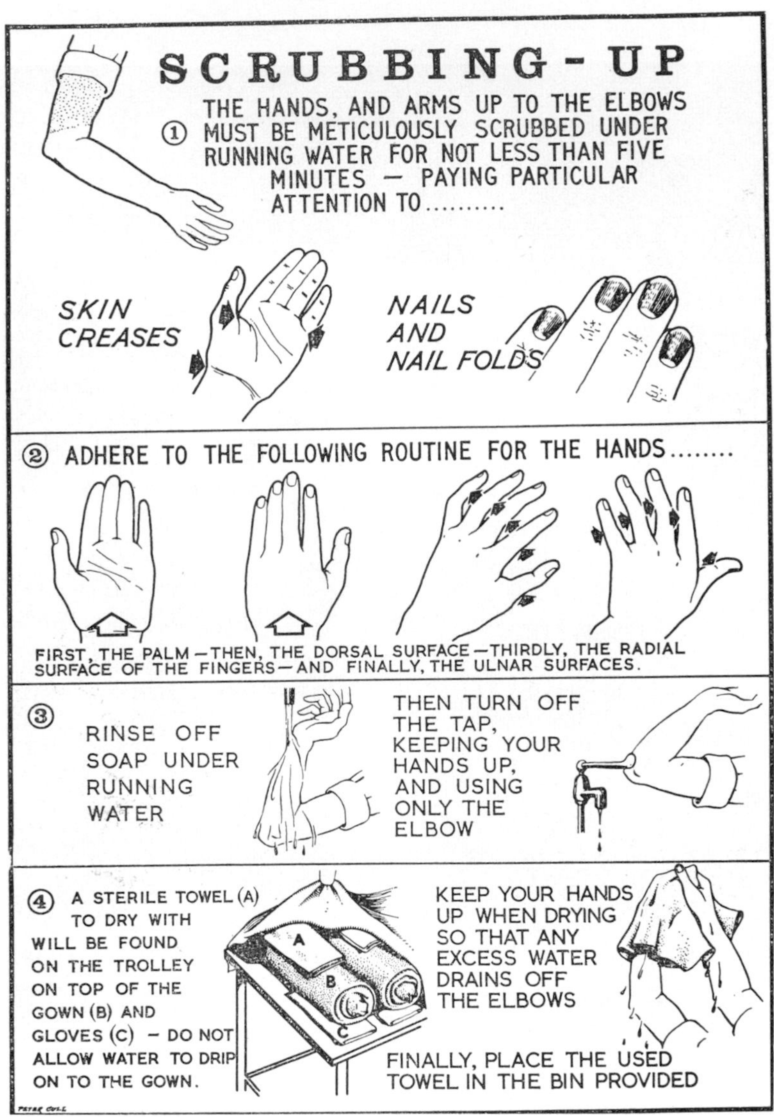

Fig. 108. Preparation of the hands and arms for the operating theatre.

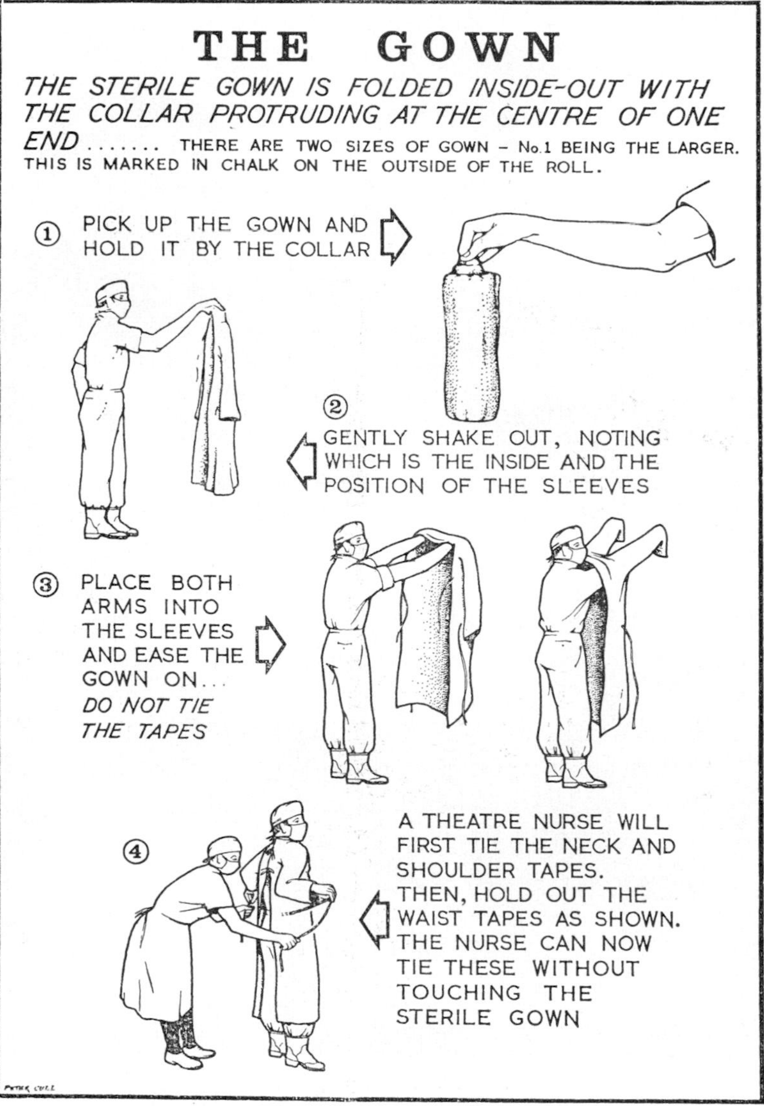

FIG. 109. The surgeon and the theatre sister use the same method when putting on the gown.

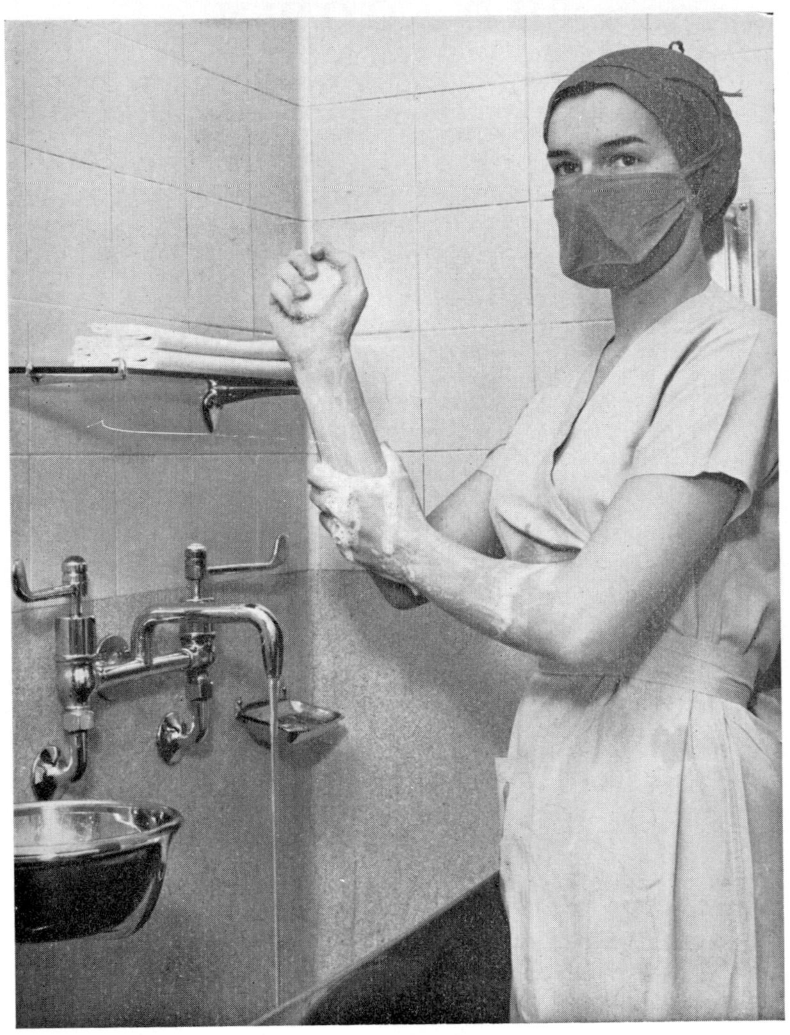

Fig. 110. Hand preparation.

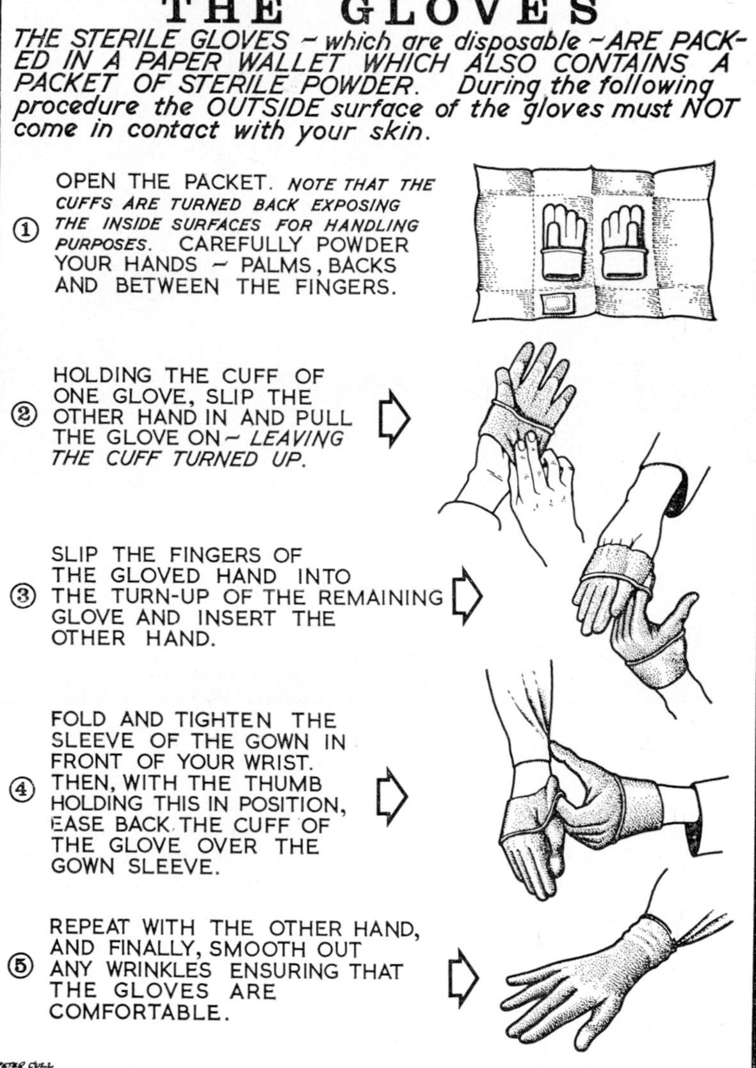

FIG. 111. Putting on sterile gloves.

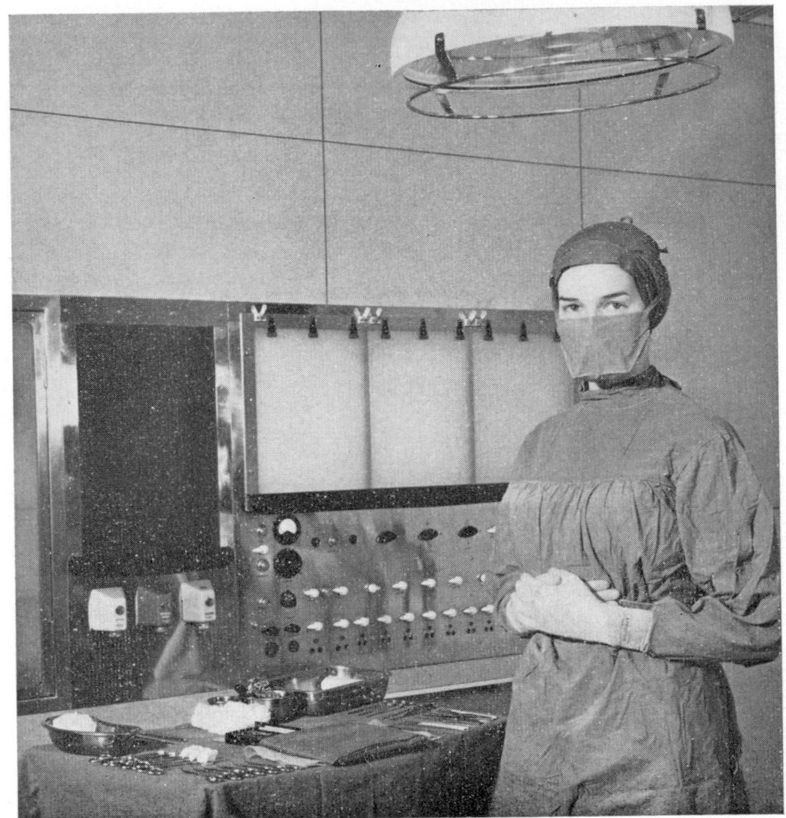

FIG. 112. The gloved hands are not allowed to drop below waist level.

The gloves must be most carefully kept from contact with non-sterile articles. The front of the gown as far as the waist is regarded as sterile, and the hands must be kept in front, and not allowed to drop below the waist level. If a nurse is unoccupied she stands with the hands clasped.

Sterilization of instruments today is by autoclaving, or by dry heat, or some other method capable of killing spores. Boiling is only used as a means of decontamination, e.g. for parts of the anæsthetist's equipment which does not come in contact with spore-forming organisms; his suction catheters and endotracheal tubes should be pre-packed and sterilized.

When using an autoclave, care must be taken in the packing to ensure that it is easily unloaded; this is especially important if the autoclave is double-ended. A Brown tube, or some similar indicator of the temperature reached during the cycle, must be included in each load, in such a position that it is available for scrutiny before the autoclave is unloaded.

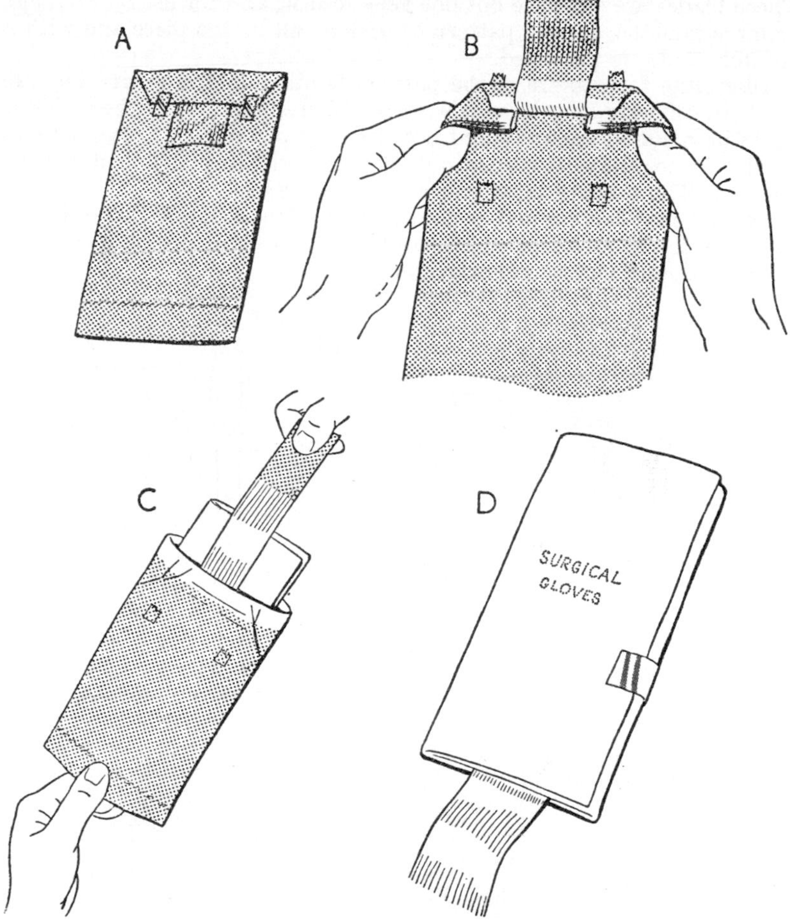

FIG. 113. A method of presenting sterile gloves. Sterile surfaces of the pack are white, unsterile stippled.

A. Gloves sterilized in a paper bag.
B. Opening the pack without contaminating the mouth of the bag.
C. Drawing out the sterile glove packet by means of a paper strip.
D. Sterile pack delivered uncontaminated to the operator.

THEATRE INSTRUMENTS

The basic theatre instruments are not very numerous, but each one has been reproduced in endless variety and size and details of structure, so that even experts cannot hope to recognize all of them. The nurse should aim to recognize the basic patterns, their use and care.

Knives. Knife handles of the Bard-Parker type with detachable blades are very widely used. There are three sizes of handle, and many different sizes and shapes of blade that can be used with them.

These blades are versatile but not very robust, and for use on cartilage or large tendons, the old pattern of scalpel, all in one piece and with a stouter blade, is preferred.

Dissecting forceps are of the pattern familiar in the wards, but are made in differing lengths, and with the blades plain or toothed. They must be handled carefully and not used for picking up heavy articles or the blades may be turned out of true and the instrument will be useless. The grooves must be scrubbed after use.

Scissors may have round or pointed tips. Mayo scissors have shaped blades with rounded tips which can be used in blunt dissection. They can be straight, curved or curved on the flat.

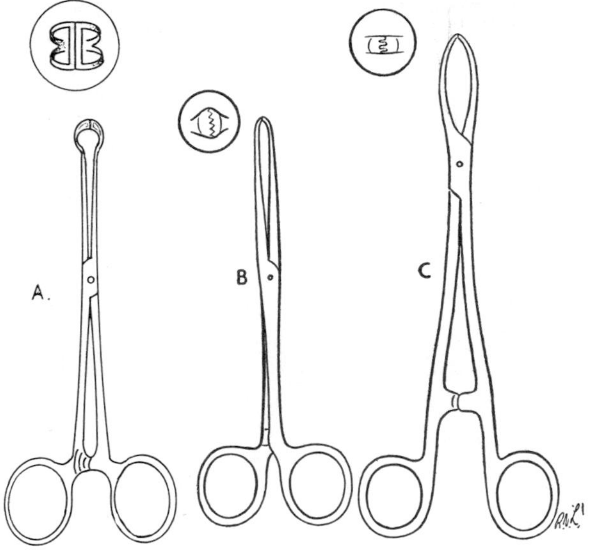

FIG. 114. Tissue forceps.
A. Babcock's. B. Allis'. C. Littlewood's.

Pressure forceps or artery forceps are used to secure bleeding vessels, and the type is the *Spencer Wells'* forceps with serrated blades which can be tightened by a ratchet near the handles. They are sterilized for theatre use fastened together in sixes, and must be accounted for in the same way as swabs are before the peritoneum is closed. After use they are scrubbed in detergent and a spot of oil may be put on the joint with a brush. Though this prolongs the life of the instrument, some authorities think it may interfere with sterilization.

Dunhill forceps are curved in the blade ; *Kocher's* are toothed at the tip. Artery forceps must not be used for clamping thick substances such as rubber tubing or the blades will no longer meet accurately.

Larger forceps are used for special functions. *Pedicle* clamps are less used than formerly, since it is now usual to dissect out vessels and structures and ligature them separately rather than enclose them all in one pedicle clamp. *Moynihan's* cholecystectomy forceps have curved

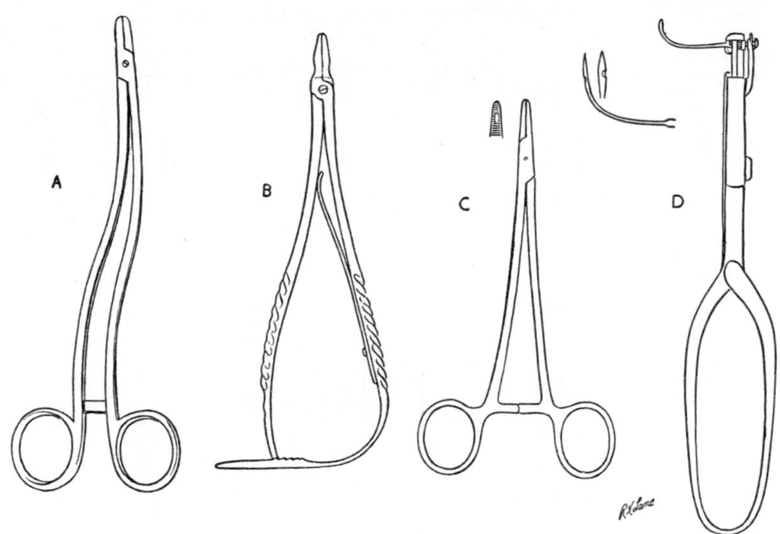

Fig. 115 Some patterns of needle-holder.

A. Bozemann.
B. London Hospital pattern.
C. Mayo pattern.
D. Reverdin.

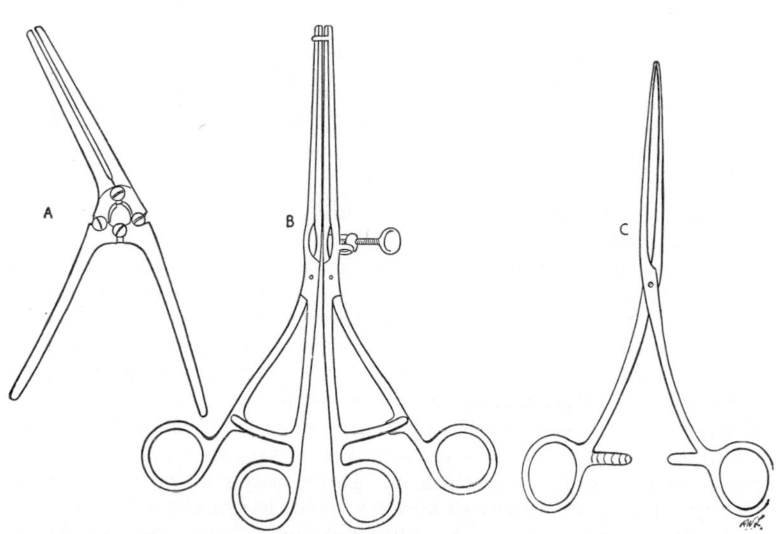

Fig. 116

A. Payr's crushing clamp. **B. Lane's twin clamps.**
C. Kocher's intestinal clamp.

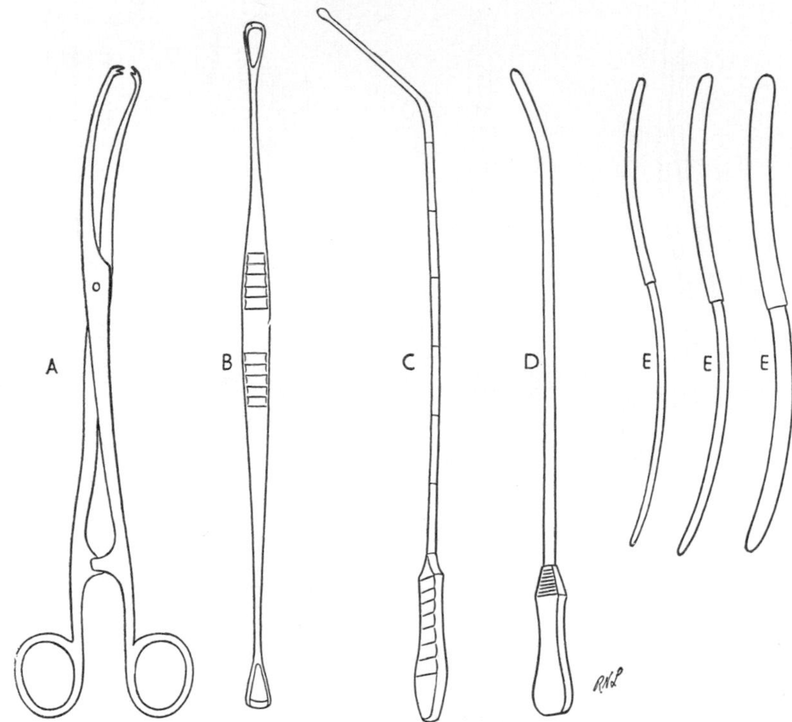

FIG. 117. Some gynæcological instruments.

A. Volsellum forceps. C. Uterine sound.
B. Double-ended uterine curette. D. Female bladder sound
E. Hegar's cervical dilators.

serrated blades and long handles to enable them to reach beneath the liver to the cystic duct.

Tissue forceps are designed to hold tissues without damaging them. Many are made with teeth which meet to grasp the tissue, others have broader ends to hold soft or vascular tissues which must not be punctured by the teeth of the first type. A special example is the volsellum forceps with a curved axis and long blades, used by the gynæcologist to attach to the cervix and draw it down into the vagina.

Retractors are needed by the eye surgeon to keep the lids open, and the thoracic surgeon to spread the ribs apart, so that the greatest variety of shape and size is required. Retractors may be self-retaining, with adjustable blades screwed to a frame, or may have a handle which is held by an assistant. The gynæcologist often uses the Auvard self-retaining speculum for operations within the vagina ; it has a broad blade which lies on the posterior vaginal wall and a weight at the other end.

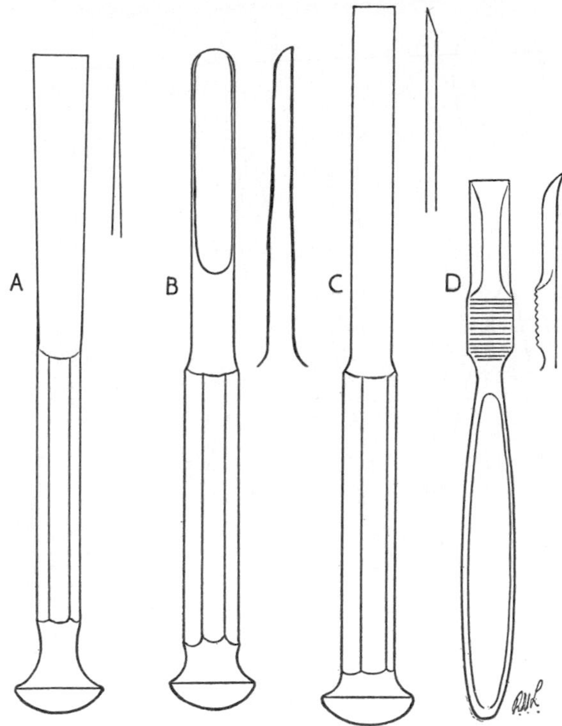

FIG. 118. Bone instruments.
A. Osteotome. C. Chisel.
B. Gouge. D. Periosteal elevator.

Probes are malleable, and often made of silver ; seekers and *dissectors* are also used to explore tissues and channels. The probe-pointed director has a groove along it down which a scalpel can be passed.

Volkmann's spoon is found in every foundation set, and is used for scraping, lifting and extracting fragments of tissue. The *lithotomy* spoon is roughened inside to make it easier to lift stones from the bladder or other organs.

Needle holders have jaws designed for holding curved needles without fracturing them, a ratchet for grasping them, and handles of various designs. Some have thumb and finger rings, in others the instrument is held in the palm. Some have a bend to allow better vision of the needle when working deep in a cavity.

Intestinal Clamps. Clamps for holding the intestine during resection and anastomosis must not damage the structures on which they are placed. The blades only meet at the tips when they are lightly closed, and the required amount of pressure can be obtained by adjusting the ratchet. Some like the blades to be protected by rubber tubing, others believe that this interferes with the efficiency of the instrument.

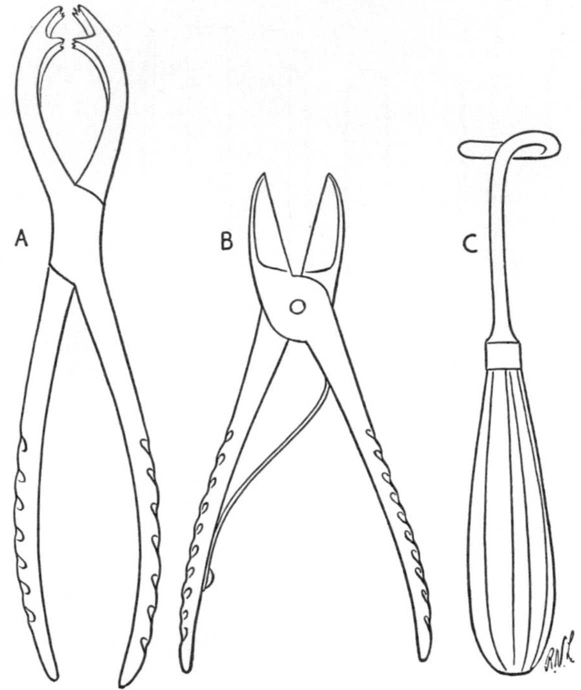

FIG. 119

A. Lion bone-holding forceps. B. Bone cutters. C. Doyen's rib raspatory.

Payr's crushing clamp is used in excision of the colon, and its name indicates its action. When not in use it should not be kept closed or the joints will be strained.

Sounds are used to explore cavities ; bladder sounds may be male or female in shape (the latter shorter and much less curved). The uterine sound is graduated, and its operative end is angled and has an olive-shaped tip. Dilators can be used to stretch urethral strictures or to dilate the cervix.

Bone Instruments. A *chisel* is flat on one side and bevelled on the other ; an osteotome is bevelled on both sides and sometimes is graduated as well. *Gouges* are similar in shape but the cutting edge is curved. *Rugines* or *periosteal elevators* are used to raise periosteum from bone. *Doyen's* rib raspatory is employed in cleaning the tissues from the ribs, while rib shears are used in resection. Lion bone-holding forceps have stout jaws for seizing bone.

Ear, Nose and Throat Instruments. *Eve's tonsil snare* is threaded with a wire loop which can be drawn tight to encircle the tonsil. A *tonsil guillotine* has the handle at right angles to the rest of the instrument, which has a hole which is placed over the tonsil, and a blade which can be pressed home to sever the tonsil. The *adenoid curette* has a stout handle, and a working end which is curved to pass behind the uvula and is armed with a cutting edge or teeth.

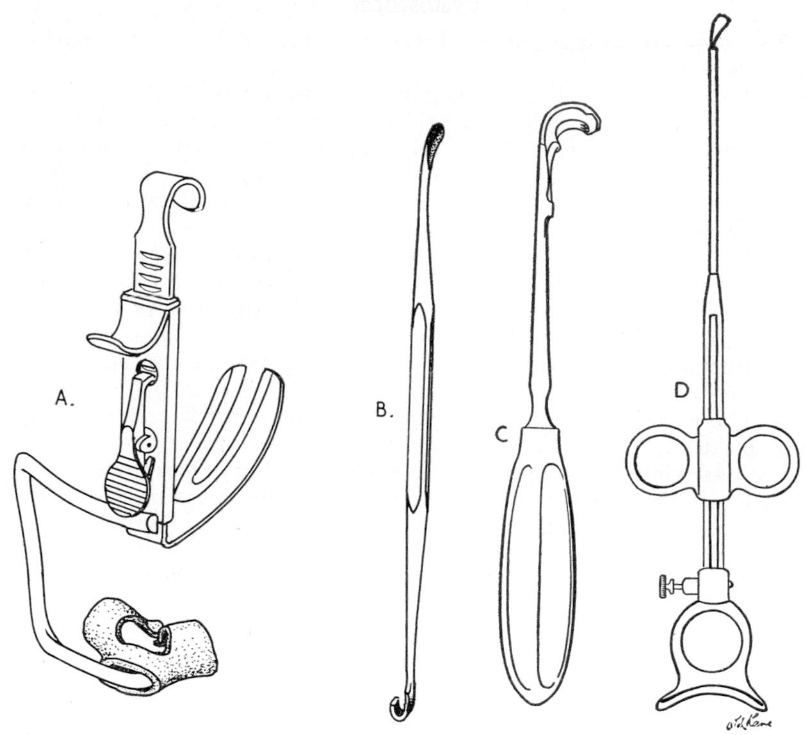

Fig. 120. Some ear, nose and throat instruments.
A. Mason's gag. B. Mollinson's tonsillar pillar retractor/dissector.
C. Adenoid curette. D. Tonsil snare.

ENDOSCOPES

The light by which the body cavities are examined is usually obtained from batteries with a maximum current of 10 volts.

The intensity can be varied by a switch, which must be moved with caution, because the bulbs used are delicate and easily blown. The battery should be connected with the switch in the " Off " position, all terminals should be screwed tight, and the switch gradually advanced until illumination is satisfactory, and the use of the maximum current is not usually needed. The circuit should be tested before the endoscope is prepared for use, and the theatre should be darkened during the procedure.

All scopes must be sterilized after use, and those which are used within bacteria-free cavities, such as the bladder, must be sterile before use. Sterilization is complicated by the fact that some electrical equipment cannot be boiled or autoclaved, and that some of the delicate optical systems are harmed by chemicals.

Cystoscopes

The ordinary cystoscope used for inspecting the bladder consists of these parts :

1. A sheath, the hollow outer part in whose tip is an electric bulb. This tip is set at an angle, and below it is an aperture through which the bladder will be seen. At the other end a valve is screwed on to the sheath, and on to this goes a compression ring, separated from it by a washer. This compression ring can be adjusted to allow a close fit between the sheath and the next part of the cystoscope.

2. The telescope fits into the sheath and contains the lens system by which the bladder is inspected. The only lenses to be seen are one near the tip, and the eyepiece at the other end, but six or more additional ones are concealed within the telescope.

3. Inlet and outlet tubes allow lotion to be run in and out of the bladder.

4. The switch, which clips on to the sheath, and is connected by flex to the battery, or the transformer from the mains supply.

Catheterizing cystoscopes vary in pattern, and may carry one or two catheters. The ureteric catheters are inserted through nozzles and the tips can be passed into the ureters under direct vision by directing them with a pinion handle.

When the light has been tested, the cystoscope is take to pieces for sterilization.

Glutaraldehyde (Cidex) is a lotion specially designed for sterilizing cystoscopes. Spores are destroyed in 3 hours. Cystoscopes are rinsed in sterile water before use.

Ureteric catheters are difficult to re-sterilize and the use of disposable pre-packed ones will solve this problem.

After use, the cystoscope is taken apart and washed, water being allowed to run through it. Spirit must not be used for cleaning the lens, as it harms the cement in the mount. If it is required again during the same operating session, pasteurization is the best method. Cystoscopes may be immersed for 10 minutes in a tank kept at 75° C. If this is not available, hibitane 0·5% in 70% isopropyl alcohol can be used.

The lotion used for filling the bladder is usually sterile water, and the lubricant must be a jelly since liquid paraffin interferes with visibility.

The *resectoscope* is similar in construction to a cystoscope but permits the passage of a diathermy terminal in order to remove papillomata or excise part of the prostate gland. Diathermy loops of various sizes must be supplied, and a diathermy button for coagulation of bleeding points.

Sigmoidoscopes

The sigmoidoscope consists of a sheath graduated in centimetres, which is closed during insertion by an obturator. When the instrument is in place, the light-carrier is inserted, and the lights in most modern instruments are near the eye end. A glass eye piece closes the end while the surgeon is inspecting, and a bellows is attached to a side opening so that the folds of the sigmoid colon may be opened out. Swab carriers, biopsy forceps and retrieving forceps are used in connection with the sigmoidoscope.

After use it is dismantled and cleaned meticulously, and since it is of metal it may be autoclaved or boiled before it is put away. It is not sterile when in use.

Bronchoscopes

The bronchoscope is a tapering metal sheath with side holes and a distal bevelled end. The light, which is very small, is on a long carrier which passes down the side of the tube. Suckers may be used down the apparatus to aspirate secretions or blood, and oxygen may be passed

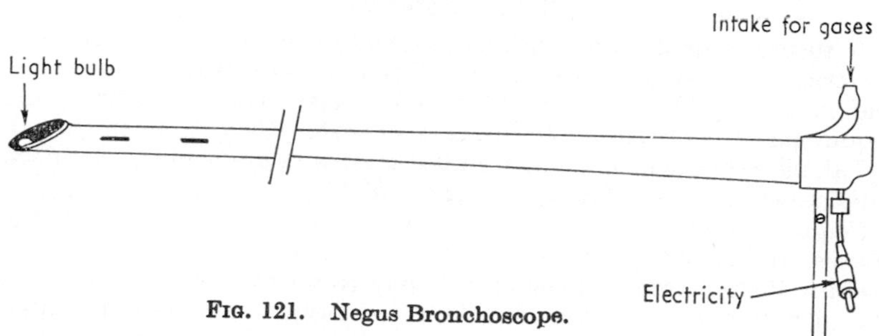

FIG. 121. Negus Bronchoscope.

through a side arm. Biopsy and retrieving forceps are usually necessary. Inspection of the various bronchi may be made with telescopes that allow forward or sideways vision.

After use the bronchoscope is cleaned inside with a long brush and is sterilized at once, since it is so often used in infective conditions. The metal parts can be boiled or autoclaved, and the light is sterilized in formalin instrument solution or hibitane. It is sterilized again just before use.

Œsophagoscopes

These are blackened on the inside, and graduated on the outside, and as the procedure is conducted in a darkened theatre a torch must

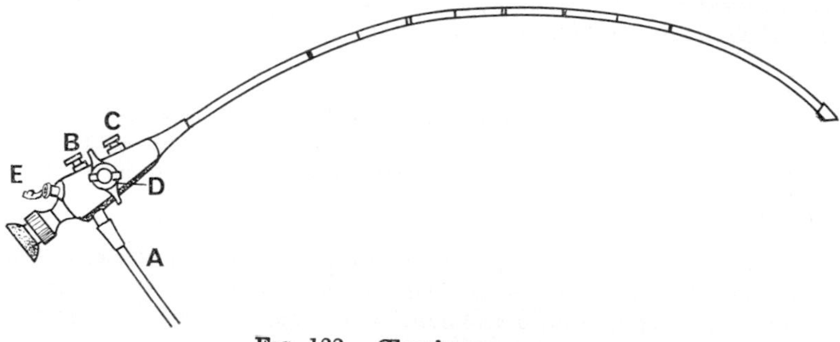

FIG. 122. Œsophagoscope.

be available to allow the figures to be read. Newest types employ fibre lighting; the light is transmitted along bundles of glass fibres from an outside source. It is sterilized before use.

Sucker and biopsy forceps are required for a diagnostic œsophagoscopy, and if it is being performed for the extraction of a foreign body, bone-cutters (to break up hard objects) and retrieving forceps will be used. Souttar's tube is sometimes introduced at œsophagoscopy in order to try to maintain a passage for fluids past a growth. Spiral metal ones are commonly used, but if radiotherapy is to be given a plastic one is inserted. After use œsophagoscopes are washed and autoclaved or boiled.

Suture Materials

A suture is used with a needle ; a ligature is used to tie off such structures as a cut vessel or ureter. The materials used are the same, and in no way do surgeons differ more widely than in their suture requirements, both in material and in size. Catgut, linen-thread, nylon, all varieties of silk and stainless steel wire are made in standard thicknesses, from 4/0 (finest) through 0 to 4.

Catgut is used internally, since it does not remain for ever in the tissues, and sometimes on the perineum where the same property is useful. Plain catgut will last from a day to about a week ; while the chromicized variety remains for about ten days, or for the time stated by the manufacturers under normal conditions. It is supplied ready sterilized in ampoules or packets.

Nylon is a very popular suture material for the skin, and for peritoneum, deep tension stitches and muscle repair. Various types of man-made fibres are in use (e.g. Teflon for arterial surgery), and these are constantly being improved and changed.

Wire has many uses, especially internally. It is difficult to handle, and must not be kinked, or it will break or damage the tissue through which it is being drawn.

Silk is widely used for sutures and is manufactured in many different forms, such as mersilk, a proofed, braided silk. Size 000 is in common use for the skin.

Linen thread can be used for muscle or internally. Silk and thread are transferred to spools, and should be wound loosely as they shrink with sterilization.

Metal clips are used for the skin.

Needles

Surgical needles are used on all structures from conjunctiva to bronchus, and on sites varying in accessibility from the skin to the depths of the pelvis. They differ, according to their uses, in these respects :

1. Size.
2. Shape. They are made semi-circular, five-eighths circle, curved or straight. Straight needles are used in general on the skin, and may be held in the fingers ; half-circle needles require a needle holder and are most used within cavities.
3. Edge. They may be round-bodied for use within the peritoneal cavity, or have a cutting edge for traversing fascia or skin.
4. Point. Lance-pointed needles have a flattened tip, while trocar-pointed ones have the shape their name implies.

5. Atraumatic or eyeless needles have a special slot which holds the suture by its end, so that the double strand associated with threading an ordinary needle is avoided. They are especially used for intestinal and vascular anastomoses and other situations where the injury inflicted by the passage of the needle and suture must be minimal, but are replacing other types of needle for general work.

6. Some needle holders, such as Reverdin's, have a needle incorporated in the instrument.

Swabs

Gauze swabs for mopping are usually bought ready made to save labour by the theatre staff, and may have a radio-opaque thread in them so that they can be easily identified by X-ray in the unlikely event of one being left within a body cavity. Large swabs often have a black tape attached to make them more readily visible within the peritoneal cavity.

Swabs should be tied with tape in bundles of a convenient number and five is a standard one. As the theatre sister brings a bundle into use she discards the tape and counts them. As soiled swabs are discarded, they are picked up with forceps and hung on a swab rack so that the number can be checked, and the surgeon can also obtain an estimate of the blood loss. In some centres the swabs are weighed after use to find the blood loss accurately, and this is useful unless lotion or wet swabs are being used.

The swabs used and those still remaining on the sister's trolley should be counted and totalled before the closure of the peritoneum and any organ (such as the bladder or uterus) that has been opened, and at the end of every operation, and the surgeon told that all have been accounted for. Small swabs should be held in pressure forceps, as it is easy to mislay them when they are soaked in blood.

The Theatre Table

The theatre table is capable of very fine adjustment to meet the needs of the patient and the surgeon. Its position is movable, and there is a brake to stabilize it when it is in place. The height from the ground can be altered to suit the surgeon. The level can be changed from the horizontal by lowering either the head or the foot, and it can also be tilted from side to side. The table can be dropped 90°, the head may be raised or lowered, or the trunk hyperextended.

Along the sides are brackets to which can be attached such equipment as a wire screen which can be draped with sterile towels to exclude the anæsthetist and his equipment from the sterile field; an instrument stand; pelvic rests; or lithotomy poles. These are used to maintain the patient in position on the table, and the following are among the commoner ones.

1. *Dorsal.* The patient lies flat on the back for most abdominal operations. For operations on the breast the arm on the affected side lies on an arm rest, and must not be abducted to more than a right angle for fear of injury to the brachial plexus. The arms must be secured at the sides by linen restrainers, or padded malleable lead strips which pass beneath the trunk at the desired level, and are bent

over the wrists or forearms. The arm rest is also used when intravenous fluids are being given.

No part of the patient must be in contact with the metal of the table, and many surgeons like to have sandbags beneath the Achilles' tendons to prevent pressure by the table on the calves (which might predispose to venous thrombosis) or on the heels of patients with vascular disease.

2. *Lithotomy*, for operations on the vagina, perineum or rectum. The bottom section of the table is dropped, the lithotomy poles are inserted alongside the break, and the legs supported on the outside of the poles by straps passing round the feet. Both legs must be flexed and brought into position simultaneously or injury to the hip joint may result. The buttocks should be brought right down to the end of the table, and pads put between the legs and the poles.

3. *Trendelenburg*. This is the head-low position, used for operations on the pelvis through the abdominal wall, especially gynæcological ones and in the treatment of shock. Obviously some means must be

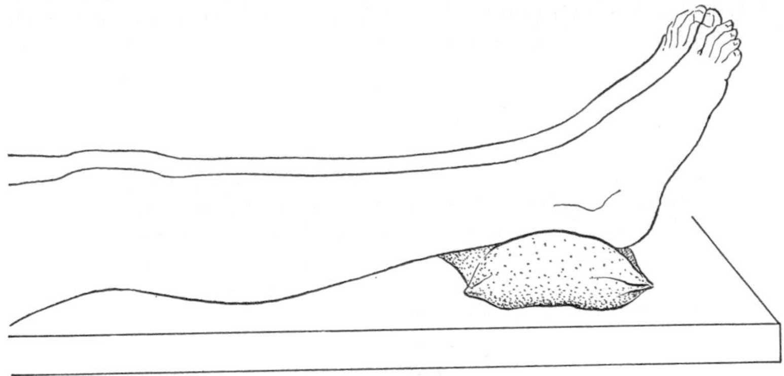

FIG. 123. Ankle pads. Pressure on the calves is relieved and the risk of venous thrombosis decreased.

used to prevent the patient slipping down the table. Shoulder rests have been much used, but may cause brachial plexus injury; the end of the table may be broken so that the knees are flexed to a right angle and the ankles are secured to the table. This puts pressure on the calves and increases the incidence of post-operative thrombosis.

The Langton-Hewer non-slip mattress avoids both risks. It is of anti-static rubber, grooved transversely, to which the bare skin of the back and calves will adhere. A small lumbar pillow similarly grooved increases the area of contact, and has straps attached for securing the arms to the mattress ; the shoulders rest against a similar pillow. It is obviously important to see that the end of the mattress is hooked over the end of the table before it is tilted.

This mattress can be kept on the table in emergency abdominal cases, since if it is necessary to lower the head of the table quickly, it can be done with the minimum of trouble. For abdomino-perineal operations a combined lithotomy-Trendelburg position is used, with the legs supported in troughs, so that the hips need not be flexed to such an extent that access to the abdomen is impeded.

4. *Kidney Position.* The kidney is exposed by an incision parallel to the lower ribs, and sometimes involving resection of the 12th rib. The patient lies on the sound side with the lower leg flexed and the upper one straight, and the table is broken in the middle, or a sandbag or a kidney bridge used, in order to hyperextend the operation site. The upper arm is supported on a rest, and the trunk and arm strapped to prevent accidental movement. If the table has a lateral tilting mechanism it is useful for kidney operations.

5. *Thyroid Position.* Operations on the neck require extension of

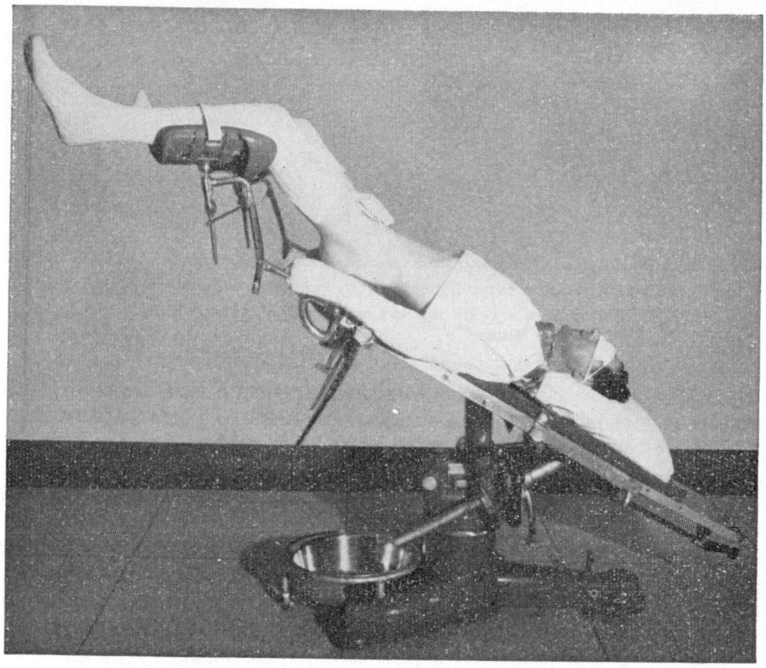

Fig. 124. Lithotomy-Trendelenburg position. It may be used for abdomino-perineal excision of rectum, and for radical excision of malignant growths of the uterus. (*Atlas of Surgery. By F. Wilson Harlow, Heinemann.*)

the head and neck, and the table is raised slightly at the upper end.

Whatever position is adopted, it must be stable ; the best possible working conditions for the surgeon must be assured ; and there must be no undue pressure on any part of the patient. This is especially true of the arms of which the nerves can easily be injured by pressure or abduction with extension.

6. *Postero-lateral Thoracotomy Position.* This ressembles the kidney position, but the left leg is straighter and there is a pad between the legs above the ankle. There is a buttress behind the lower thigh, a vertical post in front of the pelvis, a rest in front of the chest, and a pad

under the chest to open up the ribs. The upper arm hangs free, to allow the scapula to move forwards.

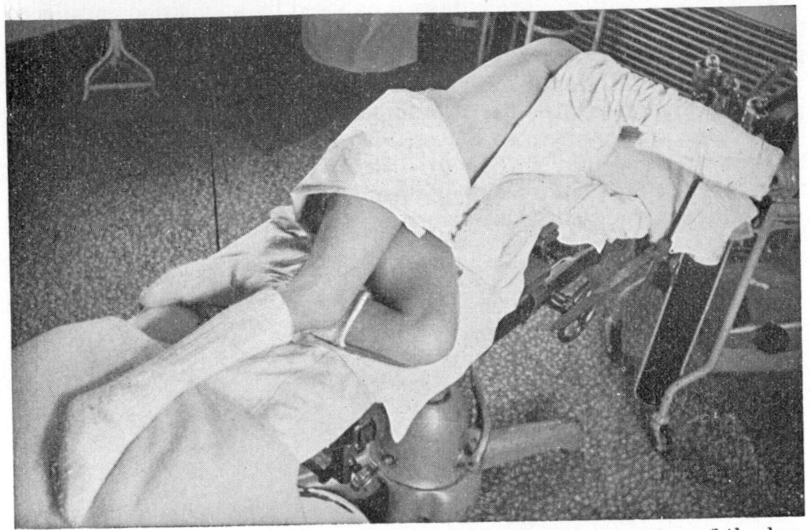

FIG. 125. **Kidney position, showing the arm rest and the position of the legs.** (*Atlas of Surgery. By F. Wilson Harlow, Heinemann.*)

CONDUCT OF AN OPERATION

When the patient is firmly and safely in position and his anæsthetic condition is satisfactory the operation site and a wide area around is cleaned by an assistant with swabs in sponge-holding forceps and the lotion of the surgeon's choice. The sterile towels are put in position by the theatre sister and an assistant, and the patient is ready for the surgeon.

He is offered the knife with the handle towards him and the cutting edge of the blade downwards and artery forceps are given to his assistant to secure the bleeding points. These are handed up closed, held by the middle and with the handle foremost. Plastic sheets (e.g. vidrape or steridrape) through which the incision can be made are often used.

The sister watches the course of the surgeon's work, trying to anticipate his needs. Swabs and artery forceps are at hand when required, needles are threaded, and instruments that have been used are rinsed in sterile lotion and put back. The operation field and trolley should be kept neat and business-like.

The surgeon's work is made as easy and speedy as possible by handing his instruments ready for use. Ligatures are held in both hands so that he can take them without looking up. Ligatures are drawn one-third of the way through the needle, and the needle holder is attached fairly near the eye end. The thread should be held while the needle-holder is being passed, so that it does not drag over the operation site. Ligatures and sutures must not be too long or they will knot and cause waste of time and temper.

In addition, she thinks constantly of her sterile technique and watches that of her assistants. Her hands are not allowed to drop below the level of the table, and if she turns away from the table she turns away from the surgeon. If two people in gloves want to change places, they should cross back to back.

As the operation draws to a close, instruments are cleared from the table, the dressing is prepared and applied, and the patient is moved to the trolley or his bed ready for transfer to the ward. He remains in the care of the theatre staff until the ward nurse appears, hears from the houseman what surgery has been performed, and accompanies her patient back to the ward. Meanwhile the theatre is being prepared for the next patient, who is already in the anæsthetic room.

Emergencies

Dangerous complications may arise suddenly in the theatre, and action must be prompt and cool. The ones with which the nurse may assist are these :

1. *Vomiting.* Vomiting, especially at the beginning or end of anæsthesia, may endanger the airway. The anæsthetist will call for the head of the table to be lowered, and the nurses must be familiar with the mechanism so that it can be done instantly. The anæsthetist may ask for a bronchoscope to aspirate fluid from the trachea.

2. *Cardiac arrest.* If the abdomen is open, the heart may be massaged through the diaphragm. If the operation has not yet begun, the procedure described on p. 516 is instituted. Syringes and needles for intracardiac and intravenous use are prepared, and the drugs that may be needed include nikethamide, 1% procaine, 1% calcium chloride, 10 ml. sterile normal saline, and 1 ml. 1–1,000 adrenalin.

3. *Hæmorrhage.* Large vessels may be cut, ligatures may slip or veins may tear. Artery forceps and packs should be ready in quantity, and the nurses should be ready to alter the position of the table as requested.

4. *Fire.* Anæsthetic explosions are fortunately rare because of the precautions taken to avoid them. If diathermy is to be used, ether should be avoided, and the ether bottle should be removed from the anæsthetic machine.

Explosions are usually initiated not by electrical equipment but by static electricity, which is generated by friction, e.g. by drawing a blanket over a mackintosh, or a theatre trolley. Theatre tables, trolleys or beds may be given a high voltage charge in this way if the wheels are of a non-conducting material, and this is discharged with the production of a spark if a person or another piece of apparatus is near. Static electricity is generated most easily in a dry atmosphere, and much thought is given to averting its formation. Tables, trolleys, anæsthetic machines, and similar equipment are earthed by the addition of a small chain which just reaches the floor and allows any charge to leak away. Alternatively the wheels are made of anti-static rubber which conducts the charge away. The floor in the theatre should always be of a conducting material.

STERILIZATION

The methods of sterilization used in surgery involve heat (dry or moist) and chemicals. Chemical sterilization tends to be uncertain and manufacturers are constantly introducing substances capable of heat sterilization to replace those which would not withstand it.

Autoclave Sterilization

This most efficient method has already been described in Chapter 19.

Boiling

Boiling cannot be relied upon to kill spores, but is effective against all ordinary bacteria, and is widely used for china and instruments for ward use. In theatre work autoclaving is rapidly replacing it. Boiling for five minutes is effective, if the water really boils throughout that period and timing is accurate and articles are completely submerged. Nothing else must be put into the sterilizer during this period.

Dry heat

The use of hot air for sterilization takes a longer time at higher temperatures than does steam. Bulky items such as dressings cannot be sterilized by hot air, neither can plastics, which are damaged by the high temperatures needed. Oils, powders and glassware can be effectively treated. The times and temperatures given here are those ruling after the required temperature has been reached.

Temperature	*Holding times*
190° C	$1\frac{1}{2}$ minutes
180° C	$7\frac{1}{2}$ minutes
170° C	18 minutes
160° C	45 minutes

In conveyor ovens, equipment to be sterilized is carried on moving belts through ovens heated (usually) by infra-red radiation. This method is only suitable for large-scale use, as the ovens are not easy to manage. Syringes are often sterilized in bulk by this method.

Ionizing Radiation

Sterilization can be effected by exposing articles to gamma rays from a radioactive source, usually cobalt 60. The size and cost of the necessary plant is such that this is almost always used by commercial firms for pre-packed articles, especially plastics. There is no risk that the articles will become radioactive.

Ethylene Oxide

Large articles such as ventilators and heart-lung machines can be sterilized by enclosing them in large plastic bags, and admitting ethylene gas 10% in carbon dioxide. Respirators should be allowed to cycle for 24 hours in the gas.

Disinfectants and Antiseptics

Most chemical disinfectants, however, are liquids, and articles are immersed in them for sterilization. A disinfectant suitable for the purpose should be chosen, and the strength and time of exposure must be known. Unfortunately, standard methods do not exist, and perhaps cannot in view of the varying textures of the articles exposed to them. The list here is of some of the better-known ones and what they may be used for.

Name	*Comments*	*Uses*
Phenol (carbolic acid).	Corrosive at full strength; not usually stocked stronger than 1–10.	1–20 for linen, excreta, mackintoshes. Phenol and its derivatives are not commonly used now.
Perchloride of mercury.	Corrosive to metals. Poisonous.	1–1,000 for gum elastic catheters. 1–10,000 for eye irrigation.
Oxycyanide of mercury.		1–10,000 for bladder irrigation.
Mercurochrome.		1% for bladder irrigation.
Formalin.	Is used as a gas or in solution.	Formalin vapour is used for fumigating rooms. Borax and formaldehyde instrument solution will disinfect metal or glass in 30 minutes.
Chloroxylenol (Dettol).	Pleasant smelling, slightly sticky.	1–20 for vaginal douches. In cream as an antiseptic hand cream.
Surgical spirit.	A good skin antiseptic; not a disinfectant.	70% for dressings; skin preparation.
Potassium permanganate.		1–1,000 as deodorant irrigating fluid.
Hydrogen peroxide.	10–20 volumes. Decomposed by light.	Oxygen is evolved on contact with organic matter. Used as an irrigant for infected wounds. Is followed by normal saline.
Iodine.	Tincture of iodine 2·5%. Betadine is less irritating than the tincture.	A good skin disinfectant to which some are sensitive. Skin must be allowed to dry before being covered.
Milton.	Electrolytic sodium hypochlorate. Liberates chlorine. Will rot wool, silk or similar materials.	1–80 hand disinfectant (30 seconds). Sterilization of babies' bottles and teats between feeds.
Chlorhexidine (Hibitane).		0·5% in 70% alcohol for skin preparation, or for emergency disinfection of instruments. Allow at least two minutes and rinse in sterile water before use.
Gentian violet. Brilliant green. Bonney's blue.	Dyes from coal tar.	Skin disinfectants. Once used for burns dressing. Gentian violet 1% for thrush of vagina and occasionally of mouth.
Cetrimide.	Quaternary ammonium compound.	Is a detergent very widely used at 1% in surgical dressings.

Name	*Comments*	*Uses*
Bradosol.	Quaternary ammonium compound.	A detergent. 1–2,000 for skin lotion.
Roccal (Benzalkonium chloride).	Quaternary ammonium compound.	Tincture (1% for skin preparation). 1–10 for 30 minutes for instruments. 1–20 as hand lotion and for bowls, basins, baths. 1–40 for rubber articles, disinfecting soiled linen ; floors, walls, etc.
Hexachlorophane		Soap with hexachlorophane 1% if used constantly reduces bacterial skin counts. pHisoflex is hexachlorophane and detergent, and is used in sterilizing the hands before donning gloves in the theatre.
Sudol	Phenol derivative. Damages plastic materials.	Strengths and uses are similar to Lysol; is not corrosive. 1–20 for disinfecting baths; swab thoroughly and leave five minutes. 1–40 for six hours for grossly infected linen. 1–80 for four hours will disinfect enteric stools.

CHAPTER 29

BANDAGES AND BANDAGING

BANDAGING is a skill over which the student nurse is very likely to suffer disillusionment. During her preclinical period she spends some considerable time in learning the theory and practising bandages for all parts of the body, but soon after entering hospital she finds that only a small proportion of these patterns are used regularly, while others are needed so seldom that when they are required she is no longer familiar with them. Some are never used, and have become embalmed by tradition as examination techniques, while in out-patient departments where bandages are most used, a proprietary brand of stockingette bandage is used almost exclusively.

This position is the result of three factors. The technique of bandaging was evolved at a time when most patients stayed in bed at rest, and there was no need to put on bandages which would withstand movement. Secondly, adhesive materials are much improved in design, and the lighter dressings now favoured have brought them into extensive use. Thirdly, the greatly increased scope of nursing has made the saving of time and labour imperative, so that the rapid and efficient results that can be achieved with Tubegauz have gained wide recognition. The details of applying bandages by this means to all parts of the body can be obtained from the manufacturers, and a useful one for a finger is illustrated.

MATERIALS

These are the more common materials from which bandages are made :

1. Cotton. Heavy weaves are used for slings ; thin porous ones form open-wove bandages which are cheap and light but whose edges fray and which cannot be laundered. Firmer ones with a fast edge can be washed repeatedly.
2. Domette. This woven material with a slightly fluffed surface makes a firm supporting bandage, which has some resilience but can be used to give firm support.
3. Flannel. Strips are used for dressing splints like Thomas's and Braun's.
4. Crepe. These bandages are elastic and the degree to which they are stretched in applying determines the amount of pressure they exert. They are very widely used.
5. Plaster. Plaster muslin is the basis for making plaster of Paris bandages, which are described on p. 379.
6. Stockingette, the use of which has already been mentioned.
7. Proprietary tubular material, such as Tubegauz or Netelast.

BANDAGE SHAPES

1. *Manytail.* Five lengths of 5-in. domette bandage are laid overlapping each other by a third of their width and stitched together at their centre over a piece 8-in. of domette. This is the standard abdomi-

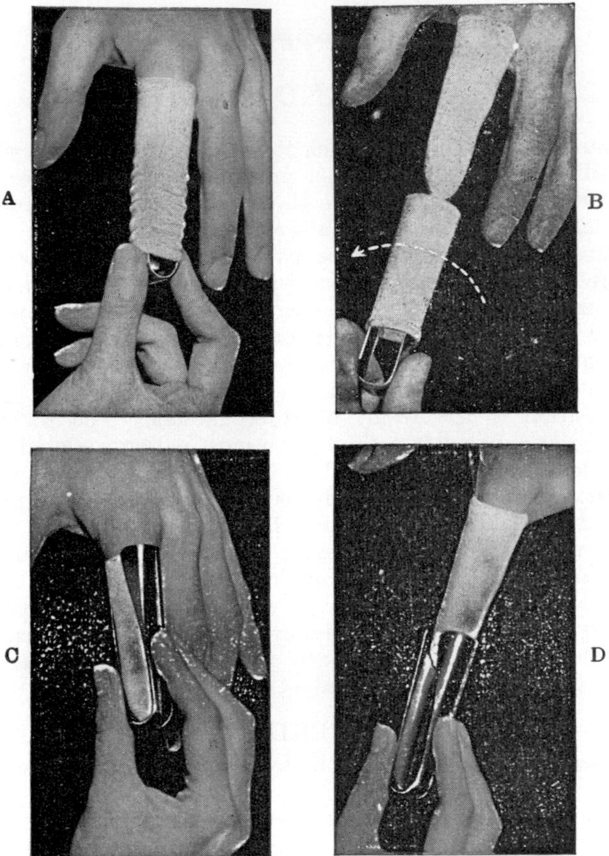

FIG. 126. Finger bandage using Tubegauz.

A. Cut off length of Tubegauz, a little more than twice length of finger. Gather on to the applicator and place over finger.
B. Lightly hold Tubegauz in position at base of finger ; withdraw the applicator to the extremity and twist one complete turn.
C. Move applicator forward again and the Tubegauz doubles back and applies the second layer.
D. Withdraw applicator leaving bandage complete, and secure with adhesive plaster.

(*Reproduced by courtesy of The Scholl Manufacturing Co. Ltd.*)

nal bandage, if one is used at all, since it will cover an incision anywhere on the abdomen and can be applied and undone with the minimum of disturbance. When preparing for application, both ends are rolled up to the centre and put behind the patient so that the tails to be used first are the lowest. Two nurses can apply it more evenly and firmly than one, and each in turn folds a tail firmly over the abdomen, overlapping her partner's turn. The last tail is carried transversely across the abdomen and fastened with safety pins. If the bandage tends to ride up it can be secured by groin straps, which are lengths of 4-in.

open-wove bandages folded into three. These are passed behind the thigh, at the level of the gluteal fold and the ends brought together in front and secured with a pin to the bandage.

A standard length for manytails is 56 in., but ward sisters order them to suit the size of patient they habitually nurse. Domette shrinks in washing, and too small a bandage is ineffective.

2. *T-bandages.* These are used to retain perineal dressings in place, and are made of a piece of domette large enough to encircle the waist and tie in front. To the centre back is stitched a double length of domette, the two ends of which are brought between the legs and tied over the belt at the front.

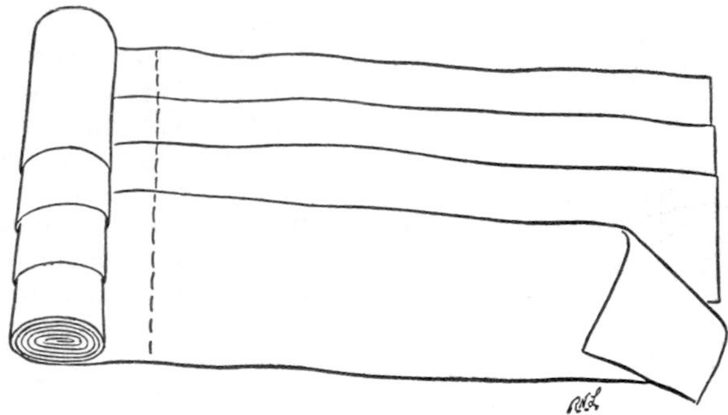

Fig. 127. Manytail bandage.

3. *Triangular.* The chief use in hospital is as a sling, but triangular bandages are much used in first aid to cover temporary dressings, either open or folded into bands of varying width.

When applying a sling, one corner is laid over the sound shoulder, with the right-angled corner just above the level of the elbow on the injured side. The remaining corner is brought across the forearm, adjusted so that the hand is supported at a slight upward slope, and tied with a reef knot which lies in the hollow above the clavicle on the sound side. The right angle is folded forward and pinned to enclose the elbow, all edges are folded neatly under, and a pad is put under the knot if it seems likely to cause pressure. Finally it is inspected to see that the wrist is supported, and the shoulder in a natural position.

4. *Roller.* Roller bandages are of different materials and of widths from one inch upwards. When applying them the nurse selects an adequate number of well-rolled bandages of a width appropriate to the part, and takes them in a tray with pins to her patient. These principles apply to bandaging any part of the body.

(*a*) The part is exposed, put in a good position and supported if necessary. If a dressing is used it must be neatly applied first.

(*b*) Begin with a fixing turn, and work from below upwards and within outwards.

(*c*) Each turn overlaps two-thirds of the previous turn.

(*d*) Turns must lie parallel, and the pattern be kept regular.

(*e*) The dressing must be completely covered.

(*f*) The tension is adjusted to the purpose

(*g*) The pin should be on the outside of a limb, or in a position where it cannot cause inconvenience.

The following patterns can be made :

1. **Simple Spiral.** The bandage makes ascending spiral turns. Unless a crepe bandage is used, the turns will only lie flat on parts of a uniform shape, so that the fingers are the only parts that are efficiently bandaged with spirals.

2. **Reversed Spiral.** This pattern is elegant and will fit a shaped limb, but is unstable and will only remain in place if the limb is at rest. It might be used for a forearm kept in a sling, if no pressure was required.

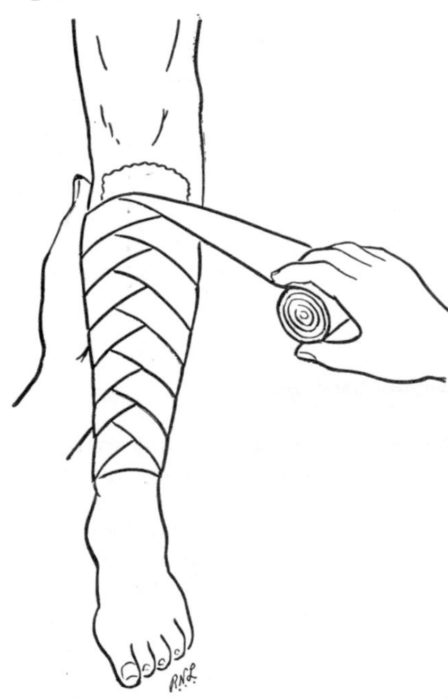

Fig. 128. Reversed spiral of leg.

With the back of the patient's hand towards you, take a fixing turn round the wrist and carry the next turn upwards at an angle of 45°, turn the bandage over to cross itself at a right angle, and bring it round the limb ready for the next turn. The reverse must be made without tension, and the pattern kept up the centre of the pronated forearm.

3. **Figure of 8.** This is much the most useful pattern. It can be used to apply pressure over an extended joint, or to bandage a leg, foot, hand or arm if movement is allowed. To use it on the leg, take a fixing turn, then carry the bandage upward across the front of the limb at 45°, round behind it at the same level and downwards over the front to cross the first turn at a right angle. Repeat the turns until the limb has been sufficiently covered.

4. **Divergent Spica.** This pattern encloses a flexed joint or projection, e.g. knee, heel, or elbow. It merely covers the dressing and exerts no pressure.

To apply it, pass the first and second turns over the centre of the joint. Succeeding turns pass alternately above and below these turns, forming a pattern at each side of the joint.

"Spica" means an ear of wheat, and refers to the type of pattern made in all bandages that bear this name.

BANDAGES FOR VARIOUS PURPOSES

Bandaging the Eye. Stand facing the patient, who is asked to hold the eye pad in position till the bandage includes it. Begin from the affected side to the good across the forehead and round the head in a

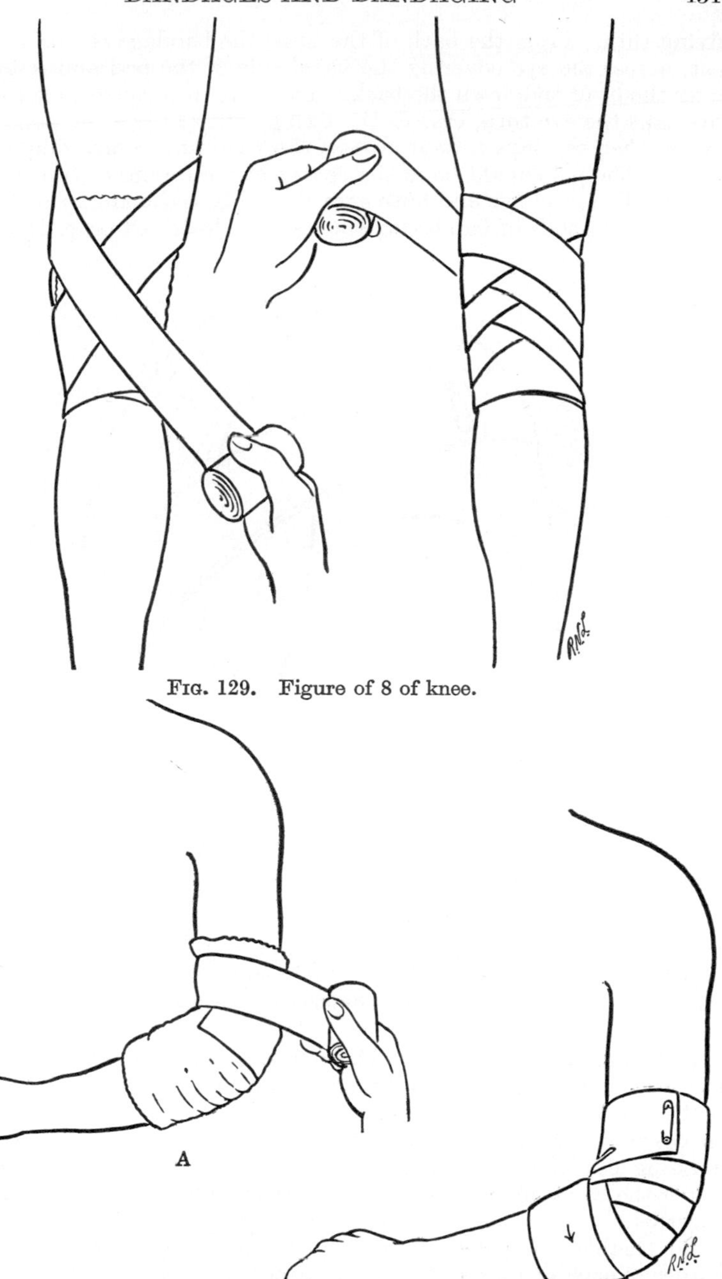

FIG. 129. Figure of 8 of knee.

FIG. 130. Divergent spica of elbow.
A Commencement. B Completed.

fixing turn. From the back of the head the bandage comes under the ear, across the eye covering the nasal side of the pad and straight on over the head and down the back. The next turn comes under the ear, overlaps the eye turn, crosses the fixing turn at the same point as the other, then overlaps it as it crosses the head and comes round to the front. The pin should be in the centre of the forehead, transfixing all turns. The good eye and both ears should be quite unimpeded.

Other methods of bandaging the eye are described on p. 333.

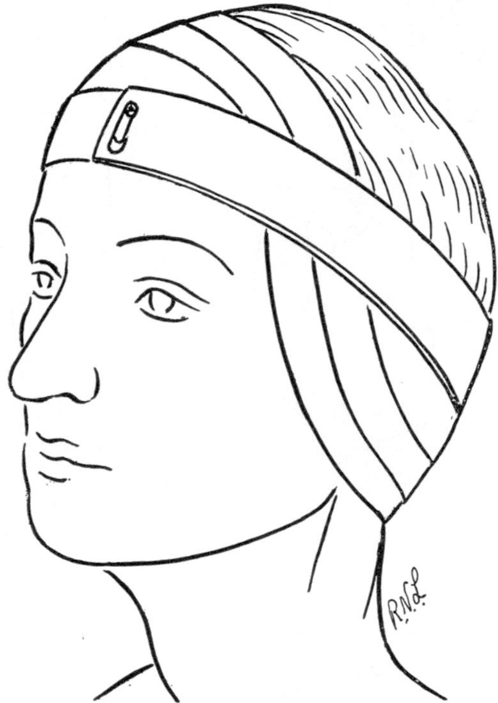

FIG. 131. Single ear bandage.

Ear Bandages. (*a*) Single. The dressing must be adequate for the purpose, and is secured by a fixing turn round the head. The pattern is then as described for the eye, but three or four turns will be necessary to cover it. A crepe bandage is most convenient, and to keep the dressing clear of the eye an 8-in. length of narrow tape may be inserted under the bandage at the angle of the eye and tied to keep all the turns together.

(*b*) Double. A piece of tape is laid over the head at the outer corner of each eye for securing this bandage, which is not very stable, after finishing. The fixing turn round the head takes in the upper margin of each dressing, then passes behind the right ear, up in front of it, is reversed at the corner of the eye, crosses the forehead, reverses again and passes down over the front of the left ear and across the occiput ready to begin the next series of turns. A crepe bandage is advised, and two finishing turns round the head ; the side tapes must be firmly tied.

Jaw Bandage. A fractured mandible can be temporarily immobilized by a " barrel " bandage. False teeth must first be removed. A 4-ft. length of firm bandage is passed under the jaw and tied in a

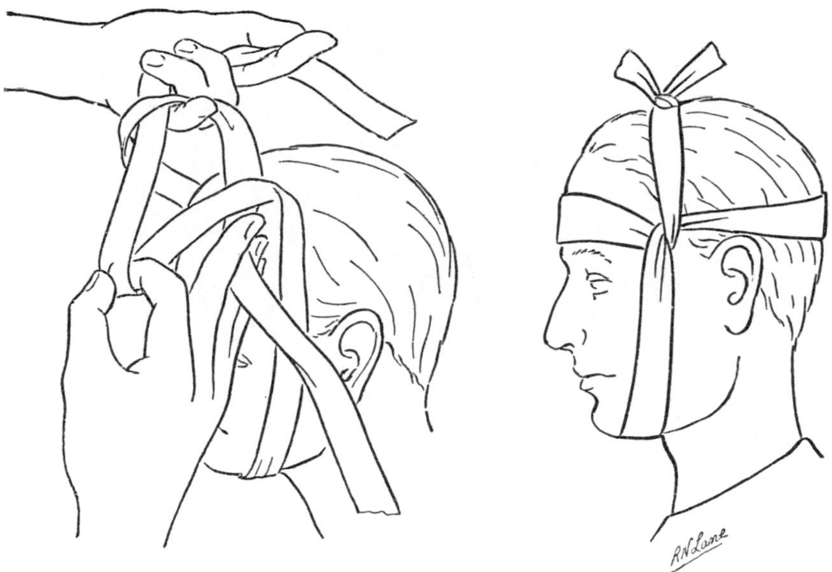

FIG. 132. Barrel bandage for jaw.

half-knot on the vertex ; the two halves are separated, one being pushed behind the occiput and the other on to the forehead. The two free ends are brought up and tied firmly on the vertex over a pad.

The old four-tail jaw bandage is dangerous and can impede the airway by drawing back the jaw. Patients who have sustained a jaw injury and had such a bandage applied should not be left alone for fear of vomiting.

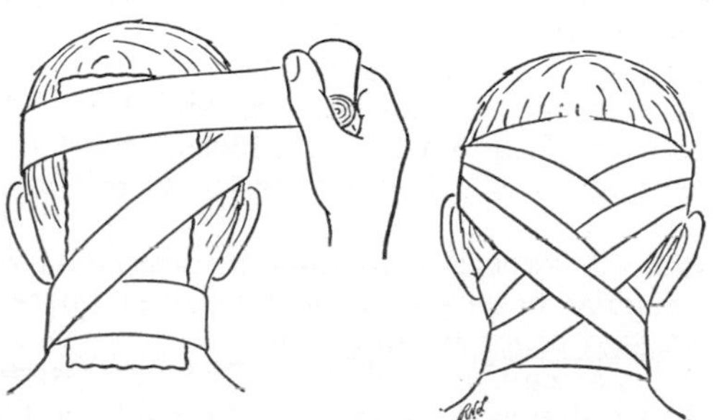

FIG. 133. Bandage for carbuncle of neck.

Neck Bandages. (*a*) Carbuncle. Plenty of dressing should be used, to support the inflamed tissues, absorb discharge and enable a good bandage to be applied. The bandage is a figure of 8 with the turns going alternatively round the neck and the forehead. The neck turns should gradually ascend to cover the dressing, but the turns across the forehead should coincide. (*b*) Glands of neck. Elastoplast is now generally used to retain the dressing after excision, since bandaging involves

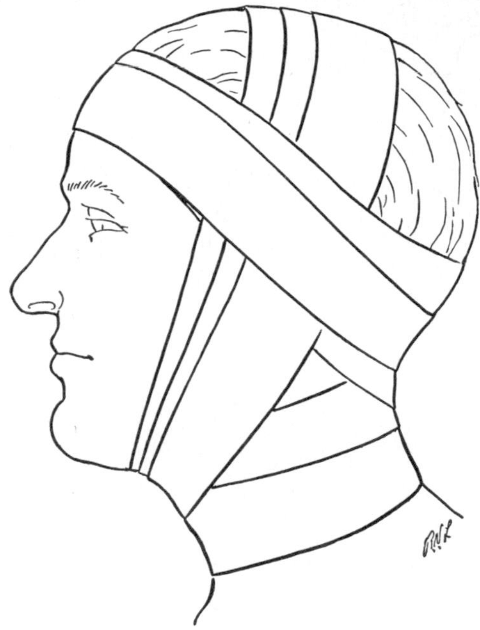

Fig. 134. Glands of neck bandage.

including the head. If a bandage is necessary, use crepe ones and proceed as follows :

1. Take a fixing turn around the head, from the affected to the unaffected side.
2. The bandage passes down behind the occiput and round the lower edge of the dressing.
3. Up behind the good ear, across the vertex in front of the other ear.
4. Under the chin, across the occiput and round the forehead. These last three turns form a triangle which is filled in to cover the dressing by repeating turns 2, 3 and 4 two or three times. Fasten on the forehead.

Head Bandages. A Tubegauz bandage is most effective and rapidly applied or a triangular bandage can be used. The capelline bandage is executed with two roller bandages stitched together at their free ends, with the rolls facing the same way. The nurse stands behind the patient and with a roll in each hand starts by applying the back of the bandage to the centre of the forehead. Each bandage is carried round

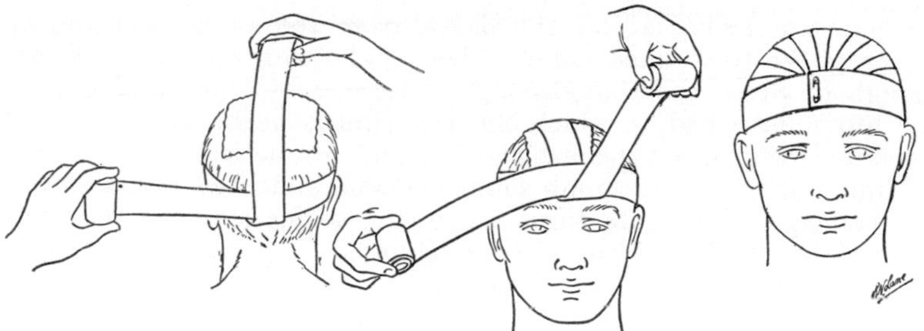

FIG. 135. Capelline head bandage.

its own side of the head to the occiput, where they are crossed. The upper bandage now crosses the head to the forehead, while the other goes round the side of the head again to the forehead to cross the other once more. The bandage circling the head continues to do this, while the other crosses it from forehead to nape and back in diverging overlapping turns, being caught in place by the circling bandage each time it turns. Both finish by being fastened together on the forehead.

The bandage crossing the vertex must not be drawn too tight, or it will pull the circling bandage up off the head.

Fractured Clavicle Bandage. The aim in treating this fracture is to draw back the shoulders to prevent overlapping of the fragments and to hold up the arm which has lost the support of the shoulder girdle. This can be achieved with three slings; two of these are folded around a strip of brown wool and passed under the axillæ and over the point of the shoulders and knotted. The free ends are now fastened to the opposite side tightly enough to brace back the shoulders, and wool inserted under knots. The arm is supported in the third sling.

Shoulder Spica. A wool dressing is placed in each axilla, and a fixing turn made round the arm, on the affected side. The bandage is carried across the back to

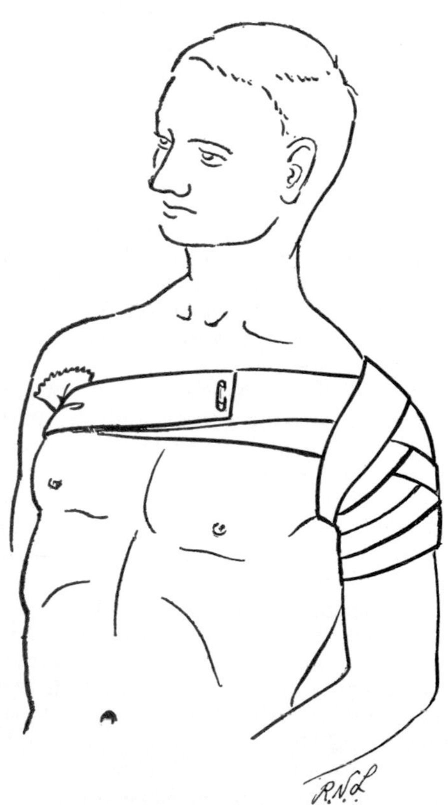

FIG. 136. Shoulder spica.

the opposite axilla, across the chest, over and round the arm and so across the back once more. These two turns are repeated often enough to cover the shoulder. A " descending " spica of shoulder and hip is described, in which the spica turns begin at the top and move downwards, but the result is ugly and impractical.

Thumb Spica. The thumb should be well abducted before starting the bandage. Alternate turns are made, as for the shoulder, going alternately round the wrist and the thumb.

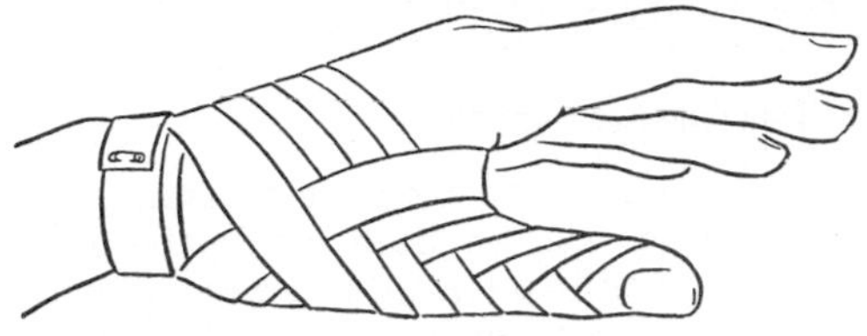

FIG. 137. Thumb spica.

Finger Bandages. If the finger tip is to be included, it should be covered with recurrent loops which are held in place with a circular turn which progresses in simple spirals to the base of the finger. If several fingers are to be bandaged, a spica turn can be taken round the wrist between each. The bandage starts with the finger nearest the little one, and should cross the back of the hand, not the palm, to reach the wrist. Tubegauz makes an excellent finger bandage.

Breast Bandages. After breast amputation, there is a long incision reaching from the anterior border of the axilla across the chest, and it is the axillary portion which presents difficulty in coverage. Wide crepe bandages should be selected, and the bandage begun around the lower border of the ribs, working from the affected side to the good one. Two to three spiral turns can be taken round the trunk, and then a spica turn is made round the arm by bringing the bandage across the back, round the shoulder and beneath the axilla, back across the shoulder to the chest. Two spica turns round the shoulder are usually necessary to cover the axilla, and between each an ascending spiral round the trunk is included.

A single breast bandage to support an inflamed or infected breast is begun by a fixing turn round the trunk, working from the affected side. The bandage then travels up below the affected breast to the opposite shoulder and diagonally back to begin another turn round the chest. These two turns alternate until sufficient support has been afforded. A double breast bandage is rarely needed and not very comfortable ; a binder or a manytail bandage with shoulder straps is more practical.

Hip Spica. This bandage was the one used following hernia operations, but the immobility it produced is not now favoured. The spica turns went alternately round the thigh and the trunk until the groin was adequately covered. A double hip spica is still less often used ; the sequence is as follows: (1) a spica turn round one thigh ; (2) a turn round the body ; (3) a spica turn round the second thigh ; (4) the bandage passes across the back of the trunk to reach the first thigh. These four turns must be repeated three or four times.

Bandaging the Ankle. Ankle strains are frequently treated by an

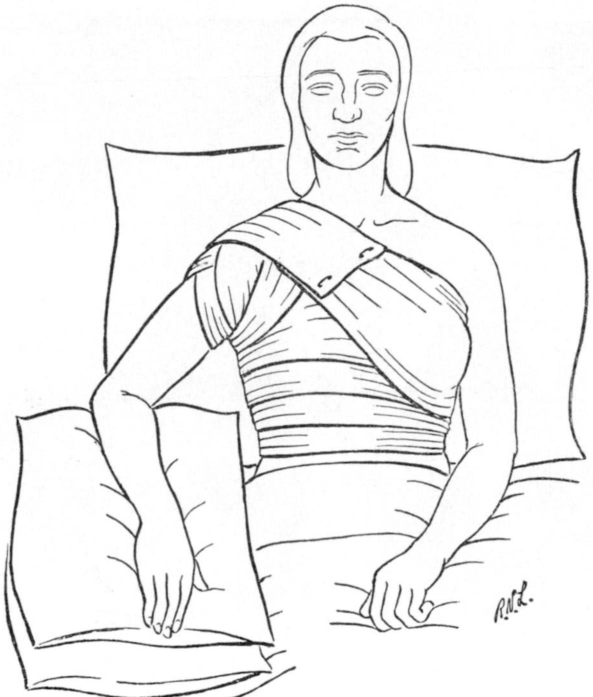

Fig. 138. Bandage after breast amputation.

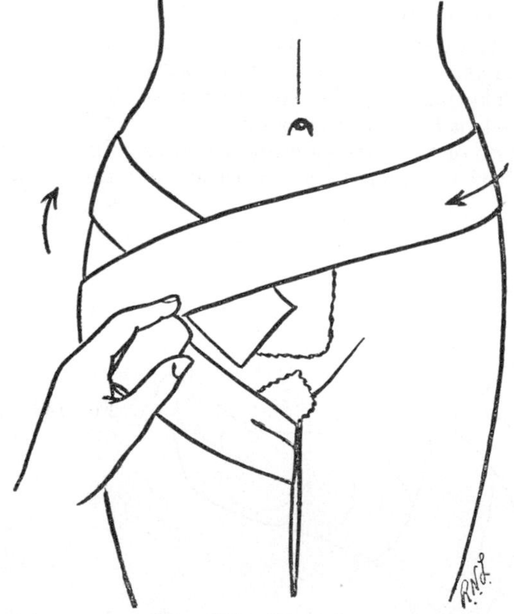

Fig. 139. Hip spica.

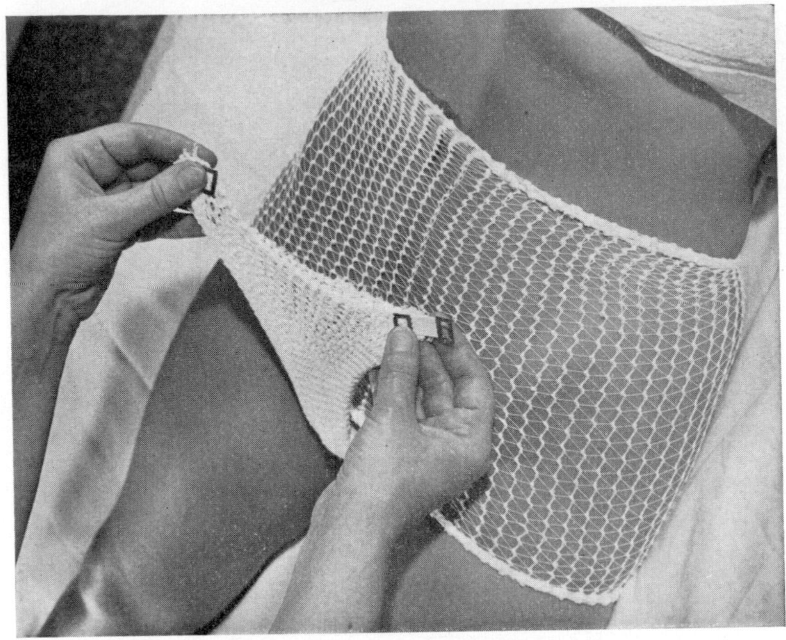

FIG. 140. A method of retaining abdomino-perineal dressings, using " Netelast ".

adhesive elastic or crepe bandage, and it is one at which the nurse should be proficient. It must reach to the base of the toes if swelling is to be avoided, and the foot must be in a good dorsiflexed position. The nurse stands facing the patient and takes a fixing turn around the ball of the foot. The bandage then passes across the dorsum of the foot around the heel (*not* the ankle) as low down as possible. These turns are repeated two or three times more depending on the size of the foot, and the bandage is finished by a turn around the ankle. The spica

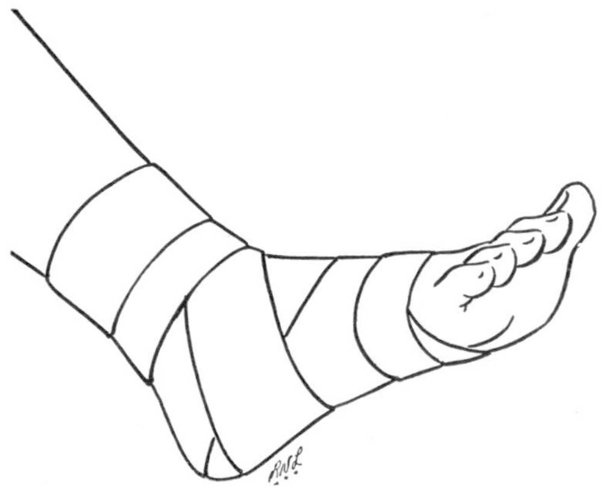

FIG. 142. Figure of 8 of ankle.

pattern lies up the centre of the foot, and the turns around the heel and ankle should be perfectly parallel.

Knee Bandages. A divergent spica for the knee is not usually needed, but a figure of 8 is commonly used after knee operations to keep pressure on the joint and avoid effusion.

Bandaging the Leg. Varicose veins may be supported by a leg bandage, and such a bandage forms part of the treatment for six weeks after operation. Crepe or nylon net bandages are used, and should be applied before getting up when swelling is minimal. They must be firmly applied, beginning at the web of the toes, and the heel must be included ; the first turn off the foot should go over the point of the heel. One or two simple spirals may be used above the ankle and then a figure of 8 is used for the rest of the leg. Bandages should be washed each time they are taken off, not only for hygienic reasons but because they are easy to apply well when freshly laundered, and patients who have been taught to apply their own should be given a spare set.

Bandaging an Amputation Stump. Treatment aims at preventing the formation of œdema and producing a firm conical stump well suited to the support of an artificial limb, and at mobilizing the patient at an early opportunity, so the bandage used should be a crepe one applied in a figure-of-8 pattern. If the amputation is a mid-thigh one, it will be necessary to carry the bandage around the hips for a turn or two in order to keep it on.

CHAPTER 30

NURSING INFECTIOUS DISEASES

An infectious disease is one that can be conveyed from one person to another by one of the following routes :

1. **Inhalation.** Diseases in which the respiratory tract is mainly involved—measles, scarlet fever, diphtheria—have long been thought to be spread by droplets of moisture and bacteria coughed or sneezed into the air. This is now being questioned and some bacteriologists think that infection is mainly through hands and articles contaminated by infectious discharges.
2. **Ingestion.** The organism enters by the digestive tract. The enteric fevers (typhoid and paratyphoid), cholera and dysentery are spread in this way. Although the number of diseases thus spread is small, they are of great social importance, since contamination of a food or water supply may lead to a wide-spread epidemic. The amount of alimentary infection in a country is a fair index to its hygiene level. In England cholera is unknown today, enteric fever is rare, but food poisoning is regrettably common, and indicates the possibility of achieving better results through teaching hygiene.
3. **Inoculation,** in which the infecting organism enters through a break in the skin surface. This break may be a wound, as in the surgical infections tetanus and gas gangrene ; an insect bite, as in plague, malaria and typhus ; or a minute abrasion, as in syphilis.

The sources of the infection are the (1) *acute* case, and the prevention of spread from such a case to other patients, staff and the general public is the concern of the hospital nurse. (2) *Fomites*, which are infected articles which harbour the bacteria, and may release them into the air or contaminate the hands if the fomites are handled or disturbed. Disinfection of such articles is undertaken by hospitals and local authorities. (3) *Carriers*. The carrier is a person who is immune to a disease, having had a clinical or a subclinical attack, but still harbours the organism and can transmit the disease to others. This method of transmission is of great importance in some diseases, of which typhoid is the outstanding example. Carriers must be identified and, if it is not possible to cure the state, he must be taught how to avoid conveying disease to others.

In no field of health have the benefits of preventive medicine been more strikingly demonstrated than in connection with communicable disease. In all countries with a modern health programme, the incidence and the mortality from infectious disease have fallen markedly.

Those aspects which are important to nurses include the following :

1. Active immunization against many diseases is possible. Smallpox and diphtheria are outstandingly successful examples. There seems every hope that diphtheria will disappear from most of Europe and North America following inoculation, but it must be remembered that

if immunization is not kept up, a susceptible population will develop among which a diphtheria epidemic might prove very dangerous. Whooping cough, tetanus and poliomyelitis are more recent additions to the list of diseases which it is hoped to prevent by active immunization.

2. Passive immunization by means of serum is of more limited application, but may be used to prevent disease appearing in a person exposed to infection for whom an attack would be undesirable. In treatment of disease and mitigation of severity immune serum still has a big part to play.

3. Health teaching makes available the benefits of medical knowledge to the general public, and health visitors and home nurses and midwives are important in inducing those with whom they come in contact to avail themselves of immunization, to understand the means by which diseases are spread, and simple methods to avoid contracting them or infecting others.

4. Social programmes like better housing contribute indirectly to lowering the incidence of infectious diseases, which is always at its highest among the under-privileged, poorly educated and badly fed. Others, such as pasteurization of milk, and the extension of tubercle-free agricultural areas have an obvious and direct effect.

5. Medical advances have been great. Many diseases already have a specific cure, while in others (such as measles) for which no drug has, as yet, been found, the serious complications can be prevented.

6. Barrier techniques for effectively isolating the acute case have improved greatly with our knowledge of the methods of spread. Such methods must be intelligently and meticulously applied, and their efficacy is in direct ratio to the conscientiousness with which they are used.

BARRIER NURSING

Barrier nursing is the term used to describe the nursing technique by which a patient with a communicable disease is prevented from infecting others. Many different problems are presented and must be intelligently solved ; diphtheria, for instance, is transmitted through the air, typhoid through the excreta ; smallpox is so highly infective to the unvaccinated that cases are usually nursed in special units, while glandular fever has a very low infectivity rate. Where infectious conditions are being nursed in special wards, such routines as the boiling of all crockery and bedpans will avoid the laborious necessity of keeping china and sanitary utensils apart for individual patients. Premises, too, are better adapted to the needs of the situation. From time to time, however, every general hospital ward admits an infectious case, and nursing precautions are instituted to prevent an extension of his disease to others.

Bed. If the infection is an airborne one, the bed must be in a separate room or cubicle ; any other form of isolation is quite illogical. The patient with an intestinal infection may be nursed in a general ward, preferably in a corner near the service rooms, to which bedpans can be taken by the shortest route. Screens round the bed in no way help to limit the spread of infection, but will remind staff and other patients of the precautions necessary. If the diagnosis is known before admission, a mattress of a type that can be disinfected without harm should be selected.

Articles Needed. Within the isolation area should be collected those articles needed for the patient's personal and sole use. They will include washing materials and bowl; thermometer and feeding utensils. They should be kept in a cupboard or on a covered trolley, and should be as few in number as is consistent with good nursing care or the unit will always be depressing in appearance. Paper-back books or magazines are useful for a patient well enough to read. A bedpan may be kept on a marked shelf in the sluice room, and the cover used should be metal and not of cloth.

Gowns. While attending to the patient, a gown should be worn, of which the outside and the fastenings are considered contaminated or "dirty," while the inside that comes into contact with the uniform is "clean." It will be understood that this distinction is rather fragile, and can only be maintained by a most meticulous technique in putting the gown on and off, and by using only a clean, dry gown. If it becomes wet or soiled it must be changed at once, and in any case every twenty-four hours.

A gown should be put on a coathanger (which is "clean") right side out, and should hang on a hook or stand inside the infected area. The inside of the gown should not be visible, and if two gowns hang on the same hook they must be face to face.

Method of Putting On the Gown. The hook is taken in the right hand and held with the back opening of the gown towards the nurse. The left arm is slipped into the gown, the coathanger transferred to the left hand and the right sleeve put on. The hanger is returned to its hook, and the nurse fastens up her gown. It will be seen that neither the coathanger nor the interior of the gown was contaminated.

Taking Off the Gown. Once the service to the patient has been completed, the gown must be removed without contaminating the interior. The tapes or buttons are undone, and without removing the gown, the hands and arms are well soaped and washed, the nails and fingers are scrubbed, and dried on a "clean" towel. The coathanger is taken in the right hand, inserted at the neck into the left sleeve, and the arm carefully withdrawn without touching the "dirty" outside of the gown. The coathanger is changed to the left hand, the free end inserted into the right sleeve, and the right arm similarly withdrawn. The hanger is put on the hook and the gown adjusted. If it is necessary to touch the outside while doing this, the hands must again be well washed before leaving the unit.

Masks are used in connection with infectious disease for quite a different purpose from the more usual one. When doing a dressing or performing a sterile procedure, a mask may be used to prevent contamination of the sterile field from the nurse's respiratory tract. In the present instance it is used to protect the nurse from the patient's infecting organism. It will be seen at once that this protection is only relative, since the nurse must breathe the air of the patients' room around the sides of the mask, but it does protect her from a heavy

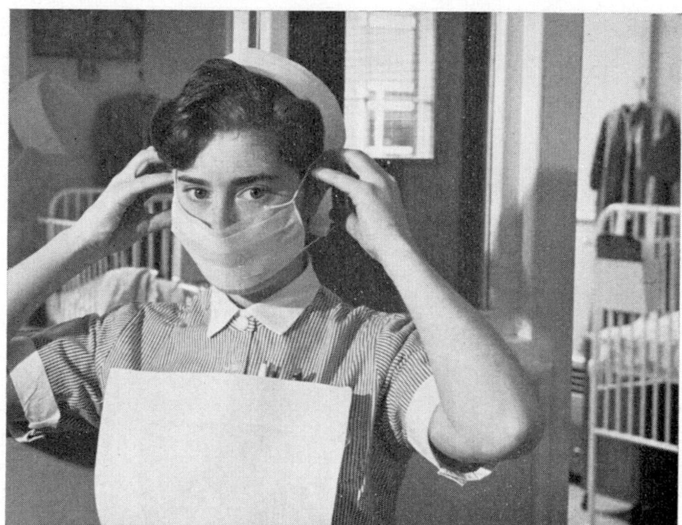

Fig. 142. The mask is put on outside the unit.

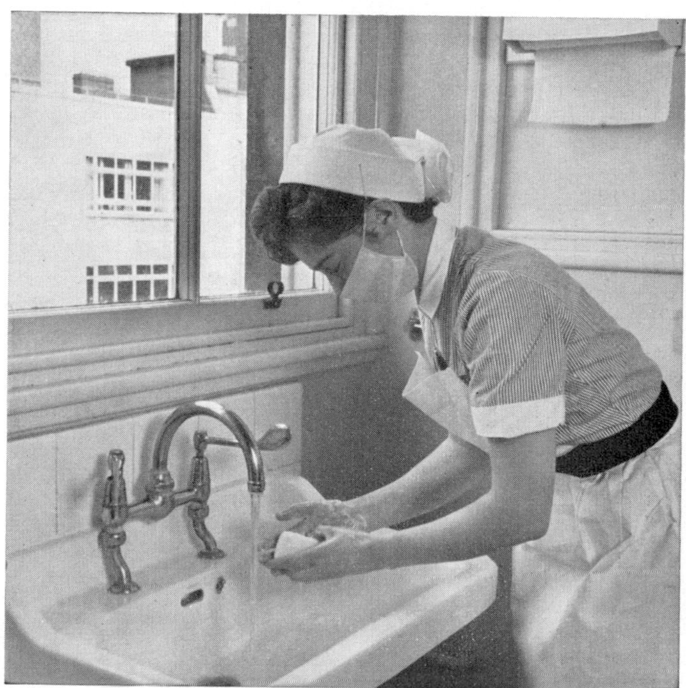

Fig. 143. The hands are washed.

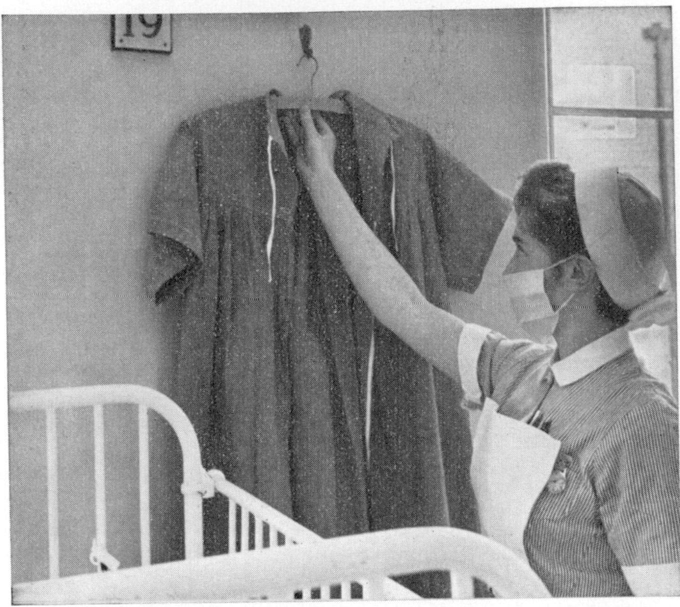

Fig. 144. The gown is lifted by the coathanger, which is " clean ".

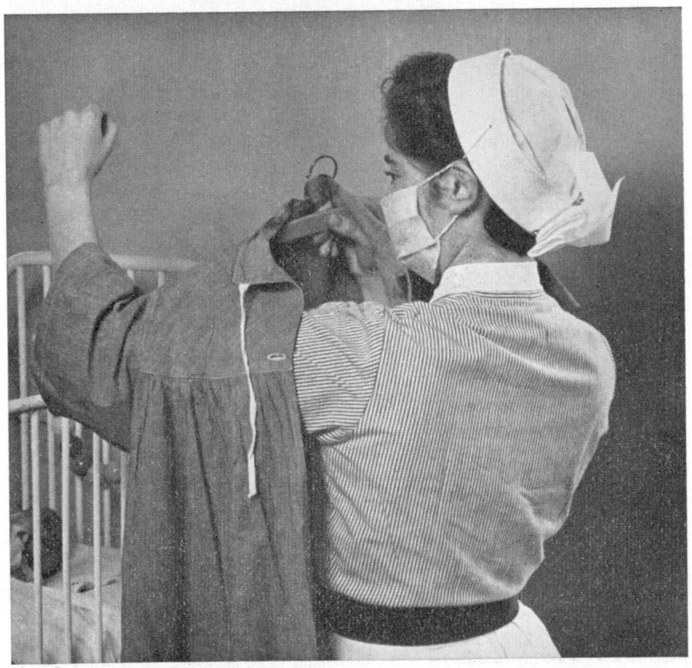

Fig. 145. The left arm is slipped into the gown.

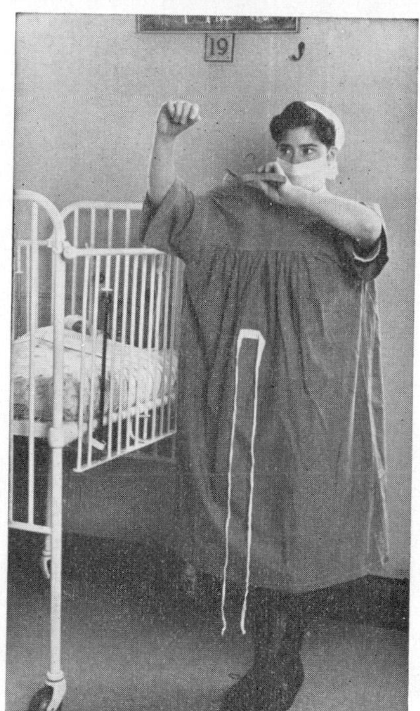

FIG. 146. The coat hanger is changed to the left hand, and the right sleeve put on.

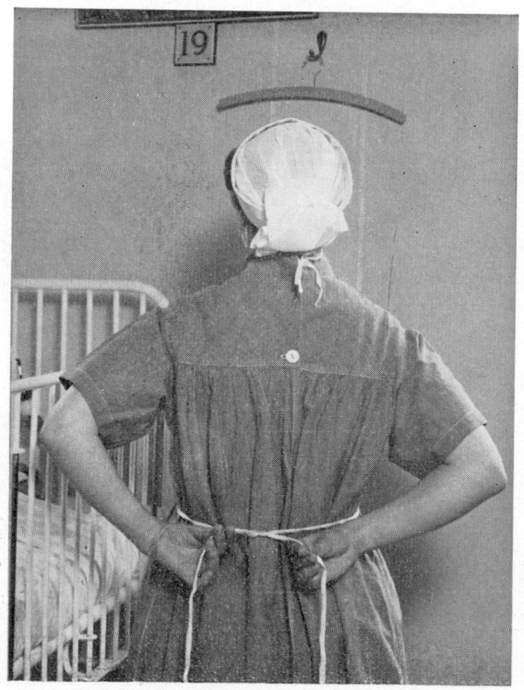

FIG. 147. The coat hanger is replaced, and the tapes of the gown fastened.

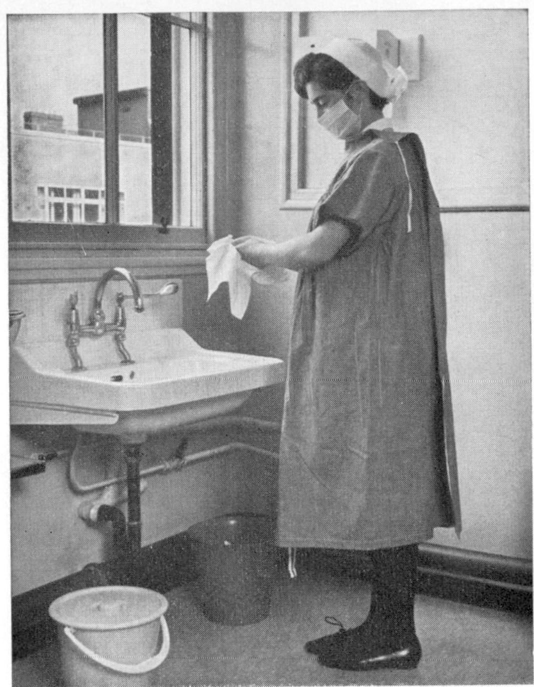

Fig. 148. When the task is finished the tapes (which are "dirty") are unfastened and the hands are washed and dried.

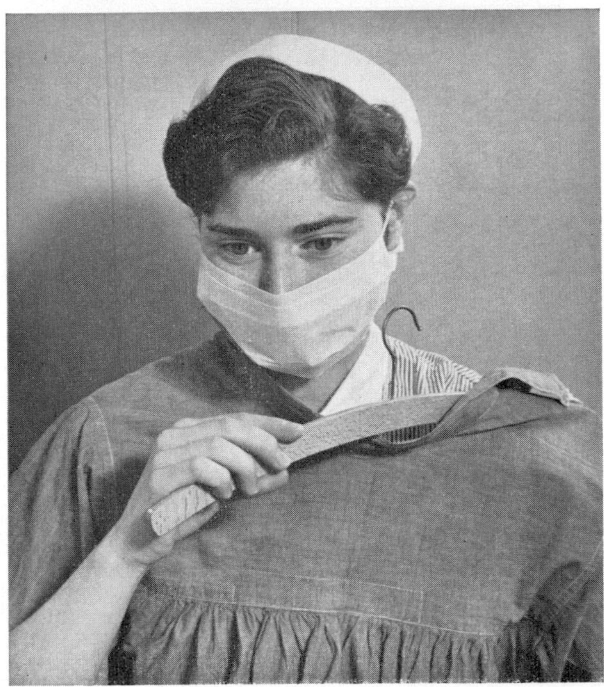

Fig. 149. To remove the gown, insert the coat hanger into the left sleeve and slip the arm out. Change the coat hanger to the left hand, and take out the right arm.

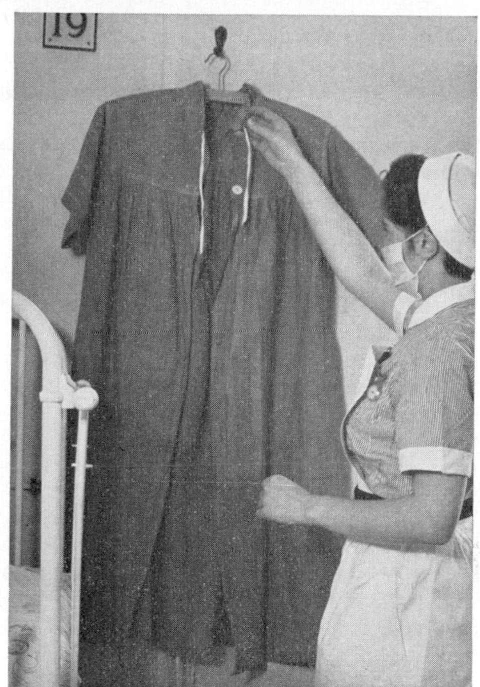

Fig. 150. The gown is hung up and adjusted; the hands are washed again.

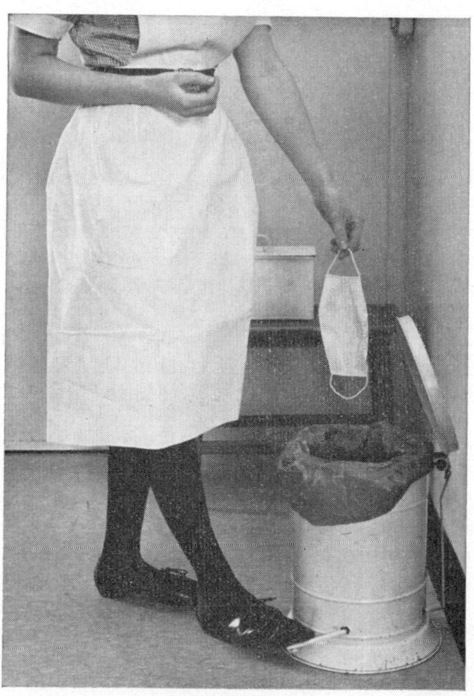

Fig. 151. The mask is removed, handling it only by the strings, and dropped into a covered bin.

discharge of bacteria should the patient cough in her direction, or while she is treating the mouth or throat.

In cases of droplet infection, a supply of clean masks should be kept outside the room, and one is put on before entering. On coming out the mask is removed, handling it only by the tapes, and discarded. The use of disposable masks is general now, since fabric ones are tedious to launder and disinfect.

Notes and X-rays of infectious patients should be kept outside the room and should remain clean. They can be inspected before entry or after the final hand-cleansing.

Waste. Foodscraps, magazines, paper handkerchiefs, mouth swabs and similar articles should be put on a thick piece of newspaper, firmly rolled up, and put in a bin whose contents are burnt.

China Disposable crockery and cutlery for the infectious patient are a great convenience. Where all ward china is boiled after use, no special precautions are necessary.

Dusting. The floor is swept with a marked brush, and the dust rolled up in newspaper for burning. Dusting should be done with old sheeting which can be burnt after use. It is important to see that domestic staff who may perform these duties are well aware of the routine to be followed.

Excreta. Most wards are equipped with bed pan cleansers which have a steam as well as a cold flush, and although the makers do not claim that these are " sterilizers," bacteriological tests indicate that in practice they are. The only patients for whom special precautions have to be taken with regard to the excreta, are those with an intestinal infection. The bedpan should be filled with Sudol 1%, and left for an hour.

Terminal Disinfection

When bacteriological tests show the patient to be no longer infectious, she should be taken to the bathroom, where she discards the infected night attire on to a sheet of paper, so that it can be returned to her room for disinfection. After a bath and shampoo she goes in clean clothes to a new bed, and the room she has vacated and its contents are disinfected.

Sterilization by heat is the safest method, but for some articles chemical disinfection is necessary. A routine that is simple, economical and effective is required, and that given here fulfils these conditions, and does not entail stocking a large number of chemicals. Other disinfectants can of course be used just as effectively.

Baths. Add 30 ml. of hypochlorite (10% available chlorine) and 90 ml. of liquid detergent to a few gallons of hot water in the bath, and mop its sides thoroughly.

Beds. Wearing gloves, mop the frame with hypochlorite (1% chlorine).

Sheets and Cotton Blankets. These can be laundered after the patient's discharge, having been disinfected in a formalin chamber. Woollen blankets can also be disinfected in formalin vapour, but over-frequent laundering will cause deterioration.

Bowls can be swabbed with hypochlorite 1%. **Cheatle Forceps** for sluice-room use should be stood in Sudol 1%.

Electric pads and blankets should be disinfected in a formalin chamber.

Floors can be washed with hypochlorite 1% with added detergent.

Hair brushes can be stood in hypochlorite 1% for 15 minutes, unless the back seems likely to be harmed by disinfectant, when they should be given formalin treatment.

Hand basins can be disinfected like baths. **Nail-brushes** do not need disinfection if hexachlorophene soap is used. They can be kept dry.

Lavatory brushes should be stood in Sudol 1%.

Mattresses of foam rubber, or those in plastic covers can be swabbed with hypochlorite 1%. Others should be treated in the formalin chamber.

Electric razors can only be safely sterilized in ethylene oxide.

Rectal or **vaginal electrodes** should be wiped with hypochlorite 1%. The same can be used for X-ray **Cassettes**.

Clinical thermometers should be stored dry, and disinfected by immersing in 70% methylated spirit for 15 minutes.

Once the room has been stripped, local custom will decide what follows. Some still like to close the room and disinfect it with formalin vapour. Others wash the walls, bedstead and locker with antiseptic and thoroughly air the room. The bacteriologist will advise on the method, having regard to the nature of the infection, its severity and the path of transmission.

Finally the nurse discards her gown with the infected linen and scrubs her hands and arms. Circumstances may well indicate a bath and a change of uniform for her as well.

THE SPECIFIC FEVERS

This group of diseases have in common a certain pattern which they follow, sometimes in a remarkably consistent way, though they differ from each other in the length of time which the disease takes to run its course, and in their severity. Each is produced by a specific organism. In no field of medicine have more spectacular advances been made than in the prevention of the specific fevers, their cure, and avoidance of their complications.

The course of each is as follows :

1. **Infection.** Entry is by one of the methods and routes described above.

2. **Incubation.** For a variable time from the entry of infection no symptoms occur, and the time up to the onset of symptoms is called the incubation period. The majority of diseases in temperate climates vary between a few days and three weeks.

3. **Onset.** During the incubation period the body's resistance is being overcome and the organism is establishing itself. The signs of onset depend on where the infection is, but fever, anorexia, headache and constipation are usual. Droplet infections commonly produce also sore throat, sneezing, and lacrimation.

4. **Fastigium.** This word refers to the height of the disease, when the signs are florid and the clinical picture fully developed. A rash is seen in fevers in which a skin toxin is present.

5. **Defervescence.** As the antibody level in the blood rises in response to the infection, the severity of the disease declines and a fall in the temperature is accompanied by abatement of all the other symptoms.

6. **Convalescence.** Once the temperature is normal and the patient free from infection, there follows a time in which appetite is regained and loss of weight made good ; muscle tone is improved after the period in bed and the patient regains normal health.

These fevers are " specific " in that infection by one provides no protection against another. Indeed, the reverse may be the case if a child convalescent from one infection is exposed to another. There follows a brief account of the main fevers ; many of these are still common ; others are rarely seen but could easily become a menace again if precautions against them were relaxed.

Diphtheria

Organism. Corynebacterium diphtheriæ (Klebs-Lœffler bacillus).

Mode of Infection. Inhalation. Carriers are of some importance where this disease is still common.

Incubation Period. Under one week (two to seven days).

Signs and Symptoms. Sore throat, dysphagia, slight fever, marked rise in pulse rate and toxic pallor. Examination of the throat shows injected fauces and a patchy greyish membrane over the inflamed surfaces. In severe cases the membrane may spread on to the larynx and into the trachea.

Treatment. A swab is taken from the throat and nose, and treatment with anti-diphtheritic serum is begun at once by intramuscular and/or intravenous injection. Three dangerous complications may occur. (1) Laryngeal obstruction. If the air entry is impaired, preparations for tracheotomy are made so that it may be performed as soon as it becomes necessary. (2) Cardiac failure, as shown by tachycardia, restlessness and cyanosis. All cases should be nursed flat to try to avert this complication and patients should remain in bed for at least three weeks, during which time they are fed, washed and spared all exertion. Should the heart fail, an oxygen tent is useful. (3) Paralysis. The palate is commonly first affected, and regurgitation of fluid through the nose while drinking is often the first sign, occurring about the 4th week. Paralysis of the eye muscles, pharyngeal and respiratory muscles may follow, and require treatment in a respirator (p. 461).

If the patient recovers from the acute stage, the cardiac and paralytic complications will completely disappear. The prognosis is grave in young children, and in the uninoculated of all ages. Prophylactic immunization is most successful, but unfortunately as the disease becomes rarer people tend to neglect immunization. All health workers must urge its importance to mothers of young children.

Scarlet Fever

Organism. Streptococcus hæmolyticus.
Mode of Infection. Inhalation.
Incubation Period. Under one week (one to seven days).

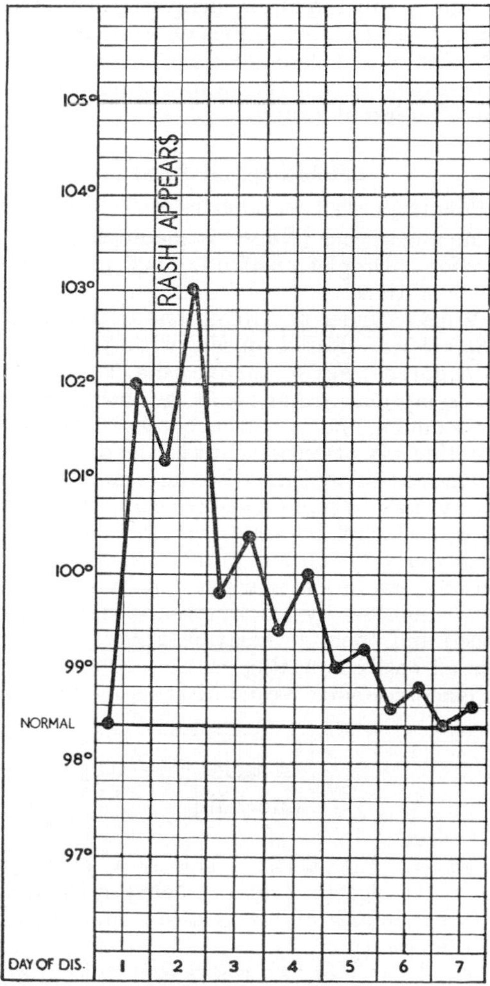

FIG. 152. **Temperature chart in scarlet fever.**

Signs and Symptoms. Vomiting may occur at the onset, followed by fever, sore throat and headache. The fauces and tonsils are much inflamed, the rash appears on the second day as a bright red punctate flush. The area around the mouth is spared, and the circumoral pallor stands out against the scarlet cheeks.

Complications. Cervical adenitis, otitis media, bronchitis, pneumonia, acute nephritis and rheumatic fever can occur about a month after infection. Scarlet fever itself is a very mild disease in Britain, but its complications must be prevented by early treatment to ward off the septic complications, and careful observation to detect the onset of the others.

Treatment. Penicillin is usually reserved for the cases which develop complications, but a sulphonamide drug is often prescribed. Anti-streptococcal serum is available, but is only needed for the infrequent severe case. Nurses should remember that acute tonsillitis in no way differs from scarlet fever except that a rash is not seen, and the general public finds the term less alarming.

Cerebro-spinal Fever

(Meningococcal meningitis, spotted fever)

Organism. Meningococcus (Neisseria meningitides).

Mode of Infection. Droplet. Infection is favoured by close contact in ill-ventilated conditions.

Incubation Period. Under one week (one to five days).

Signs and Symptoms. Rapid onset, with rigor in an adult and convulsions in children. Fever, tachycardia, vomiting and the other general febrile symptoms occur, and headache is usually severe. Photophobia is common, and in the early stages the patient lies curled on his side, resenting any attention, but as the disease progresses, neck rigidity and retraction of the head becomes marked. A rash caused by small capillary hæmorrhages appears about the third day on the trunk and limbs, and may be very profuse in severe cases. In the untreated or unfavourable case the patient sinks gradually into coma ; incontinence occurs, wasting is marked and hyperpyrexia is common. Early diagnosis (supported by examination of the cerebro-spinal fluid for meningococci) and effective treatment have materially improved the prognosis in all but fulminating cases.

Treatment. Penicillin is effective against this organism, and is generally used.

Measles

(Morbilli)

Organism. A virus.

Mode of Infection. Inhalation. This is a very common, highly infectious disease, the biggest incidence being in children between two and ten. It is rare in infants of less than nine months, who retain some of the mother's immunity.

Incubation Period. One or two weeks (ten to fourteen days).

Signs and Symptoms. The condition starts like a heavy cold, but the fever, red eyes and brassy cough often indicate the true diagnosis. Between the second and fourth day, small white-headed spots appear on the inside of the cheeks opposite the molar teeth. These are Koplik's spots, and they are of great diagnostic importance. On the fourth day the temperature rises and the rash appears, first behind the ears, then spreading to the face and limbs. When fully developed it is a red, maculo-papular, patchy rash which is highly characteristic. It begins to fade in a few days.

Complications. Otitis media ; bronchopneumonia ; encephalitis.

Treatment. Temporary (passive) immunity can be conferred by preparations of immune serum which must be given within five days of contact if it is to be effective. If given later, a modified attack of

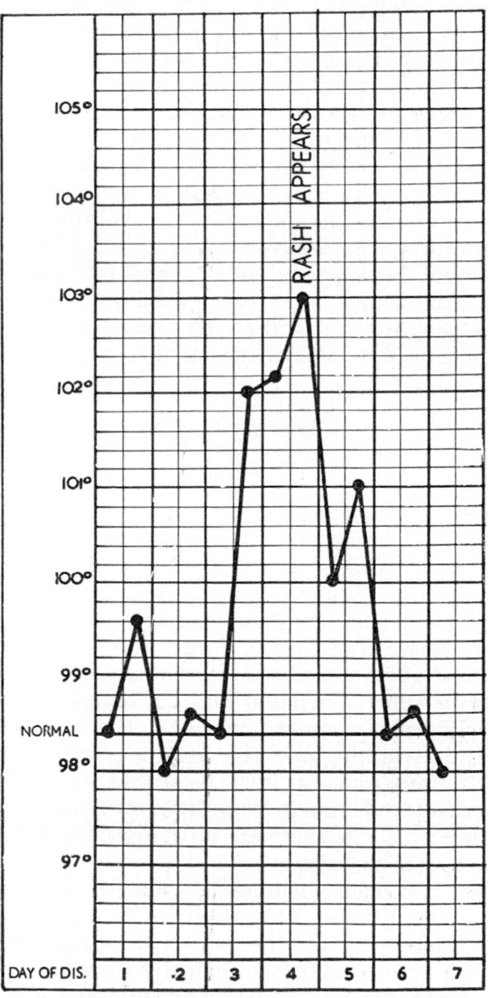

FIG. 153. Temperature chart in measles.

measles occurs which will confer active immunity. Protection of all children by active immunization is now widely given, and measles should become increasingly uncommon.

The child should be put to bed in a warm but ventilated room and paper handkerchiefs used to dry the secretions. If the cough is hoarse and painful, a steam kettle often gives relief. The eyes should be bathed with warm boracic solution and bright light is excluded. The fluid intake must be adequate and most children are thirsty enough to drink well. Since fever will be present for a week or more, milk, egg custard, mince, pounded fish or scrambled egg should be given when the appetite allows, or convalescence will be prolonged. The night clothes should preferably be of cotton, and not of a shape or size to chafe between the legs or under the arms. Calamine lotion may be dabbed on the rash if it is very irritable and a daily warm bed bath given. Mouth washes are welcome to older children and younger ones may have the tongue swabbed with old linen dipped in glycothymoline.

Pain in the ear, indicating otitis media, and a rise in the respiration rate and temperature which may herald the onset of broncho-pneumonia are the signs for which most careful watch must be kept. Some doctors like to prescribe an antibiotic for children with measles in order to prevent these complications.

The child should be kept in bed for a week after the fever has subsided, unless the attack was a very mild one, and a convalescent period with fresh air, sunlight and a high protein diet is necessary.

Active immunization is increasingly used.

Whooping Cough

(Pertussis)

Organism. Hæmophilus pertussis.

Mode of Infection. Inhalation.

Incubation Period. One to two weeks (six to eighteen days).

Signs and Symptoms. General feverish signs and catarrh with cough occur in the first week. The coughing tends to be paroxysmal and to be followed by vomiting. By the second week the fever has gone, but the type of cough that gives the disease its name now appears. Bouts of coughing occur in which the child sits up, clutching the sides of its cot, coughing with ever-increasing violence ; the face is congested, the eyes injected and streaming and the tongue protruding. Finally the child manages to draw some air into the larynx with a long effort that produces the whoop. There is very little sputum, but vomiting is common. Between attacks there are no symptoms, but the child fears the onset of each new paroxysm.

Complications. Broncho-pneumonia, which may later lead to bronchiectasis ; convulsions ; ulceration on the under surface of the tongue through friction against the teeth while coughing.

Treatment. Chloramphenicol is clinically effective, but in view of its causing an occasional fatal aplastic anæmia is not now prescribed. Tetracycline may be used if the severity of the case warrants it. The most important nursing point is the maintenance of nutrition, especially if vomiting is troublesome. Meals should be small and frequent, and a feed should always be given after vomiting has occurred.

Whooping-cough is at present one of the most serious infectious diseases of children, especially among infants and active immunization is well worth while. Administration of the vaccine can be combined with diphtheria immunization.

Typhoid Fever

Organism. Salmonella typhi (Bacillus typhosus).

Mode of Infection. Alimentary. The organism is excreted in the fæces and/or urine of a carrier and reaches some food or water supply through imperfect sewage disposal or faulty hygiene on the part of the carrier. Acute cases are of course important sources of infection but nursing precautions in socially developed communities usually prevent cross-infection, and the carrier has been the cause of most epidemics in such countries. Water, milk, ice-cream and oysters have provided the starting-points for outbreaks. The incidence of typhoid in a country reflects fairly accurately the standard of its public health administration.

Incubation Period. One to two weeks (five to twenty-one days).

Signs and Symptoms. As with lobar pneumonia, the classical course of typhoid is now rarely seen where antibiotic treatment is available. In the unmodified case three phases may be seen, each lasting about a week. During the first there is the stage of onset, usually insidious, with headache, backache, epistaxis and bowel upsets with either constipation or diarrhœa. The temperature shows a gradual rise, falling in the morning but advancing a little higher each evening, while the pulse rate shows a much smaller rise. At the end of this week a rash appears, usually scanty, and consisting of pink papules. The organism may be cultivated from the blood at this stage.

In the second week the infection localizes in the lymphoid tissue of the small intestine, where ulceration and sloughing may occur. Continuous pyrexia is present, diarrhœa is usual, and the patient is toxic, wasted, often delirious and with a very dry mouth. Culture of the urine and stools shows that the bacillus is now being excreted.

During the third week there may be a gradual return of the temperature to normal by lysis and steady improvement of other symptoms. In unfavourable cases, the toxæmia increases and the patient becomes comatose. Whether treated or no, relapse and a repeat of the infection is not rare.

Complications. Pneumonia and heart failure, as in all severe infections. Acute parotitis, if mouth hygiene is ineffectively performed. Venous thrombosis and pulmonary embolism. Hæmorrhage from an ulcer is quite common, and is indicated by a sudden fall in temperature and blood pressure, with sweating, pallor and a rise in the pulse rate. Perforation of an ulcer is shown by abdominal pain and rigidity, a subnormal temperature and a rapid deterioration. Both these serious complications occur in the third week. Arthritis and typhoid abscesses may be encountered as late sequelæ.

Treatment. Chloramphenicol is effective in typhoid and has vastly improved the outlook in this highly dangerous disease, and where it is available, the classical course of typhoid will not be seen.

The principal nursing duties fall under three headings :

(*a*) *Supportive.* A high-fluid, high-calorie, low-residue diet must be given, and much perseverance and skill may be necessary to induce an ill patient to take it. Milk and eggs form a valuable basis, and ice-cream with casilan, junket, jelly and cream, very thin crustless bread and butter with honey or cream cheese and soups are valuable in the early stages. The mouth requires constant care, and the prevention of pressure sores and footdrop is undertaken. A blanket bath is given daily, especially while there is fever.

(*b*) *Anti-infective.* All the measures described under barrier nursing must be conscientiously used. All excreta, which are the source of infection, must be disinfected before being put down the drain, and the bed linen which is always heavily infected should be adequately dealt with. While attending to her patient in a gown, the nurse must constantly think of her technique, and avoid touching her face, hair, handkerchief or any part of her person. The patient remains isolated until three negative stools have been obtained and terminal disinfection is carried out with care and thoroughness.

(*c*) *Observatory.* All changes in the condition must be noted and reported, but it is especially in the third week that vigilance must be exerted so that hæmorrhage or perforation may be detected and treated promptly. Bleeding is treated in the same way as that from a peptic ulcer (p. 213), while a perforation is repaired surgically.

The points which are important in the prevention of typhoid are: (*a*) the detection, cure or control of carriers ; (*b*) the maintenance of a high public health standard with regard to water supplies, sanitation and the inspection of food; (*c*) the active immunization of those exposed to infection, e.g. soldiers, and visitors to areas where typhoid is endemic.

Paratyphoid Fever

This infection closely resembles typhoid fever in its course and treatment, though toxæmia is less marked and complications less common. The term " enteric fever " comprises typhoid and the three strains of paratyphoid that are encountered.

Smallpox

(Variola)

Organism. Virus.

Mode of Infection. Inhalation, and probably alimentary. This disease is very highly infectious among the non-vaccinated, and fomites may be important in transmission.

Incubation Period. Very constant at twelve days (ten to twelve days).

Signs and Symptoms. The onset is sudden, with headache, vomiting, abdominal pain and marked pyrexia, but these symptoms may abate somewhat before the rash appears on the third or fourth day. This begins on the forehead and wrists, and spreads to the head, arms, trunk and legs, and passes through the papule and vesicle stage to pustule formation by about the tenth day. At this stage toxæmia is profound and may be fatal, but in a favourable case the pustules dry and the scabs separate, leaving deep " pock " scars which are permanent.

A minor form of smallpox (variola minor) is occasionally seen, and the vaccinated with not quite enough antibody to resist the disease may have a mild modified form of smallpox.

Complications. Encephalitis, pneumonia, otitis media. Hæmorrhagic forms are often fatal.

Treatment. No drug has any effect on the virus, but penicillin may be useful in limiting secondary infection. The most important nursing duties are the care of the mouth and eyes and skin, and the giving of an adequate fluid diet. Potassium permanganate 1 in 10,000 can be used for bathing the rash, which should afterwards be dried and dusted with powder.

Smallpox is endemic in many countries of the Middle and Far East, but vaccination has in others caused it to disappear except for the occasional case or minor epidemic brought in with travellers. As fear

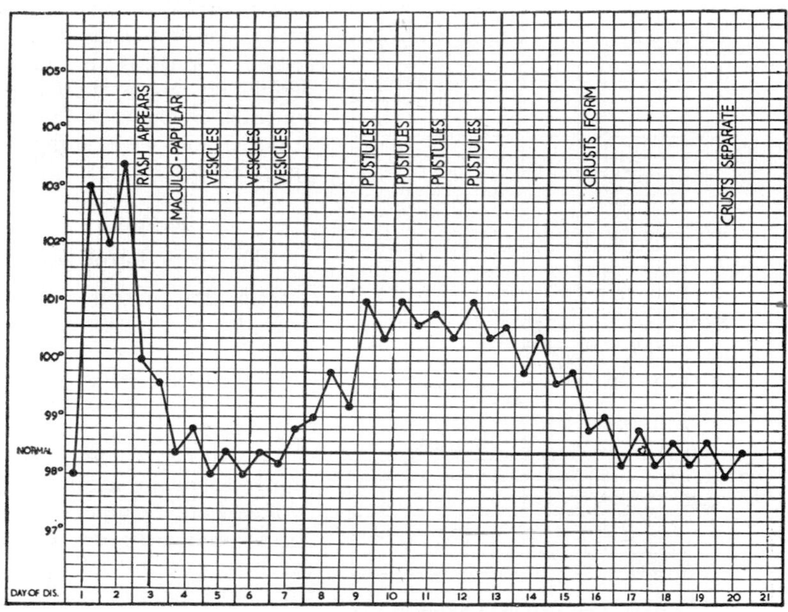

Fig. 154. Temperature chart in smallpox.

of smallpox declines, the numbers of the unvaccinated grow, and nurses should tell mothers the advantages of infant vaccination, which causes only a trivial upset, whereas if vaccination has to be undertaken in adult life because of one's profession or travels, it is a more painful affair. All contacts with a smallpox case should be at once vaccinated or re-vaccinated.

Chickenpox

(Varicella)

Organism. Virus.
Mode of infection. Inhalation and by fomites.
Incubation Period. Over two weeks (eleven to twenty-one days).

Signs and Symptoms. After a few hours of malaise, headache and mild fever the rash appears, commencing on the trunk and spreading to the extremities. It passes through vesicular and pustular stages like smallpox, but successive crops of lesions appear, unlike the rash in that disease. Constitutional upset is slight unless the rash is very profuse. Scarring will be slight unless itching causes scratching and secondary infection.

Treatment. There is no medical treatment, and nursing is concerned with alleviating the symptoms. Calamine lotion with carbolic 1% is useful in decreasing skin irritation.

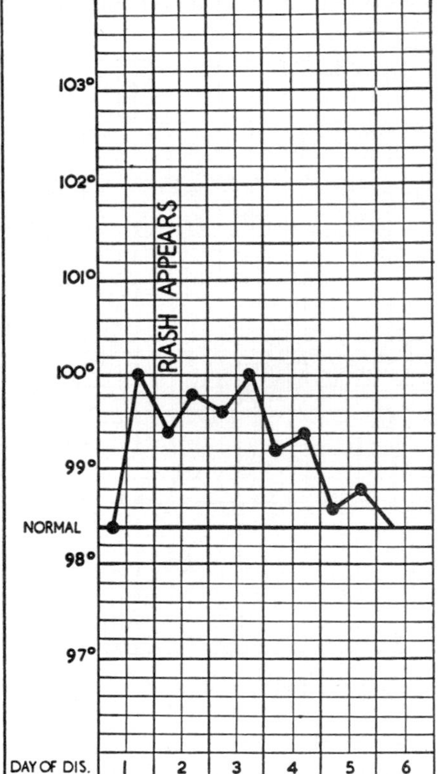

FIG. 155. Temperature chart in varicella (chickenpox).

A point of interest about this disease is that the virus is capable of causing herpes zoster (shingles) in older people, so that a child may contract chickenpox from a grandparent with shingles, and vice versa.

Mumps

(Epidemic Parotitis)

Organism. Virus.

Mode of Infection. Inhalation.

Incubation Period. Over two weeks (twelve to twenty-eight days).

Signs and Symptoms. Commonly there are a few days of increasing headache, sore throat and stiffness of the jaw before one or both parotid glands start to swell. As the enlargement disappears the temperature falls again.

Complications. Although the parotid is the most obviously affected gland, others are often involved. Of these the most important is the testis, and orchitis is a very painful condition which in a boy past the age of puberty may end in fibrosis of the testis, fortunately very rarely bilateral.

Treatment. Drugs are not usually given, though tetracycline may be used if orchitis is present in the hope of modifying it. A supporting bandage and analgesics will also be indicated. The most important point in nursing mumps is to provide a soft bland diet, remembering that sharp flavours and fruits provoke a painful spasm in the swollen gland as secretion is stimulated.

German Measles (Rubella)

Organism. Virus.

Mode of Infection. Inhalation.

Incubation Period. Over two weeks (sixteen to eighteen days).

Signs and Symptoms. There is little constitutional upset apart from headache, coryza, and enlargement of the occipital lymphatic glands. The rash, which is a red punctate one, sometimes profuse, appears on the first or second day, and all symptoms subside quite quickly.

Treatment. No special medical or nursing problems are presented by this disease. Its main importance lies in the fact, first investigated in Australia, that the baby of a woman who contracts this disease in the second or third month of pregnancy is more liable than usual to have certain congenital defects, especially cataract and deafness. It is, therefore, desirable that girls have this mild disease during childhood, and that those who have never had it should avoid exposure to it during pregnancy, especially in its early stages. Active immunization is being developed.

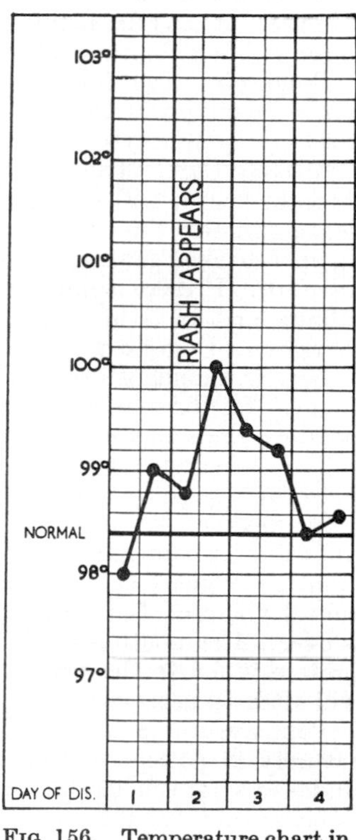

FIG. 156. Temperature chart in rubella (German measles).

Anterior Poliomyelitis

Cause. A virus.

Mode of Infection. The virus is present in the fæces and in the pharynx of infectious cases, and the former is probably the more important factor in spread.

Outbreaks occur most commonly in the late summer and autumn, and may affect countries with a generally high standard of public hygiene. The popular name " infantile paralysis " indicates that children are the main victims, but in such countries there is a comparatively high number of adult cases. Liability to infection is increased following tonsillectomy, and if inoculation of any kind is given during the incubation period, there is increased liability to paralysis in the limb used. Insufficiently chlorinated swimming baths are thought to be dangerous.

Incubation Period. This is probably four to twelve days.

Signs and Symptoms. The early signs are fever, loss of appetite, headache, nausea and vomiting. This relatively minor illness lasts two or three days. Following this there may be recovery, and these abortive cases may not be recognized except in an epidemic when doctors are on their guard.

The virus in unfavourable cases passes into the anterior horn cells of the spinal cord, and the result will depend on how severely these are affected. Two types of case are seen :

(*a*) Non-paralytic. Headache, neck rigidity, photophobia and backache and pyrexia occur but paralysis does not develop and in a few days the patient begins to improve and is usually recovered in two weeks. Lassitude is often well marked afterwards ; progress must not be hurried, and convalescence is necessary.

(*b*) Paralysis occurs in the limbs, trunk, respiratory or swallowing muscles. It may be slight or extensive, and expert care is needed to preserve life and minimize subsequent disability.

Diagnosis. The fully developed case is readily diagnosed, but lumbar puncture is necessary in others, and will show a raised protein level and lymphocyte count in the cerebro-spinal fluid.

Nursing Care. The patient should be supported by a full-length fracture board, and a footboard at the end will keep the feet dorsiflexed and hold the bedclothes from the feet. The patient is dressed in an open-backed gown and lies flat with a small pillow under the head if an adult. If there is limb paralysis, the limbs must be supported with pillows and pads in a position of rest. Paralysed hands must be straightened over a pad.

Barrier nursing is used for all cases, and is usually continued in this country for three weeks. In special units, group isolation technique is possible, since all are suffering from the same complaint.

The observations necessary include a four-hourly temperature, pulse and respiration chart ; whether retention of urine is present ; pain, weakness or paralysis of the limbs ; the colour ; any respiratory difficulty ; whether there are voice changes or difficulty in swallowing. Routine hygiene care is indicated, but in the acute stage handling causes pain and bed bathing can be omitted until the sensitive stage is over. The mouth is tended, and an adequate soft diet with plenty of protein is fed to the patient by his nurse. Analgesics and sedatives will often be necessary.

Poliomyelitis is a word that terrifies patients and relatives. The severely ill patient is too exhausted to be anything but glad to be under care ; it is in the later stages when the slow road to convalescence is being taken or the possibility of permanent invalidism being faced, that the patient most needs the encouragement of his nurse. Visitors must be shown how to don a mask and gown, and are warned against touching the patient or his surroundings in the acute stage. Natural behaviour is very difficult under such circumstances, and much kindly support will be needed.

During the acute stage active physiotherapy is not given. The patient is turned regularly, and painful spasm of the muscles may be treated by hot wet packs (p. 228). Once this is over, treatment is begun to re-educate the muscles.

There are three types of paralysis which threaten life :

1. Bulbar paralysis.
2. Respiratory paralysis.
3. A combination of both these.

Bulbar Paralysis

The patient is unable to swallow, so that secretions collect in the mouth, the voice is nasal, and regurgitation of fluid occurs. It is a condition highly alarming to the patient, but if prompt and adequate measures are undertaken, complete recovery may occur.

As soon as the symptoms manifest themselves, the end of the bed should be raised and the mouth and pharynx cleared by a sucker. The chief nursing problem is to keep the airway clear, and once a good airway is established, the patient's fear diminishes. Nasal oxygen may be helpful, and in severe cases tracheotomy may have to be performed on admission.

A Nelson postural drainage bed is useful except for small children, and the patient must never be left alone. Secretions can be swabbed out of the dependent cheek, and the sucker must be used when necessary, but not without real indication or soreness will result. Nasal feeding must be instituted if inability to swallow lasts more than a day or two and must be done with all vigilance.

When swallowing is once more possible, spoon feeding of small quantities of fluid is begun, and carried out very slowly so that fatigue is not caused. It is best done with the patient sitting up, and if choking occurs the head-down position must be promptly instituted.

Respiratory Paralysis

Inability to maintain adequate chest movement was formerly treated by enclosing the whole patient, except for the head, in a cabinet-respirator. The pressure inside the tank was varied by a motor, and as the pressure fell the chest was expanded and air was drawn down the air passages. The great disadvantage of these machines was that access to the patient for nursing duties was very limited, and it was almost impossible to turn the patient and give the physiotherapy to chest and limbs that is now thought so vital.

A respirator of the type described here would be used.

Intermittent Positive Pressure Breathing

Artificial ventilation of the lungs may be necessary in the following circumstances.

1. *Respiratory failure*
   (*a*) due to central depression, in (e.g.)
   carbon dioxide poisoning
   cerebral injury
   narcotic poisoning
   (*b*) due to peripheral paralysis, in (e.g.)
   myasthenia gravis
   poliomyelitis
   tetanus
   chest injuries
   (*c*) due to lung disease, e.g.
   pneumonia

2. *Nebulization treatment*, which enables the patient to inhale a fine mist of antibiotic or bronchodilator.

A positive pressure ventilator inflates the lungs, which deflate by elastic recoil, and the machine takes over the task of breathing until the primary cause of the respiratory difficulty has been cured. This may take only a matter of hours or days, and a cuffed endotracheal tube can be used. If treatment takes longer than three or four days, tracheostomy is performed, and the machine connected to a cuffed tracheostomy tube.

In either case, the nose is by-passed, and its action in warming, moistening and filtering the incoming air must be supplied by the ventilator. Unless the air is moistened, the secretions of the bronchi become viscid, and cannot be expelled, and if a sterile technique is not adopted, lung infection readily occurs.

The East-Radcliffe ventilator, the use of which is here described, is in common use. The air is supplied by bellows, which are compressed by weights, and expanded by a lever, driven via a cam by the motor. Air is drawn into the machine through a filter, oxygen is added, the mixture is blown through a heater-humidifier, and then through tubing to the catheter mount and the tracheostomy tube or endotracheal tube. Condensed water collects in the tubes, and runs down to water traps, from which it can be emptied when necessary. The repiratory pressure is measured by a gauge, and the expired tidal volume by a respirometer. These figures must not vary beyond the limits determined by the doctor for the individual patient.

Management. The nurse must watch not only the machine but the patient. Chest movement and colour must be observed, since the ventilator will go on compressing the bag even if the machine has become detached from the patient. The blood pressure; temperature and pulse, respiration rate as shown by the chest movement; the respiratory pressure and the expired tidal volume—all these must be recorded hourly, but observed constantly. Observations of the *patient* include the temperature and pulse; the respiration rate as shown by the chest movements; the colour; blood pressure, intake and output. The observations of the *ventilator* are the pressure (maximum and minimum) and the expired tidal volume. If these vary beyond the prescribed limits, the anæsthetist must be informed.

The respirometer which shows the expired tidal volume is a delicate instrument which is damaged by condensation, so it is not set to record continuously, but only when a spring-loaded receiver is raised.

The tubing is lifted at intervals to drain the condensed water back to the water traps. These must be emptied when half full, and if it is done quickly and dextrously there is no need to detach the patient from the ventilator. The respiratory trap must be pushed tightly home, or air to the patient will leak out and cause a drop in respiratory pressure.

The humidifier is on the lower shelf, and should be checked hourly. The temperature is kept by a thermostat at 50–60° C, which feels hot to the touch. The water vapour cools in the tube on the way to the patient. The catheter mount should be felt frequently, and should feel warm but not hot to the hand. There is an automatic cut-out device on the humidifier, and this may have to be pressed to reset it.

In some models, the humidifier can be taken out of circuit when it needs refilling by pressing a lever. If there is no such mechanism, the patient must be hand-ventilated while refilling. Distilled water is used, in order to avoid deposition from hard water on the elements. The humidifier is filled by a funnel to the maximum mark, but no higher, or water may be forced into the tubing or even into the patient's respiratory tract.

"Fighting the ventilator" means that the patient is making respiratory efforts out of rhythm with the machine. It is often a sign that the bronchi are becoming filled with secretion, and suction will remedy this. Sometimes it is due to under-ventilation, which will necessitate adjustment of the machine by the anæsthetist. The tracheostomy tube must not be allowed to ride forward. Persistent leakage around the tracheostomy tube may mean that the cuff requires inflation, or that the tube needs changing.

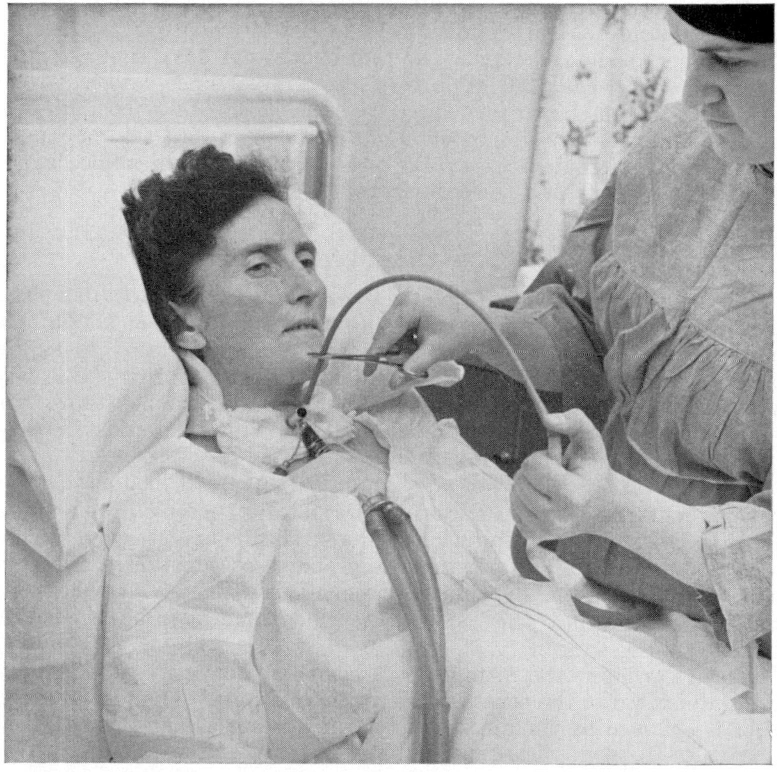

Fig. 157. Tracheo-bronchial suction for a patient with a tracheostomy and a ventilator. The catheter is being compressed with the left thumb against the connection, while the right hand introduces the catheter with an aseptic technique.

Nursing care of the patient. Speech is impossible with a tracheostomy or a cuffed tube, and a patient who regains consciousness and finds himself in this situation will be terrified. He must be talked to, and his needs foreseen as far as possible, so that he does not need to ask for anything. Some nurses become adept at lip reading, and some patients are well enough to write messages.

Movement and coughing must be encouraged, and the patient turned hourly from one side onto his back, and then to the other side. Hourly mouth care, daily bed baths, and attention to the pressure areas must be given. Tube feeding by a naso-gastric tube is necessary at first, but as the condition improves, soft foods can be given. These must be eaten slowly and quietly, or choking may occur.

Suction of the secretions of the airway must be performed hourly, or as often as necessary, and a sterile technique for its performance is described on p. 325.

In any emergency, the patient is detached from the ventilator at the catheter mount, an Ambu bag is attached, and the patient ventilated by hand until the anæsthetist arrives. The mask is applied to the face with the chin supported, and the bag is squeezed rhythmically to inflate the lungs with air. Difficulty is only likely to arise from squeezing the bag nervously and rapidly, so that it does not have time to fill.

Prevention of chest infection is of major importance, and it is usual to change the machine every three days, and disinfect it with ethylene oxide. The patient's life depends on his machine, but the machine is only a mechanical device, and depends on the constant skilled supervision of the nurse and the anæsthetist.

Bulbo-spinal Paralysis

A patient who can neither breathe nor swallow has the most dangerous paralysis of all. In an emergency, a cuffed endotracheal Magill tube may be passed and the positive-pressure apparatus used to supply oxygen through it. This allows time for preparation for tracheostomy, when a cuffed tube may be passed through the tracheostomy, and linked to the positive pressure apparatus. The head must be kept slightly lower than the trunk.

Nursing care is that for any other patient with poliomyelitis in routine matters. An indwelling plastic nasal catheter allows artificial feeds to be given, and aspiration of the trachea is necessary as often as secretions collect. The pressure gauge must be constantly observed, and watch must be kept for escape of air from the trachea that might indicate that the cuff of the endotracheal tube needed re-inflation.

At regular intervals the foot of the bed is further raised, and clapping is administered to the chest by the physiotherapist. The tracheostomy tube is changed by the anæsthetist when he deems it necessary.

Prevention

Active immunization against poliomyelitis is possible and all children should be given this protection.

VENEREAL DISEASE

The venereal diseases are those which are contracted by intercourse with an infected person, and in the temperate zones the commonest are syphilis, gonorrhoea and non-specific urethritis. These diseases are associated with poverty, overcrowding and ignorance; they are always common during wars, and among immigrant communities in which housing is poor and emotional insecurity high. Since effective treatment is available for syphilis and gonorrhoea, the prevention of these diseases is a social rather than a medical problem. It is therefore all the more disturbing that many countries have to report an increasing amount of venereal disease and that these include some of those with the highest living standards. The United States in 1961 reported a " sharp and consistent rise " in early syphilis from 1958 onwards, and in Canada the situation is similar. England and Sweden are alarmed at the incidence of gonorrhoea, and all these countries are especially worried at the number of teenagers involved.

All thinking members of the community have a duty to help with this situation in every way they can, and nurses have an especial responsibility. Our duty is not only to cure, but if possible to educate to avoid further illness. Many are innocent victims of circumstance, and we have no right to apportion blame and should not desire to do so. The prevention of infection is our chief duty, especially as children born of infected mothers can be afflicted.

Gonorrhœa

The causative organism is the gonococcus, which infects the mucous membrane of the genito-urinary tract, and the incubation period is from three days to three weeks. The initial lesions are urethritis, with scalding, painful micturition, and cervicitis, accompanied by profuse purulent discharge. Bartholin's glands are frequently enlarged and tender, and the vulva is swollen and painful. If the patient is untreated, the acute condition slowly subsides and a chronic infective state with slight discharge persists. Salpingitis may occur in women, epididymitis in men, while arthritis and iritis occur as remote effects.

If a woman with gonorrhœa has a baby, its eyes may become infected during passage through the birth canal, and the resulting ophthalmia may cause blindness if treatment is not early and effective. The decline in the number of children so tragically affected is falling due to preventive measures. These include ante-natal examination designed to detect infection and treat it ; cleaning the lids of the baby at birth, before its eyes are open ; and in areas where gonorrhœa is endemic, the installation of penicillin eye-drops.

Penicillin is generally effective against the gonococcus, and if the organism becomes resistant there are others as efficient ; it is usually possible to render a patient non-infectious in forty-eight hours, though observation must naturally continue longer. Should a patient be admitted with gonorrhœa, barrier nursing is used and gloves should be worn for local treatment. It is not a disease that is dangerously infective, except venereally, and provided the gloved hands are well washed in soap and water before the gloves are removed and dropped into antiseptic before sterilization, there are no exceptional precautions. It is most important not to touch the eyes while the hands are infected, but this is not a thing that a nurse instructed in the technique of barrier nursing would be likely to do. After gloves and gown have been removed, the final washing of the hands should be a careful one.

Syphilis

Syphilis is caused by a spiral organism (treponema pallidum) whose effects are felt throughout the body for many years, and which can cause death in many ways.

Acquired Syphilis

(*a*) Early infectious syphilis. About four weeks after infection (between 9 and 90 days) an ulcer appears, usually on the genitalia, at the site of infection. In men it is commonly on the glans or the shaft of the penis; in women it is often on the labia minora, but may appear on the cervix where it is unnoticed. The glands in the groin are swollen but not tender; general symptoms are usually absent, and the serum tests, such as the Wassermann, are negative. In this primary stage diagnosis is made by finding the spirochaete in the discharge from the sore or chancre. Even if untreated the ulcer usually heals.

Six to eight weeks after the appearance of the primary sore, appear the general symptoms and signs of the secondary stage. There is fever, headache, anæmia, lymphadenitis and hoarseness due to ulceration of the fauces. Sodden masses of heaped up epithelium appear around the anus and spread on to the vulva. Rashes of many kinds affect the face, trunk and limbs; they do not irritate, and are often symmetrical and reddish-brown in colour. All the moist lesions are highly contagious and the serum tests are strongly positive. These infectious patients are not often seen in a general hospital.

(*b*) Latent syphilis. This stage, in which signs are absent, may last for years, but the serum remains positive, and reactivation of the disease process may occur even after a long interval.

(*c*) Late non-infectious syphilis. The characteristic lesion of the third stage is the gumma, which is an area of necrosis surrounded by an inflammatory zone. This forms a lump which if near the surface breaks down to form a chronic ulcer. Gummata may affect many tissues, such as skin, subcutaneous tissue, mucous membrane, viscera or bones. Later still other general conditions occur.

(*d*) Congenital Syphilis. In untreated children, gummatous lesions like those of adults may appear.

Serological Tests

The Reiter Protein Complement Fixation Test is similar to the older Wassermann and Kahn Tests, and is more reliable than they are. The Fluorescent Treponemal Antibody Test is also used.

Treatment

Acquired. In early cases a course of penicillin followed by bismuth injections is given. For the late stages, the same treatment preceded by a course of bismuth is used.

Congenital. Penicillin (e.g. 200,000 units per lb. body weight) given over a period of 10 days is effective. The general medical and nursing care necessary for an ill baby is given to those with marasmus.

Congenital Syphilis

Babies born to a syphilitic mother are afflicted with congenital syphilis. They are underweight and fail to grow, and soon after birth a brownish rash may appear, sometimes covering the whole body. There is nasal catarrh and ulceration of the nasal bones may lead to their collapse. Cracks at the angles of the mouth heal with scarring, and when the central incisors appear they are notched (Hutchinson's teeth). In late childhood and adolescence the child is at once recognizable as syphilitic by the saddle nose, angular mouth scars, notched teeth, bossed forehead and hazy cornea. In untreated cases, the late stages of syphilis may supervene before the patient is 20.

Such infection can be prevented by adequate antenatal care. Serological tests should be performed on those attending antenatal clinics, and treatment commenced for those who are positive.

CHAPTER 31

PULMONARY TUBERCULOSIS

There is no disease in which the social implications are more important than in tuberculosis. For centuries it has caused long years of invalidism or death all over the world, but since the nineteen thirties there has been a most heartening decline in case numbers and in mortality, and it is hoped that the improvement reached in some countries may soon extend all over the world. It is essentially a disease of the underprivileged, and both social and medical factors have contributed to the decline. These are the most important ones operative in Britain :

1. A rise in the standard of living. Wages have risen, making possible a better diet and improved housing.
2. Earlier diagnosis is the result of better methods. Mass radiography formerly found many symptom-less cases, and routine examinations in clinics and schools have similar results. If patients are seen in the early stages, treatment is more effective and the illness is shortened.
3. A certain amount of active immunity can be conferred by means of B.C.G. vaccination, and large numbers of young people are protected by it.
4. The tuberculosis clinics do excellent work in families where a patient has this disease, examining contacts and especially safeguarding the health of children.
5. Treatment is better. The principles of sanatorium treatment are well established, and the introduction of the anti-tuberculous drugs—streptomycin, isoniazid and P.A.S. (para-amino salicylic acid) has been of incalculable value.
6. Surgeons have played a big part in stimulating treatment, first by collapse therapy to rest a diseased lung, and later by resection of diseased tissue.
7. Tuberculosis of bones, joints and glands in children is largely bovine in origin, and has been much reduced by pasteurization of milk, tuberculin-tested herds, and the designation of tubercle-free areas of milk production, which will eventually cover the whole country.

Signs and Symptoms

The early signs are often indeterminate—lassitude, loss of appetite and weight, cough, slight fever in the evening, night sweats—so that sometimes they have been present for some time before the patient seeks medical advice. Coughing up of small quantities of bright blood may also occur at an early stage, and usually brings the patient to the doctor promptly. A sudden form of onset is seen in pleural effusion, in which there is fever, pain in the chest and increasing breathlessness as the fluid in the pleural cavity increases.

In more advanced cases the tuberculosis lesions which are most commonly found near the apex of the lung soften and may ulcerate into a bronchus so that the infected contents are coughed up, and cavities are left in the lung. These are difficult to heal because of the tension and movement of the elastic lung during respiration. There is marked fever and wasting, and if blood vessels are involved, there may be copious hæmoptysis. Infection may appear in other parts of the body, such as the kidney ; the larynx, due to the coughing up of infected sputum ; or the intestine, owing to the swallowing of bacilli from the lungs.

Investigations

As soon as the disease is suspected, the patient should be carefully and thoroughly investigated, both from the general and pulmonary aspects. The temperature, pulse and respiration rate is recorded four-hourly ; the weight is taken every week, and the erythrocyte sedimentation rate regularly estimated. An X-ray of the chest and possibly tomograms to investigate lesions accurately will be required. The Mantoux reaction may be tested, and specimens of sputum obtained to find if tubercle bacilli are present. If none are found, they may be sought in the stomach after gastric aspiration in the early morning (p. 133). A bronchoscopy may be deemed necessary in some cases. If a pleural effusion is present, a few millilitres will be aspirated for investigation, and should the fluid be sterile (as it usually is) some may be inoculated into a guinea pig.

A diagnosis of tuberculosis is a shock to a young patient, but the more hopeful prognosis in this disease is now known to the general public as well as to medical people. Contacts in the family will be investigated, and the tuberculosis visitor will call to see what help and economic advice can be usefully given. Treatment may be undertaken at home in suitable cases, but sanatorium or hospital treatment is usually more satisfactory.

Treatment

The principles of treating the tuberculous patient which enabled many to recover before the introduction of the anti-tuberculous drugs, are still basic. Of these, the most important is rest. Physical rest in bed decreases the depth and rate of respiration and so diminishes the movement of the affected lung. Mental rest is just as important, and physicians have long recognized that freedom from anxiety and the ability to relax mental tension have a favourable effect on the outcome in this condition. It is not difficult to appreciate the anxiety that the patient feels about his family and his financial situations, but in addition to these there are many minor irritations and frustrations felt by the long-term patient which the nurse can help to minimize by patience, tolerance and humour. In a sanatorium these frictions result from the prolonged stay in a rather segregated community ; in a general hospital the patient may feel himself isolated by his disease, and irked by the barrier nursing which divides him from his fellow patients and emphasizes to him the infectious nature of his disease. He must be enabled to make a good adjustment, accept the fact that treatment may be lengthy, and look forward to the future with hope.

Once healing has begun, graduated exercise slowly builds up his confidence to resume full activity without fear of lighting up the infection once more.

A good full diet is important, but in the early days when the spirits are low the appetite is apt to be slight. High calorie, non-bulky foods must be given, and opportunities taken to give fortified milk drinks. If the patient is awake in the night a glass of hot Horlicks or Ovaltine will provide extra calories as well as inducing sleep.

Direct sunlight is not beneficial in the active stage of tuberculosis, but open-air conditions are desirable. High temperatures in ill-ventilated rooms induce night sweats with all their discomforts.

Some form of occupation for hand and mind is desirable as soon as the doctor allows activity, and handicraft is especially popular as everyone likes to see the product of his exertions. Those who have the ability can be encouraged to learn a new language, or to continue to study the subjects of their particular interest, so that at the end of their stay they have benefited mentally as well as physically.

Drug Therapy

The three drugs most often used are streptomycin, isoniazid, and P.A.S. (para-amino salicylic acid), either alone or more usually in combination. Tubercle bacilli often become resistant to streptomycin given alone, but the onset of resistance is delayed if P.A.S. or isoniazid is given with it.

Streptomycin is given by intramuscular injections for pulmonary tuberculosis, but intrathecal injections may be used for tuberculous meningitis. The dose for an adult is in the region of 1 G. a day, and it is supplied as a sterile powder in ampoules which is dissolved in distilled water when it is to be used. If the container is a multi-dose one, the solution must be stored in a refrigerator and used within a few days. It is a drug which has a reputation for producing such symptoms as vertigo, deafness, rashes and fever, but the reputation is based mostly on experience of earlier impure forms, and the more serious complications are not commonly seen now. Complaints of giddiness or affection of the hearing must, however, be reported before the next dose is given.

Streptomycin is a potent sensitizer when applied to the skin, and nurses must take every precaution to avoid contaminating the fingers with solution or the face with spray. Gloves are worn throughout ; the same needle is used for mixing, drawing up and giving ; the amount is levelled off with the needle point still in the phial ; and the needle and syringe are washed afterwards with the gloves still on.

P.A.S. is given by mouth in doses of from 10–20 G. daily. It is very nauseating, and some patients find the utmost difficulty in swallowing it, and it must be given with a pleasant-tasting drink. Few patients are entirely free from nausea and diarrhœa while taking it. More serious complications include fever, vomiting, leucopenia and vitamin B deficiency.

Isoniazid is less toxic than the other two in its usual dosage of 4–8 G. per kilo body weight. It may produce such signs as drowsiness and drying of the mouth like the anti-histamine drugs, and some patients complain of an undefinable unease while taking it. It is seldom used alone for pulmonary tuberculosis, but is the drug of choice for lupus vulgaris, or tuberculosis of the skin.

Whenever these drugs are being given the temperature is recorded four-hourly, a fluid chart kept, and the cell count regularly estimated. Vitamin tablets are given, and any complaints reported at once.

Nursing Precautions

Patients with " open " tuberculous lesions vary in their infectivity The bacteriologist who reports on the sputum may indicate this on the Gaffky scale ; a Gaffky count 1 means that only one bacillus has been found on a slide, while a count of 12 means that innumerable bacilli are seen in every field.

The precautions to be adopted depend on whether the patient is in a sanatorium ward where all patients have the same disease or in a general hospital where others must be protected from his infection. Since the sputum is the source of danger, these precautions are the most important in a general ward :

1. A single room is necessary.
2. Ventilation must be excellent.
3. The patient is taught not to cough unguardedly, and is given paper handkerchiefs which he puts into a paper bag for burning.
4. The sputum is expectorated into a covered container. This may be a waxed carton which can be weighed and burnt, or metal sputum mugs which can be steam sterilized or boiled. The hands must be thoroughly washed after dealing with sputum.
5. Washing and eating utensils must be reserved for the patient's sole use, unless all those in the ward are sterilized.
6. A gown and mask should be worn for all tasks involving close contact with the patient or disturbance of the bedclothes.
7. All bed linen is treated as infectious before being sent to the laundry, as described on p. 448

Protection of Staff

Young students often feel some alarm about tuberculosis, which they feel to be a threat to their age group, and this is especially so in general hospitals where only the occasional case is seen. Their seniors have a duty to see that they understand the routine which will protect them, and follow it conscientiously. They must also understand that they have the duty to conserve their own health by such measures as taking regular meals, having enough sleep and open-air exercise. The sister in charge of the nurses' health should see them regularly, record their weight and listen to any complaints.

The most important single factor in the protection of the nurse is that she should have some resistance to tuberculosis before beginning her career. Those students who are Mantoux negative on entry to hospital should be given B.C.G. vaccination on admission to the School of Nursing, and any who have not become tuberculin-positive before starting work in the wards should not be allowed to nurse infected patients until they have.

Rehabilitation

Men or women cannot be said to be recovered from tuberculosis until able to maintain their place in society and at work. The long and disabling course that the disease used to run sapped the self-confidence as well as the physical strength of the sufferer, and there was much fear of infection among less well-informed people. Papworth Village Settlement has done notable work in providing an environment where those unable to compete in the open labour market might work and live until they were able once more to face the world with confidence.

Today the course of the disease is so much shorter that the crippling psychological effects so often seen are not common, and full employment has made it possible for all patients fit enough to do so to return to work.

CHAPTER 32

ATTITUDES AND TECHNIQUES IN PÆDIATRIC NURSING

Children suffer from many of the diseases which afflict adults, from others which are peculiar to the young, and from congenital defects which surgery may remedy. There are many good textbooks on the medical and surgical conditions from which they suffer, and this chapter deals not with such diseases, but with the way in which hospitals affect children, and the way in which the nurse must adapt and modify the attitudes and the techniques which are used for adult patients.

The number of children admitted to hospital is falling steadily, and this highly commendable fact is a tribute to the preventive medicine which is done by general practitioners and public health workers. This begins with efficient antenatal care and neonatal management by the midwife. The welfare clinics to which well babies are taken to keep them healthy, the health visitor who advises on food, clothes and immunization, the doctor who performs inoculation against diphtheria, smallpox, whooping-cough and tetanus, and the school nurses and doctors who look after the school child have all made contributions of great importance.

It has long been recognized that hospitals are dangerous places for small children, who are exposed to risks of cross-infection that only the most conscientious nursing technique can prevent. It is now recognized that children from the age of about nine months to four years suffer with varying degrees of severity from separation from their mother. The ones who feel this most deeply are those of one and two to whom it is difficult to explain that the parting is only temporary. The toddler feels not only grief but a sense of rejection and abandonment by the one he loves best, and when he gets home may show behaviour upsets and severe anxiety lest he be left again.

It must be stated at once that not all toddlers suffer more than passing unhappiness if their mother can visit regularly. They may cry a bit when she leaves, but are content with the ward life, and when they go home will re-visit the ward to see the sister without signs of fear. However, many feel the experience very deeply for a long time, and anything that we can do to minimize the disturbance, we must certainly do. The parents also have a vital part to play, and will require some coaching in it.

The child should never be threatened with visits to hospital or the doctor when he is naughty ; building up the hospital into a place of fear will cause much unhappiness if he eventually has to be admitted. When a stay in hospital has to take place, he must be told about it in terms that he can be expected to grasp, not too far ahead, and not in over-explicit detail if surgery is contemplated. Hospital should be thought of as a place where children are made well, and where parents come to see them every day. Parents naturally feel fearful about it and must take care not to burden the child with their anxiety.

On admission, the child comes into the ward with his mother, who should bring any object, however decrepit, that he likes to take to bed with him. He should not be undressed at once, and a bath is a very bad introduction; probably he has had one before coming in, and to receive a second one in the middle of the day, even if his mother is present, confirms his suspicions that all is not well. He should be allowed to wander about if he will while mother talks to sister, and if there is a play room he will be interested in looking on if not joining in.

The mother should be asked if she can visit daily, and told she may come freely. If other young children keep her at home, she is urged to find someone as a baby-sitter as often as possible, or to send her husband. If she lives at a distance, perhaps there are relatives or friends near who would call and remind him of mummy, or she can send postcards to show him that he is not forgotten. Mothers often ask if daily visiting does not upset the toddler, and whether it would be wiser for her to forego the pleasure. She is told that the child will almost certainly cry when she leaves, but that this is natural and is rarely long continued. It is sad that parents' last view of their child is a tearful one, but it is better than that he should feel rejected; after all, children cry at home sometimes, and it would be too much to expect that it would never happen in hospital.

If an operation is to be performed, the surgeon's intentions are made clear and they are asked to give their written consent; it is wrong to ask them to sign an anæsthetic form as a routine if surgery is not definitely intended. They must also be given an opportunity to see the houseman, and the consultant should not be inaccessible if important decisions have to be made. The mother should promise to come back the next day as she says goodbye, if she intends to.

The first meal in hospital is rarely eaten with a good appetite, even by older children, but no fuss should be made about this even if it is refused. Unless it is necessary the child should not be undressed and put to bed, neither should examination be undertaken soon after admission; if the child is crying, little information is gained, and the foundation of a bad relation with the doctor is laid. A pleasant feature of ward life is the kindliness children display to each other in hospital, and the new one will have plenty of small comforters assuring him that it is not too bad, and that mummy will be coming back. During the first day toddlers will shed many tears, but this should be thought of as normal, and much as nurses like to have a ward of happy, cheerful children, they must not expect this always to be the case.

The attitude that the nurses adopt depends on the age of the child. Babies under nine months will not miss their mothers, but they do need affection and handling. If it is practical, they should be picked up for feeding. Older children understand as well as adults that their stay is necessary and temporary, and present few problems. Toddlers are quite different; they want a mother-figure but not a mother-substitute who usurps the place of the real mother. Since toddlers have fathers as well as mothers, the male nurse can also play an important part in their management.

A solution to the question of separation and the trauma it entails is the admission of the mother to hospital as well as the toddler. She undertakes for the child the care that she would give it at home and such other duties as the nurse can train her in. The advantages of such a scheme to the child are obvious, but not all mothers are able to abandon all other obligations completely and must not be made to feel guilty if they cannot. The nurse has an adjustment to make in this kind of situation, since she has to give all the difficult and uncomfortable treatment like injections, without any of the happier tasks that make for friendly relations. However, the toddler soon feels that his mother likes and esteems the nurse, and comes to accept her intentions as good. If such a situation seems unusual in England, there are many parts of the world where not only the child but the adult patient is regularly accompanied to hospital by most of the family.

Premises

A pædiatric ward must have an adequate number of cubicles in which can be nursed infants who have to be protected from infection and older children who must be isolated. There should be running water in each and those which are designed for babies should have space for a mother who is breast-feeding. The partitions should be of glass down to cot level so that nurses can see in and children who are in quarantine can see out. The main ward can be divided into units of about four cots so that children can be grouped according to age and temperament.

The kitchen should have a dish-sterilizer so that all crockery is boiled after use, and in all but small units, a milk kitchen with its own refrigerator and sterilizer, where infant feeds are made, is a necessity. A treatment room is a necessity, so that dressings and such procedures as lumbar puncture can be conducted in peace. A play room is of inestimable advantage, and children of all ages enjoy being able to keep shop, play at housekeeping, build, draw and paint ; it enables those who feel well enough to enjoy some activity and allows more peace and quiet in the main ward. A verandah permits those who need it to have fresh air and sunshine, but the railings, must, of course, be of a type that cannot be climbed.

Illuminated tanks of tropical fish are in vogue as a focus of interest and are always attractive to newcomers, but they must not be at too low a level and the top should be screened or very strange articles may sometimes be found among the fish.

Cots

A variety of beds and cots will be kept, and the latter should have tall sides with safety catches so that toddlers standing in them are safe from the danger of falls without the use of restrainers. These should not be used except when really necessary as accidents occasionally occur from children getting entangled in them, and they restrict chest movement.

Those who are ill lie down and should have the bedclothes made up in the same way as for adults, but a toddler who is able, always uses his cot like a playpen and walks around and stands up in it. The most rational method is, therefore, to dress the child in vest, knickers, jersey and shorts, or frock and jumper, and make up the bed only as far as the drawsheet. This implies that the ward temperature must be a comfortable one, and that a blanket is in the locker ready for throwing over the toddier when he lies down. If top bedclothes are used for a child who does not want to lie under them they will be constantly rumpled and often wet.

Small children usually sleep outside the bedclothes and usually face downwards and there is no need to try to keep them covered if the ward is warm, but if nightgowns are open-backed it is wise to put on a vest. Laundries which wash the children's ward woollies without shrinking them are rare, and it is quite usual to have jerseys and cardigans washed by the ward orderly, and if this is so a drying cupboard or a spin-dryer is a necessity.

EXAMINATION AND OBSERVATIONS

The doctor's examination of all except the urgent and ill cases should be postponed until the child has had a few hours to become accustomed to the ward, and may be performed with the child in bed, or sitting on the nurse's knee if it is a toddler. The more unpleasant parts—such as examination of the throat, ears or rectum—should be left to the end, and an opportunity must be found to examine the abdomen while the child is quiet, as it cannot be done while he is crying. When the throat is to be examined, the pillow should be drawn down under the shoulders so that the head and neck are extended, and if the child cannot co-operate the nurse will hold both its hands with one of hers and use the other to control the head.

The *blood pressure* can only be taken efficiently if the child consents, and explanation may ensure its co-operation ; normally after the first time no further difficulty is experienced. It is not an observation made as often as in the adult wards. The appropriate size of sphygmomanometer cuff must be used, and the manometer should be kept turned away from older children, who display the same desire to know their blood pressure as adults do.

The *weight* should be ascertained on admission and babies should be re-weighed daily or every other day if there is no contra-indication. Toddlers can be weighed weekly unless they are having cortisone, when daily record is kept.

The *temperature* is taken per rectum in babies ; the rectal thermometer is lubricated and passed into the anal canal while the baby lies on its back on the nurses's knee or in the cot, and it must be held until it is withdrawn. Toddlers should have the thermometer put in the axilla or groin, and must not be left alone ; older children can be treated in the same way as adults. The temperature in children is much more labile than in grown-ups, fluctuating more rapidly and rising to greater heights in the presence of infection.

Practice is needed before the *pulse* can be estimated in babies and toddlers with confidence ; the rate is higher and it is very easily compressed. Babies, especially, must be quiet, and must not have had a feed within the last fifteen minutes or an unduly high rate will be recorded. Variation of the pulse rate with respiration (pulsus paradoxus, or sinus arrhythmia) is occasionally met with during the course of infections and if the breathing is very rapid, the pulse may appear quite irregular to the inexperienced.

Observation of the *stools* is of great importance, especially in infants. At birth the intestinal canal is filled with meconium, a dark green sticky substance which is voided in the first few days after birth. As soon as milk is being taken the stools gradually assume the normal consistency and mustard colour of infancy. Small, dark-green stools may indicate underfeeding ; loose, pale-green stools are the result of infection ; undigested curds are seen after digestive upset. The stools of breast-fed babies are usually soft and plentiful, while those of bottle-fed babies are often paler and more constipated. If the stools are frequent, the amount of fluid loss must be observed.

The *skin* and the subcutaneous tissues readily show the effects of the dehydration that may result from such loss, the skin becoming dry and losing its elasticity. Pallor around the nose and mouth often accompanies colic.

The collection of *urine* specimens presents no difficulty in children who are old enough to have bladder control. For baby boys from whom a specimen is required, a test tube should have two lengths of strapping attached round the top ; it is put into place and kept there by attaching the strapping to the groins. Girls have a special plastic bag taped over the vulva. If there is no great hurry, a specimen can usually be obtained in a day or so by sitting the baby regularly on a " pot."

If it is desired to examine the urine for organisms, a clean specimen can be obtained from boys. Girls are supplied with the plastic bag mentioned above, and the urine is decanted into a sterile jar as soon as possible after it is passed. Catheterization is not desirable for children on any grounds; it is impossible to explain to small ones what it is all about, and older ones feel it to be highly distasteful and embarrassing.

CHILDREN'S TOILET

Bathing an Infant

A baby with fever, low temperature or constitutional disturbance should not be bathed until it is fit to withstand undressing and immersion ; the face and hands are washed and the buttocks cleaned, but the exposure and disturbance that must accompany a bath are avoided until the condition improves.

Newborn babies are often admitted to pædiatric wards with congenital abnormalities, and if it is necessary the nose, eyes and ears of such babies are cleaned with swabs dipped in warm water, since the orifices are especially liable to infection. No attempt must be made to introduce swabs deeply into the nose or ears ; it is harmful and unnecessary. After two or three weeks a clean face cloth can be used, which must be kept for the face alone.

Requirements. Soap.
Bath towel.
Face cloth.
Bath, or bath-sink of water at 100° F. (38° C.)
Clean napkin.
Bucket for used napkin.
Baby cream if liked.
Powder
Clean clothes.
Covered pail for used clothes.

Small babies are nursed with a gown and mask technique, which in its operation is exactly the same as that used in barrier nursing (p. 441) but for opposite reasons. It is used to protect the baby against infection from other sources in the ward.

The nurse puts on a mask, enters the cubicle and puts on one of the gowns hanging up inside. The bath or bath sink is filled with water at 100° F. (comfortably warm to the bend of the elbow when it is immersed) and the articles needed are assembled. The clean clothes are laid over a radiator or chair with outer ones at the bottom and the napkin folded ready for use on the top. The baby is picked up and the nurse sits with the bath towel on her lap and puts the baby on her knees. The nightdress and vest are discarded, and the towel wrapped round the baby to enclose his arms. The face and ears are washed and dried, then the baby is tucked under the left arm, the head is soaped with the right hand and rinsed off while being held over the bath. The head is dried, then the towel is unfolded and the napkin removed. The nurse soaps her hands and lathers the trunk and limbs with special attention to the flexures, draws the baby on to his side towards her so that she can soap his back. He is now picked up and put into the bath, and as he is wet and soapy a firm and careful hold must be used. The left wrist is behind the shoulders supporting the neck, while the left hand holds the baby's left upper arm. If the baby is a small one he is held by the lower legs; if he is larger the right wrist is passed beneath the thighs and the hand grips the far thigh. The left hand remains in place to support the head and shoulders, and the right one rinses off the soap. The baby is lifted out, placed face downwards in the lap and the towel folded over him and used to pat him dry. He is turned (rolling him towards the nurse to avoid the risk of dropping him off the knee), drying is completed, and the skin is powdered. The wet towel is discarded and the baby dressed, the cot is made and the baby put back.

Pressure Areas

Nurses in general training sometimes believe that children need no treatment of the pressure areas to prevent soreness. This is far from being the case, and in all ill children, and those immobilized in splints or plasters, care should be given to ensure cleanliness and good circulation in all parts exposed to pressure. Spirit is not advised for tender skins, but the principles of treatment are the same as for adults.

Mouth Hygiene

Ill children need mouth care as adults do, and older ones can be treated in the same way. Pressure forceps and not mouth sticks should be used for holding swabs. For small ones forceps and swabs dipped in normal saline are best.

Thrush is an infection of the mucous membranes to which babies and toddlers are prone, and which is easily transferred if sterilizing techniques or barrier nursing is faulty. Especial care should be taken with regard to the cleanliness of teats. The infection appears as milky-white patches on the tongue and inside of the cheeks. Gentian violet is an old remedy but messy for babies, and merthiolate 1 in 1,000 is better, since the effects of its action can be better observed.

Treatment with broad-spectrum antibiotics which sterilize the intestine is sometimes complicated by thrush, which may spread down the whole of the intestinal tract. If a baby has a sore mouth from thrush it is sometimes felt that it would be helpful to give it its feeds by an œsophageal tube passed through the mouth, but if this is done the infection will inevitably be passed further down. Nystatin is used for these widespread infections.

Toilet Training

Regular toilet rounds should be made of toddlers from a year upwards, but if he objects strenuously it should not be made the subject of a struggle. It makes a great difference to the physical atmosphere of a ward if clean habits can be maintained, and it is a great disappointment to mothers if they send a well-trained infant into hospital and find that he has relapsed when he comes home.

FEEDING CHILDREN IN HOSPITAL

BREAST FEEDING

Since milk is secreted to supply the physiological needs of the baby and is sterile, the advantages of an initial period of breast feeding are very great indeed. The danger of gastro-intestinal infection in a breast-fed infant is negligible, and it is very rare for breast milk not to agree with a baby. The comfortable physical contact at feeding times is very satisfactory to mother and baby, and establishes their psychological relation on a good basis. Whether bottle or breast feeding is practised depends on cultural, economic and social patterns as well as physical ones. In countries where milk is in short supply breast feeding is universal and will continue until the baby can support himself on other foods. As economic standards rise, there is a tendency for breast feeding to be abandoned earlier, or not to be used at all, as can be seen in North America today.

In England breast feeding is common among mothers delivered in hospital, and midwives aim to send their patients home with a good supply of milk and their feeding routine well established. A young baby needs $2\frac{1}{2}$ fl. oz. (75 ml.) per lb. of its optimum body weight in every twenty-four hours; that is, an 8 lb. baby should have $8 \times 2\frac{1}{2} = 20$ fl. oz. (600 ml.). This amount could be taken in five feeds of

4 fl. oz. (120 ml.) each, and these could conveniently be given at four-hourly intervals (perhaps at 6 a.m., 10 a.m., 2 p.m., 6 p.m. and 10 p.m.), which is satisfactory spacing for a thriving baby.

Once it was thought that a feeding schedule should be a fixed one, and that to feed a baby before the prescribed time produced dire physical and temperamental results. Such a belief has obviously no physiological basis, and a swing of the pendulum introduced " on demand " feeding, when the baby is fed when he asks for it. This eventually results in time spacing very much like that given above, and is very successful with an experienced or placid mother. It is not easy, however, for a young or anxious mother to manage. Whenever the baby cries she fears he is hungry and feeds him at over-frequent and irregular intervals, until the baby has chronic wind and bad temper, and the mother has sore nipples and is short of sleep. In these circumstances it is more satisfactory to give her a schedule which is meant to be elastic. She need not feel guilty if she feeds a crying baby half an hour before his time, or if he wakes at night, and she need not rouse him at the appointed hour if he is asleep.

If a baby who is being breast-fed must be admitted to hospital, it is valuable if his mother can come in too and continue to feed him. It is an additional burden on a sick infant to cope with a new feeding system as well as an illness and it is worth a sacrifice of other interests by his mother if breast milk is made available. This is especially the case with babies with congenital hypertrophic pyloric stenosis, which is often treated by incising the thickened sphincter at laparotomy. Feeding with small quantities, preferably of expressed breast milk, begins immediately after operation, and in a day or two the baby can return to the breast.

ARTIFICIAL FEEDING

Bottle feeding may have to be introduced at birth for a variety of medical and social reasons, or it may be introduced later if the mother is no longer able to continue breast feeding. There is no doubt whatever about the excellence of breast feeding, but nurses in hospital are less aware of the difficulties in maintaining it in some home conditions than are district midwives and health visitors. In hospital the newborn is *test-fed*; i.e. the nurse weighs him before and immediately after feeding, so that she knows how much he has taken, and if he cries later is able to assure his mother that he is not hungry. At home the mother lacks this comfort, and has, besides, to cope with household tasks and her husband, who may be feeling relegated to the background. Breast feeding is undoubtedly a drain on the physical resources, and anxiety and fatigue may make bottle feeding seem desirable.

In these circumstances she must not be made to feel guilty over what she may regard as a failure, since artificial feeding conducted with regard to hygiene and the baby's dietetic needs is quite satisfactory. The points to be considered are :

A. The type of bottle. Upright ones with a teat at one end and no valve are convenient to store, but are slightly less easy to clean than the other, and air can only enter through the hole in the teat, so that the baby must learn to stop sucking occasionally, or the teat must be withdrawn from his mouth. The boat-shaped bottle has a valve at the end for air entry.

B. Cleaning and sterilizing bottles and teats. Both should be rinsed in cold water immediately after use. The inside of the bottle is thoroughly cleaned with a bottle brush, soap or detergent, and hot water, then put into hot water and boiled for three minutes. Teats are brushed inside and out with salt and boiled for two minutes. Alternatively, both can be immersed in Milton 1 in 80 until the next feed is due. If dried milk is being used, a measuring jug and spoon should be similarly treated.

C. Type of feed. Cow's milk and human milk are of quite different content. In approximate figures that are easy to remember, the values are these :

	Cow's Milk	Human Milk
Protein . .	4%	2%
Fat . .	4%	4%
Carbohydrate	4%	6%

Not only are they dissimilar quantitatively, but in quality as well, because the protein in cow's milk contains much more caseinogen than the more easily digestible lactalbumin. Babies of three months or over may be given unmodified cow's milk or dried milk, but up to that time a formula must be found for a suitable mixture. There are many of these, and the one selected should be simple and free from ambiguity that may give rise to error.

Dried milks are simple to use, and are made up by mixing 1 scoop of powder to 1 oz. of boiled water for every oz. of feed required. The powder is measured into a jug, a little water is added and mixed in with a sterile spoon to form a cream, the boiled water is stirred in to make the correct quantity. Feeds should be put up individually ; if they are stored in bulk, it is very difficult to ensure that the mixture is homogeneous, and feeds may vary in constituents, and digestive upsets can be traced to this cause sometimes.

D. Feeding technique. The milk should be at blood heat, and can be tested with the hand on the bottle. The baby lies in the lap, comfortably supported in a semi-upright position with one arm. The teat is put on the baby's tongue, so that it can be compressed between the tongue and the hard palate, and the bottle is held well up so that the baby does not suck air from it. The rate at which air bubbles are entering is observed and if it is not satisfactory, the teat is taken out of the mouth occasionally. Half way through the feed the bottle is set down and the baby supported upright to enable him to bring up wind ; his back may be gently patted or rubbed to encourage him. At the end of the feed this is repeated, and if necessary the napkin is changed.

The time taken should not exceed twenty minutes and is normally less. Slow feeding may be due to too small a hole in the teat, and it can be enlarged with a sterilized needle. Sometimes the baby enjoys sucking just as much as feeding, and is willing to prolong the pleasure. He should be gently stimulated into action by movement of the teat or a change of position.

Vitamin Supplements

Vitamin C should be given daily as orange juice, or rose hip syrup, from about the age of six weeks, whether the baby is breast or bottle fed. It is given with a spoon and is enjoyed by all babies. Vitamin D, the anti-rachitic vitamin, is required to the amount of 750 units daily, and breast-fed babies should have it as cod liver oil or halibut liver oil. This vitamin is added to dried milks by many firms, and the doctor should be asked about the dose for babies fed on them. Overdosage with vitamin D is harmful, producing overconcentration of calcium in bones and leading to kidney stones. The circumstances in which the baby is being reared affect the amount required; if he can spend time in the open air in the country he can make some vitamin D for himself from the action of ultra-violet light on the ergosterol in the skin.

MIXED FEEDING

The age at which food other than milk is given has been advancing, and it is customary now to introduce such food to the baby at two to three months. The first teeth begin to erupt at about six months, and mixed feeding should be well established by then, as the infant will not take kindly to it when his gums are sore.

The only feeding reflex present at birth is sucking, and the baby has to learn the techniques of drinking and chewing, so that the first foods introduced must be fluid in consistency. Milky cereal, broths and thin vegetable purées are the first foods introduced, and cereal is begun by giving a few spoonfuls before one of the feeds. The baby is allowed to suck them from the spoon, which should be placed on the tongue and not between the lips. The baby ought to enjoy the new food, and will if the consistency is correct. When it is being taken with pleasure, it should be given before the 10 a.m. and 6 p.m. feeds as well, and the quantities given increased steadily. When spoon feeding is well established, milk should be given with a cup and spoon, and the bottle should be unnecessary by the time the baby is nine months old, or earlier. The 10 p.m. feed is omitted as soon as the baby will sleep through the night without it.

Crisp foods such as toast can be given when the teeth begin to appear, and by the time he is a year old the infant should be having meals constructed on these lines :

On waking.	Orange juice and rusk.
Breakfast.	Cereals in variety.
	Crust or toast with butter; honey or jelly.
	Lightly boiled or scrambled eggs.
	Cup of milk.
Mid-morning.	Drink of milk or fruit juice.
Lunch.	Vegetable purées and gravy or broth.
	Lightly cooked eggs or steamed fish or finely minced meat.
	Milk puddings, custards, baked or raw apple.
	Fluids as desired.
Tea.	Bread or toast with butter ; marmite.
	Jelly or custard.

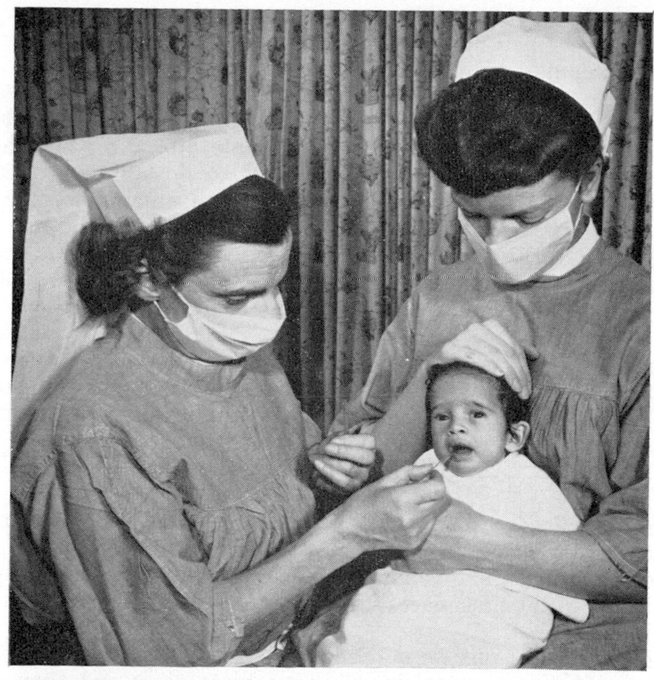

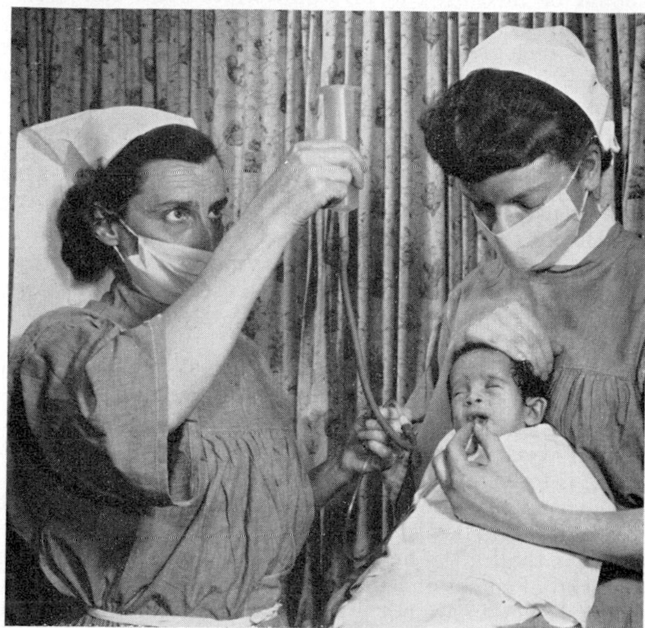

Fig. 158. Giving a stomach washout to a baby, showing the method of holding the baby.

	Plain biscuits or sponge cake.
	Cup of milk.
Before sleeping.	Cup of milk.
	Many enjoy this feed in a bottle.

Feeding toddlers in hospital does not differ from feeding them at home. They are protected with an adequate bib, and when they are old enough to feed themselves and want to do so, they should be allowed to under supervision. Cot boards from which meals are taken should have a washable surface.

In the case of the sick toddler, the maintenance of the fluid intake is all-important, and is one of the most exacting tasks in the children's ward. Nurses in general training who are accustomed to trying to keep up a fluid intake of five pints a day must remember that 30 fl. oz. is sufficient for a toddler, and that attempts to give large amounts at a time to a sick, tired child, will not succeed. Cups or mugs should be small, feeds are given at frequent intervals and an accurate chart is essential.

PROCEDURES

Giving Medicine. Medicines for children are best dispensed in liquid form, for swallowing pills and capsules is not easy, and if pills have to be crushed and given in liquid, they should have been dispensed as a mixture in the first place. Unpalatable substances can be made up as elixirs or syrups.

A bib should be put on a toddler before giving him his medicine, which should be measured in an appropriate glass and then poured into a teaspoon. If it is not willingly taken, the child should be sat on the nurse's knee ; she can keep the child's near arm under hers, and hold the other hand, and is then in a position to give the medicine, which can be followed with a sweet or a spoonful of rose hip syrup. Medicine glasses or minim measures must not be used for the actual administration, for an enraged toddler will readily bite a piece off.

Powders and crushed tablets can be given with a spoonful of fluid, but it is not generally wise to put them in food or a drink, or the child may be suspicious of all that is offered. Drugs in suppository form should be avoided if possible, for their administration is felt to be an assault on dignity. Capsules should not be given to an unwilling child. If the child does not think he can swallow it, a different form of presentation should be used.

Injections. The needles used for giving hypodermic or intramuscular injections to a child should be the same size as those used for adults, but the depth of penetration must be intelligently judged. Two people should always be present, one of whom controls the part where the injection is to be made, and restrains the hands if necessary. Even children who want to co-operate may be unable to control a start as the needle is put in. The best site for intramuscular injections is probably the front of the thigh ; the buttock is not very large, and children may be more fearful of something they cannot see being done.

Enemata. Enemata are not prescribed very freely for children, who not unnaturally dislike them. Doctors and nurses are more tolerant of occasional failures of bowel regularity under hospital conditions than they used to be and there are better aperients on the market now than there were once. Glycerine suppositories are as effective as enemata if an aperient is not favoured, and can be more rapidly administered.

Stomach Washout. Gastric lavage may be required for quite small infants, and two nurses are required, one to give the washout, and the other to hold the baby, who is wrapped in a blanket. His nurse sits, with the baby supported against her, and one hand over his forehead presses his head to her chest. A tube of adequate size should be selected, or milk curds cannot be successfully evacuated, and care is taken to syphon back all the fluid given before pouring in more. The lotion is allowed to flow in until it is nearing the bottom of the funnel, which is then lowered below the level of the stomach until fluid and stomach contents rises into the funnel, so that the nurse is assured before she inverts it over the bucket that she has syphoned back all the lotion she put in, and is in no danger of over-distending the stomach. 1,000 to 1,500 ml. of normal of normal saline may be needed before the washout returns clear.

Rectal Washout. Normal saline should be used, since, if water is left behind in an infant, it is absorbed and upsets the electrolyte balance. The amount syphoned back into the funnel should be checked in the same way as for a stomach washout.

Lumbar Puncture. Pre-medication is given, and if possible this procedure should be done in the treatment room on a couch of a height convenient for the operator. One nurse should be solely concerned with keeping the child in position, which she maintains by standing facing the patient with one arm behind the shoulders and the other around the knees.

Unless a toddler feels ill it cannot be induced to lie down after a lumbar puncture, yet it is very uncommon to notice any signs suggestive of headache such as an adult might contract in similar circumstances.

Intravenous Infusion or Transfusion. Pre-medication is given to toddlers or older children, who cannot fail to be alarmed over this procedure. Pædiatricians will have different opinions about a suitable drug, but pethidine is a very satisfactory way of producing euphoria without narcosis.

It is more often necessary to cut down on to the vein than in adult patients, but with practice a needle can be used even in infants receiving fluid into a scalp vein. When transfusion has to be repeated, it is highly desirable to use a needle, or else suitable superficial veins will become scarce. Fine needles will have to be used, and the standard needle and connection supplied in the adult transfusion set is too clumsy for an infant. For small children a presterilized small needle with polythene attached is used; for larger ones, an intracath is suitable.

The needle is secured with strapping over the flange. Scalp vein needles can be held in place with one or two collodion swabs.

Subcutaneous Infusion. This used to be rather an unhappy business before the introduction of hyalase, but absorption with it is so quick that the small amounts needed by an infant can be readily given. The arms should be splinted by applying corrugated paper around the elbows and bandaging it into place.

Oxygen Tents. Small children with pneumonia, or others who require oxygen, must be nursed in an oxygen tent since a mask is not suitable. The tent resembles an adult one except that the canopy tucks inside the cot rails to enclose the whole of the mattress. Nursing attention has to be quite frequent so that the necessity of taking the patient out of the tent for short intervals (as in the adult wards) does not arise here. Mechanical and wind-up toys should not be put inside the tent because of the risk of a static spark causing a fire.

SOME TYPES OF PÆDIATRIC ILLNESS

Children with Malignant Disease

Cancer is usually thought of as a disease of the elderly, but it occurs quite frequently in infants and toddlers, while leukæmia, which may also be placed in the same category, is met more often than we could wish. The prognosis for these children is only fair, though advances in radiotherapy and in the use of cytotoxic drugs are still being made.

The problem in nursing these children is two-fold ; the care of a very sick child who is possibly going to die, and the relations with the parents who can hardly believe that they may lose the child.

Small children do not, of course, realize that they are going to die, but older ones, though they rarely envisage death, do often appear to understand that they are not going to get any better. Deep X-ray treatment is often given, and while, fortunately, radiation sickness is uncommon, the usual skin reactions will occur, and the precautions described on p. 502 must be taken to prevent them. If the treatment involves lying very still, sedation will be necessary, such as trimeprazine (vallergan), while if the treatment is for the eyes, a general anæsthetic may be administered. When treatment stops over the weekend, it may be possible to allow the child to go home with its parents if conditions are suitable there are no nursing problems.

The parents will be allowed free access to the child in the ward, and will often need much help. If they allow their grief to appear, the child will be unhappy, and it is a great strain to spend long periods daily with him and always to appear hopeful and cheerful. All aspects of treatment should be fully discussed with the consultant, but it is the ward sister who will have to sustain their morale from day to day in very grievous circumstances.

Diabetes Mellitus

Children who have diabetes will always need insulin treatment if they are to grow and thrive, and since when they leave hospital the parents must take on the responsibility of his daily diet and injections, this is another situation in which the parents must be helped.

The dietitian who prepares his food must understand children as well as diets. They must be given food that they will eat, and it must compare favourably with what the other children in the ward are having for dinner. Very strict adherence to a diet cannot be expected with toddlers, who will get sweets off their companions.

Children can easily be taught to give their own injections if they are of average intelligence, and they are proud to do it. A mature eight-year-old will learn to draw up and give insulin, and by ten years all may be expected to. Urine testing by tablet methods is easy to perform, and children will keep their own charts to bring to the clinic or their doctor.

Hypoglycæmia may be signalized not only by the usual symptoms, but by any unusual behaviour. It is shaking to the self-confidence, and should not be allowed to happen often. Diabetic coma used to be a great danger to children, especially before they were diagnosed, but it is not now frequently seen, and the young diabetic can look forward to a long and healthy life if he has the support of his parents during his early days.

Children in Splints or Plaster

One of the reasons for which children may be put into plaster before continence has been attained is for congenital dislocation of the hip and the most important nursing point is to keep the plaster dry. Sand bags beneath the pelvis and thighs to keep the child clear of the bed permit the use of a receiver to catch the excreta.

A welcome and marked reduction in the incidence of tuberculosis of bones and joints has decreased the number of children immobilized for long periods in plaster, but there are still many children who for various reasons are treated in this way. They are astonishingly active in circumstances that would render adults helpless. They also insert, accidentally or on purpose, all kinds of foreign bodies, and complaints of pain may be due to coins or similar objects.

Strapping extension (p. 372) when used for children slips very readily because of their activity, and it should be examined daily to see if adjustment is wanted. Foot supports are not used, but movement is maintained by daily exercises. A gallows splint may be used for children under two for whom traction in the legs is needed. Skin extension is applied to both legs, and the legs are suspended at right angles to the trunk from the upper part of the splint with weights enough to lift the buttocks just clear of the bed. This solves the nursing problem of how to keep the bandages dry and clean. Toddlers are normally in constant movement, and the extension must be adjusted at least every other day.

Congenital Hypertrophic Pyloric Stenosis

Babies with congenital hypertrophic pyloric stenosis are often treated surgically, and the operation is sometimes performed under local anæsthesia. To keep the baby still but comfortable on the operating table, he is bandaged to a crucifix splint. The requirements are:

Padded crucifix splint
Cotton wool pads in gauze
2 in. × 4 in. cling bandages
Jacket or open-front vest
Bootees, mittens and cap
Small blanket

A clean napkin is put on, and tucket in, not pinned. The baby is dressed, and laid on the splint. A pad is put over the elbow, and first one arm and then the other bandaged to the splint. Next both legs are bandaged (both together) on to the splint with pads over the knees.

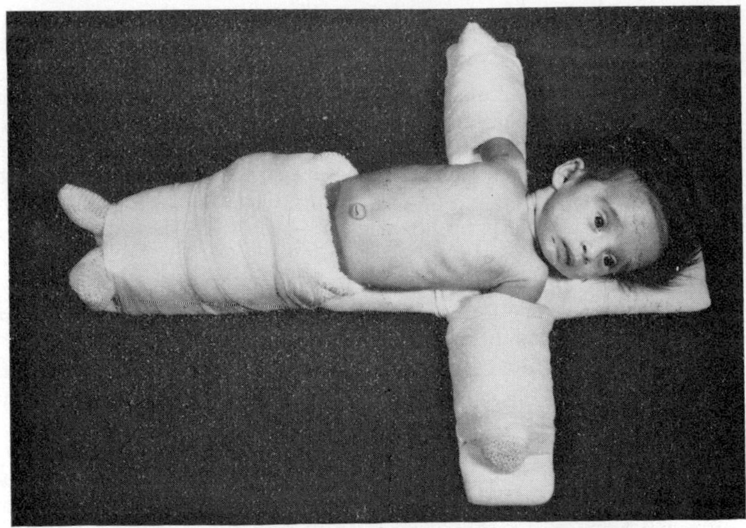

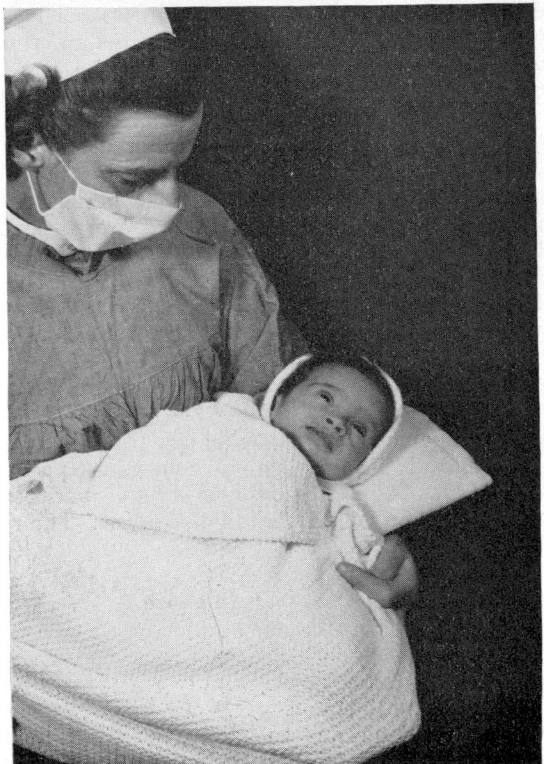

Fig. 159. A baby prepared for an abdominal operation.

CHAPTER 33

ELEMENTS OF PSYCHIATRIC NURSING

THE amount of mental disease in this country can be gauged from the fact that half the beds of the National Health Service are for the mentally ill. In addition, there are 60,000 certified mental defectives in hospital and many thousands more awaiting admission. These are the people whom the general public regards as mentally affected, but there are many thousands of others who come for medical advice with some mental or personal disturbance. Most general practitioners agree that nearly a third of the patients who consult them have nervous complaints, while if those whose physical illness has a nervous element are included, the proportion rises to about half.

It is customary to speak of disease as *organic* when some pathological change such as inflammation, injury or new growth can be demonstrated, and as *functional* or psychological when no such change occurs. Some patients fall readily into one category or another ; a patient with cancer of the stomach, complaining of abdominal pain and lack of appetite, obviously has a grave organic disease. Another may complain of the same symptoms, and possibly others like sweating, palpitation and anxiety ; his complaint is functional, and his symptoms are occasionally experienced by everyone in moments of fear. Yet another may have a duodenal ulcer—a condition which is certainly organic, but which is classed as a *psychosomatic* disorder—one in which the mind and personality play a powerful part in initiating and maintaining the disease.

The attitude of the general public to mental illness is quite different from the attitude to physical disorders, and has a strong emotional tone. Mental patients are regarded with uneasiness often amounting to fear, and mental disease is thought to be incurable. The reason for the fear is the quite mistaken belief that all psychiatric patients are dangerous to themselves or others. Violence and heedlessness of safety is sometimes shown by such patients, but it is not common, and many mental wards are as quiet as a ward in a general hospital.

The belief that mental illness is incurable is no more true than that physical illness is incurable. The proportion of patients discharged completely well from a general ward is not 100% ; many are merely relieved or have had their disease arrested, or have received palliative treatment. Yet most of these are able to adapt to life outside hospital although restricted in activity. With mental patients the situation is rather different. Many are cured and can leave with hopes of a completely normal life. Those who are not completely cured, but only relieved, cannot, however, in many cases, return to live a life of restricted activity outside hospital. A comparatively small ment disability may prevent them from being reabsorbed into their famil community, and the hospital has to provide a sheltered environmen them, often for many years. It is these long-stay patients, and n ones discharged as cured, who are the cause of the sinister feeling with which the public surrounds its concepts of mental disease.

Nurses in general hospitals have a very limited experience of major mental illness, and so are sometimes apt to react as other citizens do in thinking of mental illness, but must remember that they have a function to lead and teach the public in this respect. Everyone needs the support of the social group in which he lives, and those convalescent from mental illness need it more than others. Nurses can play an important part in their professional and private capacity in eradicating this outworn but general fear of psychiatric disorder.

DEFINITIONS

A *psychiatrist* is a fully qualified medical man with post-graduate experience and certificates in mental illness. Many fields of work are open to him in hospital and private work, and in preventive as well as curative medicine.

A *psychologist* has a University degree in psychology, and is mostly concerned with the activity of the normal mind. He may sometimes be a member of a hospital team, usually in connection with the measurement of intelligence.

The *psychiatric social worker* is concerned with the family and social problems of the mental patient. She is connected with a psychiatric department or hospital and investigates and seeks to solve the domestic difficulties of her patients. Since the mental patient's hopes of successfully re-entering social life depend greatly on the environment he is to live in, and the attitude of his family, the psychiatric social worker is of great importance in his future.

A *psychosis* is a major mental illness, of the sort that raises the question of treatment in a mental hospital. The patient is normally lacking in insight into his illness, and his personality is often broken down by the pressure of his illness, whether temporarily or permanently.

A *psychoneurosis* or *neurosis* is a mental or emotional disturbance but one in which the personality is well preserved, and insight into the illness is present. This patient may have more severe symptoms than many a psychotic patient, but he realizes he is ill and in need of help, and that his anxieties and obsessions are irrational. Unfortunately for him, it is this very fact which often makes people regard him with impatience and even scorn. He is asked why, if he knows his fears are groundless, he does not " pull himself together " or " snap out of it." The signs and treatment of psychoses and neuroses are discussed later.

A *delusion* is a system of belief unsuited to the patient's education and circumstances, e.g. that he is being subjected to electrical influences by invaders from another planet.

A *hallucination* is a false sensory impression, e.g. hearing voices that are not present.

A *nervous breakdown* is a term used by the public to denote any kind [illegible] mental illness. It is of no real meaning to doctors or nurses.

Mental subnormality is a state of arrested development of the mind [illegible]h has existed from birth or from an early age. The intelligence [illegible]ent, expressed as a percentage of the average level in the community, is 70–75. There is no hard and fast line between the upper evels in this group and less-gifted people who are classified as normal

The Mental Health Act, 1959, recognizes two grades of subnormality. In the upper group are those who can be trained to simple tasks and may be self-supporting. The *severely subnormal* (I.Q. below 50) include some who can be toilet-trained and form some kind of relation with other people, and others who are totally dependent, and cannot guard themselves from physical danger.

Mental subnormality may be caused in the uterus by chromosome abnormalities, by maternal rubella, or the results of Rhesus incompatibility; from birth trauma; or by causes arising in infancy, such as hypothyroidism or phenylketonuria. Some of these conditions are preventable, and some can be improved by early detection. Phenylketonuria, for instance, may be detected in infancy by testing the urine with Phenistix, and a suitable diet may lead to normal development.

8 in 1,000 of the general population are mentally subnormal, but only a quarter of these will require hospital care. Education in hygiene; social behaviour is given, and those capable of performing simple work receive training which may enable them to work in the community.

CAUSES OF MENTAL DISEASE

Many factors appear to precipitate mental illness, and often more than one are operative in the same patient.

1. **Organic causes,** e.g. general paralysis of the insane, senile dementia.

2. **Toxæmia.** Delirium may occur in acute infections like lobar pneumonia, and such conditions as chronic alcoholism.

3. **Heredity.** A family history of mental disease is not unusual.

4. **Endocrine Causes.** Psychoses occur not uncommonly following childbirth, at the time of the menopause in women and a similar age in men.

5. **Personality Pattern.** A history of difficulty in accepting or giving affection, feelings of inadequacy and inferiority, inability to hold employment, etc., are often forthcoming.

6. **Social circumstances,** e.g. divorced parents, broken marriages, financial insecurity.

SIGNS AND SYMPTOMS OF PSYCHOSES

1. **Emotional.** Changes of mood—depression, agitation, mania, poverty of feeling, feelings of guilt and unworthiness.

2. **Intellectual.** Failure of memory, delusions, hallucinations, blocking of thought.

3. **Motor.** Hyperactivity, or the reverse, suicide attempts, stereotyped speech, retention or incontinence of urine and fæces.

SOME PSYCHOSES

The following are some of the commoner psychoses:

1. **Schizophrenia.** This term means "split mind," and refers to a disease usually arising in young adults and adolescents. It is charac-

terized by emotional disturbances, disordered thinking and conduct, and hallucinations. Acute attacks may occur, with complete or partial recovery between but sometimes there is a progressive breakdown of the whole personality.

2. **Manic-depressive** psychosis. The mood swings between depression with feelings of guilt, unworthiness and despair, and elation with intense excitement, mental and motor. In most cases one or other mood is dominant and characteristic, and well-marked alternations are less often seen. The prognosis is not unfavourable in many cases.

3. **Involutional Melancholia.** This severe form of depression is seen in patients of both sexes of about 50 years old. The patient's depression is often an agitated one, with delusions about unpleasant bodily symptoms. Many patients make a striking recovery with treatment.

4. **Paranoia.** The prominent feature of paranoia is delusions of persecution. These may be complicated and bizarre, but logical, within themselves. Sometimes they dominate the patient's whole life until he cannot live outside a mental hospital.

5. **Senile Dementia.** This is a degenerative condition, in which there is a progressive intellectual failure, with loss of power of thought and attention. Emotion is shallow but violently expressed, sleep is poor, and the patient is often especially confused and restless at night. A cure cannot be expected in this condition, but nursing care may do much to maintain nutrition and preserve the patient from harm.

6. **Acute Alcoholic Psychosis** (Delirium tremens). The patient passes into a tense, agitated, busy delirium with terrifying hallucinations. It is apt to arise in alcoholics suddenly deprived of their alcohol, and so is sometimes seen in hospital in patients (more often men) admitted for some other medical or surgical condition and so cut off from their drug of addiction. Relatives are not anxious to disclose such a history but should be questioned as to the patient's habits if his appearance or manner suggest that he is an alcoholic. An acute attack may be arrested by the prescription of a maintenance dose of alcohol.

METHODS OF PSYCHIATRIC TREATMENT

1. **Environmental.** Someone who is mentally ill with a psychosis at home has to support not only the strain of his own illness, but many others, especially the grief and anxiety of his relatives. In hospital most of these pressures are at once relieved. He is surrounded by people who expect nothing of him, and are not upset by his behaviour. He has no decisions to make or responsibilities to shoulder, even at the simplest level, until he is able to do so. Even if his personality has completely degenerated, he can be given a routine of regular meals and toilet training, and from this he may possibly be slowly built up again. The importance of a stable and peaceful routine cannot be overestimated.

Safety is a vital consideration in the care of the mentally ill. Those who are depressed may have suicidal thoughts, and must be protected from this risk by removing potentially dangerous articles from their neighbourhood, and maintaining sympathetic vigilance. Elderly or confused patients may endanger themselves and others by heedlessness.

Fire is a serious risk in mental hospitals. Smoking may have to be controlled and supervised, and day rooms should be inspected when patients have gone to bed for the night. Bathrooms must be made as safe as possible, with non-slip mats in baths, and precautions to prevent scalding from unguarded hot taps.

It is sometimes felt by relatives that unless some active treatment is being undertaken, nothing is being done, while nurses in general hospitals occasionally think of mental nursing as being mostly custodian duties. Neither view is true. Someone with an infection may be admitted to a general ward to limit the spread of infection in the community, and in the ward the nurse takes precautions to prevent other patients being affected, and strives to build up her patient's physical powers to resist the disease. In much the same way a patient may be admitted to a mental hospital, which will prevent the spread of his emotional disturbance through his family group and the nurse strives to conserve his mental energies to deal with his emotional situation. The nurse-patient relation, and the doctor-patient relation are vital factors in recovery, and it follows that the doctor and nurse must have good personal communications to establish a consistent method of management.

2. **Psychotherapy.** In interviews with the psychiatrist the patient may be led to express his feelings, receive sympathetic support, and gain insight into his own illness. *Psychoanalysis* is the method of psychotherapy designed by Freud to bring to consciousness repressed material and reorientate the personality. The sessions may last for years and many shorter techniques have been introduced. *Hypnosis* may be used, i.e. a state of heightened suggestibility in which ideas may be introduced and instructions given. Psychotherapy is extensively used for psychoneurotics.

3. **Drugs.** Sometimes specific treatment is available, e.g. *penicillin* for general paralysis of the insane, or other antibiotics for toxic states.

Apart from these, however, there are many new drugs, the use of which has profoundly influenced the management of the mentally ill. The ones in use are constantly changing, since finding out how these drugs do their work and how well they do it is difficult. Animals do not appear to suffer from mental illness, and to compare degrees of depression or excitement in patients receiving different drugs can never be an objective test. Drugs acting on the nervous system are powerful, and many undesirable side effects are met.

Drugs used for their psychological action fall into two main groups, (*a*) sedatives and tranquillizers, (*b*) anti-depressant drugs.

Sedatives and tranquillizers. The barbiturates have been used for many years in this way; their effect is enhanced by taking alcohol, and disturbed anxious people must be especially warned about this. Newer drugs include diazepam (Valium), chlordiazepoxide (Librium) and nitzazepam (Mogadon).

A more powerful group, the *phenothiazine* derivatives, includes chlorpromazine, which is extensively used in general hospitals. Chlorpromazine is given by mouth in doses of 25–150 mg. It is used to relieve distress from pain in inoperable carcinoma, and for agitated and disturbed behaviour in psychiatric patients, and controls agitation and distress. It is invaluable in the control of symptoms in chronic schizophrenia. Trifluoperazine (Stelazine), promazine, perphenazine (Fentazin) and prochlorperazine (Stemetil) are other members of the group. Jaundice, rashes and agranulocytosis are serious side effects that must be watched for. These drugs depress the vagus nerve, so constipation and dry mouth are sometimes complained of.

Anti-depressants. Monoamine oxidase is an enzyme which breaks down adrenalin and similar substances in the nervous system. The monoamine oxidase inhibitors prevent this breakdown, and so increase alertness and responsiveness. Tranylcypromine (Parnate), phenelzine (Nardil) and isocarboxazid (Marplan) are examples. These powerful drugs may cause severe headache due to fluctuations in the temperature. All patients must be warned verbally and in writing not to take cheese, Marmite or Bovril while taking these drugs, since they contain a substance which interacts with monoamine oxidase inhibitors and causes hypertension, with severe headache and a risk of subarachnoid hæmorrhage.

4. **Electro-convulsive Therapy.** An electric current is passed briefly through the frontal lobes of the brain causing unconsciousness and an epileptiform fit. The fit is usually modified by giving thiopentone and oxygen as a short anæsthetic, and a curare-type drug to abolish the actual convulsion. Treatment is repeated once or twice a week on six to twelve occasions. The reason for the success of this treatment, especially in depression, has not been adequately explained yet.

5. **Abreaction Techniques.** Traumatic experiences, real or imaginary, may be repressed into the subconscious, but may continue to give rise to symptoms. If these are recalled to consciousness, the patient may relive the experience with much emotion and distress, but with insight into the cause of his symptoms. The psychiatrist may use inhalant anæsthetics or intravenous injections to produce a drousy susceptible state which facilitates recall.

6. **Pre-frontal Leucotomy.** The frontal lobes are disconnected from the rest of the brain by cutting the connecting white matter through burr-holes. This operation is not commonly performed, except for great tension and agitation, since it causes personality changes.

7. **Group Therapy.** Patients are encouraged to talk of their own difficulties in groups, under the guidance of the psychiatrist. They are cheered to discover that their difficulties are not unique, and much emotional tension may be relieved in a group.

8. **Occupational Therapy.** This should not be thought of only as a way of passing the time. It turns the patient's thoughts outwards, increases his morale and his motor skills.

9. **Case Work.** The psychiatric social worker may help to relieve stress on the patient by helping his family to understand him, giving advice on personal and economic problems, and in all ways helping to reduce strain in his environment.

PSYCHONEUROSES

Psychoneurotics are people who are sane, but are mentally badly adjusted to life, and who suffer from physical symptoms as a result of that maladjustment. These symptoms do not need direct treatment ; they will disappear when the mental conflict is resolved. The reason why these patients prefer to admit to physical rather than mental disorder lies in the unconscious part of the mind. Within this part lie desires and instincts which when socially and mentally well directed are a source of energy and purpose in life, but some people repress into their unconscious painful ideas, thoughts and associations, which are not available for conscious examination, but disturb the patient's mental life, often very severely. The commoner kinds of psychoneuroses are these :

1. **Anxiety neurosis** is the commonest neurosis seen today, perhaps because modern life often gives cause for anxiety, even in the well balanced. The patient is overcome with panic, and experiences the normal bodily accompaniments of intense fear—sweating, shivering, palpitation, gastric and intestinal upsets, dry mouth. Sometimes the fear arises in specific situations, and is then called a *phobia*, e.g. fear arising in enclosed places is *claustrophobia*. Fatigue, due not to bodily exertion but to emotional conflict, is often felt, and patients complaining of it were formerly said to be suffering from *neurasthenia*, but this is a distinction not now usually made.

Often the patient directs his attention to one specific aspect of his overactive sympathetic nervous system, e.g. the heart or stomach. He then sometimes arrives in a general hospital for investigations to exclude organic disease. His complaints of pain appear exaggerated to his nurses—" terrible," " dreadful," " unbearable " are the kind of words he uses—and she compares him unfavourably with patients with " real " complaints. He is likely to be told the re is nothing wrong and discharged, and may take himself to another hospital where the experience is repeated. He is not, however, a ma ingerer—he is not pretending illness—and is as much in need of treatment and sympathy as any other patient.

2. **Obsessional Neurosis.** The patient cannot escape from some thought, that he is impelled constantly to repeat, or the urge to commit some act. He may, for instance, constantly feel that he must wash his hands, or may be unable to sleep unless he has performed some intricate ritual. Symptoms of obsessional neurosis may be exceedingly severe, interfering greatly with normal life.

Everyone can recognize in themselves a glimpse of this neurosis—walking in the squares on the pavement, crossing the fingers or touching wood in order to stave off by magic some disaster.

3. **Hysteria.** Physical signs, sometimes gross, are exhibited, but have been unconsciously assumed for some mental reason. Paralyses, slight or severe ; anæsthesia ; loss of voice and blindness, are examples of such signs. Sometimes the mechanism is quite clear, e.g. a soldier in battle is smitten with hysterical blindness, and is removed from the fighting. He has solved his emotional problem, and displays a bland disregard (" belle indifférence ") of his disability. Hysteria of this major kind is not likely to be displayed by people of the highest intelligence, who are more likely to react with anxiety.

Hysteria is a condition whose manifestations are changing as the general public becomes more sophisticated about nervous illness. The hysterical " fits " with screaming and flamboyant motor signs once associated with this syndrome, are now rarely seen.

Hysterics are usually easily cured of their symptoms by suggestion, and contribute some of the spectacular cures at " healing " sessions. The underlying disposition, however, is not easily changed, but the aim of treatment must be this, rather than the mere displacement of physical symptoms. Indeed, a patient suddenly deprived of his protective illness may find himself defenceless against his circumstances.

It will be seen that the neuroses are exaggerations of normal mechanisms and character traits. Everyone has at some time had a headache that prevented her from performing some unpleasant or boring duty, or been unable to walk under a ladder, or returned to make sure that the front door really was locked. The neat, meticulously clean person absorbed in details of routine has a valuable contribution to make to society, but it only needs some exaggeration of his character to cause the development of obsessional neurosis.

Treatment is directed towards making the patient realize the source of his symptoms, and gain some insight into their cause, and the outlook is good in a big majority of cases. The nurse's main problem in looking after them in hospital is to give them sympathetic support without being monopolized with over-lengthy accounts of physical signs, the reiteration of which cannot help the patient. She should also remember that though his complaints are of " terrible " pain, the dose of analgesic that he will need to relieve it is no greater than normal, and may well be less. He must not be encouraged to dwell overmuch on his physical symptoms, but neither must these be dismissed as imaginary. " Neurotic " is used as a term of derision by the lay public, but the nurse knows the amount of real suffering that underlies the word.

The serious nature of neurosis is well seen in *anorexia nervosa*, a condition usually met in young women, in which the patient completely loses her appetite, and if forced to eat will vomit. She rapidly becomes emaciated, and death from starvation is not unknown, unless treatment in hospital is undertaken. The doctor's task is to find the cause of this neurotic illness and give the patient insight into it. The nurse's task is constant perseverance in the administering of very small tempting high caloric meals at regular intervals. Intravenous therapy is occasionally needed.

NURSING CARE OF MENTALLY DISTURBED PATIENTS IN GENERAL HOSPITALS

Patients with a psychosis are not often seen in general hospitals, but an acute illness may arise suddenly in any ward. Normally such a patient would be taken to a mental hospital for observation and treatment, but sometimes there is a medical or surgical contra-indication. In such cases, the following points are important.

1. *Position of the Bed.* The other patients' peace must be considered, but a confused patient must not be kept in a sideroom unless he has a special nurse, since he must not be left alone. Bedsides are usually necessary.

2. The risk of *suicide attempts* must be borne in mind. This applies especially to depressives at the onset of their illness, sometimes before its gravity is realized, when they are not too sunk in apathy to take action. Knives and forks should not be given for meals, a razor is not allowed, and windows should have a safety catch. Patients who are actively suicidal should be removed from a general hospital. Neither the premises nor the training of the nurses is designed for the continuous observation needed to avert tragedy.

3. *Nutrition* must be maintained. Depressed patients feel they are too unworthy to eat, excited ones cannot fix their attention on it. Dehydration will lead to acidosis, with still further clouding of the mind, and tube feeding must be used if necessary.

4. Detailed instructions should be obtained from the doctor as to the *drugs* to be given, and the frequency with which they may be repeated. It may be very difficult to induce sleep in excited patients.

5. *Retention of urine* and *constipation* must not be allowed to occur in the depressed and incontinence can sometimes be avoided in excited patients by regularly offering a bedpan or urinal.

6. The nurse will find that it is useless to argue with a patient about delusions ; these cannot be removed by logic and argument only serves to disturb nurse-patient relations. It is unwise, however, to agree with such delusions, or phantasies will grow unchecked.

7. A florid psychosis is easily recognized, but the early signs are sometimes overlooked. The nurse spends more time with her patient than does the doctor, and has the opportunities to observe and report changes that may be of great diagnostic importance. Depression, suspicion, agitation, or delusions must be reported at once, even if mild. These are of especial importance in new patients, those with infections, and in women following delivery.

8. The other patients in a general ward often feel the usual reaction of the lay public to mental disturbance, and may show unease and even fear. The nurse must do her best by her example of calm sympathy and serenity to dispel this reaction. Neither must the nurse permit the mood of a disturbed patient to affect her other patients. A depressed tearful patient may lower the morale of the rest, while noisy, rude and abusive behaviour may alienate them. It is difficult for people to understand that such conduct is a sign of illness, just as much as pain or vomiting. The nurse's understanding reaction to such signs will influence all the other patients.

CHAPTER 34

SOME FORMS OF THERAPY

RADIOTHERAPY

The electro-magnetic waves with a wave-length shorter than that of ultra-violet light include X-rays, the gamma rays of radium and radio-active isotopes, all of which have a therapeutic use in medicine. They have a destructive action on all living cells exposed to them but this action is greatest on cells undergoing division, so that it may be possible to destroy malignant growth without doing real harm to the tissues around. The relative speed with which the cells are destroyed by irradiation is known as radiosensitivity. Some cancers are very radiosensitive but so, unfortunately, are some normal body tissue cells, such as those of the bone marrow and the sex glands. The sources of the therapeutic waves in use are:—

(1) X-rays which are produced by high voltage electricity.

(2) Radium: The oldest radio-active material known and a naturally occurring one.

(3) Radio-active Isotopes.

Radio-active forms of most ordinary elements can be produced in an atomic pile ; the most medically important include iodine, phosphorous, cobalt, gold, strontium, cæsium, sodium and potassium. Research into the possibilities of their use in medicine and industry is proceeding rapidly. Some already have been proved of value, both in medical research and therapeutics.

Dangers of Radio-activity

Many of the pioneer workers in this field found to their cost that constant exposure over a long time resulted in sterility, chronic radio-dermatitis of the skin which might proceed to skin cancer, and blood diseases especially anaplastic anæmia and leukæmia. The results of sudden severe radiation were tragically seen in the atomic bomb results in Japan, and scientists also warn us that long-term effects may result to humanity at large through mutation of genes from all the radio-activity now being produced in so many ways.

Workers in X-ray departments and isotope laboratories are exposed to greater dangers than other members of the public, and precautions for their health are continually strengthened. Their hours of work are restricted, blood counts are made at regular intervals, film badges are worn which measure the exact amount of any exposure, monitoring is undertaken to check the amount of radio-activity on such premises, and intelligent adherence to all safety precautions is expected.

Nurses who are concerned in the transport or handling of radio-active materials in the wards or theatre must also observe the rules that are laid down for their protection. The precautions necessary have been laid down in a code of practice issued by the Ministry of Health, and the guidance of the physicist or radiotherapist should be sought and observed in connection with all new methods of treatment.

X-rays

Although X-rays are used for a number of innocent conditions, their chief therapeutic value is in malignant disease. Their effectiveness depends partly on the extent of the growth, but mainly on how sensitive the tumour is to such treatment. Some very rapidly advancing growths, such as chorion epithelioma, may be radio-sensitive, and very successful results are sometimes obtained from X-ray therapy. The greater the voltage by which the rays are generated, the greater their power of penetrating deeply without undue harm to the skin through which they have to pass.

X-ray Therapy may be classified as:—

(1) Superficial X-ray therapy up to 140 kV. for treatment of conditions of the skin and accessible mucous membranes.

(2) Orthovoltage or Deep X-ray up to 300 kV. for the treatment of relatively superficial cancers, such as those of breast and lymphatic glands.

(3) Megavoltage Radiotherapy which implies treatment with voltages over 1 million volts. This will include Cobalt Bomb Therapy (1·3 MV) and such apparatus as linear accelerators which operate between 4 and 15 MV.

The ways in which X-rays can be used are as follows :

1. As the treatment of choice in a few conditions, such as rodent ulcer of the face, for which cure with minimum scarring can usually be expected.

2. In conjunction with surgery, in order to cover the lymphatic field, or deal with any outlying malignant cells that may have been left after operation. About 80% of patients with carcinoma of breast suitable for this treatment will be alive and well five years later.

3. As treatment for diseases of the reticulo-endothelial system such as lymphadenoma or reticulo-sarcoma. A cure is not obtained, but comfort during the remainder of life is much increased.

4. As a palliative treatment for recurrences, or growths too advanced for surgical treatment.

Not all growths are suitable for such treatment ; some are not radio-sensitive, and some are situated in organs which cannot be irradiated, e.g. the liver, of which the large and rapidly dividing cells are as easily destroyed as the tumour.

Nurses who work with patients undergoing such treatment have two main problems. One is the pessimism they sometimes feel over the prognosis when they only see patients being treated in wards. These are the ones who are too ill to come up from their homes, and were the nurse able to see the many who come up as out-patients for their treatment without undue discomfort, she would be much cheered. The other problem is the amount of information that ought to be given about their condition to those with malignant conditions. It is especially the young nurse on whom this presses heavily ; as she gains experience of people and life, some of the difficulties disappear. Of course it is necessary to adopt the policy of the surgeon or physician in charge; some feel that all patients should be told the nature of their complaint, others would only give such a diagnosis in exceptional circumstances. Probably no hard and fast rule can be made that applies to everyone. Many patients with conditions that they feel to be malignant never ask to have their fears confirmed ; they do not want to face the emotional implications of such a diagnosis and it seems unkind to force it on them. Neither should it be presumed that all who ask really want to know the truth, and experience soon enables the surgeon to detect those who are only asking for reassurance, and it is usually possible to give them comfort without resorting to untruth. Whatever policy is adopted towards the patient, at least one responsible relative should be aware of the true situation.

Depression among patients is less than might be expected, and can justly be ascribed in many cases to the physical effects of treatment, and the courage and fellow-sympathy they display is remarkable. The physical problems that may arise during treatment are principally these :

1. *Nutrition.* People with advanced malignant disease, especially if there is an ulcerated area that is infected, are anæmic, toxic and undernourished. Appetite may be poor, swallowing may be difficult in certain conditions, diarrhœa may cause fluid loss. It is essential to measure the fluid intake and to ensure a sufficient calorie allowance. Protein is especially valuable because tissue breakdown occurs during treatment, and if appetite is lacking, milk, eggs and casilan should be given.

2. *Nausea.* Radiation sickness is often a problem, and increases the difficulty of maintaining nutrition. On return from the department patients should rest in bed if they are prone to nausea, and meal times may be adjusted. Sedatives such as dramamine, avomine or chlorpromazine may be effective, while vitamin B6 (pyridoxine) is said to have a specific action.

3. *Skin Reactions.* The skin reactions produced by megavoltage (e.g. cobalt) therapy are minimal, but with orthovoltage (deep X-ray) they still occur. The principles of the care of the skin in such cases are to avoid injury, irritation and infection. Soap is forbidden, and friction of any kind is harmful. Nightclothes should be of soft material, and if the beard area is being treated, shaving must be abandoned, though clippers can be used occasionally to improve the appearance. If a perineal pad has to be worn during pelvic irradiation, it is kept in place with a soft bandage. Zinc oxide or Elastoplast strapping on the treatment area is especially harmful.

Reddening of the skin is universal, and in the later stages of treatment dry branny peeling is usual. Moist desquamation is sometimes seen, and is very painful ; the radiotherapist will prescribe treatment, and nothing should be applied without his approval. Ointments containing metal (such as zinc cream) increase skin damage by becoming secondarily irradiated and must never be used while treatment is in progress. Cleanliness can be achieved by gentle cleaning with surgical spirit and applying a starch dusting powder, but care should be exercised in retaining the markings on the skin which the radiotherapist has painted to guide him in his treatment. Ulceration or X-ray burns should not be experienced with modern control of dosage.

4. *Dryness of Mucous Membranes.* If the mouth and neck are being treated, soreness and dryness of the mouth is painful and inter-

feres with swallowing. A little liquid paraffin or butter held in the mouth may be useful, and every effort is made to maintain a good fluid intake, or thickening of the saliva will be caused by dehydration. Aspirin mucilage or benzocaine emulsion before meals may help to make drinking possible. If enough fluid intake cannot be taken by mouth, rectal infusion at night is valuable.

5. *Blood Changes.* Anæmia and leucopenia results from depression of blood formation by the bone marrow, and regular blood counts are made to ensure that this effect does not become dangerous.

6. *Metastases.* Secondary growths may manifest themselves in other parts of the body, especially in the brain, lungs and bones if spread is by the bloodstream. Complaints of cough, breathlessness, blood-stained sputum, pain in the limbs or headache should be reported.

7. *Obstruction of the Airway or Œsophagus.* Treatment of the throat causes œdema, and this may be sufficient to prevent swallowing or to make breathing difficult. A tracheotomy will have to be performed if the airway is much impeded, and the surgeon may feel that feeding by gastrostomy should be undertaken if swallowing is impossible.

The troubles experienced by patients having deep X-ray treatment are many, but all can be lessened by careful management and sympathetic thought for detail. The problems are of the kind that nurses learn to solve so successfully by considering all the causes of discomfort and striving to alleviate each of them.

Radium

The discovery of radium by Mme. Curie is one of the romances of science known to everyone. The tendency today is to use radium rather less frequently than formerly ; it is very expensive, and though its effectiveness for practical purposes does not diminish with age, substances like radio-active cobalt, whose activity decreases markedly in a few years, are replacing it to a certain extent. It is used in these ways :

1. Interstitial; needles may be platinum, containing 0·5 mg. of Radium upwards, and can be introduced directly into and round the growth.

2. Intra-cavity; in special containers, the most common indication for which is in the treatment of cancer of the cervix and body of the uterus (p. 293).

3. From the surface; (*a*) needles may be incorporated in applicators of orthopædic felt, dental wax or Perspex; (*b*) a beam can also be directed from a large amount of Radium (10 G.) or Cobalt 60 up to 2,000 curies in the same way and under the same conditions as X-ray treatment is given. (Telecurie Therapy).

Radium Precautions

Applicators are loaded and needles assembled by the radiographer from behind a two-inch screen of lead, and the table on which the work is done has a lead top. Long-handled forceps are used, and the radium never touched by hand. It is carried in lead containers with a long handle, and must be signed for by the head of the theatre or ward that receives it. If the radium is to be taken out in the ward, or if interstitial needles are used which may become loose, a lead box is provided to receive it.

If applicators are being used, they are put on by senior staff in rotation, and while it is perfectly safe to perform all normal nursing duties for patients wearing one, long periods should not be spent at the bedside for social purposes. Once the treatment is finished, the radium curator signs for the radium and takes it away in its lead box. The precautions taken against loss depend on the site, and as an example of the nursing problems that may arise, a description is given of the treatment of carcinoma of tongue by radium needles.

Radium Treatment of Carcinoma of Tongue

Hemi-glossectomy was once the standard treatment for cancer of tongue, and at present there is a tendency to revive the operation again, but many cases are still treated by radium needles. The radiotherapist calculates the dose needed and works out a pattern of needle insertion for the surgeon and indicates the time for which they should be worn.

The mouth must be as free from sepsis as possible; all decayed teeth are removed, and treatment given to clean the mouth. The patient must understand that while the needles are in place he will be unable to speak and that some swelling is to be expected, but that this is part of the reaction which will cure his ulcer. When the needles are inserted, they are threaded with a double loop, on which there is a knot or a bead to facilitate counting, and these threads are brought out of the angle of the mouth and fastened together. Zinc oxide strapping must on no account be used on the cheek or a burn will result.

The bed may be in a sideroom if that is possible, or if in a ward must not be close to the others. Beside the bed is placed a feeder of water with polythene tubing on the spout, a pad and pencil, a bell, and apparatus for mouth treatment. This may consist of a reservoir and tubing and kidney dish for irrigating the mouth, or a mouth tray with a dental syringe. The nursing staff are instructed in the precautions to be adopted which are these :

The mouth is inspected to see that all needles are in position every time the mouth is treated, and at change of duty for every shift. If a needle has come out and is lying in the mouth the nurse fetches the lead box, Spencer Wells forceps, a pair of scissors and a kidney dish of water. She picks up the needle with forceps, cuts the thread and releases it, rinses the needle and puts it in the box, which is closed. The time of removal is noted, as this influences the dose.

The number of needles is checked and recorded by the senior nurse in each shift before she goes off duty, and mouth wash should not be thrown away without permission from a senior nurse who has inspected it. A bin may be kept for laundry, and one for the room sweepings, and these are not emptied until the radium has been safely returned. If there is at any time a discrepancy in the needle count, the radium curator is at once informed. A signal is often put on the end of the bed to indicate that radium is in use.

The patient must be able to summon help with a bell or signal light if he needs it, and must be given paper and pencil to write to the nursing staff. Pain and discomfort must be relieved by suitable analgesics, and there will be two serious nursing problems. One is nutrition ; solid food cannot be taken, and even swallowing of fluids is difficult once the tongue is swollen. Milk and beaten eggs are given, but the principal need is for fluid, and if enough cannot be taken by mouth, the rectal route can be used, or intravenous dextrose saline administered.

The other problem is the care of the mouth. It cannot be closed because of the swelling, and the surface of the tongue will become coated with thick offensive saliva unless adequate measures are taken. Rubbing with swabs may dislodge the needles, and the most effective measures are irrigation with a catheter from a reservoir of glyco-thymoline, or syringing with a dental spray.

The needles commonly remain in place for about a week, and are then removed under anæsthesia. Cleaning of the tongue can now proceed unhindered, and glycerine will be found the most effective agent. Swelling diminishes rapidly, and the patient is given soft high-calorie foods to make up for the period of deprivation. The courage and cheerfulness displayed by the old gentlemen who are usually the victims are remarkable in face of this very trying treatment.

In 1913 it was discovered that some substances can exist in two or three forms with different atomic weights. These different forms are known as *Isotopes*. Many elements have naturally occurring isotopes, and in addition, many artificial isotopes can be made, most of them unstable and therefore radio-active. Many uses exist in industry and in medicine, both in research and in treatment.

Radio-active Isotopes

These substances can be used either in diagnosis or in treatment. The doses used in the former are much lower than the latter, but precautions must be taken in disposing of the excreta of such patients, in order to avoid contaminating the area with radioactive material that will interfere with other tests. The amounts used in treatment are large, and may constitute a radiation hazard to staff unless they follow the instructions given by the isotope department.

Diagnosis

Radioactive iodine is used in the diagnosis of thyrotoxicosis. I^{131} is given intravenously and I^{132} by mouth. I^{132} loses half its radioactivity (i.e. has a *half-life*) of two hours, and is therefore suitable for women in the childbearing age, and children. Careful preparation is essential for good results. Antithyroid drugs must not have been given for two months, nor Lugol's iodine for two weeks. No radio-opaque X-rays, which may involve use of iodine, are given, and for three days beforehand the patient must have no diuretics, and no fish to eat. All oral doses must be given on an empty stomach. The urine is collected for 48 hours into two Winchester jars. Gloves are worn, and a funnel is used to prevent spilling. Lost specimens and spills must be reported, or the result of the test will be misleading.

Cobalt^{58} is used for labelling vitamin B12 (cyanocobalamine), and is given by mouth in investigating pernicious anæmia. A 24 hour urine specimen is saved, and the stools are saved for a week. Vomitus must also be saved, if the patient is sick after taking the dose. Several other substances are helpful in investigating the physiology and pathology of the circulation, for instance $Iron^{59}$, and $Chromium^{51}$, which is used to determine the red cell volume.

$Crypton^{85}$ is an inert gas which can be used during cardiac catheterization (p. 129) to diagnose congenital heart abnormalities, especially abnormal communications between the right and left sides of the heart.

Radioactive isotopes are increasingly used to scan various organs for changes in function, or for the presence of tumours and other lesions. The patient receives a dose of an isotope which the organ under examination will retain, and after the appropriate interval he is placed under the scanner, which travels to and fro over the part to be examined, recording the radiation emitted as a series of dots. The pattern thus formed will be denser in abnormal tissues than in normal, while non-functioning areas remain blank.

The brain, kidney, liver, lung, thyroid and pancreas may be scanned for abnormalities. Technetium ($TC99^{m}$) is often used, especially for brain scans, because its radioactivity is comparatively short lived, being negligible after 48 hours. Preparation is minimal; a dose of potassium perchlorate is often ordered to inhibit thyroid activity, and restless patients undergoing brain scan require a sedative to enable them to lie still. The examination is quite painless.

Treatment

Since the thyroid gland does not distinguish between the isotopes of iodine, it will take up I^{131} if this is provided. Patients with thyrotoxicosis can thus be induced to fill the gland with radio-active material which depresses thyroid function. It is normally only used for middle-aged or elderly patients, in case malignant changes are induced later. It is given by mouth, and excess will be excreted in the urine, which is collected in Winchesters for the next 48 hours. If a big dose has been given, the technicians will provide a lead screen for the jars. Gloves are worn, and spills avoided or reported.

It was hoped when I^{131} was first used that cancers of the thyroid would take up I^{131} and stock themselves with material that would destroy them. Unfortunately, few such cancers store iodine, but if a therapeutic dose has been given, the patient should be kept in a single room for 48 hours, and staff should not spend undue periods in close proximity (e.g. not more than two hours at a distance of 1 metre). The urine is collected and kept behind a lead screen until the Isotope Department directs otherwise.

$Phosphorus^{32}$ is most effective in polycythæmia rubra, a condition in which the red cells are present in excess. Phosphorus is taken up by the bones, inside which the red cells are made in the marrow. No special hazard exists, but the urine is collected with the usual precautions for 48 hours.

PHYSIOTHERAPY

Physiotherapy means treatment by physical means ; these measures are used to relieve pain and to restore or improve function. They are especially directed at the nervous and muscular systems of the body, and to its joints. The techniques by which these treatments are given require very specialized knowledge, but the nurse will want to know something of them when she sees them ordered for so many different types of patient in and outside hospital.

Remedial exercises. These form the major part of treatment used. Exercise is the only way to retrain muscle endurance or to increase the strength of muscles, and exercises have to be specially devised for their purpose. A detailed knowledge of anatomy and physiology and of the patient's condition is needed by the physiotherapist, however simple these exercises may seem to the onlooker.

Resisted exercises are used to build up muscle power, and as this power grows the resistance can be increased. The resistance can be manual, for greatest accuracy, and weights or springs can also be used. For instance, the patient who has had a knee operation may practise straightening the knee and lifting a weight attached to the foot. These kind of exercises must be carefully supervised.

Gait training is re-education in walking, and is an important part of treatment following fracture, dislocation, amputation of a leg, or spinal injury. People with disseminated sclerosis and other nervous diseases benefit from gait training. A patient who has had a stroke may be permanently bed-ridden if he is not given correct re-education. The same is true of children with cerebral palsy. Paraplegics must be taught to walk by swinging their paralysed legs along with trunk and arm muscles.

Free exercises are mainly used in the stage of recovery, when there is a fair range of movement which needs enlarging. Such exercises can be given individually or to groups. Some people benefit from group activity and are encouraged to greater efforts. Leg, trunk and breathing exercises may be done in unison by patients in a surgical ward. Antenatal classes are given to pregnant women to train them for labour.

Breathing exercises are an essential part of the treatment of asthma, chronic bronchitis and emphysema, and of the rehabilitation of the patient who has had a chest operation. These exercises retrain the diaphragm, re-establish the rhythm of respiration and permit relaxation and control. Postural drainage is the accurate positioning of a patient to help get rid of sputum ; it is always combined with breathing exercises and chest " clapping " or percussion.

Manipulation and traction, or stretching, is usually applied to the cervical or lumbar spine to relieve pain in nerve roots. It is not used if active or severe disease is present.

Heat

Before heat is used in treatment, the skin sensation in the appropriate area should be tested, or injury may result. Infra-red irradiation (radiant heat) is produced by a lamp, and the rays cause superficial heating. It is used to ease pain, relieve muscle spasm, and to help the healing and drying of wounds.

Short-wave diathermy produces deep warmth in all the tissues of the field exposed to treatment. It is ordered for joint conditions, deep muscle injuries, extensive pressure sores, and chronic salpingitis, among other disorders. There must be no metal (e.g. safety pins) in the area, or the skin may be burned, and for the same reason any dressing must be a fresh dry one.

Wax baths are given by immersing the hand or foot in paraffin wax, kept in liquid at a temperature of 120–130° F. Usually the limb is dipped ten to twelve times in the wax until a thick coat is formed. It is then wrapped in a plastic sheet and blanket to retain heat, and kept covered for about twenty minutes. The wax is then peeled off and exercises are given immediately.

Ultrasonics are sound waves which, as their name implies, are beyond the audible range. They cause warmth, and also appear to produce other changes in the tissues. The treatment is applied directly to the lubricated skin with an applicator, or is given through lukewarm water in a bath, the applicator being moved constantly during treatment to prevent concentration of the ultrasonic beam, which might damage the tissues. It is used to promote absorption of exudate in œdema, or of blood from a hæmatoma. Recent muscle and tendon injuries, tenosynovitis, gravitational ulcers and other similar conditions of the soft tissues may also benefit from it. Skin sensation must be normal before this treatment is ordered.

Stimulating Currents. Muscle can be made to contract by passing a suitable current through it. If its nerve supply is normal, a muscle is stimulated by a surging *Faradic* or *Sinusoidal* current, which causes sustained contraction. Muscle whose nerve supply has been interrupted can be stimulated by a series of single shocks from a modified direct current.

Faradism is used to restore normal control to a muscle when following injury or operation the patient has lost the ability to feel a muscle, and so cannot use it. It is most commonly used for the quadriceps extensor group on the front of the thigh after knee operations, or in foot strain for the small muscles of the foot. Individual muscles or groups can be stimulated accurately by Faradism.

Sinusoidal current is used for large muscle groups to cause a widespread increase in circulation. If given under pressure bandages it will cause absorption of exudate. An important use is in the retraining of the sphincter muscles of incontinent patients.

Radio-active Gold. Colloidal gold in saline is injected into the pleural or peritoneal cavities to control malignant effusions, and if no large malignant masses are present may be successful in limiting the effusion. The cavity should be tapped beforehand, and after the injection the patient should be turned from side to side every thirty minutes for six hours to ensure as even dispersal as possible.

Following successful therapy, the rate at which effusion accumulates is much reduced and the need for frequent tapping eliminated. The gold remains within the serous cavity, so precautions about the urine are unnecessary. For the first week while radio-activity is high, neither staff nor visitors should spend long periods close to the patient. The maximum permitted dose would be received by spending an hour a week within a yard of the bed. If tapping has to be performed within two weeks of injection, the fluid should be treated as radio-active and the isotope department consulted. Palliation can be hoped for, but not cure.

Ultra Violet Radiation. The source of such radiation is arc lamps, either of mercury vapour or phosphor. The rays are absorbed by the skin and have a local bactericidal effect, form Vitamin D and perhaps increase antibody formation. The nature of the tonic effect felt is not fully understood. General treatment is given to people with psoriasis and rickets, and local treatment is beneficial for acne, alopecia, and some other skin conditions.

Occupational Therapy

Muscles that need strengthening can be trained by the physiotherapist, but they can also be exercised in other ways, and it is these methods that are used by the occupational therapist. Basket making exercises the fingers, weaving at a loom uses the muscles of the shoulders and chest, and patients will pursue such occupations that produce a finished article for longer periods than they can practise an exercise without boredom.

The occupation selected must be one suited to the patient's needs and temperament, and for in-patients must be one that can show results before discharge, so that short-stay patients do not generally require this kind of therapy. Again, if the patient is confined to bed the occupation must be one that can easily be performed there, and does not need equipment too bulky to be conveniently stored at hand. Basketry is popular because it uses the fingers, is not difficult to do well, and can be completed in a short time. Rug making, marquetry and tapestry work are other examples.

Long-stay patients such as those in sanatoria and orthopædic hospitals benefit greatly from occupational therapy, which can help them to overcome boredom and even despair. The man who has fractured his spine finds that his hands and arms are still useful, and if he can learn something like typing which is relevant to earning a living, he may begin to foresee a future for himself once again.

Once patients can get up and go to the occupational therapy department, a bigger range of crafts is available and scope for using more muscles is possible. Feet and legs can be exercised as well as hands and arms with a lathe or a treadle fret-saw. Out-patients can attend for sessions, and a busy department is full of an atmosphere of activity and interest

For people in mental hospitals occupational therapy has a two-fold importance. The physical one is that health is increased by muscular activity, and that the depressed patient may be roused from his wretchedness to participate, while the excitable and aggressive one may work through his anger. Other methods than those of the conventional occupational therapy department may be found stimulating. Some have a " factory " in which piece-work for some industrial processes is done, and patients in mental hospitals which have tried it are eager to clock-in and begin work which seems to them like normal life. This indicates the second value of occupational therapy, its mental one, which is of the greatest importance to those who are disabled either mentally or physically.

In this connection, art therapy has been a very successful occupation in sanatoria and mental hospitals. Undiscovered talent may come to light, and a new world of experience may be opened to people. The psychotic patient may work out emotions that he finds impossible to express in words, and may also by his pictures or models indicate to the psychiatrist the course that the disease is taking.

The nurse has a contribution to make in this field. She should recognize the occupational therapist as a trained colleague who is not teaching handicrafts as a way of passing the time, but assisting in the return of the patient to full mental and physical wholeness. Nurses should not feel impatience if the bed and locker are not as tidy as usual while the patient is working, and above all must not make men feel that there is anything unusual or undignified in doing tapestry work or making mats.

CHAPTER 35

FIRST AID IN EMERGENCIES

THE accidents that occur daily in large numbers in any industrial civilization occasion death, disablement, painful illness and loss of working hours. In all countries deaths and injuries from road accidents increase yearly, factory hazards are many and accidents in the home to the young and the aged are very numerous. Many of these are preventible, and nurses in their capacity as citizens drive cars and manage homes, and may help to reduce the incidence of injuries. As industrial nurses and health visitors, they have a similar responsibility. In hospital, too, accidents may be prevented by fastening guard rails on cots, keeping disinfectants locked away, the use of care with corrosive fluids, close watch over disturbed patients, by refraining from putting cleaning liquids in cordial bottles for storage, and many other ways that will occur to students.

In factories, mines, and other places where injuries occur, teams of workers are trained in first aid of a kind suitable to their needs, and they possess equipment such as Thomas's splints which would not be available in other circumstances. This kind of knowledge is not what the nurse needs. First aid consists in applying that treatment which the patient should have received before being brought to hospital and without any equipment other than might be obtained in the home or street. Nurses tend to think of first aid in terms of blood transfusions, stomach washouts and Ryle's tubes, but such help is not the kind which, as a member of the public, she may be able to supply in case of an emergency.

The principles of first aid here to be considered are :

1. To save life by removing danger—extinguishing fire, removing the patient from water or electric wires. All of us hope that if faced with such an event we would display courage and the necessary knowledge.

2. To treat urgent symptoms. The two foremost are cessation of breathing and severe bleeding, since if either of these continues for any time death will result. These are the emergencies with which every nurse should feel competent to deal, since although such knowledge will never be frequently used, it is vital to be proficient on the occasion when the need arises.

3. To prevent extension of injuries. Fractures must be temporarily splinted or a simple one may be converted into an open one ; burns must be covered to prevent infection. Whatever is done should not prejudice professional treatment later.

4. To avoid doing harm by undertaking treatment beyond one's scope. For instance, a foreign body embedded in the cornea cannot be removed without anæsthetic drops and an instrument, and efforts to do so may make the damage worse. Nurses are usually diffident about exceeding their capabilities because they are too well aware of the dangers involved, but someone armoured with a little knowledge is

liable to rush in where the professional would fear to tread. It is worth mentioning that death should not be presumed without medical opinion, and restorative measures should be continued until they are pronounced useless.

5. To use intelligence in the application of the rules of first aid. Such maxims as " send for medical aid " stand at the head of many

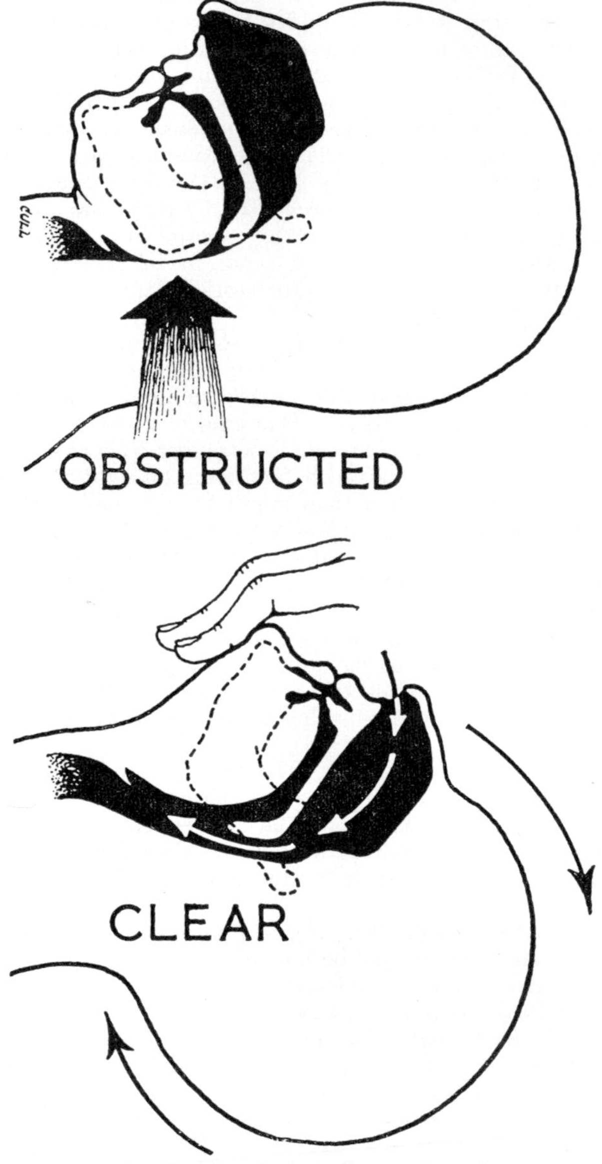

Fig. 160. Raising the jaw allows a clear airway.

lists, but it is often more appropriate to get the police and an ambulance so that the patient can be transferred to hospital without delay. Those with trivial injuries can appropriately be sent to the doctor or hospital, but the first-aider should never recommend the patient *not* to visit the doctor. Her diagnosis that the injury is insignificant may not be correct.

Respiration will be inhibited if the airway is obstructed. This obstruction may be external, as in suicidal attempts by hanging, but

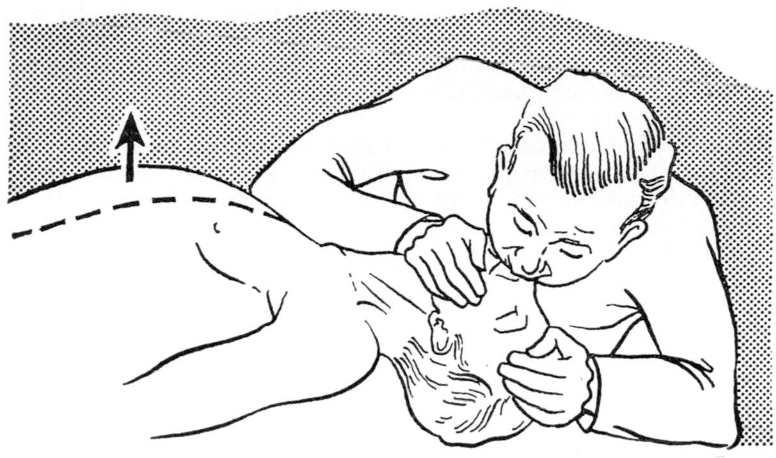

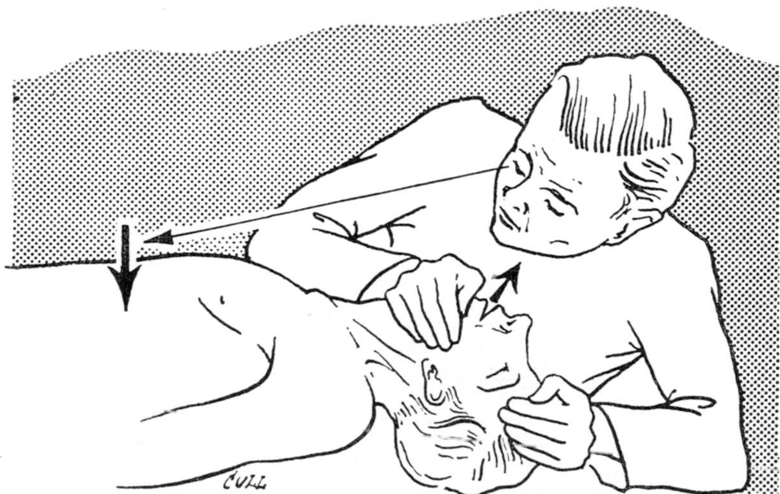

Fig. 161. Mouth to nose respiration. The chest should inflate as the rescuer blows into the airway, and fall when he withdraws his mouth.

usually it is internal, and is caused by the tongue blocking the larynx, or by blood, vomit or mucus. Such a block is especially common after road accidents, and unless speedy action is taken, the victim will die.

An external obstruction must be removed ; internal blocking of the airway is cleared :

(*a*) By supporting the jaw and extending the head and neck so that obstruction by the tongue is prevented.

(*b*) The jaw is opened, and blood or secretion cleared with a handkerchief or swab.

Breathing will often begin again after this, and the patient should be turned into the semi-prone position, so that neither tongue nor secretions can cause further obstruction. This is especially important if the jaw is broken, since this will deprive the tongue of its main support.

If the patient does not start to breathe again, artificial respiration is begun. The method most favoured now is expired air ventilation (" mouth-to-mouth," " mouth-to-nose," or in popular terms the " kiss of life " method). Expired air contains 16% of oxygen, which is enough to oxygenate blood in an emergency, and the rescuer inflates the patient's lungs by blowing air into them through the nose or mouth, following which they deflate by elastic recoil.

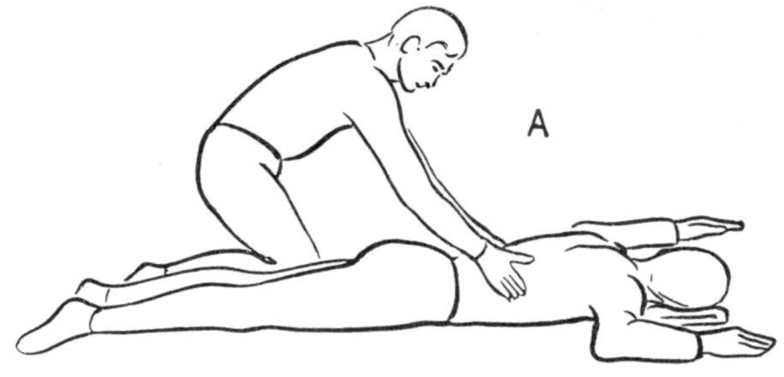

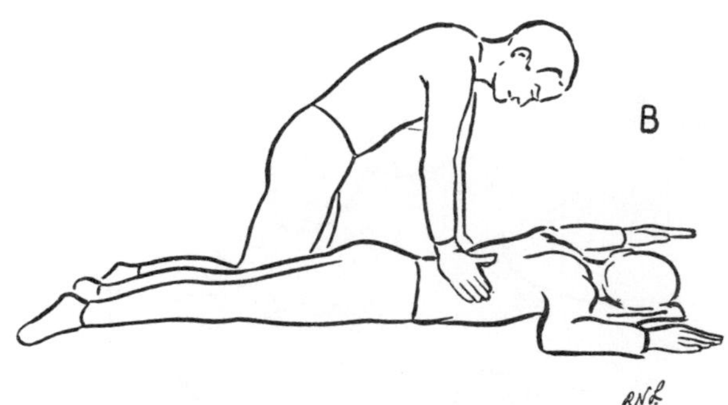

Fig. 162. **Schafer's method of artificial respiration.**
A. Inspiration. B. Expiration.

The airway should be cleared if obstructed, and the patient placed on his back. The head is well extended on the neck and the jaw supported. Air may be blown into mouth or nose, but the nose is preferable if it is uninjured. The rescuer closes the patient's mouth with the hand that supports the jaw, spreads the lips to cover the patient's nostrils, and blows firmly into them. If he is operating effectively, the chest will expand and the rescuer should remove his mouth and allow the chest to recoil. Too-forceful blowing will open the œsophagus and cause regurgitation of stomach contents. The rate should be twelve to fifteen times per minute.

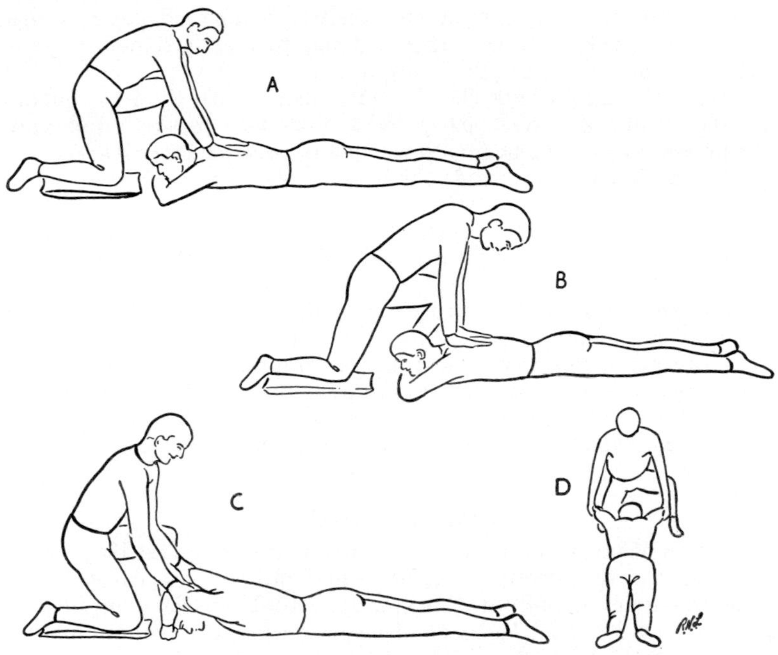

Fig. 163. Holger Nielsen method of artificial respiration.
A. Preparatory position. B. Expiration.
C. and D. Inspiration.

If there are facial injuries, this method may not be applicable, and in such a case, the next method may be used. It can be employed by a rescuer single-handed, and without extreme effort.

Schafer's Method. The patient lies prone, with the head turned to one side, and the shoulders abducted to a right angle and the forearms above the head. The airway must be clear. The operator kneels at one side with the knees at the level of the patient's hips, and puts the hands over the small of the back with the thumbs parallel to the spine and close together. The movements are :

(*a*) Swing forward with the elbows straight so that pressure is made over the abdomen and the diaphragm is thrust up to empty the chest. Count two seconds.

(*b*) Without moving the hands, relax the pressure and swing back until sitting on the heels. Count three before recommencing. The cycle is repeated twelve times a minute.

The advantages of this long-established method are that the prone position allows a clear airway, so that a single worker can operate, and that it can be continued without undue fatigue. Care has to be taken not to exert too heavy pressure on a small patient, and if abdominal injuries are present it is not suitable.

Holger Nielsen Method. The casualty lies prone, with his forehead supported on his flexed forearms, and the operator takes up a position on one knee at his head. The foot is level with the patient's shoulder and the knee behind and slightly to one side of the head. Change from one knee to the other will help to avert fatigue.

The movements are :

1. Place the hands over the shoulder blades with thumbs touching and fingers spread. With extended elbows lean forward and apply light pressure to the chest for 2½ seconds to produce expiration.

2. Release the pressure, slide the hands up the arms to just above the elbow.

3. Lean backwards with straight arms until the arms and shoulders are raised, but the chest is not lifted off the ground ; count 3 for 2½ seconds.

4. Lay the arms down, return your hands to the shoulder blades and prepare to recommence.

The process is repeated nine times a minute, and good movement of the chest is produced ; the advantage of a positive manœuvre to cause inspiration is obvious. It can be used if the chest is injured by omitting the expiratory pressure, and is, perhaps, the best all-round method.

Cardiac Arrest

Cessation of breathing may be accompanied or followed by stopping of the heart ; the colour becomes livid blue, and the carotid pulse beside the inner border of the sternomastoid muscle alongside the larynx cannot be felt. In cases of electrocution, drowning, and such medical causes of sudden death as coronary thrombosis it may be possible by external cardiac compression to maintain a flow of oxygenated blood to the brain until the heart begins beating once more.

Massage must be started within four minutes of the heart stopping if normal brain function is to survive. The principle is to compress the heart between the sternum and the spinal column, so that blood is forced out through the valves into the arteries. It is only a means of keeping up the circulation and must usually be continued until the patient reaches hospital.

The patient should be placed flat on his back on a firm surface, such as the floor. The palm of one hand is placed on the lower third of the sternum, and the other placed on top of it. Firm sharp pressure is applied, enough to depress the sternum 1 inch or 1½ inches, 50 to 60 times a minute. It is important that pressure is applied only to the sternum, or injury to the liver or the ribs will result. It is quite hard physical work, especially if the operator must also perform artificial

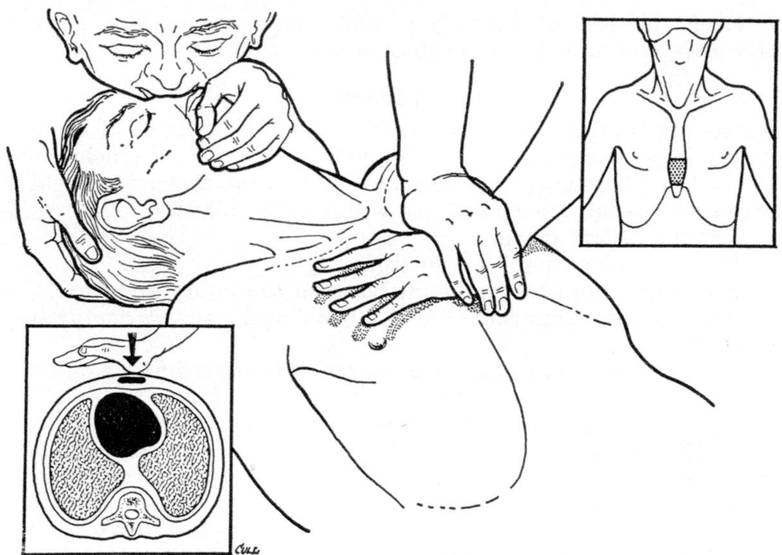

FIG. 164. External cardiac massage. The large figure shows the way the hands are applied ; the smaller ones show the part of the sternum which is compressed, and the way in which this can stimulate the heart.

respiration himself. If there are other helpers, an ambulance must be summoned, and the patient's legs raised to help the return of blood to the heart.

Hæmorrhage

The kind of bleeding for which first aid is required is usually primary, and may come from an artery, a vein or capillaries. The latter is rarely dangerous unless a large area is involved in injury, but is sufficient to alarm and dismay both patient and bystanders. Arterial or venous hæmorrhage may well endanger life unless treated promptly and efficiently.

Capillary Bleeding

The patient should always be sat down in order to avoid fainting, and if the bleeding is from a limb it should be elevated. A dressing and bandage is usually sufficient to check bleeding, and if gauze is available, it is more suitable than old linen because its open structure encourages clotting. Cold water or hot water at 120° F. are efficient styptics, and if the wound is of the nature of a graze will remove dust and grit.

Venous Bleeding

The volume of blood welling from the wound shows that vessels larger than capillaries have been cut.

1. Lay the patient down.
2. Elevate the limb if this is the part involved ; this reduces the bleeding at once.
3. Apply a pad and firm bandage.

4. Keep the patient recumbent and under observation until a doctor arrives or transfer to hospital is arranged.

Arterial Bleeding

Nurses are familiar with this type on a small scale, as all of us have seen arterioles severed in the theatre spurting a jet of blood synchronous with the heart beat until they are secured, and can understand that if a large artery is cut, life may be lost within a few minutes.

1. Lay the patient down.
2. If a limb is bleeding it is elevated.
3. Apply pressure over the point between the injury and the heart where the artery concerned crosses bone and can be compressed against it.
4. If an assistant is available a large pad is bandaged firmly over the wound.
5. Get the patient to hospital as soon as possible.
6. The tourniquet, as a means of checking hæmorrhage, has fallen into disfavour because, unless it is put on tightly enough, it constricts thin-walled veins before the arteries and increases the blood loss, while if it is applied too tightly, it will damage the nerves and remove the skin. Even if it is efficiently applied, there is a danger that it may not be removed in time and that gangrene of a limb may result. Tourniquets are especially dangerous on the upper arm, where the nerves are less protected by muscle than in the leg. However, there are exceptions to all rules, and if it is necessary to apply one a scarf or large handkerchief is folded and passed round the limb, a pencil or stick is knotted into it and rotated to increase the pressure until bleeding just stops. It must be loosened every fifteen minutes, and if bleeding does not recommence, should not be tightened again. If one has been applied, a label should be pinned on the coat giving the position of the tourniquet and the time for which it has been applied. The most dangerous time to put on a tourniquet is when many casualties are being treated, as in a railway accident, when its presence may escape notice until irreparable harm to the limb has been done.

Arterial Pressure Points

The points at which arteries can be compressed against bone in order to interrupt their blood flow are these :

1. *Common Carotid.* The artery runs alongside the trachea, and can be compressed against the transverse processes of the cervical vertebræ at the level of the lower border of the larynx.
2. *Subclavian.* This artery is pressed against the first rib from the hollow above the clavicle, with the patient's head flexed to the affected side. It is not easy to do, and is painful.
3. *Brachial.* Pressure is made beside the inner margin of the biceps muscle (at about its middle) against the humerus. It is easy to practise compressing this artery and to check effectiveness by feeling the radial pulse.
4. *Radial and Ulnar.* Press them against the radius and ulna at their lower end just proximal to the wrist joint.
5. *Facial.* The facial artery crosses the mandible an inch in front

of the angle of the jaw. Communication between the facial and temporal arteries is free, and compression of one artery alone may not be sufficient to stop bleeding.

6. *Temporal.* This artery can be felt pulsating as it crosses the zygomatic process of the temporal bone. Nurses frequently use this artery as a means of taking the pulse, and should be familiar with its position.

7. *Occipital.* The pressure point is four fingers' breadth behind and a little below the external auditory meatus.

8. *Femoral.* This great artery leaves the pelvis for the thigh in the middle of the groin where pressure can be made by both thumbs. Considerable pressure is needed, and is transmitted from the shoulders by keeping the arms straight. This is one of the points that every nurse should be able to locate without hesitation, since compression of it may possibly be required in hæmorrhage following leg amputation.

Hæmorrhage from Common Sites

Epistaxis or nose bleeding. Bleeding from the nose following a head injury may indicate fracture of the skull, and the need for medical care. Simple nose bleeding, such as is common in adolescents, is a capillary, and is treated as follows :

1. Sit the sufferer at a sink or with the head inclined over a basin.
2. Ask him to pinch the nose to compress the bleeding area.
3. Apply cold swabs to the nose.

The efficiency of the old country remedy of applying the front door key to the back of the neck indicates that bleeding usually ceases without rational treatment. If it does not, treatment may be needed in hospital, as described on p. 320. The patient must not be allowed to keep the head back and swallow the blood or vomiting will follow.

Bleeding Tooth Socket. (1) Give iced water mouth washes. (2) Fill the socket with an adequate plug and ask the patient to bite on it, or to keep a finger pressed on it if it is at the front of the mouth.

3. Ring the dentist, since this almost invariably follows dental extraction.

Hœmatemesis. Vomiting blood necessitates hospital treatment. While awaiting the ambulance, the patient is kept lying flat and under observation. Such symptoms as rising pulse rate, pallor, yawning and nausea show that bleeding is still continuing and more vomiting will occur. An accurate estimate of the amount of blood lost is a helpful observation.

Hœmoptysis. The patient who is coughing up blood should lie with the head and shoulders slightly raised and inclined towards the affected side if this is known. If it is caused by chest injuries, any wounds should be firmly covered to prevent air entering the pleural cavity. It is a condition that naturally alarms the patient, who needs reassurance while awaiting transport to hospital.

Bleeding from a Varicose Vein. Such bleeding may be very severe, and recently a tragic case was reported of death from a wound $\frac{1}{3}$ in. long in a varicose vein, which had been treated by applying a tourniquet.

1. Lay the patient flat, and elevate the limb as much as possible.

2. Apply a firm pad with pressure over the area. Blood flow in a varicose vein is usually reversed, i.e. towards the ankle, and simple elevation checks the hæmorrhage very markedly.

Foreign Bodies in Wounds. If large foreign bodies are present in wounds, caution should be exercised in removing them, and if bleeding is not great they should be left for attention in hospital. In superficial injuries fragments of glass or gravel may be taken out, and pressure must not, in any case, be made over a wound with foreign bodies in it. If bleeding is considerable it is controlled by compressing the artery supplying the part against the nearest pressure point.

Poisoning

Poisoning may occur :

1. By accident. Children will eat any tablets which may be sugar coated, or drink from any bottles within their reach, while adults occasionally drink from bottles of medicine without looking at the label. Children especially require protection against these accidents, and the medicine cupboard should be out of their reach. Tablets which adults consider harmless (such as iron) can cause death to children if taken in quantity.

2. In suicide attempts. Barbiturates are the commonest drugs taken, and aspirin is next. Gas poisoning is also not infrequent.

3. In murder cases.

If a poison has been taken by mouth, the symptoms will depend on the variety of substance swallowed, and these may be classified as follows :

1. *Corrosives.* The lips and mouth are swollen and burnt and there may be a characteristic odour on the breath. Such cases are not often seen in England today, except as the result of accidents.

2. *Irritants,* such as arsenic or mercury. Colic and vomiting are characteristic.

3. *Narcotics.* Barbiturate poisoning is a very common example.

4. *Deliriants,* e.g. atropine. The berries of the deadly nightshade (atropa belladonna) are very attractive to children, and in places where this plant grows, occasional cases of poisoning occur in late summer. Widely dilated pupils and delirium are diagnostic.

5. *Convulsants,* e.g. strychnine.

Treatment. Removal to hospital is urgent, and any tablets or bottles that may contain the poison should be sent along as a help in diagnosis. If the poison is corrosive, vomiting will cause further harm to the stomach and œsophagus and must not be induced. Milk is soothing and harmless and may be given to dilute the poison, while if its reaction is known, an effort may be made to neutralize it by giving dilute vinegar or lemon juice for corrosive alkali poisoning, or chalk or milk of magnesia for acids. In all other cases, vomiting should be induced. Putting the fingers down the throat is usually effective, and if the first-aider is doing this herself, she should first hold the jaw with one hand and with the thumb push the patient's cheek between his teeth to prevent the operative hand being bitten. The emetic that is most readily available is two tablespoons of salt in a tumbler of water. Specimens of vomit should be saved.

Poison	Common Source	First-aid Treatment
Arsenic.	Old-type weed killers, rat poisons, sheep dip.	Induce vomiting.
Aspirin.	Household medicine cupboards.	Induce vomiting. Give dilute soda bicarbonate.
Atropine.	Deadly nightshade berries, eye drops.	Induce vomiting. Give black coffee.
Barbiturates.	Sleeping tablets.	Induce vomiting. Give black coffee.
Corrosive acids.	Industries, garages.	Do not induce vomiting. Give plenty of water if possible with magnesium oxide, chalk or milk of magnesia added.
Corrosive alkalis.	Industries.	Do not induce vomiting. Give plenty of water, if possible with vinegar or lemon juice added.
Ferrous sulphate.	Anæmia tablets.	Induce vomiting. Give soda bicarbonate.
Mercury.	Corrosive sublimate.	Give white of egg in water to precipitate mercury, then induce vomiting.
Phenol, lysol.	Disinfectants.	Do not induce vomiting. Give plenty of water, and a teacup of liquid paraffin.

Coal Gas Poisoning

This occurs accidentally as the result of faulty fittings, or turning on the gas and forgetting to light it, and in an attempt at suicide. If a casualty has to be rescued from a gas-filled room, a few deep breaths should be taken before entering and opening or breaking a window and dragging the victim out. Artificial respiration is begun at once, and continued on the way to hospital.

Other Forms of Asphyxia

Carbon monoxide poisoning from exhaust fumes may occur in closed garages, in mines and in ill-ventilated rooms from stove fumes. The treatment is the same as for coal gas poisoning.

Hanging causes death by suffocation, and anyone finding a person hanging should support his weight and shout for help to assist in cutting him down. Artificial respiration must be tried.

Choking on a foreign body, such as a sweet, coin, or button, is not uncommon in children. Small ones can be picked up and turned upside down ; larger ones must be made to bend down and be struck smartly between the shoulders. If this fails, inducement of vomiting by stimulating the back of the throat usually dislodges it.

Drowning

Immersion results in the air passages filling with water and cessation of breathing, and as soon as the patient has been rescued he should be laid prone. The first-aider stands astride his hips and raises the pelvis to allow the water to drain out, or if the patient is a child, inverts it to empty the air passages. If the ground is sloping, the patient should be laid with the head down the slope so that any more water expressed by artificial respiration can run out. Artificial respiration is begun without loss of time and is continued until breathing starts again or a doctor says that it is useless. The time for which one should go on in the absence of expert advice depends on the length of time of immersion, the colour and similar factors. Recovery has been recorded after long periods of apnœa, and efforts should not be abandoned for an hour or even two.

If there is additional help, the wet clothes can be gradually removed and dry coverings substituted, and when breathing starts again, the patient should be kept flat until transport to hospital has been arranged.

Fractures

A break in a leg bone may cause the loss of a pint of blood into the hæmatoma around the fracture, so that shock is always considerable. It will be increased by movement and the attendant pain, so such fractures should be temporarily immobilized before the patient is moved. Treatment may be summarized as :

1. Do not move the patient until inspection shows that there are no major fractures.
2. Immobilize fractures of large bones on the spot.
3. Keep flat and warmly covered.
4. Arrange ambulance transport.

Clothing should not be removed from the broken limb unless bleeding shows that there is a wound that should be covered with the cleanest dressing available.

In works where first-aid teams operate, Thomas's splint is used in the immediate treatment of fracture of the femur, and is a safe and comfortable appliance. It is not, however, likely to be available in most accidents, and broomsticks, hazel rods, or other improvised material will have to be used on both sides of the injured leg, reaching, if possible, from the hip to below the foot. Splints for shorter bones are easier to find, and slings for the arm can be devised from scarves or any lengths of material.

Elderly people sustain a fracture of the neck of the femur with so little violence that bystanders often fail to realize the extent of the injury, and try to help the victim to his feet. External rotation of the leg after a fall suggests that such a fracture has occurred, and that the patient should be carefully moved on to some firm support before being lifted.

Fracture of the spine carries the risk of injury to the cord or cauda equina, and it is often suggested that, if it is suspected, the patient should be placed in the prone position for transport. If he is already lying on his face this is the safest position, but if there are other fractures, turning is not advisable. He should be kept flat, and lifted on to an improvised stretcher as gently as possible, with a pad under the lumbar area to keep that part of the spine extended. The most dangerous manœuvre is to carry him by the shoulders and legs with the spine flexed.

Sprains and Strains

Injuries to the ligaments of the ankle and knee often occur in walking and climbing accidents, and the joint should be firmly bandaged or supported as soon as possible to keep down swelling. The boot should not be removed. When shelter is reached the leg should be elevated, and bandages may be kept wet with cold water. The doctor will decide whether an X-ray is necessary to exclude fracture.

Foreign Bodies

Children will readily insert small objects into the nose, and less commonly into the ear, but there seems no good reason why attempts should be made at first-aid extraction. Warnings are often given against syringing the ear if it contains a foreign body that might swell, but this could hardly be accounted a first-aid measure and nurses are unlikely to undertake it without medical advice. The patient should be taken to a doctor, and the relatives reassured.

Foreign bodies in the eye are usually lodged either in the lower fornix, or within the upper lid. The lower fornix should be inspected first, and the fragment removed with the corner of a handkerchief or a moist wisp of wool if seen. If it is adherent to the upper lid, drawing this lid down over the lower one may dislodge it, but if it does not, the upper lid may be everted as described on p. 337, and if the mote is there, it may usually be removed quite easily. If it is embedded, or if it is in the cornea, a good-sized pad and a bandage should be applied, and the patient taken to a doctor or to hospital.

Splashes of acid or alkali in the eye require prompt attention. The principle of first-aid treatment is to dilute the irritant as quickly as possible with large volumes of water. In the first-aid departments of factories where chemical processes take place, reservoirs of lotion are kept filled for such a purpose, but if an accident occurs elsewhere, a jug should be filled with water and poured over the eye and into both fornices. Undines or wet swabs are not appropriate, and no time should be wasted in searching for a substitute to neutralize a corrosive.

Electric Shock

All measures should be taken in the home to avoid the risk of electric shocks, which can produce severe burns or death. Electric appliances should always be earthed and in good repair ; re-wiring should be done by an expert ; portable electric fires must not be stood on the edge of the bath ; switches should not be touched with wet hands ; the back should not be taken off the television set without disconnecting the current ; if a fuse blows as soon as it has been replaced, the electrician should be called ; and above all, householders should know the position of the main switch that cuts off the current.

A severe electric shock may render the victim unable to let go of the object that has caused it, and the current must be switched off at once if this is feasible. If not, he must be dragged clear, and the rescuer must be insulated before attempting it. Thick rubber gloves are kept in electricity departments ; rubber soles to the shoes are a protection, or several thicknesses of material (such as a folded coat) can be used over the hands and the victim grasped by his clothes. Breathing is usually suspended, and artificial respiration must be begun at once.

Burns to the hands from live appliances are always worse than their first appearance suggests, and they should be covered with a clean, dry dressing and seen by a doctor even if apparently slight.

Burns

Burns are caused by electric currents, as discussed in the last paragraph, by heat, and by corrosive chemicals.

If someone's clothing is on fire, he should be tripped up if he is running, covered if possible with a rug to smother the flames, and rolled to extinguish them. If cold water is at hand, the burnt area should be soaked with it to remove heat still in the skin. No attempt should be made to remove burnt clothing.

Corrosive chemicals are washed off with copious amount of cold water. Acid burns should in theory be treated with dilute alkalis (e.g. sodium bicarbonate) and bases by dilute acid (e.g. vinegar), but on no account should the water treatment be delayed while an antidote is sought, and if there is any doubt in the first-aider's mind as to the substance to use, he should use water only.

Burnt areas should be covered with clean linen, e.g. laundered sheets, and no ointment or other dressing is used. The patient is kept lying flat until the ambulance arrives.

Superficial burns, such as sunburn, can be covered with powder or calamine lotion. Burns involving skin loss should always be seen by a doctor.

Fits

The commonest cause of a fit in an adult is epilepsy. Fits occur with little warning and in all circumstances, some of them dangerous to the patient, they follow a regular pattern.

1. *Aura.* The patient has a premonitory feeling specific for each individual, but not lasting long enough for him to remove himself from any danger. He often gives a cry, due to the onset of stage two.

2. *Tonic Phase.* All the muscles, including those of respiration, become rigidly contracted, so that breathing is suspended and the face darkens.

3. *Clonic Phase.* Alternate relaxation and contraction occurs, so that there is violent movement of the trunk, limbs and jaw. The contractions gradually become shorter and weaker until they cease, and the patient lies unconscious. The tongue is often bitten if it gets between the teeth and involuntary emptying of the bladder, and sometimes of the bowel, occurs. If left undisturbed the patient will sleep after the fit is over.

The nurse who sees an epileptic fit will not feel the alarm that the ordinary spectator feels. The most urgent first-aid is to see that no harm comes to the patient from his external surroundings, for many epileptics are burnt or sustain fractures because of a fit. It is usually felt that something must be inserted between the jaws to prevent biting of the tongue, and if a pad of material can be pushed between the teeth, this can be done, but attempts to lever open the jaws in the tonic stage will lead to breaking the teeth, and there is never time to wind something round the handle of a teaspoon, as writers often suggest. It is worse than useless to insert articles like pencils that will be bitten through.

Efforts to restrain the limbs during the clonic phase may produce fractures ; the most helpful thing is to ensure that there is no furniture or similar objects near, against which he can injure himself. When the fit is over, an improvised pillow should be placed under the head and the collar loosened, the face is dried and the mouth mopped out. If the fit happens in some public place, an ambulance will take the patient to hospital, but this is not necessary if it is in his home and his history is well known. It is advisable, however, that he see his doctor in case his dose of sedative should be adjusted.

Unconsciousness

The circumstances in which one finds an unconscious person—a road accident, a gas-filled room—may at once indicate the cause of the coma. In others, however, the nurse who is called on to render first aid must rely on the evidence of her senses and her professional knowledge to supply a provisional basis on which to give assistance. The points to which she will give attention are these :

1. *Signs of injury*—wounds, especially of the head ; hæmorrhage ; blood or cerebro-spinal fluid coming from the nose or ears.
2. *Pulse*—its rate, rhythm and volume.
3. *Respiration*—volume, rate, whether accompanied by an unusual sound.
4. *Skin*—whether flushed cyanosed or pale ; hot or cold ; sweating or dry.
5. *Pupils*—dilated or contracted, equal or unequal.
6. *Odour of breath*—a smell of acetone, disinfectant, alcohol.

Apart from injuries, there are three not uncommon causes of unconsciousness that should be considered, but the nurse should not give an opinion on the diagnosis ; her object is to find the appropriate first-aid treatment. It is easy to see the harm that would result from stating that a patient was drunk when he was in fact suffering from hypoglycæmia.

1. *Cerebro-vascular Accident.* Cerebral thrombosis is the commonest cause of apoplexy or stroke. The onset is fairly rapid and causes coma with slow full pulse, flushing, stertorous breathing, and perhaps an obvious paralysis of one side of the body. Most patients are elderly, but younger adults are not entirely immune.

The clothes round the neck should be loosened, and the head and shoulders supported. Vomiting sometimes occurs, and the patient must be kept lying on one side if this threatens, to prevent inhalation.

2. *Hypoglycæmia* (insulin overdose). Diabetic patients of any age and either sex may lapse into unconsciousness as a result of a fall in the blood sugar. Sweating is marked, the pulse is rapid and usually of good volume, and muscle tremors or actual convulsive movements can be observed. Search in the pockets may produce a card stating that the patient is a diabetic and giving the name of his doctor or clinic.

If the swallowing reflex has not been lost, sugar in water or any sugar-containing fluid such as milk or fruit juice can be given. If the coma is deep enough to make this dangerous, all that can be done is to safeguard the airway while awaiting the ambulance.

3. *Poisoning.* Narcotic poisoning, especially by the barbiturates, is a not uncommon occurrence, and the victims are usually found in bed. The first-aid treatment is suggested on p. 520.

The commonest cause of coma is undoubtedly alcoholic poisoning. The signs of slight alcoholic overdose are familiar—incoherence, muscle imbalance, emotional instability—but the patient in deep coma is less often seen and presents an alarming appearance. The face is pale, often with a tinge of cyanosis, sweating is marked, the skin cold, the pupils contracted and the temperature subnormal. Vomiting is common and may endanger the airway if no one is present.

Vomiting should be induced, and the face sponged with cold water. If improvement does not occur, medical help will be necessary. The diagnosis of alcoholic poisoning can be made confidently in many cases where the circumstances are known, but if the patient is a stranger found by accident, the greatest caution should be exerted in presuming drunkenness. Many people who feel ill take a drink in the belief that it will make them better, and are subsequently found unconscious and smelling of drink. Nurses are aware that drunk persons collected by the police are not confined until they have had medical treatment and the diagnosis confirmed.

Fainting

Simple fainting or syncope is a very common cause of transient unconsciousness. It is caused by a fall in the blood pressure which renders the blood supply to the brain insufficient to maintain consciousness, and is signalized by pallor and sweating and the feeling so aptly described as "faintness." Fainting is most common in young people, and occurs especially in hot, oppressive atmospheres and in emotional circumstances—in church, in crowds, after unpleasant sights or minor trauma, such as squeezing a finger or having an inoculation.

If possible, the victim is laid flat, as this position quickly restores the circulation to the brain. Fresh air is welcome, and such a stimulus as smelling salts or sal volatile in water are useful in rousing the patient. If circumstances make this position difficult, the head should be bent down towards the knees to compress the abdominal area and drive the blood out of it towards the brain.

Every student nurse fears that she will faint on first visiting the operating theatre, but this is, in fact, quite unusual, since interest and excitement operate against such an attack. It is important not to stand quite motionless if faintness is experienced, but to contract the muscles of the calves and thighs which otherwise may allow the blood to pool in them and so precipitate fainting.

Transport

In cases of accidents on roads or in the home, the quickest way of obtaining transport to hospital is by calling the police, who are able to send an ambulance. Everyone must be impressed by the speed with which the police arrive at the scene of accidents and take the necessary action.

CHAPTER 36

THE AGED IN HOSPITAL

The effects of increasing age vary from one person to another, but the factors that affect the health and well being of the old may be considered under these headings:

1. *Social.* Retirement from work leads to a drop in income, and a fall in the standard of living. It may be necessary to move to a smaller house, perhaps in a different area, which means that friends are left behind, and the elderly may lack the inability that gives opportunities to make new ones. Difficulties in sight or hearing make reading the papers or watching the television difficult, so that they become progressively divorced from current affairs. Children move away, or become absorbed in their own family difficulties, and may visit less frequently. The old people feel unwanted, and they complain of neglect and loneliness, and querulousness may alienate visitors, and increase the loneliness of which they proclaim.

2. *Musculo-skeletal.* Old people lose height because of thinning of the intervertebral discs and often by bowing of the spine. Calcium is lost from the bones, muscles waste and become stiff, so that the aged may suffer fractures from quite small stumbles and trips, because they are not agile enough to regain their balance as young people do. Osteoarthritis of the spine, hips and knees affects most people to some extent as they get older, and even if it does not cause pain, makes it increasingly arduous to do housework or shopping.

Decalcification of the jaw means that dentures no longer fit, and if they are left out, nutrition may become inadequate. Stiffness and decreasing manual dexterity makes bathing and care of the feet arduous, and may lead to self-neglect.

3. *Cardio-vascular.* Hardening of the arteries may restrict the blood supply to the legs, so that there is cramp in the calves after walking a short distance, and if the disease is advanced, gangrene of the feet may be caused. A rise of blood pressure may cause heart failure.

The most important effect of arterial disease is interference with the blood supply to the brain. Clotting may occur in diseased arteries, and if extensive will cause hemiplegia. Small clots cause minor " strokes " and if these are repeated noticeable deterioration in the mental state results. Confusion, loss of memory, muscular stiffness, shuffling gait and incontinence of urine are the result of cerebral arteriosclerosis.

The thinning of the intervertebral discs mentioned in the last section has an effect on the blood supply to the brain, since the vertebral arteries which supply half the blood to the brain pass up through the transverse processes of the cervical vertebræ. These arteries will become kinked as the neck shortens. If the patient extends the neck, this effect is increased, and interference with the blood supply to the brain and cause giddiness or fainting.

Cerebral blood supply which is just adequate to maintain normal function may become insufficient in certain circumstances. Infections such as bronchopneumonia; anæmia; and conditions such as coronary thrombosis which cause a fall in the blood pressure will lead to mental confusion and hallucinations.

4. *Temperature-regulating.* Most old people have little subcutaneous fat, and so are badly insulated against the cold. Muscular activity, which is the main method of making heat, diminishes with age. Old people may find it difficult to afford the money necessary for adequate heating, and these three circumstances combine to produce the well-known susceptiblity of the aged to cold. Hypothermia (an abnormally low temperature) is quite common, and a low-register thermometer may be necessary to find the true temperature.

5. *Respiratory.* The normal respiratory movement is restricted by muscle weakness, and increasing rigidity of the rib cage, and this makes the old highly susceptible to bronchitis and bronchopneumonia.

6. *Digestive.* The old normally retain a good appetite, if meals are cooked and served for them, but apathy and lethargy may hinder them from looking after their own nutrition. Constipation is very common, perhaps due to poor muscle tone, and if attention is not paid to it may lead to impaction of fæces. Sphincters become weak with age, and it may be difficult to retain fluid fæces, so that occasional incontinence may result.

7. *Urinary.* The ability to retain urine in the bladder until it is convenient to release it is important socially, and it is a landmark in a child's life when it gains this ability. It is an equally important event in an old person's life if it is lost. Sphincters become weak, the bladder becomes intolerant of large quantities of urine, and failing mental power may diminish voluntary control. Abnormalities and circumstances that lead to incontinence will be considered in the nursing section below.

Preservation of Health in Old Age

Preventing deterioration of mental and physical well-being as old age approaches is a means of avoiding much personal misery, waste of man and woman power in caring for neglected people who with forethought and help may be kept independent. The chief factors that cause decline are as follows.

1. *Loneliness.* Lack of company and social stimulus is a prime cause of apathy and self-neglect that will eventually necessitate institutional care. In villages and small communities old people are known, their needs for social contacts met, but in large cities total isolation is a possibility. The value of good neighbours who will call regularly for a few minutes' chat to see that all is well is beyond price.

Identification of those in need is important. Health visitors attached to a general practice will know the old people on the doctors' list and can call with advice on health, on prevention of accidents, or on old people's clubs. Churches and similar bodies have welfare schemes, and one of the most heartening features of the present social scene is the work done by sixth formers in visiting the old regularly to talk and perform small tasks.

2. *Poverty.* Those on small fixed incomes are vulnerable to the ever-rising cost of living that seems a permanent feature of the economic scene. Though pensions rise, they always lag behind inflation. Housing, food and clothes of a level that the pensioner can afford may therefore be below his needs.

Not all people are aware of extra benefits to which they are entitled, and the health visitor may offer advice on supplementary pensions, rate rebates, and in certain areas on cheap travel on corporation buses, or inexpensive holidays for old age pensioners. Those who have never been able to save to make some extra provision for old age are of course in the greatest need, but those who have been able to do so may find savings whittled away, and are unaware of the means by which the state will help them.

3. *Bad housing.* Those in financial need are obviously most likely to be badly housed, but there are also old people who find themselves in homes which once were not unsuitable, but who now cannot manage stairs, carry coals or keep a house in repair. Rehousing of the old in smaller premises or ground floor flats may be possible, and there are local authority and charitable trusts to provide flats and bungalows where the old can have supervision and communal meals.

4. *Minor defects.* Senile cataract, poor hearing and painful feet may increase isolation by limiting communications with others and the ability to get about. Age is not a bar to cataract operations, deafness may be alleviated by provision of hearing aids, and local authorities may provide free chiropody services.

5. *Bereavement.* Old couples may support each other, but if one dies the other may deteriorate rapidly, and unless support is given at this point may need admission to a geriatric hospital. Neighbours, the district nurse, the health visitor, the home help, the Women's Royal Voluntary Service who provide meals-on-wheels can all help to maintain independence in such crises.

Most old people want to remain in their own homes as long as possible, and though this takes money thought and care, the cost is small in comparison with nursing an old patient in a geriatric ward, and the gain in human happiness is great.

Nursing the Aged Sick

Old patients admitted to hospital fall into two groups. First there are those who have some acute condition not particular to age, or an illness amenable to treatment. Age is not a bar now to operations for cure of cataract, or prolapse, or nailing of a fractured neck or femur. Many of these can be cured, and if they are going to the care of relatives, may be sent home. Others, however, will not be fit to return to living alone without treatment on the lines suggested for the next group.

This consists of those with some incapacitating chronic condition such as hemiplegia or arthritis. A recovery cannot be expected, and without energetic and imaginative treatment he may well spend the rest of his life in a chronic ward, sinking ever further into apathy. The doctor will examine him and assess his physical and mental possibilities, the nurses will care for his hygienic and dietetic needs and encourage him to look forward with hope; the physiotherapist re-educates him in walking and the use of his muscles; the occupational therapist rouses his interest, trains the faculties he still possesses, and sees how she can fit him for life at home again.

Geriatric nursing can be both demanding and rewarding, but it is only the former unless premises and accommodation are adequate, the staff ratio is high enough. It is often supposed that less nurses are required for geriatric than for acute wards, but this is rarely the case, and unless sufficient nursing attention is available, old people will be kept in bed, deprived of sensory stimulus, prone to relapse into apathy and incontinence. Visitors may be few, and the nurse's presence and conversation may be the patient's only link with the outside world. It is the duty of administrators to see that the nurse has the circumstances and the time to give her patients what they need.

Old people who have been quite alert and competent in their own homes may become confused by new and strange surroundings, and give a false impression of their mental powers. Visitors, to keep them in touch with reality, should be welcomed, and if there are none nurses should find time for conversation, and should see that spectacles and hearing aids if required are kept in order and worn.

On admission, the doctor assesses the patient's condition, to determine if improvement can be made, perhaps to a level that will allow him to live again in the outside world. The medical and nursing staff will have the following aims:

1. To improve the personal hygiene, if necessary. Hair and skin may have been neglected through illness, and pressure sores may have occurred if the patient was bedfast. These must be healed by taking the weight from the affected areas. It will be difficult to heal skin loss if the patient is incontinent, so that the next section will be important in relation to the care of the pressure areas.

2. To maintain or institute continence. If mental function is normal or nearly so, the commonest cause of fæcal incontinence is impaction of fæces. It has already been noticed that constipation is common in the old, and if bowel function is neglected, fæces accumulate in the rectum, becoming hard and dry as water is absorbed from them. The resultant hard masses initiate the rectal mucosa, causing outpouring of mucus, which dissolves some of the fæces. This dark-stained fluid leaks through the lax sphincter, so that the patient and even the nurses may believe that there is diarrhœa. Incontinence of small fluid stools is very frequently a sign of fæcal impaction, and this can be at once diagnosed by rectal examination. If impaction is present, and severe, digital evacuation of the rectum may be necessary, but usually a course of enemata or suppositories is sufficient to effect a cure. It must be continued long enough to ensure that the entire colon is empty. Once normal defæcation has been established, it must be maintained by a diet with adequate roughage, a good fluid intake, offering a bedpan, commode, or a visit to the toilet after breakfast, and recording of the bowel actions. If fæcal incontinence still occurs, disease such as rectal or pelvic carcinoma must be excluded.

Continence of urine is often precarious in the old; the bladder must be emptied at frequent intervals, by night as well as by day, and without delay. Admission to hospital may be enough to upset this slender hold on continence. The patient is confused by strange surroundings, does not ask for the nurse's help, or may be some way from the lavatory. Infections like pneumonia, by increasing the mental confusion may precipitate incontinence.

Incontinence of urine is a factor of great importance in the care of the chronic sick. It renders the patient more liable to bedsores, lowers his morale, prevents his attendance at occupational therapy, creates an unpleasant atmosphere in the ward, and is a burden to the nursing staff. In a number of patients with impaired consciousness or failing cerebral power control is impossible, but in many cases it may be regained.

Infections such as pneumonia that cause mental confusion must be treated. A specimen of urine is examined for organisms, since cystitis, by decreasing the capacity of the bladder and increasing the irritation of the mucosa, may cause incontinence. Impaction of fæces is a common cause, because the distended rectum presses on the bladder. Enlargement of the prostate gland and prolapse of the uterus are other organic causes. Regular offering of bedpans, commodes, or visits to the lavatory are the most effective guard against incontinence. Those who are only wet at night may be given propantheline (Pro-Banthine) to relax the bladder and increase its capacity, but this drug should not be continued if it produces no improvement, since it also causes constipation.

If treatment is unsuccessful, men may usually be kept dry by an appliance with a urinary bag fastened to the thigh. Apparatus of a similar kind for women is not available, for anatomical reasons, and the patient is up and about, a pad and protective clothing must be worn. Those who are responsible for incontinent patients living at home will find much useful information in a book published by the Disabled Living Foundation: *Incontinence: Some problems, suggestions and conclusions.* Price 15/6.

3. *To clear infection.* It has already been noticed that pneumonia may have profound effect on the mental state and thence on the functions. The onset of a general infection is quite often announced not by fever, as in younger people, but by mental confusion, which may be apparent before the temperature starts to rise.

4. *To improve nutrition.* Diet is especially important for those who have been living alone on a restricted intake. Since fruit is expensive, vitamin C is often in short supply, and may be given as ascorbic acid or as orange juice. Meals are a very important event in an old person's day, and much enjoyed.

5. *To improve locomotor power.* It is the aim of the geriatrician to keep as many of his patients ambulant as possible. Confinement to bed may lead to contractures, as well as rendering the patient more liable to pressure sores and hypostatic pneumonia. The physiotherapist re-educates the patient in walking and the use of his muscles.

6. *To adapt home circumstances to make discharge possible.* An increasing number of old people are being rehabilitated to a level at which discharge to the care of relatives is possible, and these are given advice and help. The hazards of stairs, loose rugs, worn carpets and unguarded fires should be explained. A bedroom near the lavatory is

the best one, or a commode by the bedside may prevent accidents. The ability to perform small household tasks is treasured, and helps to keep up morale. Some councils run a laundering service to assist the relatives of the incontinent.

THE DYING

Sudden death from pulmonary embolus, coronary thrombosis or hæmorrhage occurs occasionally in hospital, but in many cases the event can be foretold for some hours or even days beforehand from nursing observations, which experience brings skill in interpreting.

If the condition of an acutely ill patient is deteriorating, serial observations of the pulse, temperature and respiration should be made, and an attempt made to decide if the pulse volume or respiratory excursion is decreasing, the colour or the state of consciousness changing. A fall in temperature of a feverish patient is not a good sign unless accompanied by a parallel fall in the pulse rate.

In patients suffering from incurable disease the end approaches quietly. The temperature usually falls below normal (though in a few conditions such as meningitis there may be a rise up to the time of death). The pulse volume diminishes, and as the circulation fails in the extremities, they become cold. Sweat appears on the skin, which is too cold to evaporate it. The amount of respiratory movement decreases and the rhythm alters so that the usual slight pause after inspiration disappears and the length of time between each breath increases. Frequently the sternomastoids and the sides of the nose move with each inspiration. Unconsciousness becomes deeper until the failing heart and lungs are no longer able to support life.

Ministers of religion are regular visitors in hospital wards, so that the dying patient need find nothing unusual in seeing the priest of his own faith, who should be told of his approaching end. It is especially important that Roman Catholic patients be given the opportunity of receiving the last rites of the church. Relatives need comfort too as well as the patient.

Relatives should be kept fully and truthfully informed as to the progress of the patient's illness. It is better not to make prophecies that may not be fulfilled, e.g. that consciousness will not be regained. Access to the patient should be as free as possible, as long as it does not interfere with treatment, and allowance must be made by those of Anglo-Saxon temperament for Mediterranean or Jewish families whose custom it is to gather in numbers on such occasions with overt expressions of grief. When the end appears near, relatives must be asked if they wish to be present, if they want to stay the night when this is indicated, or to be informed by telephone.

As death approaches, a nurse should remain with the patient. She should see that the pillows are smoothed, the lips moistened and that the general atmosphere is one of peace. Signs such as noisy breathing may be alleviated by a slight change of position, and if oxygen is being used, the mask should be removed towards the end. When the patient has died, the nurse should indicate this to the relatives, and may leave them with him for a minute if this seems desirable, then escort them away and sit them in a quiet place to collect their thoughts while the houseman verifies that life is extinct. They must then be told to return at a suitable time to see the Steward or Secretary about the patient's effects and burial, and they may be asked for special instructions especially about wedding rings. She offers them the sympathy that circumstances dictate, and sees that they are fit to leave before returning to her patient.

LAST OFFICES

An assistant is required, and if a senior nurse has a student who has not been present on this occasion before, she must show her that her natural fears are unnecessary. While the patient was alive there was no service that she shrank from performing for him, and this last one differs in no way from the others. It should be done with the gravity appropriate to preparations for burial, but not with emotion that she may communicate to others, especially the other patients.

If the patient is of the orthodox Jewish faith, he must not be touched by nurses after death, and if some essential attention must be paid, rubber gloves should be worn. Porters should remove him to the mortuary chapel, and the ministers of his faith will arrange the subsequent proceedings.

All pillows are removed, and the body laid flat, and all top clothes except the sheet are taken off. The jaw must be supported, and a flock pillow laid across the chest beneath it is the best way; bandages round the head are not advised, since if firm enough to be effective, they may mark the face. A wet swab is put on each closed eyelid, and then the sheet is drawn over the whole bed. All equipment like oxygen, fluids or mouth tray should be removed, the door is closed, and it is usual to complete the proceedings an hour later. Meanwhile the following equipment will be collected :

Trolley. Bowl of warm water.
Patient's soap, towels, flannels, brush, comb and nailbrush from his locker.
Resection tray with :
2 pairs dissecting forceps.
1 pair scissors.
White wool, 2 pieces 1 in. × 2 in.
1 piece 8 in. × 12 in.
1 piece 8 in. × 4 in.
Brown wool, 1 piece 1 in. × 2 in.
6-in. open-wove bandage.
(If necessary, dressings cut to size and elastoplast.)
Shroud.
Clean top sheet and if necessary drawsheet.
Receiver.
Fine combing requisites if necessary.

Everything that is wanted should be at hand ; it must not be necessary to leave the bedside once the nurses have begun, neither should they take there anything that is not needed. The wool, for instance, must be cut ready and not taken in a roll. The door is kept closed or curtains drawn. Fine combing requisites are taken if the patient has only recently been admitted and there is reason to think they may be needed.

The face and front aspect is washed, the nails being trimmed, then the patient is turned on the side and the back washed. Using forceps, the nurse packs the anal canal first with a small piece of absorbent white wool, then with a piece of brown. The second small piece of white wool is for the vagina if necessary. There is no need to pack the nostrils unless there is a discharge, and if such a pack is used it should be minimal, and not noticeable externally.

The drawsheet is changed if it is not immaculate, and if there is a wound it is dressed and sealed with elastoplast. If there is a cavity to be packed a gauze roll rather than pieces of gauze should be used. The 8 in. × 4 in. piece of wool is folded into a square and placed between the ankles, which are tied together with a length of the open-wove bandage. The shroud is put on, the last piece of wool is laid around the neck to support the jaw and the neck of the shroud is adjusted around it and fastened. The hands must be laid at the sides in hospital, where post-mortem examination is common, but in private practice the patient wears his own clothes, and the hands may lie on the chest, clasped or holding a rosary or similar object.

The toilet of the hair is completed last to look as natural as possible, and the nurse makes a final inspection to ensure that when the relatives visit the mortuary chapel their last impression will be one of peace and serenity. The bed, including the top rail, is entirely covered with a clean sheet, and the locker is cleared except for a small vase of flowers.

The arrival of the porters for transport of the body to the mortuary should be screened from the view of other patients. All effects are listed in duplicate and neatly packed, money, watch and jewellery being packed separately. The bed is stripped, washed and remade, and the nurse returns to the service of her other patients.

INDEX